Gastrointestinal Cancer 1

Cancer Treatment and Research

WILLIAM L. McGUIRE, *series editor*

Volume 3

1. R.B. Livingston, ed., Lung Cancer 1. 1981. ISBN 90-247-2394-9.
2. G. Bennett Humphrey, Louis P. Dehner, Gerald B. Grindey and Ronald T. Acton, eds., Pediatric Oncology 1. 1981. ISBN 90-247-2408-2.
4. John M. Bennett, ed., Lymphomas 1, including Hodgkin's Disease. 1981. ISBN 90-247-2479-1.

series ISBN 90-247-2426-0.

Gastrointestinal Cancer 1

edited by

JEROME J. DECOSSE
Memorial Sloan-Kettering Cancer Center, New York

and

PAUL SHERLOCK
Memorial Sloan-Kettering Cancer Center, New York

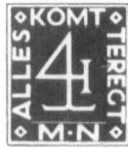

1981

MARTINUS NIJHOFF PUBLISHERS
THE HAGUE / BOSTON / LONDON

Distributors:

for the United States and Canada

Kluwer Boston, Inc.
190 Old Derby Street
Hingham, MA 02043
USA

for all other countries

Kluwer Academic Publishers Group
Distribution Center
P.O. Box 322
3300 AH Dordrecht
The Netherlands

Library of Congress Cataloging in Publication Data   CIP

Main entry under title:

Gastrointestinal cancer.

  (Cancer treatment and research; v. 3)
  Includes index.
  1. Digestive organs–Cancer. 2. Gastrointestinal system–Cancer. I. DeCosse, Jerome J.
II. Sherlock, Paul. III. Series. [DNLM: 1. Gastrointestinal neoplasms. W1 CA693 v. 3/WI 149
G265]

RC280.D5G36   616.99′433   81-38397
                                          AACR2
ISBN-13: 978-94-009-8257-4   e-ISBN-13: 978-94-009-8255-0
DOI: 10.1007/978-94-009-8255-0

Contents

Cancer Treatment and Research

Foreword

Where do you begin to look for a recent, authoritative article on the diagnosis or management of a particular malignancy? The few general oncology textbooks are generally out of date. Single papers in specialized journals are informative but seldom comprehensive; these are more often preliminary reports on a very limited number of patients. Certain general journals frequently publish good indepth reviews of cancer topics, and published symposium lectures are often the best overviews available. Unfortunately, these reviews and supplements appear sporadically, and the reader can never be sure when a topic of special interest will be covered.

Cancer Treatment and Research is a series of authoritative volumes which aim to meet this need. It is an attempt to establish a critical mass of oncology literature covering virtually all oncology topics, revised frequently to keep the coverage up to date, easily available on a single library shelf or by a single personal subscription.

We have approached the problem in the following fashion. First, by dividing the oncology literature into specific subdivisions such as lung cancer, genitourinary cancer, pediatric oncology, etc. Second, by asking eminent authorities in each of these areas to edit a volume on the specific topic on an annual or biannual basis. Each topic and tumor type is covered in a volume appearing frequently and predictably, discussing current diagnosis, staging, markers, all forms of treatment modalities, basic biology, and more.

In Cancer Treatment and Research, we have an outstanding group of editors, each having made a major commitment to bring to this new series the very best literature in his or her field. Martinus Nijhoff Publishers has made an equally major commitment to the rapid publication of high quality books, and world-wide distribution.

Where can you go to find quickly a recent authoritative article on any major oncology problem? We hope that Cancer Treatment and Research provides an answer.

WILLIAM L. McGUIRE
Series Editor

Preface

In this first volume of *Gastrointestinal Cancer,* the editors have deliberately sought topics within the broad field that are characterized by recent advances, development, importance and clinical utility. By intent, the subject matter does not encompass the totality of gastrointestinal cancer. A future volume will address additional areas.

We have selected a worldwide authorship who have made important contributions to their respective areas. We have requested the authors to develop a scholarly and well-referenced presentation of their subject. The authors have responded in an outstanding manner. We believe that their contributions are of great importance for a better understanding of the biology of gastrointestinal neoplasia and that numerous contemporary principles for current diagnosis and management are well presented.

Our modern concepts of the relevance of cell kinetics in the genesis of gastrointestinal neoplasia have been developed by Deschner and Salmon from Memorial Sloan-Kettering Cancer Center in New York. The genetic aspects of gastrointestinal cancer with its precursor states are thoroughly discussed by McConnell from Liverpool, England. Bartholomew and Schutt from the Mayo Clinic have presented our current understanding of the systemic expression of gastrointestinal malignancy with a clear delineation of the various skin, joint and chemical clues.

The extraordinarily high incidence of esophageal cancer in Iran provides the data base for a thoughtful, well-referenced paper by Sorouri, formerly from Teheran. The epidemiology of gastric cancer continues to yield clues as to its etiology as outlined by Correa from New Orleans. Although decreasing in the United States, gastric cancer continues to present a worldwide problem and Kobayashi from Tokyo discusses the radiologic and endoscopic clues which will result in early detection and more curable disease. The problem of gastric stump cancer, of note particularly in European countries and occurring 15 or 20 years after gastric resection, is discussed by Dahm from Germany. The role of bacteria and bile salts in the pathogenesis of large bowel cancer as discussed by Hill from London is an example of metabolic epidemiology. His chapter is followed by a detailed statement by Williams, also of London, on the current role of colonoscopy in the diagnosis and management of large bowel cancer and its precursors. Concepts have been changing regarding both the diagnosis of cancer superimposed on ulcerative colitis as well as the surveillance in patients with inflammatory bowel disease and this is well outlined by Bayless and Yardley from Baltimore. Colacchio and LoGerfo from New York describe the current role of carcinoembryonic antigens (CEA) in the management of large bowel cancer and indicate its importance in determining recurrence.

Weingrad and his colleagues from New York have analyzed a historic experience with primary lymphomas of the gut, delineating diagnostic, prognostic and management principles. Hormone-producing tumors of the gut, which may be slow-growing but extensive in their clinical effects, are discussed in detail by Friesen and Petelin from Kansas City. Sun-Tsung-tang and associates from China discusses hepatocellular carcinoma with its interesting epidemiologic relationships, its immunologic marker and the potential for cure when diagnosed early. Finally Neefe and Schein from Washington, D.C. have reviewed in detail the current chemotherapeutic management of gastrointestinal cancer emphasizing combination chemotherapy and multimodality therapy with an optimistic note for the future.

We believe each chapter to be the definitive statement about the respective topic. We hope the reader will share our enthusiasm.

List of Contributors

BARTHOLOMEW, Lloyd G., Mayo Medical School, Mayo Clinic and Mayo Foundation, Rochester, MN 55901, U.S.A.

BAYLESS, Theodore M, Johns Hopkins Hospital, Baltimore, MD 21205, U.S.A.

COLACCHIO, Thomas A., Columbia-Presbyterian Medical Center, New York, NY 10032, U.S.A.

CORREA, Pelayo, Louisiana State University Medical Center, New Orleans, LA 70112, U.S.A.

DAHM, Klaus, University Hospital of Hamburg, Martinistrasse 52, 2000 Hamburg 20, F.R.G.

DECOSSE, Jerome J., Memorial Sloan-Kettering Cancer Center, New York, NY 10021, U.S.A.

DESCHNER, Eleanor E., Memorial Sloan-Kettering Cancer Center, New York, NY 10021, U.S.A.

FRIESEN, Stanley R., University of Kansas Medical Center, 39th & Rainbow Blvd., Kansas City, KS 66103, U.S.A.

HILL, M.J., Central Public Health Laboratory, Colindale Avenue, London NW9, U.K.

KOBAYASHI, Seibi, Aichi Cancer Center Hospital, Nagoya, Japan.

LIEBERMAN, Philip H., Memorial Sloan-Kettering Cancer Center, New York, NY 10021, U.S.A.

LOGERFO, Paul, Columbia-Presbyterian Medical Center, New York, NY 10032, U.S.A.

McCONNELL, Richard B., Broadgreen Hospital and Department of Medicine, University of Liverpool, Royal Liverpool Hospital, Liverpool, U.K.

NEEFE, John R., Vincent T. Lombardi Cancer Research Center, Department of Medicine, Georgetown University, Washington, DC 20007, U.S.A.

PETELIN, Joseph B., University of Kansas Medical Center, 39th & Rainbow Blvd., Kansas City, KS 66103, U.S.A.

SALMON, Remy J., Institut Curie, Paris, France.

SCHEIN, Philip S., Vincent T. Lombardi Cancer Research Center, Department of Medicine, Georgetown University, Washington, DC 20007, U.S.A.

SCHUTT, Allan J., Mayo Medical School, Mayo Clinic and Mayo Foundation, Rochester, MN 55901, U.S.A.

SHERLOCK, Paul, Memorial Sloan-Kettering Cancer Center, New York, NY 10021, U.S.A.

SOROURI, Parviz, Department of Medicine, National University, School of Medicine, Tehran, Iran. Present address: 900 Hillside Road, Wilmington, DE 19807, U.S.A.

STRAUS, David J., Memorial Sloan-Kettering Cancer Center, New York, NY 10021, U.S.A.

TSUNG-TANG, Sun,Cancer Institute, Chinese Academy of Medical Sciences, Beijing, China.

WEINGRAD, Daniel N., Memorial Sloan-Kettering Cancer Center, New York, NY 10021, U.S.A.

WILLIAMS, Christopher B., St. Mark's and Bartholomew's Hospitals, London, U.K.

YARDLEY, John H., Johns Hopkins University School of Medicine and Johns Hopkins Hospital, Baltimore, MD 21205, U.S.A.

YUAN-YUN, Chu, Qidong Liver Cancer Institute, Kiangsu, China.

ZHAO-YOU, Tang, Liver Cancer Research Unit, Zhongshan Hospital, Shanghai First Medical College, Shanghai, China.

1. Cell Kinetics of Gastrointestinal Cancer and its Precursor States

ELEANOR E. DESCHNER and REMY J. SALMON

1. INTRODUCTION

Normally there exists in the gastrointestinal mucosa an equilibrium between cell renewal and cell loss through intraluminal exfoliation and cell death. In precancerous and cancerous states, this fine balance or steady state is disturbed. This condition may sometimes be recognized by an elevation in the number of cells involved in DNA synthesis, a faster cell turnover time, or an abnormal location of the proliferative compartment. An alteration in some aspect of normal cell kinetics may reveal the presence of an abnormality even before any microscopic pathology is visible. Certain aspects of cell proliferation can in some instances then be employed as an early marker for the involvement of the mucosa in a disease state such as tumor formation.

Likewise, the effect of an imbalance in hormonal levels and its relationship to the development of a disease state may be elucidated by an analysis of cell proliferation. The stimulating effect of gastrin on parietal cell proliferation and its inhibitory effect on DNA synthesis in the rat antral mucosa[1], for example, is compatible with the increase in fundic mucosal height, increased fundic mucosal area and diminished antral size observed in patients with Zollinger-Ellison syndrome[2].

The purpose of this chapter will be to provide the reader with information concerning cell proliferation in the gastrointestinal tract under both normal and diseased conditions. One can fully appreciate that the accumulation of data concerning the mucosa of man is far from complete and that much of our background must be provided by animal studies. Over the last decade there has been a surge in kinetic research along new pathways. Animal models for the evaluation of all types of gastrointestinal neoplasia have been established and it is now possible to grow, manipulate and observe tumors of human origin in immunodeficient nude mice. *In vivo* cellular kinetics at different stages of tumor growth, following the effect of both chemothera-

J. J. DeCosse and P. Sherlock (eds.), Gastrointestinal cancer 1, 1-26. All rights reserved.
Copyright © 1981 Martinus Nijhoff Publishers, The Hague/Boston/London.

peutic agents as well as substances which may modify or repress tumor growth are all areas which should provide us with a better understanding of carcinogenesis and therapy.

2. TECHNIQUES

Measurements of epithelial cell proliferation have been carried out using a variety of techniques. Radioactive precursors of DNA such as tritiated thymidine have been employed and injected into patients with limited life expectancy and biopsies taken at stated intervals over an extended interval, i.e. 2–3 days. By following the wave of labeled mitoses which emerges, it has been possible to obtain values for the duration of the various phases of the cell cycle.

In patients other than those terminally ill, information concerning the gastrointestinal mucosa has become available using *in vitro* procedures with biopsy specimens incubated in nutrient media to which radionuclides such as tritiated thymidine (^{3}HTdR) are added. This technique will provide one with a labeling index (L.I.) or ratio of labeled cells to total cells which is a measure of the proliferative activity of the tissue. In addition, it will clearly demonstrate the location of the proliferative compartment.

An *in vitro* procedure termed the double label technique not only provides the duration of S phase or the phase during which DNA is synthesized but allows one to estimate the total cell cycle time. Different populations of labeled epithelial cells are formed with the use of two doses of ^{3}HTdR a low (l) and a high dose (h) or two types of labeled thymidine, i.e. ^{3}H and ^{14}C, separated by an interval of time (t). A value for S phase (T_s) can be derived:

$$\frac{N_h}{N_l} = \frac{S}{t}.$$

Knowing the S phase duration and having obtained the L.I. at 1 hour, the total cell cycle time (T_c) can be estimated:

$$T_c = \frac{T_s}{\text{L.I.}} \times 100.$$

3. ESOPHAGUS

3.1. Histology and Kinetics in Normal Tissue

The esophageal mucosa is a stratified non-keratinizing squamous epithelium, which when it abruptly ends at the distal end is replaced by the

Table 1. Proliferative parameters of epithelial cells in human and rodent stratified squamous epithelium of the esophagus.

	L.I. (%)	M.I. (%)	S phase (h)	T_C (days)	Ref.
Man					
in vivo: basal layer	8.7	0.69			[4]
entire mucosa	0.95	0.08			[4]
In vitro: basal layer	10.0	0.85	10.6	4.5	[7]
Rat	3.7				[3]
			4.8–5.5		[6]
Mice basal cells	1.8	1.2	9.1		[5]

columnar epithelium of the cardia. Proliferating epithelial cells are located in the basal layer of the squamous epithelium. Migration occurs progressively to the lumen where cells become extruded from the surface of the mucosa. Mitotic figures are seen only in the deep basal layer since these are the cells synthesizing DNA. Repeated injections of tritiated thymidine ([3]HTdR) demonstrate that all basal layer cells of the esophagus have proliferative capability but they are scattered randomly [3]. The daughter cells emerging from cell division may remain as basal cells, or one or both may migrate and differentiate. Proliferation rates in man and in rodent are slow, i.e. one-third as rapid as epithelial cells in other gastrointestinal epithelium of the same species and lower in man than in rodent [3–7] (Table 1). Synthesis of DNA occurred *in vivo* in 8.7% of basal epithelial cells [4] in the mature human esophagus, while *in vitro* levels have been found to be slightly higher (9.2–11.1%) [7]. An estimate for the turnover time of the tissue in man or the average time elapsed for [3]HTdR labeled cells to migrate from the basal layer to the lumen is between 4 and 8 days [4, 7].

3.2. Kinetics in Diseased States

Approximately 70% of esophageal cancers are squamous carcinomas while the remainder are adenocarcinomas occurring primarily in the distal one third. Certainty regarding the nature of malignancy in the latter region may be difficult since the cancer may have an esophageal or cardial origin. The prognosis of this disease is poor, aggravated as it is by a constant nutritional deficiency related to stenosis and dysphagia.

Few kinetic studies have been reported in esophageal carcinoma. However, much interest has centered on two syndromes: Plummer-Vinson and Barrett's epithelium. Plummer-Vinson syndrome is associated with anemia, dysphagia, hypochlorhydria, and iron and vitamin deficiency in females 40–45 years of age. The histological findings feature a basal cell hyperplasia with nuclear

hyperchromatism and severe inflammatory changes in the underlying mucosa. These are very similar to characteristics of *in situ* carcinoma[8].

Barrett's syndrome, which also may be a precancerous condition[9], is
believed to arise from reflux esophagitis. Biopsies show patchy heterotopia of
gastric epithelium with or without parietal and peptic secreting cells. This
heterotopia can undergo changes characterized as atrophic gastritis and even
display intestinal metaplasia[8]. Studies of epithelial cell kinetics undertaken
in vitro after incubation of biopsies with ^{3}HTdR demonstrated a two fold
increase in the L.I. in columnar type Barrett's epithelium compared with the
esophageal squamous epithelium (23.3% vs 10.0%). S phase duration was
similar in both tissues (about 10 hours). Because of the lower L.I., the estimated cell cycle time for epithelial cells in normal esophageal mucosa was 4.4
days whereas it was less than 2 days for cells in the columnar type esophageal
epithelium[7]. The most abnormal finding reported involved an expansion of
the proliferative zone to the surface, which was observed in two patients with
adenocarcinoma of the esophagus and one of nine without adenocarcinoma[10].

The significance of this expanded zone in the development of esophageal
carcinoma requires further investigation, particularly in light of the response
of such patients to anti-reflux surgery[11]. Reversion of columnar epithelium
to squamous epithelium occurred following this procedure in four of ten
patients over a period of 1 to 2 years. Reflux either disappeared or was
severely diminished as measured by pH probe[11].

Epidemiologic findings emphasize the role of nutrition in the development
of esophageal cancer especially in combination with zinc deficiency and the
ingestion and/or endogenous formation of nitroso compounds[12, 13]. Animal studies report an acute inhibition of DNA synthesis in esophageal epithelial cells 4 hours after various N-nitroso compounds are injected[14]. The
responsiveness of the esophagus to low levels of some nitrosamines would
indicate both the ability of the tissue to activate or metabolize these substances as well as the sensitivity of this organ to carcinogenesis. Nutrient deficiencies have been shown to contribute to the sensitivity of the esophagus to
cancer induction. For example, in rats, zinc deficiency increased the incidence
and shortened the lag time for the induction of esophageal tumors with the
nitrosamine, methylbenzylnitrosamine[12].

An additional factor in the incidence of esophageal cancer, at least in China
where it is one of the most common cancers, is the concurrent presence of a
fungal infection[15]. A hyperplastic epithelium, thicker and growing faster
than normal esophageal mucosa, was found in the resected esophagus of
patients with this early cancer and growing within this mucosa was the
fungus *Candida*. Kinetic analyses have as yet not been reported on this type
of tissue.

4. STOMACH

4.1. Histology and Kinetics in Normal Tissue

There are three separate regions of the stomach, each of which is histologically distinct. As previously mentioned, the cardia with its stratified squamous epithelium is lined completely with simple columnar mucous epithelial cells. Those at the lower portion of the pits have as their special function the renewal and replacement of cells and the population, as a whole, the secretion of mucus.

The fundic portion is the largest and most complex area of the stomach because it contains the greatest number of specialized cell types. These gastric pits are lined with simple columnar mucous cells which extend downwards for approximately one-third of the total length to the isthmus area or zone of cell proliferation. Epithelial cells in this area are more cuboidal or low columnar in shape. Mitotic figures occur predominantly in this region.

Specialized cell types such as parietal and argentaffin cells are seen primarily below the isthmus or neck of the gastric pit. Here too the chief or zymogen secreting cells predominate. Interspersed among these are at least eleven different endocrine cells with their varied functions to synthesize, store and secrete hormones. Some of those which have been successfully characterized are the A cells, which secrete enteroglucagon, the G or gastrin secreting cells and the argentaffin cell secreting serotonin, histamine and possibly motilin.

The gastric pit of the pyloric region is deeper than in the fundic region and is lined with simple columnar epithelial cells similar to the mucous neck cell. A few parietal acid secreting cells have been demonstrated in this region; however, the major specialized cell type in the antrum is the G cell[16]. Moreover, the G cell population is statistically higher at the greater curvature than at the lesser curvature.

The reported L.I. for gastric epithelial cells has varied from 4.27 to 15.2%; however, the antrum has consistently been found to have the highest proliferative activity. The turnover time for the gastric mucosa is estimated to range from 2 to 6 days[17–19]. S phase values reported are within a narrow range (6.1–10 hours)[20].

The undifferentiated cells at the isthmus of the fundic pit and at the lower portion of pyloric pits are the cells that normally engage in DNA synthesis and replace those cells sloughed from the surface. They also act as stem cells for the parietal and some endocrine type cells[21, 22]. Zymogen cells and gastrin cells[22, 23] have been found to renew themselves slowly and continuously. An increased gastrin level in mice significantly enhanced parietal cell production[22]. However, high gastrin levels significantly decreased the labeling and mitotic indices in rat pyloric antral pits[1]. Thus gastrin acts as a tropic hormone in the body of the stomach while having an inhibitory effect on the antrum.

Normal turnover time of gastrin cells in the stomach of rodents is approximately 3 months[24]. Starvation for 4 days causes a 68% depletion of the gastrin cell population. When this condition is followed by six days of refeeding, gastrin cell numbers increase by 79%. In this case, gastrin cell proliferation is considerably increased and the turnover time drastically reduced[24].

4.2. Kinetics in Diseased States

Atrophic gastritis and intestinal metaplasia are strongly correlated with gastric cancer[25] based on at least five observations: (1) The incidence and extent of intestinal metaplasia is greater in a cancerous stomach than in one which is normal or has ulcer disease. (2) During the early stages, gastric cancer is often seen in a transitional area bordering one that is characterized by intestinal metaplasia. (3) The most frequent locations of intestinal metaplasia, the antrum and lesser curvature, are also the major sites for gastric cancer. (4) A large proportion of gastric cancers are of the intestinal type and (5) the incidence of gastric cancer in patients with a history of atrophic gastritis is higher than it is in other control groups.

Recent studies have shown that the lack of acid secretion in the atrophic mucosa provides an atmosphere conducive to the proliferation of certain bacterial species capable of acting on elemental nitrates[13]. The resulting exogenous nitrosamines added to those formed endogenously would elevate their level enhancing the probability of additional damage to the DNA of cells in this intestinalized mucosa and thereby allowing the initiation of gastric cancer.

An additional factor thought to contribute to the development of intestinal metaplasia is duodenal reflux. The contents, particularly bile salts with their detergent properties, may act to destroy the normally protective mucosal barrier lining the stomach.

Autoradiographic observations of epithelial cells of gastric mucosa of patients with atrophic gastritis reveal a cell cycle time of about 2 days, a slightly shorter interval than in the normal mucosa, which is believed to result from a reduced G_1 phase[19]. In general the higher labeling indices found in diseased gastric mucosa (Table 2) can be explained by the close resemblance it bears to small intestine not only in appearance but also in kinetic behavior.

Premalignant and malignant diseases of the gastric mucosa are also characterized by a two to five fold increased level of nuclear ploidy over that recognized in normal mucosa[31]. The presence of additional chromosomal material causes an increase in the size of nuclei such that the nuclei of gastric

Table 2. Kinetics of epithelial cells in preneoplastic and neoplastic gastric mucosa of man.

	LI (%)	MI (%)	T_{G2} (h)	T_S (h)	T_C (h)	Ref.
Atrophic gastritis						
Fundus	14.0		1–6	16	>30	[26]
	19.0					[27]
	10–17.3			6.5–7.6	37.6–75.3	[19]
Antrum	12.9					[27]
		12.9				[28]
	11.3–19.4			6.9–10.0	51.8–67.6	[19]
Gastric cancer						
Fundus	9.9	2.3				[29]
	16.4	1.2				[30]
	19.3					[27]
Antrum	15.8					[27]
	23.0	1.8				[30]

epithelial cells in patients with pernicious anemia and gastric cancer are almost twice the diameter of normal 2n cell nuclei.

Accompanying this elevated level of cell proliferation and increased chromosomal content of nuclei, these cells of the mucosa with atrophic gastritis display a faster migration to the surface [26, 32]. A high level of epithelial cell loss in gastritis patients may bring about the compensating high L.I. [33]. Enlargement of the proliferative compartment with cells in the upper regions of pits engaged in DNA synthesis has been recognized in normal appearing gastric pits as well as those involved in the early stages of gastritis [26, 34]. Histological alterations accompany the progression of the disease and less differentiated epithelial cells are seen at the surface and upper regions of the gastric pit. These cells are capable of cell proliferation and are characteristic of the mild to moderate level of gastritis present. In the more severe stages of the disease, intestinalization develops and parietal cells are reduced in number. These intestinalized pits have no homogeneous proliferative pattern; rather, they can express one of two types. One pattern is characterized by the presence of immature DNA synthesizing cells at the surface while the other displays the existence of well-differentiated intestinal type cells in this area. The latter pattern is thought to display the full extent or severe progression of the disease and the complete conversion of the gastric mucosa to a small intestinal mucosa with its full absorptive capabilities [34].

Investigation of cell proliferation in the pyloric antrum of the rat during early stages of induced N-methyl-N'-nitro-N-nitrosoguanidine (MNNG) gastric carcinogenesis has shown that pits lined with immature mucus-depleted cells can be recognized and separated into two groups, each expressing a

different proliferative pattern [35]. The one displayed a shift of the proliferative compartment in a downward direction toward the muscularis mucosa in
keeping with the future development of an endophytic tumor. The other
revealed an upward shift of proliferating cells, presumably preliminary to the
formation of an exophytic neoplasm. These patterns effectively forecast the
types of tumors, namely adenomas and microinvasive carcinomas, which later
appeared in these animals. These diverse routes for tumor induction have also
been noted in the development of DMH induced colonic neoplasia [36]. The
relative frequency of an endophytic to exophytic inductive sequence to cancer
is unknown. However, there is greater difficulty in the recognition of an
endophytic growth pattern within any mucosa. Thus there exists a lesser
likelihood for early detection of a malignancy expanding in a downward
direction and an enhanced probability of metastasis.

5. SMALL INTESTINE

5.1. Histology

The pyloric antrum leads into the first part of the small intestine, namely
the duodenum, the region into which bile and pancreatic secretions flow. The
effect of some substances on cell proliferation will be discussed later in this
section.

From the duodenum there follows the jejunum and ileum, differing only in
their basic structure from each other and the duodenum by the shape and
length of the finger-like projections or villi which are thrown up by the
mucosal surface to enhance absorptive capacity. The tubular gland or crypt of
the small bowel has the greatest number of specialized cells lining its wall.
The epithelial cells of this area include goblet cells, columnar cells, enteroendocrine cells and Paneth cells. All cell types are believed to originate from the
same precursor cell, the columnar cell of the crypt base [37]. The intermediate
cells formed are recognizable for their future role by the appearance of cellular
products in the cytoplasm. The appearance of granules predicts a future
Paneth or endocrine cell while a secretory product forecasts a future goblet
cell. Scattered at the base of the crypts are the many and varied endocrine
cells along with argentaffin cells, which have approximately the same population frequency throughout the entire small intestial tract. Other endocrine
cells have more specific distributions. A small population of G cells are
present in the duodenum but the primary endocrine cell types here are the
secretin-producing cell, the motilin-producing cells and the gastric inhibitory
polypeptide-producing cell.

The latter three specialized cells are also located in the jejunum but in
lesser numbers. The endocrine cell type found most frequently in this middle

area of the small intestine is the epithelial cell, which secretes enteroglucagon. These cells have been identified by immunohistochemistry but the kinetics of only the gastrin-producing cells has been investigated.

5.2. Kinetics in Normal Tissue

Regardless of the region in which they are present, crypts of the small intestine contain the same number of epithelial cells per gland [38]. Mitotic figures are seen at the base of crypts and their quantitation has allowed both estimations of the renewal time for epithelial cells to be made as well as theories to be developed regarding the mechanism of migration and replacement. Estimates of epithelial cell cycle time indicate a minimum of 42 hours [39, 40] and a maximum of 144 hours [18]. An L.I. of 27.4% was obtained for human jejunum [4] and correspondingly high M.I.s of 2.1–3.1% were seen [4, 39, 40].

Many factors influence or modify epithelial cell proliferation and the small intestine has usually been employed to assess their effect (Table 3). Aging, irradiation, nutritional status, genetic inheritance and many endogenously formed substances have been evaluated and found to alter cell renewal.

The effect of aging was noted on the proliferative activity of young 93-day-old mice compared with that in 940-day-old rodents. Greater variability in the duration of the cell cycle of individual cells occurs with age along with an increase in the synthesis and G_1 phases [38]. Chronic low level gamma irradiation of 12 rads/day produces a shortening of the cell cycle when compared to non-irradiated controls [41]. Even strain differences among mice of the same age reveal a variability in the durations of epithelial cell cycle times, i.e. BCF, mice, 15 hours vs CAF, 11.5 hours [41].

Work on neuro-modulation has begun to emerge in the literature because of

Table 3. Factors which influence cell proliferation in small intestine.

Factor	Accelerate	Depress	Reference
Aging		+	[38]
Irradiation	+		[41]
Adrenaline		+	[42]
Stress		+	[42]
Noradenaline	+		[42]
Sympathectomy		+	[42]
Somatostatin		+	[43]
Serotonin	+		[44]
Histamine	+		[44]
Starvation		+	[45, 46]
Bile acid	+		[47]
Pancreatic secretion	+		[52]

interest in the rich adrenergic innervation of intestinal crypts (see Chapter 13). Evaluations of adrenalin and substances that block alpha and beta adrenergic stimulation have been made on cell proliferation in the jejunum of rats [42]. Infusion of adrenaline inhibited cell proliferation by extending the mitotic and cell cycle time, a finding similar to that seen when restraint stress is employed. In the latter instance cell proliferation is also reduced presumably due to the increased levels of adrenaline released from the adrenal medulla [42]. Noradrenaline stimulated cell proliferation whereas surgical sympathectomy inhibited the process. Presumably inhibition was due to the absense of noradrenaline from local nerve terminals [42].

Somatostatin, which inhibits growth hormone and gastrin release as well as gastric acid secretion, represses DNA synthesis in the duodenal and jejunal mucosa when infused 8 hours before the time of maximal S phase activity (12–2 a.m.) [43]. Infusion during the day depresses the mitotic index suggesting that somatostatin can act at both the G_1-S and G_2-M boundaries of the cell cycle.

Two biogenic amines, serotonin and histamine, have been examined and found to influence cell proliferation. Both stimulate cell renewal in rat jejunum when injected intraperitoneally [44].

Starvation of rats causes a decrease in the number of cells in the gland and reduces the number of proliferating and mitotic cells [45, 46]. Bile acid feeding stimulates cell proliferation in small bowel, accelerates migration up the villus and shortens the cell cycle time [47]. While bile diversion had little effect on the L.I. and M.I. of the jejunum [48, 49], a significantly lower labeling index was reported in the distal ileum [50, 51]. It is of interest to note that the primary function of the ileum is the absorption of bile salts and that their absence destroys the integrity of the mucosa.

Pancreatic secretions have also been observed to influence epithelial cell proliferation and particularly villus size [52]. In general, the integrity of the small bowel mucosa requires controlled regulation of GI hormones, bile and pancreatic secretion levels. When disturbances in their balance occur, or the nutritional or physiological status of the individual is altered, these factors are reflected in the kinetics of the epithelial cell.

5.3. Kinetics in Diseased States

The response to disease in this portion of the gastrointestinal tract involves one of two alternatives. Either there is a diminution in the epithelial cell population and the size of the villi with resulting atrophy of the mucosa taking place, or the mucosa undergoes hypertrophy. The former condition involves decreased proliferative activity and shortening of the villi to produce a reduction in absorptive surface. This manifestation is observed in patients with severe pernicious anemia with concomitant vitamin B_{12} deficiency. In addition to a decreased frequency in mitosis, there is also an increase in nuclear size demontrated in small intestinal mucosa of these individuals[53]. Spectrophotometric measurements to determine the ploidy of these epithelial cells have not as yet been carried out.

5.3.1. Sprue. Another condition characterized by loss or reduction in villus size is celiac sprue or gluten enteropathy[54, 55]. Moreover, it is marked by enlarged convoluted crypts, frequent mitoses, and excessive cell loss. Patients with sprue show a characteristic malabsorption syndrome and may develop malignant lymphoma in 6–10% of cases of long-standing disease[56] (see Chapter 12).

Untreated patients with sprue demonstrate a three-fold greater proliferative activity and faster upward migration of epithelial cells than is seen in control individuals. Sprue patients have a crypt cell population which is four times that found in control biopsies[39, 40]. This increase involves not only a lengthening of the gland but also a widening of the crypt. A normal crypt may be composed of 800 cells, but in a sprue mucosa the crypt may contain 3000 cells. While the growth fraction or percentage of cells participating in DNA synthesis is between 0.72 and 0.83 in normal small bowel[39, 40], it is far lower in the sprue mucosa [0.55–0.61]. The number of proliferating cells, however, is still far greater in the crypts of patients with gluten enteropathy and the cell cycle time is extremely short, i.e. approximately 24 hours[39, 40]. Remission of malabsorption symptoms in patients on a gluten-free diet after 6–12 weeks is accompanied by a reduction in the L.I. and a slower migration rate such that it is intermediate between untreated sprue and control levels. Even over longer periods, a completely normal histologic picture is not achieved and proliferative activity remains rapid.

5.3.2. Intestinal Resection. Partial resection of the small bowel induces histological changes in the remaining mucosa[57]. Two months following removal of only 10% of lower rat ileum allowed the villi to increase in height and cell renewal to be enhanced 141% over control values[58]. Two months after 40% small bowel resection, both the total number of cells and the number of DNA synthesizing cells in the ileal rat crypts increased with expansion of the proliferative and maturation zone. The duration of the cell cycle was essentially unaltered; however, the number of villous cells was increased and the migration rate was accelerated[59]. Shortening of the cell cycle, due primarily to a reduced duration of S phase, was seen 60 days following resection of 70% of the small intestine[60].

Within 3 days after acute distal intestinal obstruction cell proliferation increased by a factor of three in crypts proximal to the obstruction. There were also changes in the length and width of crypts as well as in villous height and the width of villi at their base [61]. It has been suggested that a systemic factor is involved in regulation of the size of the villous cell population [62]. Gastrin and also glucagon have been suggested as effecting this compensatory proliferative response. Glucagon administered at physiological doses stimulated DNA synthesis throughout the intestine in contrast to gastrin, which had no remarkable effect on small bowel but stimulated DNA synthesis in the colon [63]. This study suggests that the major effector of post-resectional intestinal hyperplasia is glucagon. The significance of increased DNA synthesis in an area adjacent to the obstruction, which may be a tumor, is that further malignancy in transformed cells here would be expressed faster and increase the risk of local recurrence.

Patients undergoing radiotherapy in the abdominal region or receiving chemotherapeutic agents as treatment for the presence of cancer, very often are fed an elemental diet made of readily absorbable nutrients. Such a diet fed to mice for seven days brought about an increase in the length or cellularity of the villi [64]. The number of cells/villus increased by 120% but the crypt population was reduced by 35%. Unexpectedly, and in contradiction to normal feedback regulation, no alteration in the cell cycle time or S phase duration was found compared with controls. The radiation response of this mucosa was delayed by 16 hours compared with control mice and the overshoot in labeled cells normally seen following whole-body irradiation of 1000 rads did not occur. The protective quality credited to an elemental diet may be related to the increased epithelial cell population of the villi. Slower depletion of the villus cells would allow delay of compensatory proliferation in crypt cells, thus providing additional time for repair of sublethal damage in these cells.

6. LARGE INTESTINE

6.1. Histology and Kinetics in Normal Tissue

The distal portion of the gastrointestinal tract begins with the caecum and is composed of five regions, the ascending, transverse, descending and sigmoid colon and, lastly, the rectum. The mucosa in these areas is histologically similar throughout with the presence of crypts of Lieberkühn of varying depth. Columnar, mucous, enteroendocrine and Paneth cells line the cryptal walls. The latter two cell types occur only in small numbers, e.g. approximately four Paneth cells occur in every 100 crypts in the ascending colon [65]. The stem cell for all four cell types is throught to be the vacuolated crypt-base columnar cell. The intermediate cell types formed have limited capacity to replace themselves [66].

Data relative to proliferation kinetics is perhaps more available for the large bowel than any other portion of the digestive system. This is undoubtedly because of the relative ease with which biopsies may be obtained using the proctoscope and more recently the newly developed flexible colonoscope. The latter now allows sampling even from the right side of the colon.

Patients with limited life expectancy have repeatedly been sampled through a colostomy after intravenous infusion of tritiated thymidine and a percent labeled mitoses curve obtained. From this, the various phases of the cell cycle for the epithelial cells has been determined. When measurements were carried out *in vivo*, the S phase duration was between 9 and 20 hours [67–69] and the total cell cycle time between 24 and 48 hours [67, 68]. The proportion of cells in S phase for the large intestine (or L.I.) according to *in vivo* experiments varied between 12 and 25% [67, 68]. The replacement time for this tissue as calculated from these values is in the order of 4 to 8 days.

In vitro studies generally provide shorter S phase durations, i.e. 7.2–11.2 hours and lower values for labeling indices, 1.5–17% [69–74]. Consequently, estimates for the total cell time have provided longer values than those obtained *in vivo* (i.e. 77.2–129.9 hrs vs 24–48 hours) [74].

There exists no agreement in the literature concerning circadian rhythm in the gastrointestinal tract. However, if this type of biological phenomenon does exist, much of the variability in kinetic parameters expressed may be related to the time of sampling. Circadian change has been reported in all areas of the mouse digestive system including the descending colon and rectum [75, 76]. This was described when the mice were standardized on a 12 hour alternating light and dark cycle. Maximum DNA synthesis coincided with the transition period from dark to light and the lowest frequency occurred at the time of transition from light to dark. If, indeed, such a rhythm can be demonstrated in man, it may be possible to deliver chemotherapeutic agents at a time when they can be less toxic to the host's gastrointestinal and bone marrow system [76].

Evidence for neural control of cell proliferation in the large intestine as well as small intestine has been reported. Adrenergic nerves have been found in the lamina propria near the basal region of the crypts [77]. Chemically sympathectomized rats showed a decreased mitotic rate compared with controls [78]. Rats which received alpha adrenoreceptor stimulation had an increased mitotic rate while those experiencing alpha adrenergic blockade had a reduced mitotic rate. Those that received either stimulation or blockade of beta-adrenoceptors exhibited no alteration in cell proliferation [78]. Similarly neither serotonin or histamine influenced colonic epithelial cell proliferation in any measured way.

A mesenchymal–epithelial cell interaction has been postulated to exist between the fibroblasts forming the collagenous sheath around each crypt and the epithelial cells lining the crypt. The characteristic migration of epithelial cells from the base of the crypt to the lumen was reported to be accompanied by a similar migration pattern within the fibroblast population [78, 80]. The ability to undergo DNA synthesis and mitosis has recently been confirmed for the cryptal fibroblasts [81]. Labeled fibroblasts were seen along the entire cryptal wall but the predominant number were along the lower two-thirds of the gland. After three weeks little change in the distribution of labeled fibroblasts was observed, evidence that appreciable migration did not occur. An L.I. of 2.4% for these cells was determined, indicating they are a slowly renewing cell population [81].

6.2. Kinetics in Diseased States

6.2.1. Polyps. An understanding of the development of polyps and their role with regard to colon cancer has involved histological analysis of their size, appearance and proliferative activity. Histologically there are three major types, which have been studied with great intensity: hyperplastic or metaplastic polyps, tubular adenomas or adenomatous polyps and villous adenomas. The hyperplastic polyp is an independent entity not only histologically different from the two types of adenoma, but with a less aggressive nature. Hyperplastic polyps show an increased number and hypermaturity of goblet and absorptive cells [82, 83]. Epithelial cells lining the cryptal walls are of irregular size with increased numbers of tall microvilli. The variation in cell size give glands the commonly described 'sawtooth' or serrated appearance [82]. Hyperplastic polyps have a thickened, well differentiated fibroblast sheath at the surface of the crypts concomitant with a hypermature population of epithelial cells in this region [79, 80, 83]. Unlike adenomatous polyps, hyperplastic polyps are not formed by the production of new glands but grow by papillary infolding [84].

Tubular adenomas and villous adenomas are neoplastic lesions, the latter being more so than the former. These excrescences grow as a result of two operative mechanisms. There is infolding of the surface epithelium as well as new gland formation at the upper regions of the crypts. Involvement of the mesenchymal layer in proliferation along with the epithelial defects would lead to the development of villi and the formation of the villous adenoma [84].

Adenomatous polyp epithelium is composed of immature cells which are uniform in size and thin and pencil-like in shape. Goblet cells have only an extremely small size goblet and therefore sparse amounts of mucus can be present; however, the frequency of goblet cells varies from area to area [82]. Unlike the hyperplastic polyp, the fibroblastic sheath is not well developed at the surface or luminal area. It is instead similar in its immature appearance to the membrane at the base of crypts [79].

Epithelial cell renewal in hyperplastic polyps occurs in the same regions as

in normal mucosa although some enlargement of the proliferative compartment has been noted [82, 85]. In contrast, in the adenomatous polyp, DNA
synthesizing epithelial cells predominate in the upper thirds and along the
mucosal surface [71, 86–90]. No difference in the duration of S phase has
been noted between cells of the polyp and those of the normal colonic
mucosa, but a two fold increase in the labeling indices has been reported [71].
Estimates of the cell cycle time are approximately one half that of the normal
colonic epithelial cell (33 hours vs 80 hours).

When polyps are fragmented and cell separation techniques employed in
conjunction with a DNA polymerase assay with ^{3}HTTP; the growth fraction
(GF) of actual cycling cells in the total population can be determined. In the
case of adenomatous polyps and villous adenomas the GF for these tumors
was approximately 32% of the cell population [91]. It must be remembered
though that this particular assay system only follows the viable cells, those
which are not excluded by filtration as being part of a larger aggregate, and
those survivors of Ficoll-Hypaque centrifugation.

6.2.2. Mucosa Adjacent to Tumors. The histologically normal appearing
colorectal mucosa adjacent to polyps and carcinomas has been found to have
at least three different proliferative patterns (Table 4). Basically, epithelial cell
replication in the large bowel of most animals and man occurs in the lower
two-thirds of the crypts with the lower one-third the predominate zone of
DNA synthesis. Another pattern observed involves extension of the proliferative compartment to the surface (Stage I defect). This is seen in patients with
multiple polyposis, familial polyposis, some symptom-free members of polyposis families, patients with an isolated adenomatous polyp, some patients in

Table 4. Types of proliferative pattern in colorectal crypts.

Pattern	Base of gland Lower third	Middle third	Lumen of gland Upper third
Normal	————————	– – – – – – – –	
Stage I defect	————————	– –
	Extension of proliferation compartment		
Stage II defect	– – – – – – – –	————————	– – – – – – – –
		or	
	– – – – – – – –	————————	————————
		or	
	– – – – – – – – – – – – – – – – – – – –		————————
	Shift in major zone of proliferation		

——————— = predominant zone of proliferation.
– – – – – – – = area of cell proliferation.

the general population and patients with a history of a previous colon cancer [87, 90]. Although the proliferative compartment is enlarged in the Stage I abnormality, the major zone of cell replication remains in the lower third of the crypts. This defect is thought to be an early expression of loss of regulatory control over repression of DNA synthesis at the top of the middle third of the gland.

The third proliferative pattern reported in patients with a previous history of colon cancer is a shift in the predominant region of DNA synthesis from the lower third to the middle and upper thirds of the glands (Stage II defect) [90, 92]. This pattern has also been observed in mice after five weekly injections of the colon carcinogen 1,2-dimethylhydrazine [90]. It occurs at a time when focal areas of cellular atypism are beginning to appear in the upper portion of colonic crypts prior to the formation of adenomatous polyps and carcinomas [93]. When patients with the Stage I defect were surveyed, it was found that the Stage II abnormality occurred with less frequency, indicating it to be a further step in the development of a neoplasm in the mucosa [90].

6.2.3. Ulcerative Colitis. It has been reported that between 3% and 10% of all patients with ulcerative colitis develop colon cancer [94, 95] but in patients having the disease along the total length of the colon and for a period greater than 20 years, the incidence is four times higher [96, 97]. The continued ulceration and regeneration of the mucosa is characterized by alteration in chromosome number and structure. Chromatid breaks occur and cells with hypotetraploid karyotypes are present [98]. Adenomatous polyps develop in the ulcerative colitis mucosa as does adenomatous epithelium and both are believed to be precancerous. Of biopsy and colectomy specimens from patients with ulcerative colitis, 19% have been found to contain foci of adenomatous epithelium [99]. Endogenously formed carcinogens [13] or abnormal levels of promotors such as certain bile acids present in the lumen [100] may induce malignant transformation not only in such areas of neoplasia in these patients but also in any bearing adenomas.

Biopsies from patients with ulcerative colitis placed in culture and allowed to incorporate ³HTdR have revealed epithelial cells to be migrating faster toward the lumen and to be more heavily engaged in proliferative activity than cells in control material (Table 5) [101]. The duration of S phase was not significantly lengthened but the estimated turnover time for these cells is rapid (34 hours vs 90 hours for controls) [70].

Extension of the proliferative compartment to the surface of glands has been noted in ulcerative colitis material [70, 101–103], an observation previously made on histologically normal appearing mucosa adjacent to polyps [87, 88, 90]. This abnormal zone of DNA synthesis is thought to reflect an early expression of a defect in the normal regulatory controls that bring

Table 5. Histologic and proliferative characteristics of epithelial cells in ulcerative colitis mucosa.

Hypotetraploid karyotypes
High degree of adenomatous transformation
Increased L.I.
Fast migration rate
Normal S phase duration
Decreased duration of cell cycle time
No inhibition of DNA synthesis with phosphodiesterase inhibitors after U.C. >10 years
Expansion of proliferative compartment (Stage I defect)
Shift in major zone of DNA synthesis within crypts (Stage II defect)

---

about differentiation and repression of DNA synthesis. However, in ulcerative colitis mucosa, the possibility exists that this may be a response to the severity of the disease and therefore a normal component of the feedback mechanism.

The ability of phosphodiesterase inhibitors to reduce the level of DNA synthesis was tested in the colonic mucosa of patients with long-standing chronic ulcerative colitis [104]. Those with left sided and those with universal colitis for over ten years showed no inhibition of thymidine incorporation, while those with either form of the disease for less than ten years displayed normal theophylline inhibition. Similarly the mucosa of ulcerative colitis patients with colon cancer and premalignant changes in the mucosa did not reveal theophylline induced inhibition of DNA synthesis. However, this defect in the control of DNA synthesis was seen regardless of whether premalignant changes were present in the tissue and is a biochemical alteration which may precede or accompany histopatologic changes in the mucosa [104].

In addition to this defect relating to control of DNA synthesis, patients with ulcerative colitis sometimes display an abnormal distribution of S phase cells within crypts [103]. Rather than having the lower third of crypts act as the major zone of DNA synthesis, the middle and upper third of crypts have the greater number of proliferating cells. Among a group of 18 patients with ulcerative colitis ranging in duration from several months to over 20 years, approximately 39% demonstrated this shift in the major zone of DNA synthesis (Stage 2 defect); 72% of ulcerative colitis patients showed extension of the proliferative compartment to the surface (Stage 1 defect). The mucosa of patients with this shift in the major proliferative compartments is presumed to be engaged in the future development of tumor tissue in this area [103].

6.2.4. Large Bowel Cancer. Large bowel carcinoma is the second most common form of cancer found in economically well-developed countries of the West. For this reason it is this area that has had more effort applied to it to obtain kinetic information than any other region of the gastrointestinal tract. At first, observations of the kinetic properties of human colon cancer cells were made directly on the tumor following injection of ^{3}HTdR into patients with limited life expectancy [67, 68, 105]. In the sixties and seventies, much activity centered about *in vitro* measurements. Short pulse tritiated thymidine labeling indices were sought for malignant tissue using a variety of techniques [91, 106, 107]. They were obtained for clinical use to determine if there was predictive value for therapeutic treatment or a relationship with the drug of choice and clinical response. Recently studies of human colon cancer have involved the development of cell lines and observations of the nude heterotransplant system [108, 109].

Only one *in vivo* study was carried out over a long enough period to allow a complete percent labeled mitosis curve to be obtained [105]. The generation time for these colon cancer cells was 26 hours, and the duration of S phase 14 hours. The labeling index for this tissue was 23.1% and both G_1 and G_2 phases were of similar durations, 5 hours and 5.7 hours respectively.

Other L.I. obtained *in vivo* for carcinoma cells ranged from 13 to 21.7% [110]. Those reported using *in vitro* techniques often are lower, i.e. 4.5 and 6.6% [111, 112] but variability may be due to improper oxygenation of tissue for adequate ^{3}HTdR incorporation, or variability within the tumor [111]. Metastases have been shown to have a median L.I. of 5% but a range of values from 1.5 to 35% [107]. After chemotherapy with 5-FUDR, the L.I. of colon cancer tissue measured *in vitro* within 7 days changed and correlated well with the clinical effects evaluated 3 months later. A two-fold change in L.I. over time was thought to reflect an effect of therapy [107]. There may be some possibility of determining response to chemotherapy or radiotherapy early in the therapeutic schedule to delineate those resistant to treatment.

Estimated cell cycle times for tumor cells from *in vitro* studies are higher than 26 hours, the value determined by Terz [105]. They range instead from 30.2 to 244 hours [72, 73, 111]. The differences may in part be explained by the lower labeling indices and the longer S phase durations reported. Camplejohn *et al.* found normal rectal epithelial cells to have a mitotic duration of 1.2 hours while the mean value for 19 carcinomas studied was 2.3 hours [73].

Labeling indices of human colon adenocarcinomas grown in nude mice ranged from 9 to 22% [108], covering the spectrum of *in vitro* and *in vivo* values previously mentioned. Two xenograft lines, one a well-differentiated columnar cell carcinoma of the colon and the other a poorly differentiated one, examined for kinetic parameters had L.I. values of 22.2 and 19.0% respectively [109]. Carcinoma cells from the well-differentiated malignancy had a slightly longer cell cycle time than cells from the poorly differentiated one (35 vs 26 hours). The growth fraction or percentage of cells involved in proliferation was almost precisely the same for both lines (47 vs 46%). The fraction reported by Terz with his *in vivo* data was between 42 and 49% of the cells[105]; however, other estimates have been as low as 13–25% [73] in one *in vitro* study and 10.7–48.6% in another[91]. The latter two studies involved 19 and 17 colon carcinomas respectively. Varaibility in the growth fraction may be related to differences in oxygenated and anoxic areas within the tumors since fewer proliferative cells are seen in poorly vascularized tissue[113].

Tumor volume doubling times have also been found to vary considerably from study to study and compared poorly with the actual volume doubling times of 111 to 3430 days determined by analysis of radiological films[114]. Measurements of pulmonary metastases of colorectal carcinomas had a mean doubling time of 9.5 days[109]. In general estimated values derived from *in vitro* and *in vivo* studies range from 3 days[110, 111, 115] to 45 days[105], falling far short of actual measured doubling times. One factor which may play an important role in the slow growth of tumors is the rate of cell loss. This factor too has been estimated by various authors to be as high as 90% [73] but another report showed only one half the rate of cell loss[105].

Kopper and Steel measured the growth of well-differentiated and poorly differentiated colon carcinoma lines in the flank of immunosuppressed mice[109]. They determined a volume doubling of 11.8 days and a cell loss fraction of 80% for the former and a 6 day doubling time and 66% cell loss factor for the latter xenograft line. Again a far faster doubling time than has been reported in man but an extremely high cell loss fraction was indicated. The lack of resemblance between the actual doubling times for mice and man may relate to the sizes of tumors involved since doubling time often increases with increasing size and the tumors in mice are relatively small. Xenograft lines of colon carcinoma have been tested in immunosuppressed mice against several single chemotherapeutic agents, each of which altered tumor growth, regardless of the histological appearance of the line[109]. The greatest response was achieved with the use of 5-FU.

Studies of cell proliferation have been instrumental in the development and use of cell cycle specific drugs in combination with cell-cycle nonspecific agents. Improvement in leukemic cure rates is based on this approach. Of primary concern in cancer therapy has always been detection of differences in kinetic behavior between carcinoma cells and normal cells. At present, three approaches may be useful with colonic cancer and they have both come to light in experimental models.

Evidence from animal work suggests that unlike normal tissue, malignant cells do not follow a predictable synchronized circadian rhythm[76]. Thus administration of a drug or the use of irradiation at the appropriate nadir of cell proliferation in the colon may produce less toxic effect to the normal tissue and a selectively greater killing of tumor cells.

The second approach comes from research using the colon carcinogen, 1,2-dimethylhydrazine in rats. Chemical sympathectomy significantly lowered the mitotic rate in normal crypts but did not influence it in adeno-carcinomas[78]. The use of drugs releasing norepinephrine as well as alpha-adrenergic manipulation influenced cell proliferation in the normal crypts while tumor cell proliferation was unaltered. Observations such as these indicate autonomic neural control over normal colonic proliferative activity whereas it is reduced or absent in neoplastic tissue. Again selective advantage may perhaps be achieved between tumor and normal colonic mucosa by manipulation of neural response thus altering the ratio of proliferative cells in both tissues[78].

In addition to revealing the lack of neural control present in colonic tumor tissue, Tutton has demonstrated that serotonin or histamine injection stimu-lated the mitotic rate within the neoplasm but not in the normal tissue[78]. The hormone-dependency revealed in DMH-induced tumors may exist in human large bowel cancer and may be the basis for a new therapeutic strategy against its aggressive character.

It becomes evident from this brief exposition on the proliferative character-istics of normal and neoplastic gastrointestinal cells that our storehouse of information is large and growing. Kinetic data have successfully provided a rationale for chemotherapeutic usage with bone marrow malignancies but have had limited success against solid tumors, particularly stomach and large bowel cancer. Now that animal models have been developed for the induction of both gastric and large bowel neoplasia, the biological tools are available to define and describe proliferative characteristics under new and unique condi-tions, seeking always to uncover important selective differences between tumor and normal tissue growth.

REFERENCES

1. Casteleyn PP, Dubrasquet M, Willems G: Opposite effects of gastrin on cell proliferation in the antrum and other parts of the upper gastrointestinal tract in the rat. Dig Dis 22:798–804, 1977.
2. Neuburger P, Lewin M, Bonfils S: Parietal and chief cell populations in four cases of the Zollinger-Ellison syndrome. Gastroenterology 63:937–942, 1973.
3. Messier B, Leblond CP: Cell Proliferation and migration as revealed by radioautography after injection of thymidine H^3 into male rats and mice. Am J Anat 106:247–285, 1960.
4. Bell B, Almy TP, Lipkin M: Cell proliferation kinetics in the gastrointestinal tract of man. III. Cell renewal in esophagus stomach and jejunum of a patient with treated pernicious anemia. J Natl Cancer Inst 38:615–628, 1967.

5. Blenkinsopp WK: Cell proliferation in stratified squamous epithelium in mice. Exp Cell Res 50:265–276, 1968.
6. Pilgrim C, Erb W, Mauer W: Diurnal fluctuations in the numbers of DNA synthesizing nuclei in various mouse tissues. Nature 199:863, 1968.
7. Herbst JJ, Berenson MM, McCloskey DW, Wiser WC: Cell proliferation in esophageal columnar epithelium (Barrett's esophagus). Gastroenterology 75:683–687, 1978.
8. Morson BC, Dawson IMP: Gastrointestinal Pathology. Oxford: Blackwell Scientific, 1972, pp 19–75.
9. Berenson MM, Riddell RH, Skinner DB, Freston JW: Malignant transformation of esophageal columnar epithelium. Cancer 41:554–561, 1978.
10. Pellish LJ, Hermons JA, Eastwood GL: Cell proliferation in three types of Barrett's epithelium. Gut 21:26–31, 1980.
11. Brand DL, Ylvisaker JT, Gelfand M, Pope CE: Regression of columnar esophageal (Barrett's) epithelium after anti-reflux surgery. N Engl J Med 302:844–848, 1980.
12. Fong LYY, Sivak A, Newberne PM: Zinc deficiency and methylbenzylnitrosamine-induced esophageal cancer in rats. J Natl Cancer Inst 61:145–150, 1978.
13. Tannenbaum SR: Ins and outs of nitrites. The Sciences 20:7–9, 1980.
14. Mirvish SS, Chu C, Clayson DB: Inhibition of ^{3}H thymidine incorporation into DNA of rat esophageal epithelium and related tissues by carcinogenic N-nitroso compounds. Cancer Res. 38:458–466, 1978.
15. Chu-chieh H, Armstrong D, Anderson L, Tsung-tang S, I-ying I, Good RA: Relationship of human esophageal carcinoma and fungal infection of the esophagus. Fed Proc 39:885, 1980.
16. Takahashi T, Shimazu H, Yamagishi T, Tani M: G cell populations in resected stomachs from gastric and duodenal ulcer patients. Gastroenterology 78:498–504, 1980.
17. Lipkin M, Sherlock P, Bell B: Cell Proliferation kinetics in the gastrointestinal tract of man. II. Cell renewal in stomach, ileum, colon, and rectum. Gastroenterology 45:721–729, 1963.
18. MacDonald WC, Trier JS, Everett NB: Cell proliferation and migration in the stomach, duodenum and rectum of man: radioautographic studies. Gastroenterology 46:405–417, 1964.
19. Castrup HJ, Fuchs K, Peiper HJ: Cell renewal of gastric mucosa in Zollinger-Ellison Syndrome. Acta Hepato-Gastroenterol 22:40–43, 1975.
20. Hart-Hansen O, Johansen AA, Larsen JK, Svendsen LB: Cell proliferation in normal and diseased gastric mucosa. Acta Path Microbiol Scand, Sect A 87:217–222, 1979.
21. Ragins H, Winczie F, Liu SM, Dittbrenner M: The origin and survival of gastric parietal cells in the mouse. Anat Res 162:99–110, 1968.
22. Willems G, Lehy T: Radioautographic and quantitative studies on parietal and peptic cell kinetics in the mouse. Gastroenterology 69:416–426, 1975.
23. Lehy T, Willems G: Populations kinetics of antral gastrin cells in the mouse. Gastroenterlogy 71:614–619, 1976.
24. Bertrand P, Willems G: Induction of antral gastric cell proliferation by refeeding of rats after fasting. Gastroenterology 78:918–924, 1980.
25. Morson BC, Dawson IMP: Gastrointestinal pathology. Oxford: Blackwell Scientific, 1972, pp 80–103.
26. Winawer SJ, Lipkin M: Cell proliferation kinetics in the gastrointestinal tract of man. IV. Cell renewal in the intestinalized gastric mucosa. J Natl Cancer Inst 42:9–19, 1969.
27. Hansen OH, Pedersen T, Larsen JK: A method to study cell proliferation kinetics in human gastric mucosa. Gut 16:23–27, 1975.
28. Liavag I: Mitotic activity of gastric mucosa. Acta Path Microbiol Scand 72:43–63, 1968.

29. Hoffman J, Post J: *In vivo* studies of DNA synthesis in human normal and tumor cells. Cancer Res 27:898–902, 1967.

30. Tanaka J: Autoradiographic studies on the cell proliferation of the human gastric mucosa in supravital condition. Acta Path Jap 18:307–318, 1968.

31. Wiendl HJ, Schwabe M, Becker G, Kowatsch J: Feulgencrytophotometric studies of gastric mucosal smears in malignant and benign diseases of the stomach. Acta Cytol 18:222–230, 1974.

32. Bell B, Almy TP, Lipkin M: Cell proliferation kinetics in the gastrointestinal tract of man. III. Cell renewal in esophagus, stomach, and jejunum of a patient with treated pernicious anemia. J Natl Cancer Inst 38:615–628, 1967.

33. Croft DN: Cell turnover and loss and the gastric mucosal barrier. Dig Dis 22:383–386, 1977.

34. Deschner EE, Winawer SJ, Lipkin M: Patterns of nucleic acid and protein synthesis in normal human gastric mucosa and atrophic gastritis. J Natl Cancer Inst 48:1567–1574, 1972.

35. Deschner EE, Tamura K, Bralow SP: Sequential histopathology and cell kinetic changes in rat pyloric mucosa during gastric carcinogenesis induced by N-methyl-N′-nitro-N-nitroso-guanidine. J Natl Cancer Inst 63:171–179, 1979.

36. Maskens A: Histogenesis and growth pattern of 1,2-dimethylhydrazine induced rat colon adenocarcinoma. Cancer Res 36:1585–1592, 1976.

37. Cheng H, Leblond CP: Origin differentiation and renewal of the four main epithelial cell types in the mouse small intestine. V. Unitarian theory of the origin of the four epithelial cell types. Am J Anat 141:537–548, 1974.

38. Fry RJM, Lesher S, Kisieleski WE, Sacher G: Cell proliferation in the small intestine. In: Cell Proliferation, Lamerton LF, Fry RJM (eds). Philadelphia: F.A. Davis, 1963, pp 213–233.

39. Wright N, Watson A, Morley A, Appleton D, Marks J, Douglas A: The cell cycle time in the flat (avillous) mucosa of the human small intestine. Gut 14:603–606, 1973.

40. Wright N, Watson A, Morley A, Appleton D, Marks J: Cell kinetics in flat (avillous) mucosa of the human small intestine. Gut 14:701–710, 1973.

41. Lesher S, Fry RJM, Sacher GA: Effects of chronic gamma irradiation on the generation cycle of the mouse duodenum. Exp Cell Res 25:398–404, 1961.

42. Tutton PJM, Helme RD: The influence of adrenoreceptor activity on crypt cell proliferation in the rat jejunum. Cell Tissue Kinet 7:125–136, 1974.

43. Lehy T, Dubrasquet M, Bonfils S: Effect of somatostatin on normal and gastric-stimulated cell proliferation in the gastric and intestinal mucosae of the rat. Digestion 19:99–109, 1979.

44. Tutton PJM: The influence of serotonin on crypt cell proliferation in the jejunum of rat. Virchows Arch B Cell Pathol 16:79–87, 1974.

45. Hooper CS, Blair M: The effect of starvation on epithelial renewal in the rat duodenum. Expl Cell Res 14:175–181, 1958.

46. Brown HO, Levine ML, Lipkin M: Inhibition of intestinal epithelial cell renewal and migration induced by starvation. Am J Physiol 205:868–872, 1963.

47. Fry RJM, Staffeldt E: Effect of a diet containing sodium deoxycholate on the intestinal mucosa of the mouse. Nature (Lond) 203:1396–1398, 1964.

48. Fry RJM, Kisieleski WE, Kraft B, Staffeldt E, Sullivan MF: Cell renewal in the intestine of bile duct cannulated rat. In: Gastrointestinal radiation injury, Sullivan MF (ed). Amsterdam: Excerpta Medica, 1968, pp 142–147.

49. Williamson RCN, Bauer FLR, Ross JS, Malt RA: Contribution of bile and pancreatic juice to cell proliferation in ileal mucosa. Surgery 83:570–576, 1978.

50. Roy CC, Laurendeau G, Doyon G, Chartrand L, Rivist MR: The effect of bile and sodium taurocholate on the epithelial cell dynamics of the rat small intestine. Proc Soc Exp Biol Med 149:1000–1004, 1975.

51. Deschner EE, Raicht RF: Influence of bile on kinetic behavior of colonic epithelial cells of the rat. Digestion 19:322–327, 1979.

52. Altman GG: Influence of bile and pancreatic secretions on the size of the intestinal villi in the rat. Am J Anat 132:167–178, 1971.

53. Foroozan P, Trier JS: Mucosa of the small intestine in pernicious anemia. New Engl J Med 277:553–559, 1967.

54. Croft DN, Loehry CA, Creamer B: Small bowel cell-loss and weight-loss in the celiac syndrome. Lancet 2:68–70, 1968.

55. Padykula HA, Strauss EW, Ladman AJ, Gardner EH: A morphologic and histochemical analysis of the human jejunal epithelium in nontypical sprue. Gastroenterology 40:735–765, 1961.

56. Brandt L, Hagander B, Norden A, Stenstam M: Lymphoma of the small intestine in adult coeliac disease. Acta Med Scand 204:467–470, 1978.

57. Tilson MD, Sweeney T, Wright HK: Compensatory hypertrophy of the ileum after gastro-duodenojejunal exclusion. Arch Surg 110:309–312, 1975.

58. Loran MR, Althausen TL: Cellular proliferation of intestinal epithelia in the rat two months after partial resection of the ileum. J Biophys and Biochem Cytol 7:667–679, 1960.

59. McDermott FT, Roudnow B: Ileal crypt cell populations kinetics after 40% small bowel resections. Gastroenterology 70:707–711, 1976.

60. Hanson WR, Osborne JW: Epithelial cell kinetics in the small intestine of the rat 60 days after resection of 70 per cent of the ileum and jejunum. Gastroenterology 60:1087–1097, 1971.

61. Ecknauer R, Clarke RM, Meyer H: Acute distal intestinal obstructions in gnotobiotic rats. Intestinal morphology and cell renewal. Virchow Arch B Cell Path 25:151–160, 1977.

62. McDermott F, Roudnew B: Epithelial cell population kinetics of isolated ileal loops (Thiry-Vella Fistulae) after 40% small intestinal resection. Virchows Arch B Cell Path 28:179–185, 1978.

63. Fatemi SH, Cullan GE, Crouse DA, Sharp JG: Relative roles of gastrin and glucagon in the control of intestinal cell proliferation. Cell Tissue Kinet (abstract), 13:685, 1980.

64. Lehnert S: Changes in growth kinetics of jejunal epithelium in mice maintained on an elemental diet. Cell Tissue Kinet 12:239–248, 1979.

65. Verity MA, Mellinkoff SM, Frankland AB, Greipel M: Serotonin content and argentaffin and Paneth cell changes in ulcerative colitis. Gastroenterology 43:24–31, 1962.

66. Chang WWL, Nadler NJ: Renewal of the epithelium in the descending colon of the mouse. IV. Cell population kinetics of vacuolated, columnar and mucous cells. Am J Anat 144:39–56, 1975.

67. Lipkin M, Bell B, Sherlock P: Cell proligeration kinetics in the gastrointestinal tract of man. I. Cell renewal in colon and rectum. J Clin Invest 42:767–776, 1963.

68. Lipkin M, Sherlock P, Bell B: Cell Proliferation kinetics in the gastrointestinal tract of man. II. Renewal in stomach, ileum, colon, and rectum. Gastroenterology 45:721–729, 1963.

69. Shorter RG, Spencer RJ, Hallenbeck GA: Kinetic studies of the epithelial cells of the rectal mucosa in normal subjects and patients with ulcerative colitis. Gut 7:593–596, 1966.

70. Bleiberg H, Mainguet P, Galand P, Chretien J, Dupont-Mairesse N: Cell renewal in the human rectum: In vitro autoradiographic study on active ulcerative colitis. Gastroenterology 58:851–855, 1970.

71. Bleiberg H, Mainguet P, Galand P: Cell renewal in familial polyposis. Comparison between polyps and adjacent healthy mucosa Gastroenterology 63:240–245, 1972.

72. Bleiberg H, Galand P: *In vitro* autoradiographic determination of cell kinetic parameters in adenocarcinomas and adjacent healthy mucosa of the human colon and rectum. Cancer Res 36:325–328, 1976.

73. Camplejohn RS, Bone G, Aherne W: Cell Proliferation in rectal carcinoma and rectal mucosa. A stathmokinetic study. Europ J Cancer 9:577–581, 1973.

74. Galand P, Mainguet P, Arguello M, Chretien J, Douxfils N: *In vitro* autoradiographic studies of cell proliferation in the gastrointestinal tract of man. J Nucl Med 9:37–39, 1968.

75. Chang WWL, Nadler NJ: Renewal of the epithelium in the descending colon of the mouse. IV. Cell population kinetics of vacuolated-columnar and mucous cells. Am J Anat 144:39–56, 1975.

76. Scheving LE, Burns ER, Pauly JE, Tsai TH: Circadian variations in cell division of the mouse alimentary tract, bone marrow, and corneal epithelium. Anat Res 191:479–486, 1978.

77. Costa M, Gabella G: Adrenergic innervation of the alimentary canal. Z Zellforsch 122:357–377, 1971.

78. Tutton PJM, Barkla DH: Neural control of colonic cell proliferation. Cancer 45:1172–1177, 1980.

79. Kaye GI, Lane N, Pascal RP: Colonic pericryptal fibroblast sheath: Replication, migration, and cytodifferentiation of a mesenchymal cell system in adult tissue. II. Fine structural aspects of normal rabbit and human colon. Gastroenterology 54:852–865, 1968.

80. Kaye GI, Pascal RR, Lane N: The colonic pericryptal fibroblast sheath: replication, migration, and cytodifferentiation of a mesenchymal cell system in adult tissue. III. Replication and differentiation in human hyperplastic and adenomatous polyps. Gastroenterology 60:515–536, 1971.

81. Maskens AP, Rahier JR, Meersseman FP, Dujardin-Loits R, Haot JG: Cell proliferation of pericryptal fibroblasts in the rat colon mucosa. Gut 20:775–779, 1979.

82. Lane N, Kaplan H, Pascal RR: Minute adenomatous and hyperplastic polyps of the colon: divergent patterns of epithelial growth with specific associated mesenchymal changes. Gastroenterology 60:537–551, 1971.

83. Hayashi T, Yatani R, Apostol J, Stemmermann GN: Pathogenesis of hyperplastic polyps of the colon: a hypothesis based on ultrastructure and *in vitro* cell kinetics. Gastroenterology 66:347–356, 1966.

84. Maskens AP: Histogenesis of adenomatous polyps in the human large intestine. Gastroenterology 77:1245–1251, 1979.

85. Kikkawa N: Experimantal studies on polypogenesis and carcinogenesis of the large intestine. Med J Osaka Univ 24:293–314, 1974.

86. Cole JW, McKalen A: Studies on the morphogenesis of adenomatous polyps in the human colon. Cancer 16:998–1002, 1963.

87. Deschner EE, Lewis CM, Lipkin M: *In vitro* study of human epithelial cells. I. Atypical zone of H[3]-thymidine incorporation in mucosa of multiple polyposis. J Clinical Invest 42:1922–1928, 1963.

88. Deschner EE, Lipkin M, Solomon C: *In vitro* Study of human epithelial cells. II. H[3]-thymidine incorporation into polyps and adjacent mucosa. J Natl Cancer Inst 36:849—857, 1966.

89. Deschner EE, Lipkin M: Study of human rectal epithelial cells *in vitro*. III. RNA, protein and DNA synthesis in polyps and adjacent mucosa. J Natl Cancer Inst 44:175–185, 1970.

90. Deschner EE: Cell proliferation as a biological marker in human colorectal neoplasia. In: Colorectal cancer: prevention, epidemiology and screening, Winawer S, Schottenfeld D,

Sherlock P (eds). New York: Raven Press, 1980, pp 138–142.

91. Lesher S, Schaffer LM, Phanse M: Human colonic tumor cell kinetics. Cancer 40:2706–2709, 1977.

92. Maskens AP, Deschner EE: Tritiated thymidine incorporation into epithelial cells of normal-appearing colorectal mucosa of cancer patients. J Natl Cancer Inst 58:1221–1224, 1977.

93. Deschner EE: Experimentally induced cancer of the colon. Cancer 34:824–828, 1974.

94. Mottet NK: Histopathologic spectrum of regional enteritis and ulcerative colitis. In: Major problems in pathology, vol II. Toronto: W.B. Saunders, 1971, pp 63–154.

95. Greenstein AJ, Sachar DB, Smith H, Janowitz HD, Aufses AH: Patterns of neoplasia in Crohn's disease and ulcerative colitis. Cancer 46:403–407, 1980.

96. Edwards FC, Truelove SC: The course and prognosis of ulcerative colitis. In: Carcinoma of the colon, part IV. Gut 5:15–22, 1964.

97. Sherlock P, Winawer SJ: Cancer in inflammatory bowel disease: Risk factors and prospects for early detection. In: Gastrointestinal tract cancer, Lipkin M, Good RA (eds). New York: Plenum Medical, 1978, pp 479–488.

98. Xavier RG, Prolla JC, Bemvenuti GA, Kirsner JB: Further tissue cytogenetic studies in inflammatory bowel disease. Gastroenterology 64:A–189/875, 1973.

99. Fenoglio Cm, Pascal RR: Adenomatous epithelium, intraepithelial anaplasia, and invasive carcinoma in ulcerative colitis. Dig Dis 18:556–562, 1973.

100. Cohen BI, Raicht RR, Deschner EE, Takahashi M, Sarwal AN, Fazzini E: Effect of cholic acid feeding on N-methyl-N-nitrosourea induced colon tumors and cell kinetics in rats. J Natl Cancer Inst 64:573–578, 1980.

101. Eastwood GL, Trier JS: Epithelial cell renewal in cultured rectal biopsies. Gastroenterology 64:383–390, 1973.

102. Biasco G, Santini D, Marchesini F, DiFebo G, Baldi F, Miglioli M, Barbara L: Kinetics of the mucous cells of the rectum in patients with chronic ulcerative colitis. Frontiers Gastrointestinal Res 4:65–72, 1979.

103. Deschner EE, Katz S, Katzka I, Kahn E: Proliferative defects in ulcerative colitis patients. Gastroenterology 78:1155, 1980.

104. Alpers DH, Philpott G, Grimme NL, Margolis DM: Control of thymidine incorporation in mucosal explants from patients with chronic ulcerative colitis. Gastroenterology 78:470–478, 1980.

105. Terz JJ, Curatchet HP, Lawrence W: Analysis of the cell kinetics of human solid tumors. Cancer 28:1100–1110, 1971.

106. Sky-Peck HH: Effects of chemotherapy on the incorporation of ^{3}H-thymidine into DNA of human neoplastic tissue. Natl Cancer Inst Monograph 34:197-203, 1971.

107. Livingston RB, Ambus V, George SL, Freereich EJ, Hart JS: In vitro determination of thymidine — ^{3}H labeling index in human solid tumors. Cancer Res 34:1375–1380, 1974.

108. Schmidt M, Deschner EE, Thaler TH, Clements L, Good RA: Gastrointestinal cancer studies in the human to nude mouse heterotransplant system. Gastroenterology 72:829–837, 1977.

109. Kopper L, Steel GG: The therapeutic response of three human tumor lines maintained in immune-suppressed mice. Cancer Res 35:2704–2713, 1975.

110. Hoffman J, Post J: In vivo studies of DNA synthesis in human normal and tumor cells. Cancer Res 27:898–902, 1967.

111. Lieb LM, Lisco H: In vitro uptake of tritiated thymidine by carcinoma of the human colon. Cancer Res 36:733–740, 1966.

112. Wolberg W, Brown R: Autoradiographic studies of in vitro incorporation of uridine and thymidine by human tumor tissue. Cancer Res 22:1113–1119, 1962.

113. Tannock IF, Steel GG: Tumor growth and cell kinetics in chronically hypoxic animals. J Natl Cancer Inst 45:123–133, 1970.
114. Welin S, Youker J, Spratt JS: The rates and patterns of growth of 375 tumors of the large intestine and rectum observed serially by double contrast enema study (Malmo technique). Am J Roentgenol 90:673–687, 1963.
115. Baserga R, Henegar GC, Kisieleski WE, Lisco H: Uptake of tritiated thymidine by human tumors *in vivo*. Lab Invest 11:360-364, 1962.

2. Genetic Aspects of Gut Cancer

RICHARD B. McCONNELL

1. INTRODUCTION

The contribution of genetic predisposition to the origin of cancer may be much greater than has been supposed. In particular there has been gradually increasing evidence that for nearly all cancers there is at least one form which is inherited in a simple mendelian manner. In the past only certain rare tumours were known to be determined by simple genetic mechanisms and the genetic predisposition to most common cancers was considered to be vaguely polygenic, probably with genes at a large number of loci each able to make a small contribution by susceptibility to one or more environmental agents. This quantitative basis of genetic susceptibility may still underlie many sporadic cases of cancer but there is growing evidence in some of these polygenic systems that there can be one or more major genes which, when present, are able to cause cancer with only minimal environmental stimulus. Such major genes can be responsible for occasional familial aggregations of a cancer suggestive of mendelian type of inheritance. It is hoped that intensive study of this type of family will identify such major genes and their biochemical or immunological effects and thus provide insights into the nature of the carcinogenic process.

1.1. Combined Genetic and Environmental Research

The search for environmental factors responsible for human cancer has been disappointing. A considerable impetus was given to such studies 30 years ago by the smoking–lung cancer findings but they have not led to any comparable relationship being demonstrated other than in breast and uterine cancer. Apart from a vague relationship between alcohol consumption and oesophageal, liver and pancreatic carcinomas, no environmental factor of any magnitude has been established in gastrointestinal cancers. It may be relevant that a strong familial element has been demonstrated in some of these

J.J. DeCosse and P. Sherlock (eds.), Gastrointestinal cancer 1, 27-62. All rights reserved.

gastrointestinal cancers.

A combined genetic and environmental approach to cancer research should prove more profitable than separate studies. It is interesting that a genetic influence can be demonstrated in lung cancer in spite of the strength of the smoking factor. It was found [1] that the non-smoking relatives of lung cancer patients had an increased risk of lung cancer similar to that of smokers without any such family history of the disease. In addition smokers with a family history of lung cancer had a risk that was greater than the sum of both familial and smoking risks.

In a search for genes which might be contributing to this increased susceptibility to the effects of smoking, an enzyme called aryl hydrocarbon hydroxylase was studied [2]. This enzyme is inducible, membrane-bound and involved in the metabolism of chemical carcinogens found in tars. The extent of induction in cultured human leucocytes is under genetic control, there being a polymorphism in United States whites with about 10% having high inducibility and 45% low inducibility. In lung cancer patients, all of whom were heavy smokers, the inducibility was high in 30% and low in only 4%. These data suggest that susceptibility to lung cancer is associated with high levels of inducible aryl hydrocarbon hydroxylase activity and Kazazian [3] takes the view that this may be one of many inherited risk factors for lung cancer, with gradations of risk being modulated by different genes acting in combination and by different environmental factors.

1.2. Chromosomal Abnormalities

There is a vast literature on chromosomal abnormalities in tumours but it is quite uncertain if these aberrations are aetiologically significant in human carcinogenesis. Some may be directly related such as the specific deletions of retinoblastoma, Wilm's tumor or the Philadelphia chromosome of chronic myeloid leukaemia [4]. In this gastrointestinal review little mention will be made of chromosome abnormalities other than the important work of Danes in polyposis coli [5].

1.3. Genetic Mechanisms

From a genetic point of view gastrointestinal cancers can be divided into these determined by single genes and therefore inherited in a more or less simple mendelian manner and those in which the genetic influence is more complex and due to genes at several loci influencing susceptibility to environmental carcinogenic factors.

1.3.1. Single Gene Inheritance. It has been estimated [6] that there is an association with malignancy in nearly 10% of the 2 000 diseases known to have mendelian inheritance. In most of these the increased cancer risk applies

Table 1. Conditions with single gene inheritance and 100% cancer risk.

Condition	Site of malignancy
Clarke–Howel-Evans Syndrome	Oesophagus
Familial polyposis coli	Colon
Discrete colonic polyps	Colon
Cancer Family Syndrome	{ Stomach
(Adenocarcinomatosis)	{ Colon

to parts of the body other than the gastrointestinal tract.

There are only a few gastrointestinal cancers that are determined by a single gene. In some the cancer develops in nearly all the individuals carrying the abnormal gene, for instance in carcinoma of the colon with polyposis coli and in carcinoma of the oesophagus with puberty-onset tylosis (Table 1).

There are also the familial cancers ('cancer family syndrome', 'adenocarcinomatosis') which appear to show dominant inheritance, with great variability of phenotypic expression between families, suggesting considerable genetic heterogenicity. The part of the gastrointestinal tract chiefly involved in these cancer families is the colon, though there are many references in the literature to familial occurrence of cancer at other gastrointestinal sites, the explanation of which may be single gene inheritance but may equally well be chance aggregation due to an exceptional environmental load.

Other gastrointestinal cancers in which single gene inheritance plays a part are those in which an inherited condition carries a risk of cancer development, e.g. carcinoma of the pancreas with hereditary pancreatitis and malignant hepatoma with haemochromatosis (Table 2).

In some syndromes the cancer risk is mainly in organs other than those of the gastrointestinal tract, e.g. ataxia telangiectasis, in which carcinoma of the

Table 2. Conditions with single gene inheritance and increased gastrointestinal cancer risk.

Condition	Site of malignancy
Ataxia telangiectasia	Stomach
Dyskeratosis congenita ⎫	{ Oesophagus
Bloom syndrome ⎭	{ Rectosigmoid
Alpha-1-antitrypsin deficiency	Liver
Hereditary pancreatitis	Pancreas
Peutz-Jeghers syndrome	Stomach, intestines
Haemochromatosis	Liver
Wilson's disease	Liver
Multiple endocrine neoplasia I	Pancreatic islets
Severe atrophic fundic gastritis	Stomach

stomach occurs [7]. In dyskeratosis congenita and Bloom syndrome, the molecular pathology includes defective DNA synthesis and one might expect to find an increased incidence of malignancy. Indeed an increased incidence of carcinoma of the oesophagus and carcinoma of the rectosigmoid has been reported [8].

Certain single gene-determined enzyme deficiencies can lead to an increased cancer risk. For instance, alpha-1-antitrypsin deficiency may influence hepatoma development [9] in addition to predisposing to chronic obstructive airway disease in the presence of cigarette smoking.

1.3.2. Polygenic Inheritance. In the majority of patients with gastrointestinal cancer no simple pattern of inheritance is apparent. In these sporadic cases the genetic basis of susceptibility to carcinogens is probably due to several genes at different loci, most with heterozygous effect but some possibly requiring inheritance from both parents. The inheritance may be in two parts, there being considerable evidence of an inherited tendency to develop non-site-specific cancer and a separately inherited tendency to develop cancer of a particular organ. Many family studies of patients with common cancers such as gastric carcinoma, show not only an increased incidence of that cancer in relatives as compared with controls, but also of cancer at other sites.

With a common condition it can be expected that occasional families will be found in which, by change alone, several members have been affected. As well as chance, such aggregations may be due to a heavy concentration of environmental factors or to an unusual concentration of the genes of the polygenic systems, but the possibility cannot be excluded that the genetic mechanism is due to an unusual major gene. Early onset of cancer or the occurrence of multiple cancers in an organ are features favouring the major gene explanation.

Careful statistical analysis of data derived from family and twin studies is necessary before the role of genetic factors in the aetiology of common cancers can be determined. The problem of statistical controls is not easy to resolve. The incidence of cancer in the general population is important, but in stratified populations this can be misleading. With satisfactory control data, calculations can be made of the likelihood of family aggregations occurring by chance alone and an expected incidence in relatives can be approximated.

1.3.3. Polygenic Inheritance with Increased Cancer Risk. There are several conditions in which inheritance plays a part and which are associated with a cancer risk higher than that expected from general population frequencies. Examples are inflammatory bowel disease and coeliac disease (Table 3). The hereditary mechanism in this group of conditions is probably not the effect of one gene but rather is multifactorial and due to both the effect of several

Table 3. Polygenically inherited conditions with increased gastrointestinal cancer risk.

Condition	Site of malignancy
Pernicious anaemia	Stomach
Coeliac disease	Oesophagus, intestines
Crohn's disease	Intestines
Ulcerative colitis	Colon
Chronic calcifying pancreatitis	Pancreas
Cirrhosis of liver	Liver
Juvenile polyposis	Stomach, intestines

genes as well as a considerable environmental influence. The increased cancer risk in these conditions may be due to a non-specific effect of the disease or may have a genetic basis associated with the genotype of the condition. For instance, abdominal lymphoma associated with coeliac disease may be associated with the same immunological disturbance which underlies the coeliac disease. There are strong genetic influences in several immunologal defects [10].

1.4. Cancer Families

In this chapter the part played by heredity in gut cancer will be considered under anatomical headings. There is, however, an important aspect of the subject that needs to be considered separately as it can involve the inheritance of cancer at several sites in one family. Mention has already been made of an apparent inherited tendancy to develop cancer *per se*. Families are often reported in the literature in which many members have been affected by cancer of various organs. The name 'Adenocarcinomatosis' has been applied but, more often, the term 'Cancer Family Syndrome' is used.

During the past decade many cancer families have been studied by Lynch and his Omaha group and a good deal of progress has been made in subdividing this heterogeneous group into different types [11]. One of the features of the cancer families is that by far the commonest tumour has been cancer of the large bowel and, particularly, of the proximal colon [12]. In some of the families the only cancer found is in the large bowel, in others there have been, in addition, many members with carcinoma of the endometrium and ovary [13], and in yet other families the additional malignancy has been of the breast [14] or elsewhere in the gastrointestinal tract. Other features of the Cancer Family Syndrome are an early age at onset of malignancy, usually between 30 and 50 years of age, though occasionally earlier [15], and multiple primary cancers [16].

There can be little doubt that in many of these families cancer is being inherited in a dominant manner, presumably due to the presence of single genes or, possibly, one gene the expression of which varies from family to family due to other modifying genes. There have been far too many of these large families described to be merely due to chance aggregations of cancer. *In vitro* defects of cellular immunity have been demonstrated in Cancer Family Syndrome patients [17].

Though it would be unwise to exclude the involvement of environmental factors in the production of cancer in the members of these families, the evidence suggests that they are not of much importance in deciding which members develop a carcinoma.

It is not known what proportion of sporadic large bowel cancers encountered in clinical practice are due to these major genes, but the finding of a strong family history of the disease when the patient is below 50 years of age or has multiple large bowel cancers [18] suggests that single gene cancers make up as much as 10% of the total. It may be that because people have so few offspring nowadays the familial nature of the disease is often not apparent.

2. CARCINOMA OF OESOPHAGUS

There is little evidence of heredity being concerned in the majority of cases of cancer of the oesophagus. In a Danish study of 101 patients with 877 first-degree relatives and 341 healthy controls with 2572 relatives, no significant differences were found between the five cases of oesophageal cancer in the patient's relatives (0.57%) and the 13 (0.51%) in the control relatives [19].

This lack of evidence of increase in familial occurrence of cancer of the oesophagus in Denmark is in contract with the findings with cancer of other organs in which it is usual to find a site incidence in relatives about double that in controls. In China it has been found that patients with carcinoma of the oesophagus had a positive family history more frequently than controls without cancer [20]. However, in North China oesophageal cancer is the commonest type of cancer in males. In 1960, Lin county of Honan province had the extremely high prevalence rate of 67.26 cases per 100 000 population. In this county 61.4% of 935 patients were found to have a positive family history, but so had 42.9% of 375 healthy controls.

One of the most striking features of the epidemiological aspects of oesophageal carcinoma is the remarkable differences in incidence in different geographical locations. There is no other tumour with such large variations in incidence in different parts of the world. Even within Great Britain an eight-fold difference has been found between the incidence in North Wales and that in East Anglia [21]. Very much larger differences are found if

European and North American incidences are compared with those in West Kenya, Natal, the Transkei and Iran [22]. In Iran the high incidence was found both in areas populated by Iranians and in areas settled by Turkomans [23] (see Chapter 4).

The evidence suggests that in South Africa, at least the present high frequency in some locations has developed during the past half century. This suggests a strong newly-developed environmental aetiology as the genes in the population could not have changed appreciably in such a short time. Beer made from maize husks might be responsible [24]. More recent surveys in China have .revealed incidences even higher than those quoted above. In Linksien county the prevalence has been reported to be as high as 379 per 100 000 [25], and it is also of interest that a high prevalence of pharyngo-oesophageal cancer was found in domestic fowl.

One of the features of genetically determined cancer is the early age at onset compared with sporadic cancer. It is, therefore, interesting that there is a family in a village on the north-east coast of Iran, which has one of the highest prevalence rates in the world, in which 13 cases of oesophageal cancer are known to have occurred in three generations [26]. Such a family aggregation might be due to chance, But in 11 of the patients the carcinoma developed very much earlier than in patients with the same disease in other areas of north-eastern Iran. This might suggest a strong genetic factor in the aetiology of the disease in this family. Familial oesophageal cancer has been reported in three brothers in South America [27] and also in Russia [28]. There is an association with coeliac disease in which there is a strong genetic element [29].

2.1. Single Gene Oesophageal Cancer: Clarke–Howel-Evans Syndrome

The weight of evidence is in favour of the view that heredity plays little or no part in the aetiology of sporadic oesophageal cancer. It is, therefore, a surprise to find that there are families in which the disease is inherited in a simple mendelian dominant manner in association with the late onset type of tylosis (hyperkeratosis palmaris et plantaris). The first report of such families came from Liverpool [30, 31] and there has been a follow-up on them [32]. In these families at least 24 cases of carcinoma of the oesophagus have occurred during the past 50 years, all of them in members with tylosis, which is determined by a single gene. It has been calculated that members with the abnormal gene have a 95% risk of developing the cancer by the age of 65 years.

The association of tylosis and oesophageal carcinoma in these families is likely to have only one genetic explanation, and that is the existence of a single mutant gene which causes both tylosis and carcinoma of the oesophagus. This gene may or may not be at the same locus as the usual gene for late onset tylosis. A less likely, though possible, explanation is that there are two separate genes, one for tylosis and the other for carcinoma of oesophagus, so closely linked on a chromosome that no crossing-over has taken place in these large families.

Tylosis and oesophageal cancer have been reported together in other families [32–34] and it is, therefore, worthwhile to examine carefully the palms and soles of the feet of any patients who develop carcinoma of the oesophagus under the age of 50 years. Any sign of hyperkeratosis would be an indication for study of other members of the patient's family. Though prophylactic oesophagectomy is not yet a practical proposition, there is no doubt that one day it will be carried out in tylotic members of these families in the same way that prophylactic colectomy is done in affected members of polyposis coli families. In the meantime all that can be done is to tell the tylotics who are aware of their great cancer risk that they should report immediately even slight dysphagia or chest discomfort. Periodic oesophageal washings for cytology and endoscopy may be of value. The tylotics who are not aware of the risk can be told of it if it is judged that they are sufficiently stable to accept the news without the development of an anxiety state. In the Liverpool families there are few in this category, and, so far, most of the tylotics have been shielded from the knowledge of the fate that awaits them in early middle life.

In these Liverpool families with late-onset tylosis, oral leukoplakia was noted [35]. It is therefore interesting that a 25-year-old Los Angeles patient with both oesophageal cancer and oral leukoplakia had tylosis of the early childhood onset type [36].

3. CARCINOMA OF THE STOMACH

Probably there have been more investigations of the hereditary aspects of gastric carcinoma than of any other common cancer and a genetic influence has been clearly demonstrated in the increased liability of people with blood group A [37]. However, group A individuals are only about 20% more liable than people of the other blood groups. Consequently if the ABO locus represents the sole genetic factor involved it is unlikely that an hereditary component would be detected in conventional studies of the incidence of the disease in twins or other relatives.

Because carcinoma of the stomach is so common, occasional families will be found in which several cases have occurred by chance alone and it has, therefore, to be established whether or not families with multiple cases are found more frequently than can be accounted for by chance. It is, however, not enough to demonstrate significantly large numbers of familial aggregations of the disease since such familial concentrations may be due either to hereditary factors or to a common carcinogenic environment. These are, of course, the problems which have to be solved when considering the place of heredity in any common disease. However, with carcinoma of the stomach we are fortunate since there is available a considerable body of data to derive an answer.

3.1. Incidence in Populations

From the work that has been reported, it is clear that the incidence of the disease varies at least ten-fold from one country to another [38]. It is common in Japan, Finland, Poland and Chile and relatively uncommon in the white population of the United States, England and India. In addition there are smaller, but still substantial differences among ethnic, social and economic groups within countries. Gastric cancer is more frequent in North Wales than in South-East England. In industrial countries gastric cancer is more frequent among the poor, but in South Africa it is several times more frequent among the Cape Coloured as compared to the poorer Bantu workers.

It is not known whether these variations in incidence are due to genetic or to environmental differences, but with the exception of a report of asbestos in the talc used in Japan in the cooking of rice [39], specific environmental factors have, so far, escaped detection. Within Wales, varying opinions are held, from the high susceptibility to gastric cancer being a genetic character-istic of the Celtic people [40], to specific environmental factors operating and powerful enough to obliterate evidence of the ordinary genetic factors such as the increased susceptibility of blood group A people [41].

3.2. Twins

There are many pitfalls in the interpretation of twin data [42], but some reports are worthy of note [43]. A recent report concerned identical female twins who, at the age of 45, both developed adenocarcinoma of the gastric antrum [44]. Their mother had also died with a carcinoma of the gastric antrum, suggesting the possibility of gastric polyposis either of adenoma [45] or of juvenile type [46].

3.3. Incidence in relatives

Many studies have been reported in which the frequency of carcinoma of stomach among relatives of patients with the disease is compared either with the frequency in relatives of people who do not have the disease, or with the frequency of the disease in the general population. Most studies can be criticised on the grounds of biased ascertainment of the propositi, incomplete or inaccurate collection of the family data or unsuitable controls. This is particularly true of the early studies. Those published up to 1957 have been excellently reviewed [47].

Some of the investigations carried out since 1958 are open to the same criticisms as the earlier reports, but they provide further evidence for the conclusion that there is familial aggregation of carcinoma of the stomach. In addition, they tend to confirm the suspicion that the high incidence. of gastric cancer occurs in single family units (parents and offspring) rather than scattered randomly throughout all the more distant relatives. Five large cancer families have been studied in Utah, in each of whom three cases had occurred in one unit [48]. In these and 12 other families in which two or three cases had occurred, no similar concentration of cases were found in other units of the families. It was considered that this indicated that the genetic component for carcinoma of stomach is polygenic.

The families of 167 patients with carcinoma of the stomach and 145 patients with carcinoma of the large bowel were studied and the results were compared with general population frequencies in Ohio [49]. It was found that carcinoma of the stomach occurred in the relatives of patients with carcinoma of the stomach significantly more often than in the general population. Gastric cancer was about twice as common in both fathers and mothers and it was more than three times as frequent in brothers and sisters as expected. In contrast, carcinoma of the large intestine did not occur more commonly than would be expected from the frequency of the disease in the general population. In the relatives of patients with large bowel cancer, carcinoma of the stomach did not occur any more frequently than in the general population, although the number of cases of large bowel cancer was significantly higher.

There have been many other reports of the familial aspects of carcinoma of the stomach. In one from Mexico the records of 393 patients were analysed [50]. Three per cent had given a positive family history but there was such a family history in only 0.75% of the controls. More recently a detailed survey of gastric cancer in the Republic of San Marino [51] showed that gastric cancer accounted for 9.2% of deaths. Study of the families of the 36 patients who had died of the disease revealed that 25% had first degree relatives affected compared with only 5% of the relatives of age and sex-matched controls.

3.4. Incidence in Spouses

Although carcinoma of the stomach may be concentrated in some families, it does not necessarily follow that these family aggregations have a genetic explanation. Environmental factors operating on the members of some families could be responsible. An analysis of the frequency of the disease in non-blood relatives living in the same environment as the gastric cancer propositi would help to distinguish genetic and environmental factors. Two of the investigators of the incidence in blood relatives also studied the incidence in the spouses of the propositi, and in both studies it was found that the spouses had much the same incidence of the disease as the controls [52, 53].

It is thus likely that genetic factors are operating, but the results cannot be considered decisive since cancer patients and their spouses share a similar environment only during their married life. It is possible that carcinogenic factors operating in youth are important in the aetiology of the disease. These investigations do suggest, however, that important exogenous factors for stomach cancer are not present in the home environment of patients with stomach cancer during adult life.

3.5. The Genetic Basis of Gastric Cancer

Intense research during the past decade has resulted in several discoveries which suggest not only that there are a number of genes which play a relatively minor role in susceptibility of gastric cancer, such as the genes for blood group A, but also there may be genes which are able to make a major contribution to cancer susceptibility.

3.5.1. Immunologic Defects.
Isolated reports of large families with many affected relatives are not usually very informative because with such a common disease large aggregations are likely to occur by chance alone. One study, however, is worthy of particular note, not because 12 members developed stomach cancer, but because a battery of laboratory studies was applied to 16 family members in an attempt to elucidate mechanisms underlying susceptibility [54]. Evidence was found of cell-mediated immunodeficiency and a number of relatives showed antibodies to gastric parietal cells. It was suggested that a genetic defect of T lymphocytes might be involved in the concentration of cases in this family. Because of the parietal cell antibodies and the fact that several members of the family showed macrocytosis, the authors also suggested a subclinical process related to pernicious anaemia, perhaps a genetically mediated auto-immune gastritis predisposing to gastric cancer. The subject of immunological dysfunction, atrophic gastritis and gastric malignancy has been well reviewed [55].

3.5.2. Pernicious Anaemia.
Over the past 30 years it has become established that there is a strong predisposition to develop gastric cancer in both people with pernicious anaemia as well as people with severe atrophic gastritis who have not developed pernicious anaemia. The importance of heredity in these two conditions has also been demonstrated. More recently there have been important advances in the understanding of their genetic bases, which may underlie a large proportion of sporadic, apparently non-familial cases of carcinoma of the stomach.

Work in Copenhagen in the early 1950s confirmed that there is a considerable risk of gastric carcinoma developing in patients with pernicious anaemia[56]. Then more gastric cancer was found in the relatives of patients with gastric cancer than in the general population[57]. It was also shown that among these relatives there was an increased occurrence of pernicious anaemia and achlorhydria[58]. It was reasoned that the tendency to achlorhydria was possibly inherited and this in turn predisposed to both gastric cancer and pernicious anaemia.

It became certain that heredity is important in pernicious anaemia when it was shown that 20% of 106 relatives of patients with pernicious anaemia had impaired vitamin B_{12} absorption[59] and 19% of 220 other relatives had parietal cell auto-antibodies in their serum[60]. Other auto-immune conditions such as thyroid disorders, diabetes mellitus and vitiligo are also prevalent in these families[61].

A recent study in Helsinki of 68 pernicious anaemia patients, 183 of their first-degree relatives and 354 control subjects included gastroscopy with multiple gastric biopsies, testing of gastric acid output, ABO blood grouping, estimation of serum levels of gastrin, vitamin B_{12} and parietal cell antibodies and tests for intrinsic factor antibodies in gastric juice[62]. Though the overall prevalence of chronic gastritis was similar in the relatives (64%) and the controls (59%), severe atrophic gastritis of the body of the stomach, achlorhydria, parietal cell antibodies and a raised fasting serum gastrin level were significantly more common in relatives, 23 of whom had severe atrophic gastritis indistinguishable from the gastric mucosal lesion found in pernicious anaemia patients. The mean age of the subjects with slight or moderate atrophic gastritis of the body was significantly lower in the relatives than in the controls, suggesting an early onset and a rapid progression from mild to severe gastritis in some pernicious anaemia relatives. The relatives seemed to fall into two populations, one with a high proneness to severe atrophic gastritis and the other with little such proneness. It was considered that this bimodal distribution supports the participation of a single major factor, probably genetic, in the pathogenesis of severe atrophic fundic gastritis in the relatives of pernicious anaemic patients.

Other studies by the Helsinki group in pernicious anaemia families[63] have led them to conclude that severe atrophic fundic gastritis is caused mainly by a single major inherited factor, which they term the 'A-factor'. The factors causing the development of parietal cell antibodies were thought to be closely linked with this A-factor although not identical. It was concluded that parietal cell antibodies are not cytotoxic but merely an indication of altered immune response, and that circulating antibodies to intrinsic factor do not have a significant role in the development of either chronic gastritis or overt pernicious anaemia.

Serum pepsinogen I and serum gastrin levels have been measured in 171 first degree relatives of 62 pernicious anaemia patients[64]. Both a low serum pepsinogen and a high serum gastrin were found to be useful in detecting severe atrophic gastritis in these relatives, whilst tests for parietal cell antibodies were of little value. Serum pepsinogen determination had greater sensitivity but testing for both pepsinogen and gastrin levels had a specificity of 100%.

3.5.3. Severe Atrophic Fundic Gastritis. Workers in Helsinki[65] demonstrated that atrophic gastritis was associated with the development of gastric carcinoma[65]. It was found during a 10–15 year follow-up that nine of ten previously diagnosed gastritis patients had developed carcinoma of the stomach. Subsequently the genetics of chronic gastritis has been extensively investigated by this group and it has been shown that severe atrophic gastritis is largely genetically determined[66]. The liability to severe atrophic fundic gastritis was shown to be significantly higher in the first-degree relatives of patients with this type of gastritis.

Although family members tended to have similar gastric mucosal changes, patients with severe gastritis had some relatives whose fundic mucosa was normal in all biopsy specimens, even in the oldest age groups. When the liability to fundic gastritis in these subjects was measured as age-adjusted score values, it formed a bimodal curve indicating two populations, one with very high liability to severe fundic gastritis, whilst the other family members did not have this liability[67]. There is a strong probability that this liability to fundic gastritis may be due to a single factor which may be genetic rather than due to the common family environment.

The term A-gastritis has been introduced[68] for the mucosal picture of severe atrophic fundic gastritis accompanied by functional changes in the. form of achlorhydria and low vitamin B_{12} and intrinsic factor levels and immunological alterations such as high serum gastrin with parietal cell and intrinsic factor antibodies. The antral mucosa is normal or only slightly altered and A-gastritis is now further defined by having high serum gastrin and low serum pepsinogen 1 levels[64]. It would seem likely that there is a major gene underlying liability to severe fundic gastritis and that the gene is very pleotropic. Alternatively the non-histological features of A-gastritis may have separate genetic bases. There is a good deal of evidence of an hereditary basis of gastric acid output[69] and a relationship has been found between low serum pepsin activity, achlorhydria and the subsequent development of gastric cancer[70].

It has been shown that severe atrophic fundic gastritis is significantly more frequent in the relatives of patients with gastric carcinoma than in controls[71, 72]. It was found particularly when the proband had diffuse gastric carcinoma. This type of carcinoma has been shown to be associated with a much greater frequency of affected relatives than is the intestinal type of gastric carcinoma [73].

The diffuse type of carcinoma has been found to be particularly associated with blood group A and it was suggested that individual, presumably genetic, factors are of great importance in its aetiology whereas the development of the intestinal type of gastric carcinoma is influenced by environmental factors [74]. It is not known if the two histological types of carcinoma are associated within families.

Studies of first-degree relatives of patients with severe atrophic gastritis, pernicious anaemia and carcinoma of the stomach have indicated that the tendency to develop atrophic gastritis is influenced by one gene [75]. This genetically determined 'A' type of gastritis is connected with a high risk of developing gastric cancer. It is not yet known whether this severe atrophic fundic gastritis is a common precursor of sporadic, apparently non-familial cases of gastric cancer, but there is much evidence to suggest that it underlies at least some of them.

From the practical point of view the most satisfactory way to screen people for this pre-malignant type of chronic gastritis is to test their serum for pepsinogen I and gastrin levels. A low serum pepsinogen I level accompanied by the finding of hypergastinaemia, in the absence of total gastrectomy for Zollinger-Ellison syndrome, should be diagnostic of this type of gastritis [64]. A low serum pepsinogen I level would appear to be the most useful single subclinical marker of increased risk of developing gastric cancer.

3.5.4. ABO Blood Groups. The results of the investigations of the families with carcinoma of the stomach suggested that genetic factors are concerned in the aetiology of the disease, but they did not conclusively prove it. The demonstration that people of blood group A are more prone to develop the disease than people of blood groups O, B and AB proved that heredity is concerned since the ABO blood group is determined solely by what genes the individual inherits from his parents. The ABO genes are therefore concerned in determining liability to the disease and the ABO locus is probably only one of several which play a part.

The relationship between the ABO blood group genes and carcinoma of stomach was established in 1953 [76] and since then the association has been confirmed all over the world. In 1967, 71 series were summarised [77]: 55 showed an excess of group A and 14 showed little difference from the control. In only two series was there a considerable deficiency of group A and one of these was a series of only 112 cases from Jerusalem. Considering the marked heterogeneity of the ABO blood groups over quite small distances and the consequent difficulty in obtaining good controls, these data leave no doubt of the true causal nature of the relationship. The increased risk of group A people is a modest 20% over the general population risk.

Of the more recent reports, one from Amsterdam [78] analysed the data of 874 patients according to the site of the tumour within the stomach and found that group A was especially increased in the series of tumour of the antrum. Previous reports had given conflicting answers to the question of site of tumour and blood groups [77]. In a Japanese population, blood group A was associated only with the diffuse-type histology of carcinoma [79]. This is the histological type of gastric cancer that has been found to be familial in contrast to the intestinal-type in the relatives, of which no increased carcinoma of stomach incidence has been found [73].

There is no evidence that secretor character is concerned in the aetiology of gastric cancer, but a remarkable absence of Lewis negative individuals in 320 stomach cancer patients has been reported [77]. Of 1000 healthy Liverpool controls, 34 were Lewis negative. The significance of this finding awaits the tests of a series of patients in a part of the world, such as Japan, with a much higher incidence of Lewis negative in the population.

In spite of much research the reason for the blood group A association is still unknown. It seems likely that the ABO blood group genes are pleotrophic with many diffferent effects in various systems in addition to their role in determining the serological specificity of antigens on red cells and water soluble glycoproteins which are found in most body fluids including saliva and gastric juice [80]. The influence on liability for gastric cancer may be due to one of these effects and have nothing to do with the blood group antigens or it may be due to the blood group specific substance themselves. An equally high incidence of blood group A is found in series of patients with pernicious anaemia [81] and it has even been suggested that this high incidence of group A in pernicious anaemia may be the reason for the apparent excess of group A in carcinoma of stomach [82].

Work with tumour tissue involving carcinoembryonic antigens that are molecularly similar to blood group antigens has shown that changes in phenotype of blood group antigens in tumour tissue may result from altered glycoprotein synthesis by diseased mucosal cells [83, 84]. The significance of this work is not obvious: the changes may be due to the cancerous changes within affected cells.

3.5.5. Ataxia-telangiectasia. Carcinoma of the stomach occurs in immunodeficiency diseases such as common variable immuno-deficiency and ataxia-telangiectasia [2, 85–87]. Ataxia-telangiectasia (Louis-Bar Syndrome) is inherited as an autosomal recessive condition with neurological, cutaneous and immunological abnormalities [88]. A study of 27 families has been made to see if external factors could explain the increased cancer risk [89]. The malignancies are often reticuloendothelial though carcinomas of the biliary system, ovary and stomach have been described.

In one reported family [90], two sibs with ataxia-telangiectasia developed mucinous gastric carcinoma before the age of 20. Their mother had also developed gastric cancer. She must have been heterozygous for the gene for ataxia-telangiectasia. This report raised the possibility of an increased cancer risk in those who carry one dose of this gene. This possibility received some support from family studies [89] as an increased susceptibility to malignant tumours was found in heterozygotes.

Ionising radiation of ataxia-telangiectasia lymphocytes produced up to a ten-fold excess of chromatid breaks compared with normal lymphocytes [91]. A slower repair of double strand breaks was suspected. It is interesting that gastric cancer seems to be unduly frequent in heterozygotes for some other recessive defects of DNA repair [87].

Heterozygotes for the ataxia-telangiectasic gene make up about 1% of the general European population. If it is true that they share with homozygotes a high predisposition to cancer [86], their identification becomes a matter of considerable importance in cancer prophylaxis. There has been an encouraging report of laboratory identification of heterozygotes, based on the sensitivity of lymphoblastic cell lines to ionising radiation [92].

4. SMALL BOWEL MALIGNANCY

Heredity is concerned in three conditions which predispose to small bowel malignancy; Peutz-Jeghers syndrome, coeliac disease and Crohn's disease. Small bowel tumours not associated with these conditions are so uncommon that there is little data available concerning a possible place of heredity in their aetiology. Only isolated reports of familial aggregation have been made and these fall into two categories, carcinoma and lymphoma. Reports of duodenal carcinoma within families without polyposis are very rare [93], but periampullary malignancy has been described in patients with familial polyposis coli with sufficient frequency to justify its being recognised as one of the extra-colonic manifestations of the disease and be considered a variant of Gardner's syndrome [94]. Reports of abdominal lymphoma in several members of a family are also rare [95] and raise the suspicion of coeliac disease. They have however, been associated with immunological deficiency [96].

4.1. Peutz-Jeghers Syndrome

Compared with the risk in familial polyposis coli in which the development of malignancy is the rule, the cancer risk in Peutz-Jeghers syndrome is slight.

There is, however, growing evidence that the syndrome is associated with a frequency of intestinal cancer much higher than one would expect by chance. Because the polyps are hamartomas rather than adenomas it was at one time thought there might be no increased cancer risk. However, by 1957 one author had found that 13 of the 67 cases reported up to that time had developed small bowel carcinoma [97]. Since then there has been a steady flow of reports of carcinoma in the small bowel and elsewhere in the gastrointestinal tract [98–101]. The problem has been reviewed [102]. In the latest report a 56-year-old woman died of a duodenal carcinoma and her son died at the age of 29 of a gastric carcinoma [103]. It was thought that the metastasising tumours developed in hamartomatous polyps.

The genetics of Peutz-Jeghers syndrome has been reviewed [104]. There seems little doubt that it is due to a single mutant pleiotropic gene inherited as a mendelian dominant. Gastrointestinal polyps are not found in all carriers of the gene, nor is mucosal pigmentation invariably present. The cutaneous pigmentation around the mouth and eyes and on the fingers tends to fade gradually after the age of 30 years, so parents of a case may not exhibit this sign. Not only may patients be unaware of any other sufferers in the family, but even examination of the relatives may fail to reveal a few polyps or minute mucous membrane pigmentation.

Fortunately there is no clinical need to diagnose which relatives are affected as no prophylactic measures are possible to avoid the two common complications of the polyposis – chronic blood loss and attacks of intestinal obstruction due to intussusception. Several operations may be needed for the latter and surgical removal should be as restricted as possible if malabsorption is to be avoided. Even though the exact degree of risk of the development of gastrointestinal malignancy is still not known, it is certainly not high enough to warrant prophylactic resection of large parts of the bowel.

4.2. Coeliac Disease

As association between steatorrhoea and malignant lymphoid tumours of the gut was recognised 40 years ago [105] but up to 1962 the steatorrhoea was considered to be secondary to the lymphoma (also see Chapter 12). Then it was suggested [106] that the lymphoma was a complication of adult coeliac disease. This suggestion was supported by further evidence [107]. Statistical support for the concept [108] was strengthened by a significantly increased incidence of adenocarcinoma of the G.I. tract, especially in male patients. There was a particularly high incidence of oesophageal carcinoma but somewhat surprisingly adenocarcinoma of the jejunum has been reported only fifteen times [109].

Failure of a newly diagnosed patient to respond to gluten withdrawal, or the return of symptoms for no apparent reason in a patient previously well-controlled on a gluten-free diet, should raise the possibility that a malignant tumour has arisen. Rising values of serum IgA may be associated with the onset of lymphoma [110]. In a survey of the incidence of malignancy in 208 coeliacs [111], 113 had been on a strict gluten-free diet for at least twelve months and 67 had never taken the diet. In these 180 patients there had been 12 cancer deaths and six lymphoma deaths. The authors concluded that the gluten-free diet reduces the incidence of carcinomatous complications to approximately that of the normal population, but in a later report [112] the same group reported on a longer follow-up and were unable to confirm the observation.

The magnitude of the association is yet to be uncovered, mainly because it is only in recent years that it has been realised that relatively symptomless coeliac disease is not uncommon in adult life. Perhaps a gluten-free diet will become an important factor in cancer prevention. If so, an understanding of the genetic basis of coeliac disease will be important in detecting symptomless coeliacs who need to be on a gluten-free diet if they are to escape gastrointestinal malignancy.

4.2.1. The Genetics of Coeliac Disease. The genetics of coeliac disease has been intensively studied in recent years. The explanation of one incompletely penetrant autosomal gene [113] is unlikely. Discordant monozygotic twins have been reported [114]. The most informative surveys have been those in which jejunal biopsies were carried out in the relatives of coeliacs. Usually these have shown that about ten to 12% of first-degree relatives have the flat mucosa typical of coeliac disease [115–118]. However, only four of 72 (5.5% first-degree relatives of 15 child coeliacs were found to have a flat mucosa and all four were asymptomatic [119]. On the other hand 35 of 182 (19.2%) first-degree relatives of adult coeliacs were found to have a flat mucosa, and, though many were symptomless, each had at least one abnormality of red cells or other evidence of malabsorption [120].

4.2.2. Identifying Potential Coeliacs. If there is, as seems likely, a considerable cancer risk in coeliacs and if this risk can be lessened by adherence to a gluten-free diet, it becomes a matter of some importance to identify coeliacs as early as possible, perhaps even before they develop symptoms. In Western Europe between one in 250 and one in 750 of the population has been estimated to be coeliac. Therefore the early identification of coeliacs must make up an important part of any large-scale cancer prevention programme [121].

Considerable progress has been made in developing a technique for coeliac identification without carrying out jejunal biopsy but at present it is possible only in families in which one coeliac has already been identified. HLA typing of the coeliac and the first degree relatives can point to possible coeliacs who can thereafter be examined clinically and biopsied. At first the HLA type associated with coeliac disease was HLA-B8 but work on the B-cell antigens has shown that DRw3 is much more strongly associated with the disease: about 95% of coeliacs have this antigen [122, 123].

It is not known for certain whether the HLA antigen itself is concerned in the aetiology of coeliac disease or if there is linkage disequilibrium between the HLA locus and a coeliac locus. Such a major locus cannot constitute the whole genetic basis for the disease. Other loci and environmental factors, in addition to wheat gluten, must influence the age of onset of symptoms of the condition. There is a suggestion that the genes determining urinary pepsinogen phenotype, alpha-1-antitrypsin and ABH secretor character may be contributing to a coeliac genotype [124]. In cancer prevention however, merely typing for HLA-DR within coeliac families could result in the identification of the majority of the coeliacs or potential coeliacs.

4.3. Crohn's Disease

The increased risk of intestinal malignancy in patients with Crohn's disease is not yet firmly established on a statistical basis. There have been rather more reports of small bowel cancer than would be expected by chance alone [125]. Carcinoma can develop in fistulous tracts [126]. Colonic Crohn's disease has been so recently separated from ulcerative colitis that its relationship to colonic cancer may well have to wait some more years before it is clarified, although a relationship has been suggested [127, 128]. Its genetic basis is bound up with that of ulcerative colitis [129].

5. CARCINOMA OF THE LARGE INTESTINE

In this section, cancer of the colon and rectum will be considered together as they often occur within a single family, suggesting that they are not distinct entities.

Before proceeding to discuss what is known about the place of heridity in sporadic colorectal cancer, mention should be made of the genetic basis of two pre-cancerous conditions, ulcerative colitis and the polyposes.

5.1. Ulcerative Colitis

The cancer risk in ulcerative colitis may have been exaggerated in the past, but there is certainly some risk of developing colon cancer in people who have had total involvement of the colon by ulcerative colitis for a number of years [130, 131]. With Crohn's disease, the position is much less certain and consensus of opinion is that cancer is very much less liable to develop in

Crohn's colitis than in ulcerative colitis.

The most striking result of studying the families of ulcerative colitis patients is the number of relatives affected by Crohn's disease. The converse is also true with many relatives of Crohn's patients having ulcerative colitis. There is no doubt that within families there is a strong association of the two conditions [129, 133].

An association between inflammatory bowel disease and the chromosomal abnormality, Turner's syndrome, has been reported [134]. Of 135 adults with this syndrome, two developed severe ulcerative colitis and two Crohn's disease.

There has been a report of identical male twins, one of whom developed ulcerative colitis at the age of 6 and multifocal anaplastic colon cancer at the age of 22 [135]. His twin brother was quite healthy. Discordance for inflammatory bowel disease in identical twins is not unusual and there is no evidence of an inherited tendency for colitics to develop colon cancer. Rather, it is likely that the development of malignancy is related to long-standing inflammatory disease, especially if it begins in youth.

Mention will be made later of a relationship between ulcerative colitis and carcinoma of the proximal bile ducts [136].

5.2. The Large Bowel Polyposes

The cancer risk in familial polyposis of the large bowel is firmly established [137]. Prophylactic colectomy is indicated as soon as polyposis is diagnosed. Figures from St. Mark's Hospital [138] show that 50% of new patients who present because of symptoms already have carcinoma of the large bowel. On the other hand, only 9% of polyposis patients who are traced through family studies already have cancer. The comparable Swedish figures are 64 and 10% respectively [139].

In a survey of the condition in Sweden no clear-cut genetic distinction was found between families with extra-colonic manifestations (Gardner's syndrome) and those without such lesions [138]. In 12 of the 32 families with extra-colonic signs, only one member had a lesion of the Gardner type.

Conversely, families in which there have been several cases of Gardner's syndrome have been found to contain an individual with polyposis but no extra-colonic lesion. The same overlap between classical familial polyposis and Gardner's syndrome has been found in Japan [140]. In a Baltimore study [141] several cases of medulloblastoma were noted in child relatives of polyposis patients. These tumours had developed at an age before colonic polyps might have been expected.

There is therefore a good deal of evidence to support the view that Gardner's syndrome, Turcot's syndrome and other syndromes of colonic polypsis with extra-colonic lesions are not distinct entities. A genetic theory which would explain the family data so far collected is that there is one major pleotropic gene underlying the inheritance of all these syndromes, with other genes determining whether or not extra-colonic manifestations develop and also their type [142]. From the data so far published, it is not clear if these modifying genes at other loci influence the age of development of the polyps [143], though there is evidence of some genetic predisposition in younger colon cancer patients [144]. This genetic theory received some support from skin fibroblast cultures from members of Gardner's kindred 109, in which increased tetraploidy occurred in cultures derived from branches with the full Gardner's syndrome but not in cultures derived from branches showing only extra-colorectal lesions [145]. Other culture studies indicated genetic heterogeneity, which might be attributed to modifying genes [146].

Not only are the familial polyposes of adenomatous type associated with colonic cancer but so also are the inherited hamartomatous types such as Peutz-Jegher's syndrome [147] and juvenile polyposis [148], though in these latter polyposes, carcinoma of the stomach and duodenum are more frequent than large bowel cancer. To complete the versatility of the polyposes, some patients with familial polyposis of the colon have polyps in the stomach and can develop gastric carcinoma [149] and, as mentioned earlier, ampullary carcinoma occurs in both Gardner's syndrome [94] and familial colonic polyposis [150]. Another family had members with colonic polyps and with gastric polyps, and one with a medulloblastoma of the cerebellum [151]. There were sebaceous cysts but no osseous lesions in this family. Both colonic and gastric cancer had occurred. There seems to be no limit to the permutations of lesions within families and this is in keeping with the genetic theory mentioned above. Theoretically one family could have so many of the modifying genes that the various members could have skin, gastric, osseous and cerebral lesions [142].

5.3. Inherited Colon Cancers without Polyposis

In the introduction of this chapter reference was made to the Cancer Family Syndrome or Adenocarcinomatosis, in which cancers of the colon develop in some members along with uterine or breast cancers in other family members. There are in addition inherited types of large bowel cancer not associated with polyposis. The inherited polyposis conditions probably account for 1% or less of all large bowel cancers whilst the inherited types not associated with polyposis account for at least 10% and perhaps 25% of the total [8, 152].

The largest group of colon cancer families are those with Cancer Family Syndrome described previously. Families in which only colonic cancer occurs may be a variant of these, as the cancers share the characteristics of a dominant mode of inheritance, an early age of onset, and multiple cancers of the large bowel, particularly in the proximal colon [12]. A third type of hereditary colonic cancer is that in which some family members develop stomach cancer. In this hereditary gastrocolonic cancer, there may be double primaries in one individual or a combination of single primaries among relatives [152].

In Muir's or Torre's syndrome [153, 154], multiple skin tumours occur in conjunction with large bowel cancer. Some relatives may have duodenal, gastric or urinary tract malignancy and the syndrome has a dominant mode of inheritance. It may be part of the cancer family syndrome but it seems likely that it is a distinct clinicogenetic entity [152]. An isolated report of colon cancer in a family with the nail-patella syndrome raises the possibility of an association with this condition, which has a mendelian dominant mode of inheritance [155]. A man and two of his daughters died of colonic cancer.

It is difficult not to conclude that a simple major gene for colonic cancer is operating in a family in which 27 cases had developed by 1972 [156]. Of 50 deaths in the family, 22 have been due to cancer of the colon and rectum and no environmental basis was postulated because they lived in a circumscribed area and no special family quirks of dietary habit were discovered. An alternative explanation is that there exists in this type of family [157] a form of polyposis with very few polyps determined by a single gene. Consistent with this possibility is a large family in which solitary polyps were found in nearly 50% of one generation and in which a third of the previous generation had died of gastrointestinal cancer [158]. Such small adenomatous lesions of the rectum and sigmoid might easily be missed, and the cases of cancer would then be considered to be ordinary sporadic carcinoma.

5.4. Sporadic large Bowel Cancer

The incidence of large bowel cancer varies approximately ten-fold from one part of the world to another. It is common in the British Isles, North America, Australasia and Denmark, but relatively rare in countries where carcinoma of the stomach is common, such as Poland, Finland, Iceland and Japan. In Africa it is particularly rare, except in the white population of South Africa. There are no localities with extremely high incidence as is found with carcinoma of the oesophagus.

5.4.1. Incidence in Relatives. Each of the studies that have been made of the incidence of colonic cancer in the relatives of patients with the disease have showed a much higher figure than that in controls. In one survey [159] 26 of 763 relatives had died of large bowel cancer compared with 8 of 763 controls. In another [49] the finding was 31 cases in 392 relatives compared with 9.7 expected. In a painstaking survey of the causes of death in the families of 209 patients who had been admitted to St. Mark's Hospital,

London [18], the overall percentage of large bowel cancer in 430 first-degree relatives was 10.9%. The number of large bowel malignancies in the 218 males was 25 (expected 4.5) and in the 212 females it was 22 (expected 6.3). Among the 209 patients investigated, eight were aged 40 or under when their cancer was diagnosed. Of these eight, five had at least one affected relative. Of the 15 index cases who had eight or more adenomas in the specimen of bowel removed at operation, eight had a positive family history. Of the seven index cases who had two or more carcinomas in the bowel, three had a positive family history. Of the seven index cases who gave a history of previous carcinoma of the large bowel, five had a positive family history.

These findings indicate that if a patient with large bowel cancer has a positive family history, the clinician should examine the bowel carefully for neoplasms other than the presenting lesion. After operation he should be followed up because of the increased risk that he may develop a new primary tumour.

There has been an excellent survey of the individuals at high risk for large bowel cancer [161], which includes a review of the genetics of spontaneous colon cancer in rats. This rodent model develops cancer of the ascending colon resembling the human familial aggregates of colon cancer.

5.4.2. Incidence in Spouses. There has been one study that has shown a high incidence of large bowel cancer in the spouses of large bowel cancer patients [18]. Of 34 spouses who had died, death certificates were obtained for 27 and three had died of large bowel cancer. This 11% incidence in spouses was similar to the 10.9% incidence in the relatives of this study and much higher than the 3% mortality in the general London population.

These London data suggest that the increased incidence in relatives of large bowel cancer patients is due to the environment rather than genetic factors. On the other hand, in a large-scale survey of mortality of married couples in Sweden (162), it was found that 1 716 people had died of colorectal cancer in 1961. The cause of death was determined in 1 094 of their spouses (99.6% of those eligible for the survey), and it was found that the risk of colorectal cancer and other possibly aetiologically related diseases was no higher in the spouses than in a matched population. The authors concluded that if eating a diet identical with that of patients with bowel cancer is not associated with an increased risk, the current view of colon cancer aetiology may need to be revised and dietary patterns before marriage investigated. Studies of the risk in sibships would be an important approach.

5.4.3. Clinical Implications. There are certain clinical conclusions that can be drawn from these data as to whether there is a quantitative inherited tendency to develop sporadic large bowel cancer or whether large bowel cancer is mainly environmental in origin, the inherited type being found only in certain families. These clinical conclusions are that, if a patient with large bowel cancer gives a family history that includes a relative who has had bowel cancer, then the whole of his bowel must be thoroughly examined to exclude other lesions as he may well have two separate cancers at the time of first presentation. If any bowel remains after the initial operation, he must be followed up regularly in case a new primary carcinoma develops.

The occurrence of carcinoma of the large bowel in someone under the age of 40, someone who has eight or more adenomas in the operative specimen removed for carcinoma of the colon, or someone who has two or more carcinomas at presentation means that the risk in other members of his family is considerable and they should be warned to report immediately any intestinal symptoms. They also ought to undergo periodic surveillance with occult blood testing and colonoscopy.

6. CARCINOMA OF THE PANCREAS

There are marked geographically differences in the incidence of pancreatic carcinoma [163, 164]. The highest frequencies are in Western and industrialised countries, but all races can be affected. There is a considerable male preponderance. An association with heavy alcohol consumption is likely and diabetics have a two-fold increased risk of developing the disease [165]. The incidence in the United States appears to be increasing at the same time as gastric cancer has been decreasing.

Family aggregations of pancreatic cancer continue to be reported, such as four siblings [166], four brothers [167], two sisters [168] and father and son [169]. These cancers developed over the age of 60 and not at an early age as one might expect if the underlying genetic cause was the Cancer Family Syndrome or hereditary pancreatitis. It is difficult to attribute such aggregations to chance or a unique environmental agent. At one time it was considered that chronic pancreatitis predisposed to the development of pancreatic cancer [170] but recent data do not show any connection between the two conditions [165].

The only firm evidence of a genetic influence in pancreatic cancer is that there is a high risk in hereditary pancreatitis and malignant islet cell tumours of the endocrine pancreas occur in multiple endocrine neoplasia, Type I.

6.1. Hereditary Pancreatitis
Since the first report in 1952 [171], many families have been described in which chronic calcifying pancreatitis is inherited in an autosomal mendelian dominant manner, even though penetrance is not complete. Nearly thirty

large families have been reported, mainly in the United States [172] and the United Kingdom [173]. In some families the affected individuals have aminoaciduria, which may be secondary to the disease. In others, pancreatic duct anomalies are found and it is possible that the genetic abnormality is at the sphincter of Oddi rather than in the substance of the gland. Against this is the frequent finding of pancreatic calcification in members of these families who have minimal symptoms.

The disease is similar to sporadic chronic pancreatitis with the development of steatorrhoea and diabetes, but the age of onset of abdominal pain ranges from four to 14 years. The pathological features are also very similar. Though childhood onset is the rule, families with several adult-onset cases have been reported [174]. Among 300 adult cases in France, three families of this type were found [175]. Another report is of a 61-year-old man whose first attack of pain was at 17 years of age, and whose daughter and grand-daughter became symptomatic at 12 and 9 years respectively [176]. At the present time the position is uncertain, but it seems possible that there is no clear-cut genetic distinction between hereditary pancreatitis and many cases of sporadic adult chronic calcifying pancreatitis.

Attention was first drawn to the cancer risk in hereditary pancreatitis in 1968 [177]. It was thought that possibly as many as 30% developed carcinoma of the pancreas and this rate was found in another review [178]. On the other hand in three kindred reported later, only 8 of 54 deaths were found to have been due to pancreatic carcinoma [179] and none was found in 72 patients from seven families [173]. Members of hereditary pancreatitis families have developed pancreatic carcinoma without having had clinical pancreatitis [178].

6.2. Multiple Endocrine Neoplasia

Islet cell tumors are commonly familial, many of them being the gastrointestinal expression of multiple endocrine neoplasia I, MEN I, characterised by tumours in the pituitary, parathyroids, adrenal cortex and pancreas (also see chapter 00). The islet-cell lesion is the most likely to be malignant. MEN I is inherited as an autosomal dominant disorder [180]. Penetrance is nearly complete if at-risk individuals below the age of 20 are excluded. Parathyroid or pancreatic tumours are present in over 75% of affected individuals, pituitary involvement in nearly 66% and the adrenal in about 33%. The various endocrine glands are usually not affected simultaneously, so long-term evaluation is needed to assess the degree of expressivity.

The genetic entity of MEN I may not be as clear cut as previously thought as a family has been reported with features of MEN I and II [181] and a 14-year-old Japanese boy with bilateral pheochromocytoma and an islet cell tumour has been described [182].

Considerable phenotypic variability is found within individual families, but hormone radioimmunoassay has been of great help in diagnosing asymptomatic family members. When ten Zollinger-Ellison patients were studied [183], seven were found to have co-existing endocrine disease and six were members of MEN I families. During the study of 109 family members, four previously undiagnosed cases of pituitary tumour, 17 of hyperparathyroidism, seven Zollinger-Ellison syndrome and one insulinoma were found.

The proportion of cases of Zollinger-Ellison syndrome who are part of multiple endocrine neoplasia is uncertain but it is at least 40%. Patients presenting over 60 years of age, whose parents were endocrinologically normal, are probably sporadic cases and their sibs and offspring need have little concern, but any young adult patient should be considered to have the genetic form of the disease until proved otherwise. Relatives younger than the patients may not have had time to develop any facet of the syndrome and one or other parent may be affected but asymptomatic. Yearly assessment of gastric acid secretion and measurement of serum gastrin levels in those at risk should be carried out in an attempt to detect the potentially malignant islet cell lesion. Serum calcium estimation, parathormone assay and roentgenograms of the pituitary fossa are also advisable.

7. CARCINOMA OF LIVER

Malignant hepatoma in Europe and North America usually develops in a cirrhotic liver (see Chapter 14). Among the genetic causes of cirrhosis is haemochromatosis, which was though to have a dominant mode of inheritance [184]. There have been several studies of HLA antigens in patients with this disease and in their families [185]. In one large French investigation [186] it was concluded that the disease is determined by two homologous alleles giving recessive inheritance. The data from various sources are difficult to interpret but it seems likely that the genetic basis of haemochromatosis is a polygenic system with at least one major gene, which may be HLA-A3 or a gene on chromosome 6 in linkage disequelibrium with it. Some of the genes are probably responsible for increased exchange of iron from plasma to storage, and others for increased iron absorption and increased serum iron.

The early detection of affected family members and subsequent regular venesections should prevent the onset of cirrhosis and therefore of malignant hepatoma. Though malignant hepatoma is much less common in Wilson's disease than in haemochromatosis [187], hepatoma also should be preventable by effective treatment of patients with Wilson's disease with D-penicillamine. Wilson's disease has recessive inheritance.

Other inherited conditions that can result in malignant hepatoma are familial cholestatic cirrhosis of childhood [188], familial liver-cell adenoma [189] and alpha-1-antitrypsin deficiency [190]. Hepatoblastoma has been reported in infant sisters [191] and infant sister and brother [192]. In the Fanconi syndrome, it is uncertain whether hepatoma is a complication of the disease or of oral androgen therapy, but some patients have developed hepatic carcinoma without androgen treatment [193].

In cirrhosis not due to recognisable inborn errors of metabolism, there is a definite though not strong familial tendency [184], which is probably genetic rather than due to the common environment even though reports of familial hepatoma are rare [194, 195]. In a study of 254 patients who had died with cirrhosis, 24% had developed hepatocellular carcinoma [196]. HBsAg-positive chronic active hepatitis was identified as a high risk group with malignancy in 42%. In the same paper, it was noted that ten of 16 liver cancer patients who did not have cirrhosis had a family history of various cancers. The father of one of these patients had also died of primary liver cancer. In another family two HBsAg-positive brothers had had hepatocellular carcinoma but a third brother, also HBsAg-positive, has not yet developed liver cancer [197].

8. CARCINOMA OF GALL BLADDER AND BILE DUCTS

There is evidence of an association between gall stones and gall bladder neoplasms in Israel [198] and in American Indians [199]. The genetic basis of gall stones is not simple [200]. Controlled studies have shown that the incidence in sibs of patients is higher than in controls. Parents of patients affected at an early age suffered more often from gall stone disease than did parents of controls. The bile of sisters of young women operated on for gall stones was found to be more lithogenic than that of controls.

It has already been noted that a review of 103 patients with cancer of bile ducts had shown that eight had ulcerative colitis [130]. In three the carcinoma of the bile duct developed several years after colectomy, suggesting genetic factors common to the colitis and the malignancy. Seven of the eight were significantly younger than the median age of the group as a whole, but otherwise there was no other apparent difference. Though this relationship suggests a genetic basis for some cases of bile duct cancer, it should be noted that carcinoma of the bile ducts has been reported in a 45-year-old man (hepatic duct) and his 44-year-old wife (ampulla), both tumours developing in the same year [201]. This is a good illustration of the fact that familial occurrences need not be genetic.

REFERENCES

1. Tokuhata GK, Lilienfeld AM: Familial aggregation of lung cancer in humans. J Nat Cancer Inst 30:289–312,1963.
2. Kellermann G, Shaw CR, Luyten-Kellermann M: Aryl hydrocarbon hydroxylase inducibility and bronchogenic carcinoma. N Engl J Med 289:934–937, 1973.
3. Kazazian HH: A geneticist's view of lung disease. Am Rev Resp Dis 113:261–266, 1976.
4. Sonta SI, Sandberg AA: Chromosomes and causation of human cancer and leukaemia. XXX. Banding studies of primary intestinal tumours. Cancer 41:164–73, 1978.
5. Danes BS: Increased in vitro tetraploidy: tissue specific within the heritable colorectal cancer syndromes with polyposis coli. Cancer 41:2330-4, 1978.
6. Amiel JL: Mendelian genetics and cancer. Bull Cancer (Paris) 65:131–136, 1978.
7. Frais MA: Gastric adenocarcinoma due to ataxia-telangiectasia (Louis-Bar syndrome). J Med Genet 16:160–161, 1979.
8. German J, Bloom D, Passarge E: Bloom's Syndrome VII Progress report for 1978. Clin Genet 15:361–7, 1979.
9. Berg NO, Eriksson S: Liver disease in adults with alpha-1-antitrypsin deficiency. N Engl J Med 287:1264–1267, 1972.
10. Lewkonia RM: Inherited immunological abnormality and the gut. Clin Gastroenterol 2:645–660, 1973.
11. Lynch HT, Guirgis HA, Harris RE, Lynch PM, Lynch JF, Elston RC, Go RC, Kaplan E: Clinical, genetic and biostatistical progress in the cancer family syndrome. Front Gastrointest Res 4:142–50, 1979.
12. Lynch PM, Lynch HT, Harris RE: Hereditary proximal colonic cancer. Dis Colon Rectum 20:661–8, 1977.
13. Law IP, Herberman RB, Oldham RK, Bouzoukis J, Hanson SM, Rhode MC: Familial occurrence of colon and uterine carcinoma and of lymphoproliferative malignancies. Clinical description. Cancer 39:1224–8, 1977.
14. Howell MA: The association between colorectal cancer and breast cancer. J Chronic Dis 29:243–61, 1976.
15. Arthur D, Woods W, Krivit W, Nesbit M: Hereditary adenocarcinoma of the colon in childhood: association with the cancer family syndrome. J Pediatr 93:318, 1978.
16. Lynch HT, Harris RE, Lynch PM, Guirgis HA, Lynch JF, Bardavil WA: Role of heredity in multiple primary cancer. Cancer 40:1849–54, 1977.
17. Berlinger NT, Good RA: Suppressor cells in healthy relatives of patients with hereditary colon cancer. Cancer 45:1112–1116, 1980.
18. Lovett E: Family studies in cancer of the colon and rectum. Brit J Surg 63:13–18, 1976.
19. Mosbech J, Videbaek A: On the etiology of oesophageal carcinoma. J Nat Cancer Inst 15:1665–1673, 1955.
20. Li KH, Kao JC, Wu YK: A survey of the prevalence of carcinoma of the oesophagus in North China. Chinese Med J 81:489–494, 1962.
21. Ashley DJB: Oesophageal cancer in Wales. J Med Genet 6:70–75, 1969.
22. Haas JF, Schottenfeld D: Epidemiology of esophageal cancer. In: Gastrointestinal tract malignancy, Lipkin M, Good RA (eds). New York: PLENUM, 1978, pp 145–172.
23. Kmet J, Mahboubi E: Oesophageal cancer in the Caspian littoral of Iran: initial studies. Science 175: 846–852, 1972.
24. Cook P: Cancer of the oesophagus in Africa. Brit J Cancer 25:853–880, 1971.
25. Coordinating Group: Research on the etiology of oesophageal cancer in North China. Scient Sin 18:131. or Chin Med J 1:167, 1975.

26. Pour P, Ghadirian P: Familial cancer of the oesophagus in Iran. Cancer 33:1649–1652, 1974.

27. Freytes MA, Carri J: Carcinoma esofágico familiar. Rev Fac Cienc Med Cordoba 26:215–218, 1968.

28. Kasenov KU: Rol' geneticheskilch faktorov v vozniknovenii raka pishchevoda. Vopr Onkol 25:68–72, 1979:

29. Holmes GKT, Stokes PL Sorahan TM, Prior P, Waterhouse JAH, Cook WT: Coeliac disease, gluten-free diet, and malignancy. Gut 17:612–619, 1976.

30. Clarke CA, McConnell RB: Six cases of carcinoma of oesophagus occurring in one family. Brit Med J (ii):1137–1138, 1954.

31. Howel-Evans AW, McConnell RB, Clarke CA, Sheppard PM: Carcinoma of the oesophagus with keratosis palmaris et plantaris (tylosis) — a study of two families. Quart J Med 27:413–429, 1958.

32. Harper PS, Harper RMJ, Howel-Evans AW: Carcinoma of the oesophagus with tylosis. Quart J Med 39:317–333, 1970.

33. Shine I, Allison PR: Carcinoma of the oesophagus with tylosis (keratosis palmaris et plantaris). Lancet (i):951–953, 1966.

34. De Dulanto F, Martinez FC, Moreno MA, Sintes RN, Gonzalez RMR, Dulanto MC, Garcia MM, Lloret SF: Sindrome de Clarke-Howel-Evans. Actas Dermato-sifiliograficas 68:127–138, 1977.

35. Tyldesley WR: Oral leukoplakia associated with tylosis and esophageal carcinoma. J Oral Pathol 3:62–70, 1974.

36. Ritter SB, Peterson G: Esophageal cancer, hyperkeratosis and oral leukaplakia: follow-up family study. JAMA 236:1844–1885, 1976.

37. McConnell RB: The genetics of gastro-intestinal disorders. London: Oxford University Press, 1966.

38. Doll R: The geographical distribution of cancer. Brit J Cancer 23:1–8, 1969.

39. Merliss RR: Talc-treated rice and Japanese stomach cancer. Science 173:1141–1142, 1971.

40. Ashley DJB, Davies HD: Gastric cancer in Wales. Gut 7:542–548, 1966.

41. Maddock CR: Environment and heredity factors in carcinoma of the stomach. Brit J Cancer 20:660–669, 1966.

42. Clarke CA, McConnell RB: Pitfalls and problems in genetics studies. In: Selected topics in medical genetics, Clarke CA (ed). London: Oxford University Press, 1969, pp 12–16.

43. Lee FI: Carcinoma of the gastric antrum in identical twins. Postgrad Med J 47:622–624, 1971.

44. Ellis DJ: Carcinoma of the gastric antrum in identical twins. Clin Oncol 4:299–302, 1978.

45. Watanabe H, Enjoji M, Yao T, Ohsato K: Gastric lesions in familial adenomatosis coli: their incidence and histologic analysis. Human pathol 9:269–283, 1978.

46. Watanabe A, Nagashima H, Motoi M, Ogawa K: Familial juvenile polyposis of the stomach. Gastroenterology 77:148–151, 1979.

47. Graham S, Lilienfeld AM: Genetic studies of gastric cancer in humans: an appraisal. Cancer 11:945–958, 1958.

48. Woolf CM, Isaacson EA: An analysis of five 'stomach cancer families' in the State of Utah. Cancer 14:1005–1016, 1961.

49. Macklin MT: Inheritance of cancer of the stomach and large intestine in man. J Natl Cancer Inst 24:551–571, 1960.

50. Borges CC, Villalobos Pérez JJ: The epidemiology of gastric cancer. Revista de Investigacón Clin 20:11–23, 1968.

51. Jackson CE, Brownlee RW, Schuman BM, Micheloni F, Ghironzi G: Observations on gastric cancer in San Marino. Cancer 45:599–602, 1980.

52. Macklin MT: The role of heredity in gastric and intestinal cancer. Gastroenterology 29:507–511, 1955.

53. Woolf CM: The incidence of cancer in the spouses of stomach cancer patients. Cancer 14:199–200, 1961.

54. Creagan ET, Fraumeni JF Jr.: Familial gastric cancer and immunologic abnormalities. Cancer 32:1325–1331, 1973.

55. Twomey JJ: Immunological dysfunction with atrophic gastritis and gastric malignancy. In: Gastrointestinal tract malignancy, Lipkin M, Good RA (eds). New York: Plenum, 1978 pp 93–117.

56. Mosbech J, Videbaek A: Mortality from and risk of gastric carcinoma among patients with pernicious anaemia. Brit Med J ii:390–394, 1950.

57. Videbaek A, Mosbech J: The aetiology of gastric carcinoma elucidated by a study of 302 pedigrees. Acta Med Scand 149:137–159, 1954.

58. Mosbech J: Heredity in pernicious anaemia: a proband study of the heredity and the relationship to cancer of the stomach. Copenhagen: Munksgaard, 1953.

59. McIntyre PA, Hahn R, Conley CL, Glass B: Genetic factors in predisposition to pernicious anaemia. Bull Johns Hopkins Hospital 104:130–142, 1959.

60. Te Velde K, Abels J, Anders GJ, Arends PA, Hoedemaeker PJ, Nieweg HO: A family study of pernicious anaemia by an immunologic method. J Lab Clin Med 64:177–187, 1964.

61. Hippe E, Jensen KB: Hereditary factors in pernicious anaemia and their relationship to serum immunoglobulin levels. Lancet 2:721–722, 1969.

62. Varis K Ihamäki T, Härkönen M, Samloff IM, Siurala M: Gastric morphology, function and immunology in first-degree relatives of probands with pernicious anaemia and controls. Scand J Gastroenterol 14:129–139, 1979.

63. Varis K, Ihamäki T, Sipponen P: Humoral immunity and chronic gastritis in families of patients with adult pernicious anaemia. Acta et commentat Univers Tartuensis 485:53–61, 1979.

64. Varis K, Samloff IM, Ihamäki T, Siurala M: An appraisal of tests for severe atrophic gastritis in relations of patients with pernicious anaemia. Fig Dis Sci 24:187–191, 1979.

65. Siurala M, Varis K, Wiljasulo M: Studies of patients with atrophic gastritis — a 10–15 year follow up. Scand J Gastroenterol 1:40–48, 1966.

66. Varis K: A family study of chronic gastritis: histological, immunological and functional aspects. Scand J Gastroenterol 6:Supplement 13, 1–50, 1971.

67. Hovinen E, Kekki M, Kuikka S: A theory to the stochastic dynamic model building for chronic progressive disease processes with an application to chronic gastritis. J Theoret Biol 57:131–152, 1976.

68. Strickland RG, Mackay IR: A reappraisal of the nature and significance of chronic atrophic gastritis. Am J Dig Dis 18:426–440, 1973.

69. Fodor E, Vestea S, Urcan S, Popescu S, Sulica L, Iencica R, Goia A, Ilea V: Hydrochloric acid secretion capacity of the stomach as an inherited factor in the pathogenesis of duodenal ulcer. Am J Dig Dis 13:260–265, 1968.

70. Pastore JO, Kato H, Belsky JL: Serum pepsin and tubeless gastric analysis as predictors of stomach cancer. New Engl J Med 286:279–284, 1972.

71. Kekki M, Ihamäki T, Sipponen P, Hovinen E: Heterogeneity in susceptibility to chronic gastritis in relatives of gastric cancer patients with different histology of carcinoma. Scand J Gastroent 10:737–745, 1975.

72. Ihamäki T, Varis K, Siurala M: Morphological functional and immunological state of the

gastric mucosa in gastric carcinoma families: comparison with a computer-matched family sample. Scand J Gastroenterol 14:801–812, 1979.

73. Lehtola J: Family study of gastric carcinoma; with special reference to histological types. Scand J Gastroenterol (Suppl). 13:3–54, 1978.

74. Correa P, Sasano N, Stemmermann GN, Haenszel W: Pathology of gastric carcinoma in Japanese populations: comparison between Miyagi prefecture, Japan and Hawaii. J Natl Cancer Inst 51:1449–1459, 1973.

75. Varis K, Ihamäki T, Lehtola J, Sipponen P, Kekki M, Isokoski M, Saukkonen M, Siurala M: Genetic aspects of gastritis – cancer relationship. Dtsch Z Verdau Stoffweckselkr. 38:51–4, 1978.

76. Aird I, Bentall HH, Roberts JAF: A relationship between cancer of stomach and the ABO blood groups. Brit Med J, i:799–801, 1953.

77. McConnell RB: The genetics of carcinoma of the stomach. In: Racial and geographical factors in tumour incidence. Shivas A.A. (ed). Edinburgh: Edinburgh University Press, 1967, pp 107–113.

78. Van Wgyjen RCA, Linschoten H: Distribution of ABO and rhesus blood groups in patients with gastric carcinoma, with reference to its site of origin. Gastroenterology 65:877–883, 1973.

79. Haenszel W, Kurihara M, Locke FB, Shimuzu K, Segi M: Stomach cancer in Japan. J Natl Cancer Inst 56:265–274, 1976.

80. McConnell RB: Lewis blood group substances in body fluids. Proc 2nd Int Congr Human Genetics (Rome) 858–861, 1963.

81. Hoskins LC, Loux HA, Britten A, Zamcheck N: Distribution of ABO blood groups in patients with pernicious anaemia, gastric carcinoma and gastric carcinoma associated with pernicious anaemia. N Engl. J Med 273:633–637, 1965.

82. Shearman DJC, Finlayson NDC: Familial aspects of gastric carcinoma. Am J Dig Dis 12:529–534, 1967.

83. Denk H, Tappeiner G, Holzner JH: Independent behaviour of blood group A- and B-like activities in gastric carcinoma of blood group AB individuals. Nature 248:428–30, 1974.

84. Denk H, Tappeiner G, Davidovits A, Eckerstorfer R, Holzner JH: Carcinoembryonic antigen and blood group substances in carcinoma of the stomach and colon. J Natl Cancer. Inst. 53:933–942, 1974.

85. Spector BD, Perry GS, Kersey JH: Genetically determined immunodeficiency diseases (GDID) and malignancy: report from the immunodeficiency-cancer registry. Clin Immunol Immunopathol 11:12–29, 1978.

86. Swift M, Sholman L, Perry M, Chase C: Malignant neoplasms in the families of patients with ataxia-telangiectasia. Cancer Res 36:209–215, 1976.

87. Hermans PE, Diaz-Busco JA, Stubo JD: Idiopathic late-onset immunoglobulin deficiency: clinical observations in 50 patients. Am J Med 61:221–237, 1976.

88. McFarlin DE, Strober W, Waldman TA: Ataxia-telangiectasia. Medicine 51:280-314, 1972.

89. Daly MB, Swift M: Epidemiological factors related to the malignant neoplasms in ataxia-telangiectasia families. J Chronic Dis 31:625-634, 1978.

90. Haerer AF, Jackson JF, Evers CG: Ataxia-telangiectasia with gastric adenocarcinoma. JAMA 210:1884–1887, 1969.

91. Taylor AM: Unrepaired DNA strand breaks in irradiated ataxia telangiectasic lymphocytes suggested from cytogenetic observations. Mutat Res 50:407–418, 1978.

92. Chen PC, Lavin MF, Kidson C: Identification of ataxia telangiectasia heterozygotes, a cancer prone population. Nature 274:484–486, 1978.

93. Ungar H: Familial carcinoma of the duodenum in adolescence. Brit J Cancer 3:321–330,

1949.

94. Jones TR, Nance FC: Periampullary malignancy in Gardner's syndrome. Ann Surg 185:565–573, 1977.

95. Freedlander E, Kissen LH, McVie JG: Gut lymphoma presenting simultaneously in two siblings. Brit Med J 1:80–81, 1978.

96. Maurer HS, Gotoff SP, Allen L, Bolan J: Malignant lymphoma of the small intestine in multiple family members: association with an immunologic deficiency. Cancer 37:2224–2231, 1976.

97. Bailey D: Polyposis of the gastrointestinal tract: the Peutz syndrome. Brit Med J ii:433–439, 1957.

98. Williams JP, Knudsen A: Peutz-Jeghers syndrome with metastasising duodenal carcinoma. Gut 6:179–184, 1965.

99. Payson BA, Moumgis B: Metastasising carcinoma of the stomach in Peutz-Jeghers syndrome. Ann Sur 165:145–151, 1967.

100. Dozois RR, Judd ES, Dahlin DC, Bartholomew LG: The Peutz-Jeghers syndrome — is there a predisposition to the development of intestinal malignancy? Arch Surg 98:509–516, 1969.

101. Dodds WJ, Schulte WJ, Hensley GT, Hogan WJ: Peutz-Jeghers syndrome and gastrointestinal malignancy. Am J Roentgenol 115:374–377, 1972.

102. Bussey HJ, Veale AM, Morson BC: Genetics of gastrointestinal polyposis. Gastroenterology 74:1325–1330, 1978.

103. Cochet B, Carrel J, Desbaillets, L, Widgren S: Peutz-Jeghers syndrome associated with gastrointestinal carcinoma. Report of two cases in a family. Gut 20:169–175, 1979.

104. Alm T, Licznerski G: The intestinal polyposes. Clinics in Gastroenterol 2:577–602, 1973.

105. Fairley NH, Mackie FP: The clinical and biochemical syndrome in lymphoadenoma and allied diseases involving the mesenteric glands. Brit Med J i:375–380, 1937.

106. Gough KR, Read AE, Naish JM: Intestinal reticulosis as a complication of idiopathic steatorrhoea. Gut 3:232–239, 1962.

107. Austad WI, Cornes JC, Gough KR, McCarthy CF, Read AE: Steatorrhoea and malignant lymphoma. The relationships of malignant tumours of lymphoid tissue and coeliac disease. Am J Dig Dis 12:475–490, 1967.

108. Harris OD, Cooke WT, Thompson H, Waterhouse JAH: Malignancy in adult coeliac disease and idiopathic steatorrhoea. Am J Med 42:899–912, 1967.

109. Petreshock EP, Pessah M, Manachemi E: Adenocarcinoma of the jejunum associated with non-tropical sprue. Am J Dig Dis 20:796–802, 1975.

110. Asquith P, Thompson RA, Cooke WT: Serum immunoglobulins in adult coeliac disease. Lancet ii:129–131, 1969.

111. Stokes PL, Holmes GK: Malignancy. Clinics in Gastroenterol 3:159–170, 1974.

112. Holmes GKT, Stokes PL, Sorahan TM, Prior P, Waterhouse JAH, Cooke WT: Coeliac disease, gluten-free diet and malignancy. Gut 17:612–619, 1976.

113. David TJ, Ajdukiewicz AB: A family study of coeliac disease. J Med Genet 12:79–82, 1975.

114. Walker-Smith JA: Discordance for childhood coeliac disease in monozygotic twins. Gut 14:374–375, 1973.

115. MacDonald WC, Dobbins WO, Rubin CE: Studies of the familial nature of coeliac sprue using biopsy of the small intestine. N Engl J Med 272:448–456, 1965.

116. Robinson DC, Watson AJ, Wyatt EH, Marks JM, Roberts DF: Incidence of small intestinal mucosal abnormalities and of clinical coeliac disease in the relatives of children with coeliac disease. Gut 12:789–793, 1971.

117. Mylotte MJ, Egan-Mitchell B, Fottrell PF, McNichol B, McCarthy CF: Familial coeliac disease. Quart J Med 41:527–528, 1972.
118. Shipman RT, Williams AL, Kay R, Townley RRW: A family study of coeliac disease. Aust N.Z. J Med 5:250–255, 1975.
119. Stokes PL, Ferguson R, Holmes GKT, Cooke WT: Familial aspects of coeliac disease. Quart J Med 45:567-582, 1976.
120. Rolles CJ, Myint TOK, Sin W-K, Anderson CM: Family study of coeliac disease. Gut 15:827, 1974.
121. McConnell RB: The genetics of coeliac disease. Lancaster: M.T.P. Press, 1981.
122. Peña AS, Mann DL, Hague NE, Heck JA, van Leeuwen A, van Rood JJ, Strober W: Genetic basis of gluten sensitive enteropathy. Gastroenterology 75:230–235, 1978.
123. Betuel H, Gebuhrer L, Percebois H, Descos L, Minaire Y, Bertrand J: Association de la maladie coeliaque de l'adulte avec HLA-DRw3 et DRw7. Gastroenterol Clin Biol 3:605, 1979.
124. Ellis A, Evans DAP, McConnell RB, Woodrow JC: Liverpool Coeliac Family Study. In: The genetics of coeliac disease, McConnell RB (ed). Lancaster: M.T.P. Press, 1981.
125. Ben-Asher H: Carcinoma in regional enteritis. Am J Gastroenterol 55:391–398, 1971.
126. Lightdale CJ, Sternberg SS, Posner G, Sherlock P: Carcinoma complicating Crohn's disease: report of seven cases and review of the literature. Am J Med 59:262–268, 1975.
127. Weedon DD, Shorter RG, Illstrup DM, Huizenga KA, Taylor WF: Crohn's disease and cancer. N Engl J Med 289:1099–1103, 1973.
128. Fielding JF, Prior P, Waterhouse JA, Cooke WT: Malignancy in Crohn's Disease. Scand J Gastroenterol 7:3–7, 1972.
129. McConnell RB: Inflammatory bowel disease: newer views of genetic influence. In: Developments in digestive diseases, Berk JE (ed), Philadelphia: Lea & Febiger, 1980, pp 129–137.
130. Lennard-Jones JE, Morson BC, Ritchie JK, Shove DC, Williams CB: Cancer in colitis: assessment of the individual risk by clinical and histological criteria. Gastroenterology 73:1280–1289, 1977.
131. Kewenter J, Ahlman H, Hulten L: Cancer risk in extensive ulcerative colitis. Ann Surg 188:824–828, 1978.
132. Greenstein AJ, Sachar DB, Smith H, Pucillo A, Papatestas AE, Kreel I, Geller SA, Janowitz HD, Aufses AH: Cancer in universal and left sided ulcerative colitis: factors determining risk. Gastroenterology 77:295–297, 1979.
133. Kirsner JB: Genetic aspects of inflammatory bowel disease. Clinics in Gastroenterol 2:557–575, 1973.
134. Price WH: A high incidence of chronic inflammatory bowel disease in patients with Turner's syndrome. J Med Genet 16:263–266, 1979.
135. Bisordi W, Lightdale CJ: Identical twins discordant for ulcerative colitis with colon cancer. Am J Dig Dis 21:71–73, 1976.
136. Ross AP, Braasch JW: Ulcerative colitis and carcinoma of the proximal bile ducts. Gut 14:94–97, 1973.
137. De Cosse JJ, Adams MB, Condon RE: Familial polyposis. Cancer 39:267–273, 1977.
138. Lovett E: Familial factors in the aetiology of carcinoma of the large bowel. Proc Royal Soc Med 67:751–752, 1974.
139. Alm T, Licznerski G: The intestinal polyposes. Clinics in Gastroenterology 2:577–602, 1973.
140. Utsumoniya J Nakamura T: The occult osteomatous changes in the mandible in patients with familial polyposis coli. Brit J Surg 62:45–51, 1975.
141. Cohen SB: Familial polyposis coli: an analysis of 30 families. MD. Thesis, University of

Liverpool, 1979.

142. McConnell RB: The genetics of familial polyposis. In: Colorectal cancer: prevention, epidemiology and screening, Winawer SJ (ed). New York: Raven, 1980.

143. Lynch HT, Lynch PM, Follett KL, Harris RE: Familial polyposis coli: heterogenous polyp expression in two kindreds. J Med Genet. 16:1–7, 1979.

144. Utsunomiya J, Murata M, Tanimura M: An analysis of the age distribution of colon cancer in adenomatosis coli. Cancer 45:198–205, 1980.

145. Danes BS, Gardner EJ: The Gardner syndrome: a cell culture study on kindred 109. J Med Genet 15:346–51, 1978.

146. Danes BD, Alm T: *In vitro* studies on adenomatosis of the colon and tectum. J Med Genet 16:417–422, 1979.

147. Santos MJ, Krush AJ, Cameron JL: Three varieties of hereditary intestinal polyposis. Johns Hopkins Med J 145:196–200, 1979.

148. Stemper TJ, Kent TH, Summers RW: Juvenile polyposis and gastrointestinal carcinoma. A study of a kindred. Ann Int Med 83:639–646, 1975.

149. Denzler TB, Harned RK, Pergam CJ: Gastric polyps in familial polyposis coli. Radiology 130:63–66, 1979.

150. Mir-Madjlessi SH, Farmer RG, Hawk WA, Turnbull RBJ: Adenocarcinoma of the ampulla of Vater associated with familial polyposis coli: report of a case. Dis Colon Rectum 16:542–546, 1973.

151. Binder MK, Zablen MA, Fleischer DE, Sue DY, Dwyer RM, Henelin L: Colon Polyps, sebaceous cysts, gastric polyps and malignant brain tumour in a family. Am J Dig Dis 23:460–466, 1978.

152. Anderson E: An inherited form of large bowel cancer: Muir's syndrome. Cancer 45:1103–1107, 1980.

153. Muir EG, Yates-Bell AJ, Barlow KA: Multiple primary carcinoma of the colon, duodenum and larynx associated with keratoacanthomata of the face. Brit J Surg 54:191–195, 1966.

154. Torre E: Multiple sebaceous tumors. Arch Dermatol 98: 549–551, 1968.

155. Gilula LA, Kantor OS: Familial colon carcinoma in nail-patella syndrome. Am J Roentgenol Radium Ther Nucl Med 123:783–90, 1975.

156. Dunstone GH, Knaggs TWL; Familial cancer of the colon and rectum. J Med Genet 9:451–456, 1972.

157. Lovett E: Familial cancer of the gastrointestinal tract. Brit J Surg 63:19–22, 1976.

158. Richards RC, Woolf C: Solitary polyps of the colon and rectum: a study of inherited tendency. Am Sur 22:287–294, 1956.

159. Schottenfeld D, Haas JF: Epidemiology of colorectal cancer. In: Gastrointestinal tract malignancy, Lipkin M, Good RA (eds). Plenum: New York, 1978, pp 207–204.

160. Woolf CM: A genetic study of carcinoma of the large intestine. Am J Human Genet 10:42–47, 1958.

161. Lipkin M: The identification of individuals at high risk for large bowel cancer: an overview. Cancer 40 (Suppl): 2523–2530, 1977.

162. Jensen OM, Bolander AH, Sigtryggsson P, Vercelli M, Nguyen-Dinh X, MacLennan R: Large bowel cancer in married couples in Sweden. A follow-up study. Lancet 1:1161–1163, 1980.

163. Fraumeni JFJr: Cancers of the pancreas and biliary tract: epidemiological considerations. Cancer Res 35:3437–3446, 1975.

164. Malagelada JR: Pancreatic cancer: an overview of epidemiology, clinical presentation and diagnosis. Mayo Clinic Proc 54:459–467, 1979.

165. Morgan RG, Wormsley KG: Progress report. Cancer of the pancreas. Gut 18:580–592, 1977.

166. MacDermott RP, Kramer P: Adenocarcinoma of the pancreas in four siblings. Gastroenterology 65:137–139, 1973.
167. Friedman JM, Fialkow PJ: Familial carcinoma of the pancreas. Clin Genet 9:463–469, 1976.
168. Rakhu PA: Zlokachestvennaia opukhol' podzheludochnour zhelezy u dvukh sester. Vopr. Onkol 22:90–92, 1976.
169. Reimer RR, Fraumeni JFJr, Ozols RF, Bender R: Pancreatic cancer in father and son. Lancet 1:911, 1977.
170. Gambill EE: Pancreatitis associated with pancreatic carcinoma: a study of 26 cases. Mayo Clinic Proc 46:174–177, 1971.
171. Comfort MW, Steinberg AG: Pedigree of a family with hereditary chronic relapsing pancreatitis. Gastroenterology 21:54–63, 1952.
172. Malik SA, van Kley H, Knight WAJr: Inherited defect in hereditary pancreatitis. Am J Dig Dis 22:999–1004, 1977.
173. Sibert JR: Hereditary pancreatitis in England and Wales. J Med Genet 15:189–201, 1978.
174. Nash FW: Familial calcific pancreatitis: an acute epidose with massive pleural effusion. Proc Royal Soc Med 64:17–18, 1971.
175. Sarles H: Constitutional factors in chronic pancreatitis. Clinics in Gastroenterology 2:639–644, 1973.
176. Bergström K, Hellström K, Kallner M, Lundh G: Familial pancreatitis associated with hyperglycinuria. Scand J Gastroenterol 8:217–223, 1973.
177. Logan A Jr, Schlicke CP, Manning GB: Familial pancreatitis. Am J Surg 115:122–117, 1968.
178. Castleman B, Sculley RE, McNeely BU: Case records of the Massachusetts General Hospital. New Engl J Med 286:1353–1359, 1972.
179. Kattwinkel J, Lapey A, di Sant'Agnese PA, Edwards WA, Hufty MP: Hereditary pancreatitis: three new kindreds and a critical review of the literature. Pediatrics 51:55–69, 1973.
180. Schimke RN: Multiple endocrine adenomatosis syndromes. Adv Intern Med 21:249–265, 1976.
181. Janson KL, Roberts JA, Varela M: Multiple endocrine adenomatosis: in support of the common origin theories. J Urol 119:161–165, 1978.
182. Tateishi R, Wada A, Ishiguro S, Ehara M, Sakamoto H, Miki T, Mori Y, Matsui Y, Ishikawa O: Coexistence of bilateral pheochromocytoma and pancreatic islet cell tumor. Report of a case and review of the literature. Cancer 42:2928–2934, 1978.
183. Lamers CB, Stadil F, van Tongeren JH: Prevalence of endocrine abnormalities in patients with the Zollinger-Ellison syndrome and in their families. Am J Med 64:607–612, 1978.
184. Brunt PW: Genetics of liver disease. Clinics in Gastroenterology 2:615–637, 1973.
185. Eddleston ALWF, Williams R: HLA and liver disease. Brit Med Bull 34:295–300, 1978.
186. Simon M, Fauchet R, Hespel JP, Beaumont C, Brissot P, Hery B, de Nercy YH, Genetet B, Bourel M: Idiopathic hemochromatosis: a study of biochemical expression in 247 heterozygous members of 63 families: evidence for a single major HLA-linked gene. Gastroenterology 78:703–708, 1980.
187. Vachon A, Paliard P, Barthe J, Grimaud JA, Peyrol M, Gaillard L, Reiss TL: Les étapes de l'atteinte hépatique de la dégénérescence hépato-lenticulaire: lésions précoces-hypertension portale et dégénérescence cancereuse. Lyon Médical 230:591–598, 1973.
188. Dahms BB: Hepatoma in familial cholestatic cirrhosis of childhood: its occurrence in twin brothers. Arch Pathol Lab Med 103:30–33, 1979.
189. Foster JH, Donohue TA, Berman MM: Familial liver-cell adenomas and diabetes mellitus.

N Engl J med 299:239–241, 1978.

190. Kelly JK, Davies JS, Jones AW: Alpha-1-antitrypsin deficiency and hepatocellular carcinoma. J Clin Path 32:373–376, 1979.

191. Fraumeni JF, Rosen PJ, Hull EW, Barth RF, Shapiro SR, O'Connor JF: Hepatoblastoma in infant sisters. Cancer. 24:1086–1090, 1969.

192. Napoli VM, Campbell WGJr: Hepatoblastoma in infant sister and brother. Cancer 39:2647–50, 1977.

193. Mulvihill JJ, Ridolfi RL, Schultz FR, Borzy MS, Haughton PBT: Hepatic adenoma in Franconi anaemia treated with oxymetholone. J Ped 87:122–124, 1975.

194. Denison EK, Peters RL, Reynolds TB: Familial hepatoma with hepatitis-associated antigen. Ann Intern Med. 74:391-394, 1971.

195. Oon CJ, Yo SL, Chua LF, Tan L, Chang CH, Chan SH: Familial primary hepatocellular carcinoma. Singapore Med J 19:218–9, 1978.

196. Johnson PJ, Krasner N, Portmann B, Eddleston ALWF, Williams R: Hepatocellular carcinoma in Great Britain: influence of age, sex, HbsAg status and aetiology of underlying cirrhosis. Gut 19:1022–1026, 1978.

197. Johnson PJ, Wansbrough-Jones MH, Portmann B, Eddleston AL, Williams R, Maycock WD, Calne RY: Familial HbsAg-positive hepatoma: treatment with orthotopic liver transplantation and specific immunoglobulin. Brit Med J 1:216, 1978.

198. Hart J, Modan B, Shani M: Cholelithiasis in the aetiology of gallbladder neoplasms. Lancet i:1151–1153, 1971.

199. Nelson BD, Porvaznik J, Benfield JR: Gallbladder disease in southwestern American Indians. Arch Surg 103:41–43, 1971.

200. van der Linden W: Genetic factors in gallstone disease. Clinics in Gastroenterol 2:603–614, 1973.

201. McCarthy CF, Espiner HJ: Carcinoma of bile ducts in husband and wife. Gut 10:94–97, 1969.

3. Systemic Manifestations of Gut Malignancy

LLOYD G. BARTHOLOMEW and ALLAN J. SCHUTT

The familiar malignancy of the gastrointestinal tract may present some difficulty in early diagnosis but is ultimately recognized by its local effect on the organ involved, as well as by symptoms from dysfunction of adjacent viscera. Adding another dimension to the problem of diagnosis of gastrointestinal malignancies is the unusual tumor that may or may not have local manifestations but predominantly presents systemic symptoms foreign to the accepted function of the cells of the gastrointestinal tract. These aberrant symptoms may be due to the production of abnormal hormones, cellular metabolites with generalized endocrine disturbances, immunologic reactions, or other metabolic abnormalities that are even less well understood. The size and duration of the primary tumor and the presence or absence of metastasis frequently have little or no correlation with the systemic presentation. A few genetic syndromes may make their appearance known with systemic features which, if recognized, may provide early diagnostic clues heralding the presence of an underlying gastrointestinal lesion carrying a high risk of future carcinoma.

This chapter, for convenience of presentation, will be subdivided into the body systems primarily affected: dermatologic, cardiovascular, hematologic, endocrine and metabolic, neuromuscular, rheumatologic, renal, and gastrointestinal.

1. DERMATOLOGIC MANIFESTATIONS

Cutaneous changes associated with an internal malignancy are varied and common. Some are easily detected, while others are subtle and their recognition, by either the patient or the physician, is fortuitous. Because such cutaneous manifestations may be the first indication of a serious underlying disease, all physicians should be mindful of these danger signs. The major

J.J. DeCosse and P. Sherlock (eds.), Gastrointestinal cancer 1, 63-96. All rights reserved.
Copyright © 1981 Martinus Nijhoff Publishers, The Hague/Boston/London.

skin manifestations can be readily recognized, and if a physician is in doubt, dermatologic consultation should be sought immediately. Although skin manifestations often signal a poor or very serious prognosis, there are enough instances of probable cures with early recognition that one cannot take a fatalistic attitude toward their presence.

1.1. Acanthosis Nigricans

Acanthosis nigricans is a symmetric verrucous, velvety hyperplasia of the skin associated with hyperpigmentation that varies from brown to black. The lesions are located primarily in the flexural areas, in the body folds of the axilla (Figure 1), lower part of the back, neck, groin, and antecubital spaces, and on the palms and soles. When extensive, the lesions may involve the areolae, umbilicus, perineum, wrists, lips, palate, and mucous membranes. On first glance, the pigmentation may be overlooked as evidence of poor body hygiene, particularly before the lesions have become elevated from the surface of the skin.

A benign variant of acanthosis nigricans is seen in obese young adults, often with a familial background, and is also occasionally seen in patients who chronically ingest drugs such as corticosteroids and nicotinic acid. Acanthosis also may be related to endocrine disorders, including insulin-resistant diabetes, hyperlipidemia, congenital lipodystrophy, growth abnormalities, and several forms of hepatic cirrhosis.

In a study at the Mayo Clinic[1] of 90 patients with acanthosis nigricans, 17 with malignancies were noted, including 13 with adenocarcinomas and four with lymphomas. Of the adenocarcinomas, approximately one half were in the gastrointestinal tract and included often highly anaplastic lesions in the

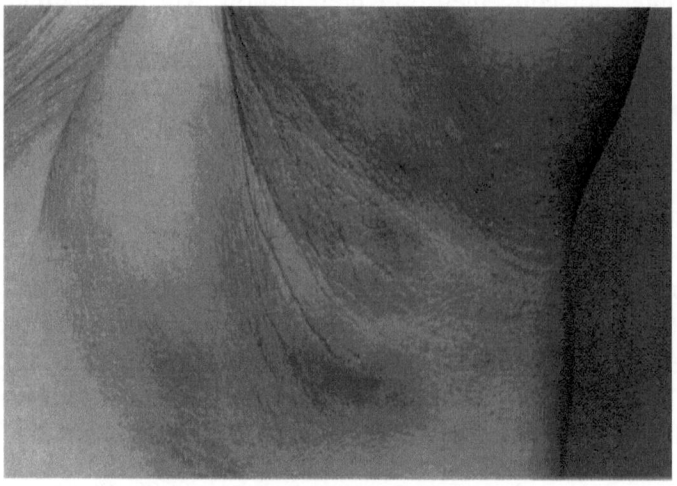

Figure 1. Acanthosis nigricans in axilla.

stomach, pancreas, and colon. Acanthosis nigricans may precede symptoms of a malignancy by months to years, as noted in 78% of patients described by Curth *et al.* [2], and may disappear when the primary tumor is removed.

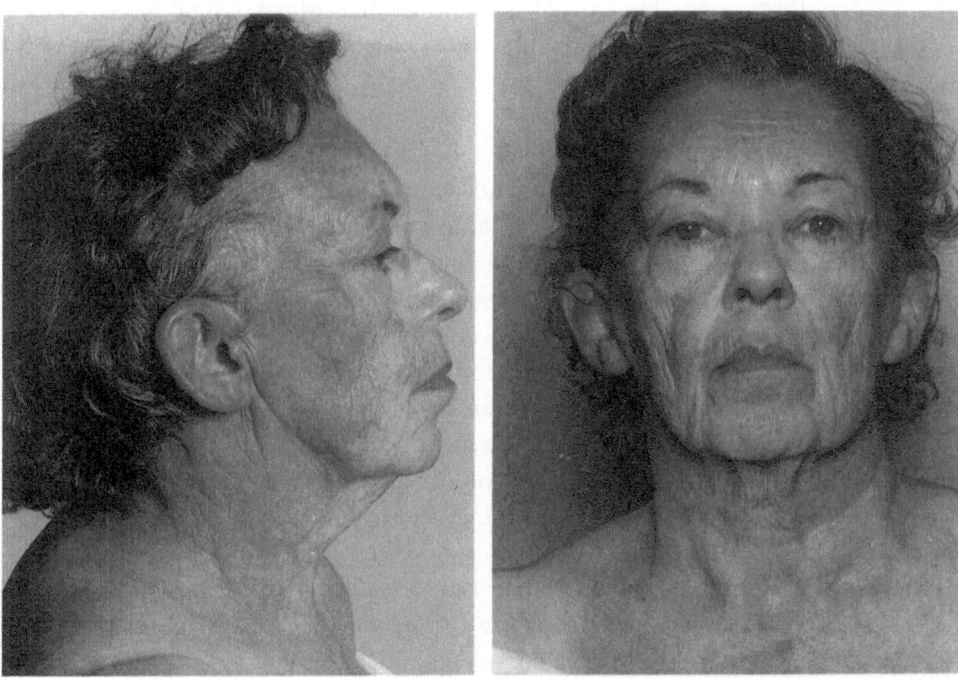

Figure 2. Dermatomyositis involving face, neck, and upper part of chest.

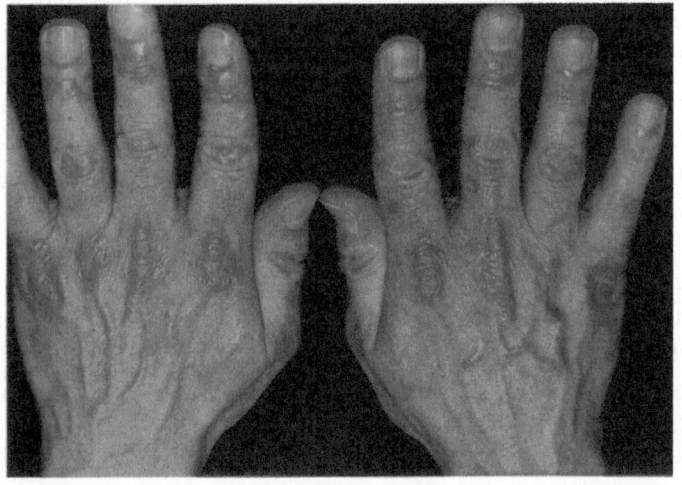

Figure 3. Dermatomyositis involving extensor surfaces of hands.

Return of the skin lesion suggests regrowth or metastasis of the malignancy. The prognosis is invariably poor in these circumstances. In most series, the average survival time of the patient after discovery of the neoplasm has been less than a year. Although the younger patient is usually considered to have the benign form, one 23-year-old patient in the Mayo Clinic series had acanthosis associated with malignancy.

1.2. Dermatomyositis

Dermatomyositis involves principally the skin, muscle, and blood vessels and has characteristic erythematous and edematous cutaneous findings associated with muscle weakness and inflammation. The proximal muscles are usually initially involved, with aching and weakness soon developing into painful and tender myositis. A violaceous hue or a purplish-red heliotropic erythema, usually seen on the eyelids, cheeks, forehead, and temples ('malignant erythema'), is considered characteristic of this disease (Figure 2). These skin changes also occur over the extensor surface of the forearms, upper back, and hands and are accentuated over the base of the nails and the dorsa of the fingers (Figure 3), especially over the joints and knuckles. When the process is healing, a telangiectatic erythema develops in areas of atrophy and scarring.

In collected series [3-5], carcinoma has been found in 15-50% of the patients. The skin changes may precede the neoplasm by days to years, with an average of 6 months. Associated malignant lesions include those of primary origin in the breast, rectum, and stomach, but the gallbladder, large bowel, and esophagus have been involved with acanthosis nigricans and the skin condition reappears with recurrence of the tumor. The mechanism of this association is unknown, but a relationship has been suggested either to a material produced by the tumor or to an immunologic mechanism. In a review by Williams [5] of 590 cases of dermatomyositis, a 15% overall incidence of carcinoma was noted. In the Mayo Clinic series of 270 patients [4], the incidence of carcinoma in all age groups was 6.7%. However, in the 18 patients with malignancy, none was less than 40 years old, giving an incidence of 17% in the group 40 years or older.

1.3. Nodular Fat Necrosis

Painful nodular lesions, particularly of the lower extremity, immediately suggest erythema nodosum, erythema induratum, and generalized diseases that are often associated with them. In the same category, a much rarer lesion is nodular fat necrosis [6, 7]. The condition may be due to excessive production of lipase from functioning pancreatic acinar cell carcinoma. This results in widespread panniculitis with nodular lesions not only on the lower extremity (Figure 4) but also on the lower abdominal wall. Although the lesions

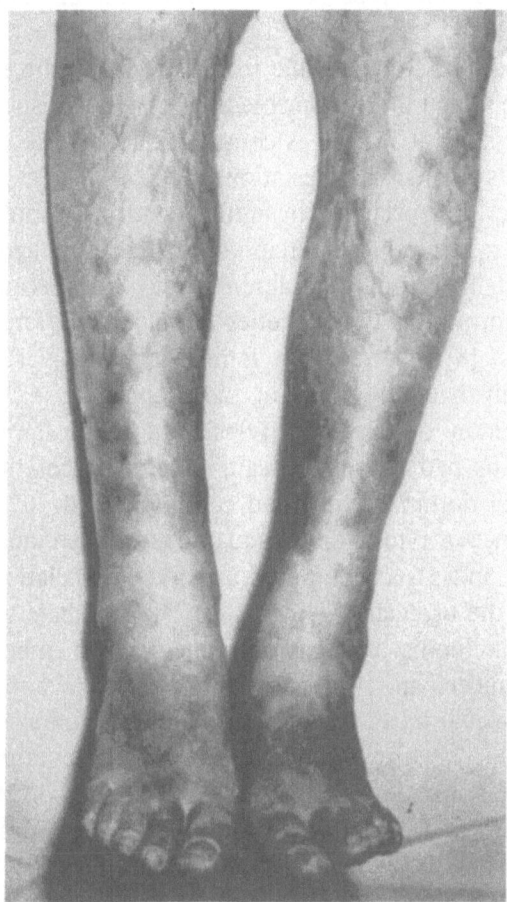

Figure 4. Subcutaneous nodular lesions of nodular fat necrosis.

resemble the other nodular erythemas, biopsy will disclose fat necrosis. The high levels of lipase seen in these situations also produce fat necrosis in the bone marrow, with resultant bone pain, polyarthralgias, and eosinophilia. The presence of persistent hyperlipasemia and nodular lesions of the lower extremity is usually associated with carcinoma of the pancreas. On a few occasions, these have been seen with recurrent and chronic pancreatitis.

1.4. Tylosis

Keratosis palmaris et plantaris is characterized by symmetric thickening of the skin of the hands and feet, generally confined to the palms and soles but with some extension onto the dorsal surfaces. Painful fissuring and local hyperhidrosis are common. 'Tylos,' from the Greek word meaning 'woody,' accurately describes the condition of the palms and soles. Two forms of tylosis are distinguishable: type A, which has a rather variable age at onset from 5 to 15 years, and type B, which is diagnosable as early as the first year of life. Type B is also distinguishable from type A by the sharply delineated edges of the lesion, a uniform thickness of the keratosis, and the relative rarity of painful fissuring. Type B is considered to be a localized disease and unassociated with systemic manifestations.

Type A, however, has occurred in families and has been associated with a high incidence of squamous cell carcinoma of the esophagus. The two types of tylosis are most likely due to different genes, and because of the serious outcome in one form, the two varieties should be differentiated. In 1958, Howel-Evans et al.[8] reported two families from Liverpool in which 18 members eventually had carcinoma of the esophagus. All 18 patients, with the possible exception of one, had tylosis. In these families, no member unaffected by tylosis had esophageal carcinoma. The condition is considered to be an autosomal dominant inherited condition, and 70% of persons with dominant inheritance of tylosis die of squamous cell carcinoma of the esophagus. Howel-Evans and associates noted a marked association between tylosis and carcinoma of the esophagus, since 18 of 48 members with tylosis developed esophageal carcinoma, whereas only one of 87 members without tylosis had esophageal cancer; and the one patient may have had tylosis. There appeared to be an equal incidence in both males and females. In 1959, Clarke et al.[9] stated that healthy tylotic persons in these families had a 95% chance of this carcinoma developing between the ages of 26 and 63 years if they had not meanwhile died from some other cause. Some of the families with tylosis have had congenitally abnormal esophagi. In one family[10], dysphagia began in early infancy, suggesting that the abnormality might be congenital, with an acquired stricture later, secondary to fibrosis and reflux esophagitis. In both these instances, the presence of gastric mucosa lining the lower esophagus was noted. In all the reports, the esophageal carcinoma was squamous cell, with no mention of adenocarcinoma (see Chapters 2 and 4).

1.5. Miscellaneous Cutaneous Reactions

Generalized pruritus, unexplained on the basis of other cutaneous lesions, is often associated with an intra-abdominal malignancy. The most common type, as far as the gastrointestinal tract is concerned, is that associated with obstructive jaundice. Other common intra-abdominal lesions associated with pruritus are lymphomas, Hodgkin's disease, and carcinoma of the stomach. Pemphigoid lesions characterized by subepidermal blisters and bullous lesions have been reported to be associated with gastric and pancreatic carcinoma.

Much controversy exists regarding the significance of herpes zoster because of its common occurrence in older people. Its diagnosis is readily apparent, but determining its significance relative to an underlying malignancy may present problems. Herpes zoster in an older person should be of concern if the patient is not in good health. Although herpes is a viral infection, its development coincidentally with a visceral malignancy may be the result of depression of the immune response in patients with malignancies such as lymphomas or leukemia. In solid tumors, including carcinomas of the breast, uterus, ovary, and stomach, herpes zoster is more commonly seen in immunosuppressed patients with advanced disease or after radiotherapy or chemotherapy. Its characteristic unilateral nerve root distribution may be the first clue to metastatic involvement of the spinal cord at the appropriate level.

Multiple neurofibromatosis (von Recklinghausen's disease) varies from a forme fruste to hundreds of soft subcutaneous neurofibromas. Most patients, however, present with a few skin tumors, and the lesions are recognized by the associated café-au-lait spots. Gastrointestinal manifestations have been recognized in association with multiple neurofibromatosis [11, 12]. These include ulceration, bleeding, obstruction, and associated malignancies. In addition to the expected benign neurofibromas of the gastrointestinal tract, other tumors, some malignant, have been noted, including neurilemmomas, leiomyomas, and leiomyosarcomas [13]. Other bowel lesions associated with this condition are polypoid ganglioneurofibromatosis of the large bowel and neurogenic fibromas.

An unusual but intriguing cutaneous clue to an underlying malignancy is acquired hypertrichosis lanuginosa [14, 15]. Lanugo refers to fetal-type hair, and its sudden occurrence should not be overlooked. It has been reported in association with malignancies of the rectum, colon, gallbladder, breast, bladder, and lung.

1.6. Genetic Disorders

Two rare but striking examples of genetic disorders involving the gastrointestinal tract are Gardner's syndrome and Peutz-Jeghers syndrome. The skin manifestations in each instance usually cause few symptoms, but they should alert the physician to potentially serious gastrointestinal disease, often before any symptoms are evident.

Gardner's syndrome [16–18] is probably a variant of familial polyposis of the colon and consists of multiple polyps of the colon and occasionally of the small bowel and stomach. Cutaneous clues to the diagnosis are its association with multiple subcutaneous sebaceous adenomas, desmoids, fibromas of the trunk and extremities, bony changes consisting of osteomas and osteochondromas, and dental anomalies. The bony lesions occur in the long bones, the facial bones along the mandible, or the pelvis. Early recognition of Gardner's syndrome is important because it invariably results in carcinoma of the colon. Such malignant transformation may occur in the young, having been seen as early as the teens. The colonic lesions may remain completely asymptomatic until malignant change has developed. Early recognition of this disease should lead to proper therapy, which in almost all instances consists of total colectomy with a permanent ileostomy. Modern surgery, however, offers some options, such as the continent pouch or ileoanal pull-through with salvage of the anal sphincter. Offering such radical treatment to a young asymptomatic patient is fraught with many difficulties, but large-bowel cancer almost always develops prematurely – the median age being about 40 years. Until recently, this type of radical surgery was believed to protect the patient with Gardner's syndrome from any future bowel malignancy. Unfortunately, in recent years[19], carcinoma of the duodenum or ampullary region has been noted in such a significant number of patients as to suggest more than a chance occurrence. Therefore, even with the best treatment available, continued surveillance of these patients, with frequent examination of the stomach and duodenum, should be considered. With the development of polyploid lesions, particularly in the duodenal area, further surgery at that time will need to be considered.

To a lesser degree, Peutz-Jeghers syndrome presents some of the problems associated with Gardner's syndrome. Peutz-Jeghers syndrome [20–22] consists of mucocutaneous melanin pigmentation on the lips (Figure 5), mucous membrane, skin around the facial orifices, and occasionally the extremities. It is associated with widespread gastrointestinal polyposis of the stomach, small bowel, and colon. Histologic study reveals that the polyps are hamartomatous, with an abnormal amount of normal tissue in its usual location. The potential for malignancy has been considered to be no greater than that of normal tissue. In more recent years, as more cases have been recognized, malignant changes in Peutz-Jeghers syndrome have been reported [23–26]. Whether

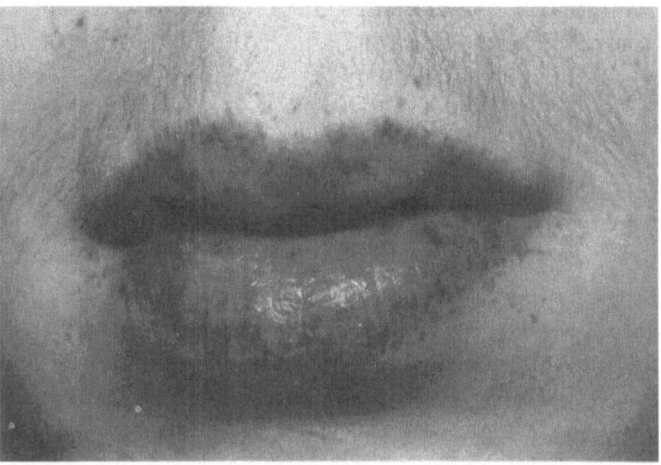

Figure 5. Melanin freckles of lips in Peutz-Jeghers syndrome.

these changes occur in hamartomatous polyps or in the surrounding mucosa, one cannot be certain. The reported increased incidence of carcinomas in Peutz-Jeghers syndrome has been in areas of the bowel where malignancy is extremely rare, for example, the duodenum and small intestine. A few malignancies have been noted in the gastric antrum and rectum. The photomicrographic material in past reports does not always give enough detail to completely convince one as to the exact origin of the malignancy. One expects the normal incidence of carcinoma in Peutz-Jeghers syndrome, so it is not unusual that a few cases have been reported.

In a recent study of 48 patients at the Mayo Clinic [27] followed up from· 1 to 47 years, with a median period of 33 years, no evidence of gastrointestinal malignancy was noted. However, six patients had malignancies of miscellaneous sites, including two with lung cancers and one each with cancer of the breast, biliary tract, kidney, and uterus. Also, women between 40 and 60 years of age but especially those less than 25 years old with Peutz-Jeghers syndrome have an increased incidence of ovarian neoplasms, varying from cysts and cystadenomas to the more unusual types such as dysgerminomas, Sertoli cell carcinoma, and the very rare sex cord tumor with annular tubules [23, 25, 28].

2. CARDIOVASCULAR MANIFESTATIONS

Hypercoagulability of the blood can manifest itself in various vascular phenomena. Spontaneous thrombophlebitis [29] in an apparently healthy person more than 50 years old usually initiates an extensive diagnostic search for an occult malignancy. The thrombophlebitis may be superficial or deep and is often migratory and multiple. Poor response to anticoagulation therapy and the development of pulmonary emboli during such therapy further suggest an undiagnosed malignancy. Other ominous signs include anemia, elevated sedimentation rate, and abnormal serum protein levels. The common primary sites of tumor origin include lungs, pancreas, and prostate and, to a lesser extent, the ovaries, stomach, large bowel, and lymphatic system.

Altered coagulability of the blood from many causes, including malignant disease, may rapidly lead to devastating vascular changes in the form currently recognized as disseminated intravascular coagulation. In these circumstances, the prognosis is poor and the disease progresses so rapidly that there may be no opportunity to search for an underlying disease.

Painless nonpitting swelling of the lower extremities may be the first sign of lymphatic obstruction secondary to a pelvic malignancy. Local inflammatory signs are conspicuously absent, and the change in size of the extremity may be all that is apparent. This syndrome may be seen with pelvic metastases from carcinoma of the large bowel, ovary, and prostate, and from pelvic lymphoma.

Transient or persistent ischemic changes [30–32] in an extremity may be associated with an altered state of coagulation, sympathetic overactivity, or peripheral emboli. These changes are clinically manifested by Raynaud's phenomenon, acrocyanosis, and ulceration and may progress to gangrene of the extremity. The development of these symptoms later in life, particularly in women with no previous personal or family history of such vascular changes, suggests the possibility of an occult malignancy. Characteristically, there is an abrupt onset, with bilateral distribution and rapid progression to digital ulceration and gangrene. The search for the cause has demonstrated primary malignancies in the pancreas, large bowel, or small bowel as well as the kidney, ovary, and lymph nodes. Usually, the sympathetic nervous system has not been infiltrated by the malignancy. Some as yet unidentified humoral or coagulation factor has been postulated as being responsible for these distal vascular changes. The prognosis is considered poor, although apparent complete remission of vascular symptoms has occurred with excision of the tumor.

3. HEMATOLOGIC MANIFESTATIONS

Cancer of the digestive tract often betrays its presence by effects on either the formed or the humoral components of the blood. Various hematologic manifestations have been associated with an underlying gastrointestinal neoplasm secondary either to quantitative or functional deficiency or to excess of elements of both the major blood cell lines and the blood proteins.

Anemia and erythrocytosis, leukopenia and leukemoid reactions, thrombocytopenia and thrombocytosis, bleeding syndromes and thrombosing tendency, hypoproteinemia or excess of one or more normal or abnormal serum proteins, and immune deficiency or hypersensitivity phenomena have all been described as systemic effects of neoplasia of the alimentary tract. These paraneoplastic effects vary in frequency from blood-loss anemia, a common diagnostic hallmark of gastrointestinal cancer, to rare hemolytic varieties.

3.1. Anemia

Anemias associated with gastrointestinal cancer can be produced by several mechanisms often acting in concert. Specific treatment for these anemias may be available when the cause is identified. Seventy percent of patients with adenocarcinoma of the right colon present with a hypochromic, microcytic anemia related to iron deficiency from chronic, insidious loss of blood. Although iron replacement may improve the anemia temporarily, the obvious treatment is surgical excision of the bleeding lesion.

Macrocytic anemia secondary to vitamin B_{12} deficiency may develop in patients who have gastric carcinoma associated with pernicious anemia or after total gastrectomy, extensive ileal resection, intestinal loop stasis with bacterial overgrowth due to surgery, radiation therapy, or chronic carcinomatous obstruction. Folate deficiency may cause macrocytic anemia when hepatoma develops in patients with cirrhosis.

Hemolytic anemia, either immune or mechanical in origin, is a rare event as a dominant syndrome in patients with malignant neoplasms of the digestive system. Coombs-positive hemolytic anemia accompanied either gastric or large-bowel carcinoma in three of 16 patients who had autoimmune hemolytic anemia associated with carcinoma reported by Spiral and Lynch[33]. Miura *et al.* [34] described a patient with localized adenocarcinoma of the colon who died of steroid-resistant Coombs-positive hemolytic anemia.

Microangiopathic hemolytic anemia characterized by the presence in the peripheral blood of a large number of schistocytes (fragmented erythrocytes with a short half-life), often with thrombocytopenia and laboratory evidence of disseminated intravascular coagulopathy, is associated with a very poor prognosis. This pattern can be seen in a number of disease states, including metastatic adenocarcinoma from the gut. The hemolytic anemia usually has an acute onset and is severe, rapidly progressive, resistant to therapy, and almost invariably fatal. The mechanism of red cell fragmentation is considered to be the mechanical forces generated by flow turbulence secondary to the intravascular deposition of fibrin strands induced by the mucin secreted by adenocarcinoma cells. In 37 cases of microangiopathic hemolytic anemia with carcinoma reported by Lohrmann and associates[35], metastatic gastric and breast adenocarcinomas were the most frequent. Other metastatic carcinomas of primary digestive tract origin included those from the colon, pancreas, and gallbladder. Microangiopathic hemolytic anemia also may be secondary to hemangioendothelioma of the liver, as reported in four cases by Alpert and Benisch[36], analogous to the thrombocytopenia seen in patients with cavernous hemangioma (Kasabach-Merritt syndrome). Presumably, the cells are fragmented in the rapid blood flow through distorted abnormal vascular channels present in these very vascular neoplasms. Shortened red cell survival also may occasionally be due to hypersplenism caused by congestive splenomegaly from obstruction of the splenic vein by pancreatic carcinoma.

The normochromic, normocytic anemia commonly observed in patients with advanced or metastatic gut cancer and many other chronic diseases has multiple causes, including reduced erythropoiesis, poor marrow utilization of iron, and low-grade hemolysis or chronic compensated disseminated intravascular coagulation. Plasma volume is increased in many of these patients, causing a falsely low hemoglobin level secondary to hemodilution. Normo-

chromic anemia may be prominent in patients who have been heavily treated
with radiation or myelosuppressive chemotherapeutic drugs, particularly those
with cumulative marrow toxicity, such as the nitrosoureas or mitomycin C.
Bone marrow infiltration with metastatic carcinoma cells may sometimes be
seen with gastrointestinal carcinoma. These patients may manifest a normochromic, normocytic anemia due to myelophthisic anemia and a leukoery-
throblastic smear.

3.2. Erythrocytosis

The only carcinoma of the digestive tract that produces paraneoplastic
erythrocytosis is hepatoma. Thorling[37] collected 64 cases of this association,
of which only one involved a female. Although erythropoietin is technically
difficult to demonstrate consistently, evidence points to its excessive production by tumor cells as the cause of erythrocytosis in these patients. While
most hepatomas are not resectable, when complete tumor resection has been
possible, the erythrocytosis has subsided. Of 448 patients with hepatoma from
four reported series, 31 (7%) had documented erythrocytosis. This compares
with an incidence of 20% in cerebellar hemangioblastoma and about 3% in
renal cell carcinoma. Because renal cell carcinoma is a far more common
neoplasm, most of the reports of paraneoplastic erythrocytosis that Hammond
and Winnick[38] collected from the literature were associated with renal cell
carcinoma.

3.3. Leukocytosis

Transient leukocytosis often is observed in patients with gastrointestinal
cancer after an acute bleeding episode. Many patients with gastrointestinal
carcinoma have persistent leukocytosis in the absence of infection, particularly
those with advanced or metastatic disease. The leukocytosis may progress to a
leukemoid reaction that resembles leukemia, although with a more orderly
progression to mature forms and a nonleukemic marrow pattern. The possibility of infection, particularly miliary tuberculosis, should always be
excluded, as it is a more common inciting factor of leukemoid reactions.
When a malignant solid tumor causes a leukemoid reaction, metastatic disease is usually present, and while the neurophilic line is most commonly
affected, eosinophilic and lymphocytic leukemoid reactions occasionally occur.
Robinson[39] studied 12 patients with cancer who had leukocyte counts in
excess of 20,000/mm^3, of whom one had a hepatoma; all 12 had levels of a
granulopoietic factor which were five to ten times normal.

Paraneoplastic eosinophilia has been noted with carcinoma of the stomach,
pancreas, and colon. Isaacson and Rapoport[40] reported that the gastrointestinal tract was the most frequent site of origin in the 12% of patients with
eosinophilia who had paraneoplastic eosinophilia. Ranke[41] described a

patient who had severe leukocytosis and 40% eosinophilia associated with hepatoma. Production of an eosinophilopoietin substance by tumor cells has been postulated (though not proved) to be a mechanism of tumor-produced eosinophilia. In comparison, lymphocytic leukemoid reactions are far less common, but they occasionally occur as a response to gastrointestinal carcinoma, as Bichel [42] reported with gastric carcinoma.

3.4. Thrombocytosis

Thrombocytosis is not uncommon in patients with advanced or metastatic gastrointestinal cancer. The condition tends to be mild, but occasionally the levels of thrombocytes increase to two or three times normal, but the thrombocytosis is almost never accompanied by hemorrhagic or thrombosing phenomena. More commonly, thrombocytosis in these patients is seen as a 'rebound' phenomenon after recovery from cytotoxic chemotherapy-induced thrombocytopenia, or it may, when mild, be secondary to iron deficiency.

3.5. Thrombocytopenia and Coagulation Defects

Spontaneous thrombocytopenia in patients afflicted with gastrointestinal cancer usually heralds invasion of the bone marrow by metastatic carcinoma cells or disseminated intravascular coagulopathy induced by metastatic disease [43]. Milder forms are more common, and frequently a balance occurs between thrombosis and fibrinolysis ('compensated disseminated intravascular coagulopathy'). When chronic and compensated, disseminated intravascular coagulopathy is characterized by elevation of soluble fibrin complexes and of fibrinolytic split products, by hyperfibrinogenemia, and, less commonly, by thrombocytopenia. In acute disseminated intravascular coagulopathy, severe coagulopathy may be present with hypofibrinogenemia, severe thrombocytopenia, prolonged thrombin and prothrombin times, and spontaneous hemorrhage or widespread thrombosis. In the series of 61 patients studied by Sun and associates [44], about equal numbers of patients had localized and advanced cancers. Most of the patients with thrombotic episodes had metastatic disease, most commonly of prostatic origin but also from the stomach, pancreas, liver, and colon.

3.6. Immunologic Disorders

Malignant diseases of the hematologic system are frequently associated with immune deficiency, both humoral and cellular, leading to severe and unusual opportunistic infection. Although immune deficiency can develop in patients with gastrointestinal carcinoma, it tends to be relatively infrequent and to occur late in patients with advanced metastatic disease who have often received prolonged or extensive antineoplastic chemotherapy, radiotherapy, or adrenocorticosteroid therapy. Lurie and colleagues [45] suggest that patients who have depression of immune parameters early during the clinical course of colon carcinoma have a poorer response to treatment, with a lessened survival, than do those who have an intact immune system.

4. ENDOCRINE AND METABOLIC MANIFESTATIONS

The endocrine cells of the gut and pancreas are believed to be embryologically of entodermal (foregut) or neuroectodermal (neural crest) origin [46]. The development of sophisticated techniques such as electron microscopy, immunohistochemical assay, and radioimmunoassay, capable of measuring minute quantities of cell products, have shown that these cells and their neoplasms share common ultrastructural, cytochemical, and functional characteristics. These endocrine cells are referred to as the APUD system, based on their properties of Amine Precursor Uptake and Decarboxylation. The gastrointestinal mucosal and pancreatic APUD-cell system is now recognized to be a very complex endocrine system. It is believed to secrete all the known polypeptide hormones and their precursors, a number of other physiologically active polypeptides, and the vasoactive amines 5-hydroxytryptamine (serotonin), 5-hydroxytryptophan, and histamine (see Chapter 13).

Those clinical syndromes secondary to hypersecretion of cell products by gastrointestinal neoplasms can be divided into two major groups. The largest group comprises patients with hormonally functioning tumors originating in gastrointestinal endocrine tissue (APUDomas), including pancreatic islet cell tumors and carcinoid tumors. The much rarer ectopic hormone syndromes are secondary to carcinomas originating in gastrointestinal tissue not ordinarily considered to have primary endocrine function. While ectopic hormone syndromes are most common in primary lung cancer (small cell) and in renal cell carcinoma (hypernephroma), hepatoma produces the widest variety and most frequently seen ectopic hormone syndromes of digestive tract origin.

4.1. Islet Cell Syndromes

Islet cell syndromes have various clinical manifestations that are produced by hypersecretion of one or more of the recognized polypeptide hormones (Table 1). These syndromes are complex, ranging from hypersecretion of a single hormone by one defined type of islet cell neoplasm to overproduction of multiple hormones by either the same islet cell neoplasm (generally a carcinoma) or multiple islet cell tumors, each producing different hormones [47]. The five major syndromes due to islet cell hypersecretion include insulinoma, gastrinoma, the WDHA (Watery Diarrhea, Hypokalemia, Achlorhydria) syndrome, glucagonoma, and polyhormonal islet cell syndrome.

Table 1. Pancreatic islet cell carcinoma syndromes.

Syndrome	Cell of origin	Secretory products	Clinical features
Insulinoma	β cell	Insulin, proinsulin	Hypoglycemia
Glucagonoma	α cell	Glucagon	Hyperglycemia, necrolytic migratory erythema
Zollinger-Ellison	δ cell (?)	Gastrin	Gastric hypersecretion, peptic ulcer, diarrhea
Verner-Morrison (pancreatic cholera or VIPoma)	Non-β cell	Vasoactive intestinal polypeptide (gastric inhibitory polypeptide, prostaglandins, secretin [?], others [?])	Watery Diarrhea, Hypokalemia, Achlorhydria (WDHA syndrome)
Wermer's (MEN, type 1), mixed pancreatic	Multipotential islet cell	Multiple pancreatic hormones	Variable
Somatostatinoma	δ cell	Somatostatin, calcitonin	Hyperglycemia, steatorrhea, achlorhydria, cholelithiasis
Multiple ectopic islet cell	Multipotential islet cell	Multiple pancreatic and ectopic hormones	Variable
Ectopic Cushing's	Multipotential islet cell	Corticotropin-melanocyte-stimulating hormone	Hyperglycemia, hypertension, hypokalemia, muscle wasting, melanosis
Inappropriate secretion of antidiuretic hormone		Antidiuretic hormone	Water intoxication
Ectopic acromegaly		(?) Human growth hormone	Acromegaly
Malignant carcinoid		Serotonin	Flushing, diarrhea
Ectopic hyperparathyroidism		Parathyroid hormone	Hypercalcemia

The symptoms produced by insulinoma are primarily of central nervous system origin, most characteristically due to subacute or chronic neuroglycopenia, rather than the acute symptoms seen with iatrogenic hypoglycemia. Diagnosis is often delayed for years. Symptoms span the spectrum of central nervous system dysfunction, from psychiatric disturbances to disordered consciousness mimicking alcoholic intoxication. Long periods of spontaneous remission may occur, but generally, a pattern of attacks of increasing severity and frequency develops, particularly before meals or after exercise. If unrecognized, chronic hypoglycemia may develop, leading to paranoid personality change and dementia [48].

Diagnosis depends on clinical suspicion, followed by demonstration of spontaneous blood glucose levels of 40 mg/dl or less, coincident with inappropriately high plasma levels of insulin. The islet cell tumor of some patients may secrete proinsulin [49], which may not be recognized by the standard insulin radioimmunoassay (a specific proinsulin radioimmunoassay has now been developed). Supplementary provocative tests (tolbutamide, prolonged fasting, glucagon, glucose, leucine, arginine, and insulin suppression with diazoxide) are sometimes helpful, though each has its limitations. About 16% of insulinomas metastasize (primarily to regional nodes and the liver) and thus are clinically malignant [50]. Islet cell carcinomas are characteristically multiple, low-grade, and indolent in progression, with a median survival of several years from the diagnosis of inoperability.

The classic manifestations secondary to uncontrolled secretion of gastrin by non-β-cell pancreatic islet cell tumor are gastric hypersecretion, severe peptic ulceration, and diarrhea. With increased physician awareness and wider use of the radioimmunoassay for serum gastrin, many cases are being diagnosed earlier, with clinical findings indistinguishable from those of idiopathic duodenal ulcer or erosive duodenitis. These early-recognized cases satisfy the criteria for the diagnosis of Zollinger-Ellison syndrome, based on levels of fasting serum gastrin and gastric hypersecretion [51]. At diagnosis, nearly two-thirds of patients have either multicentric pancreatic tumors or unresectable metastases to regional nodes or the liver [52]. The association of Zollinger-Ellison syndrome and nonpancreatic endocrine tumors – particularly parathyroid adenoma and, less often, tumors of the anterior pituitary, adrenal, thyroid, and ovary – is a feature of the Wermer syndrome of multiple endocrine neoplasia (MEN, type 1). Twenty to 30% of patients with Zollinger-Ellison syndrome have an extrapancreatic endocrine tumor [53]. Continuous suppression of gastric acid hypersecretion with long-term histamine H_2-receptor antagonists such as cimetidine now offers an alternative therapy to total gastrectomy for patients with Zollinger-Ellison syndrome [54].

In 1958, Verner and Morrison [55] described two patients with islet cell tumors and a syndrome of refractory progressive watery diarrhea and hypokalemia. By 1974[56], these same two investigators reviewed 55 cases from the literature of the syndrome now named for them but also referred to as the WDHA syndrome, pancreatic cholera, or VIPoma in view of the frequent demonstration of elevated plasma levels of vasoactive intestinal peptide (VIP). The intense hormonally stimulated gastric hypersecretion present in Zollinger-Ellison syndrome has provided enormous impetus to basic research in gastric physiology. This research produced the key to understanding and effectively managing the clinical syndromes of refractory peptic ulceration and diarrhea secondary to acid inactivation of luminal digestive enzymes. While a very rare clinical event, the Verner-Morrison syndrome, with equally striking clinical manifestations to the Zollinger-Ellison syndrome, can be considered the counterpart for stimulating research in the pathophysiology of diarrhea.

The current understanding of the genesis of hormonal diarrhea in patients with the WDHA syndrome has recently been reviewed[57]. The diarrhea of these patients is secretory, exceeding 500 ml/24 h even during fasting and often amounting to several liters daily of fluid rich in potassium and bicarbonate. Understandably, this leads to severe dehydration, acidosis, marked loss of weight, and hypotension[58]. Hypokalemia so severe as to be life-threatening may lead to hypokalemic nephropathy and renal failure[55] and is apparently largely due to secretion of potassium by the colon[59]. Water and bicarbonate are primarily secreted in increased amounts by the proximal intestine with decreased distal intestinal absorption. About half of patients with the syndrome manifest hypercalcemia in the presence of normal plasma levels of parathyroid hormone[56]. A similar incidence of diabetes mellitus has been noted for patients with the watery diarrhea syndrome. Glucose tolerance may become normal after resection of the islet cell tumor[60]. Significant elevations of both plasma calcium and glucose levels can follow infusion of vasoactive intestinal peptide in amounts sufficient to achieve plasma levels comparable to those seen in patients with the Verner-Morrison syndrome[61]. Tetany may rarely occur[55] and may be secondary to hypomagnesemia, with either normal or increased levels of serum calcium[62].

As implied by the name, vasoactive intestinal peptide produces cutaneous flushing and increases both pulse rate and blood pressure amplitude, when infused into normal volunteers[61]. Flushing was a prominent symptom in 10 of the 55 patients reviewed by Verner and Morrison[56]. Achlorhydria, reported to be a component of the watery diarrhea syndrome[63], is present in the basal state but can be moderately stimulated by gastrin and less so by histamine[64]. A wide variety of substances have been proposed as the causative agents hypersecreted by islet cell tumors to give rise to pancreatic hormonal diarrhea[65]. In addition to vasoactive intestinal peptide, these include the pancreatic peptide hormones gastrin, glucagon, secretin, and pancreatic polypeptide, as well as calcitonin, serotonin, and prostaglandins acting either singly or together.

Whereas the level of vasoactive intestinal peptide is elevated in the plasma of most patients with pancreatic cholera [66], the diagnostic value of the determination has been strongly questioned by Gardner [58], who believes that non-neoplastic causes of chronic secretory diarrhea, such as surreptitious ingestion of laxatives or diuretics [67], can be excluded on a clinical basis. He believes that the results of plasma vasoactive intestinal peptide radioimmunoassay may be difficult to interpret because of nonspecificity of antibody, variability between laboratories, and elevation of plasma vasoactive intestinal peptide levels in non-neoplastic disorders such as cirrhosis and chronic renal insufficiency. In addition, some patients have islet cell tumors and chronic secretory diarrhea but have normal levels of plasma vasoactive intestinal peptide [68]. Patients with the WDHA syndrome also have been documented to have normal levels of plasma vasoactive intestinal peptide but very high levels of pancreatic polypeptide and prostaglandin E, with the diarrhea of the latter responding to prostaglandin-inhibitor treatment [69]. Thus, vasoactive intestinal peptide may be one of the chief mediators of pancreatic cholera syndrome, but it does not act alone.

Verner and Morrison [56] found that, of 53 patients with the WDHA syndrome, 37% had malignant islet cell tumors with metastases, 30% had benign pancreatic tumors cured by surgical removal, while 20% had non-β-islet cell hyperplasia. Postoperative complications after resection of pancreatic tumors in patients with pancreatic cholera have included congestive heart failure, perhaps due to hypokalemic cardiomyopathy or to sudden loss of the vasodilatory effect of vasoactive intestinal peptide, and rebound gastric acid hypersecretion with peptic ulceration, probably due to loss of the inhibitor of gastric acid secreted by the pancreatic neoplasm [56]. Like other islet cell carcinomas, metastatic VIPoma may be responsive to chemotherapy with streptozotocin, either alone or in combination [57]. Lithium therapy may control the secretory diarrhea of the WDHA syndrome of patients not responsive to streptozotocin by inhibiting vasoactive intestinal peptide-induced increase in intestinal mucosal cyclic adenosine monophosphate [70].

The clinical hallmarks of the glucagonoma syndrome, including a unique dermatitis (necrolytic migratory erythema), stomatitis, anemia, loss of weight, mild diabetes, and hypoaminoacidemia, have been detailed by Mallinson *et al.* [71]: They collected data on nine patients, of whom eight were postmenopausal women. The glucagonoma syndrome is considered the rarest of the major islet cell tumor syndromes [72] but has been recognized with increasing frequency since specific plasma radioimmunoassay and histochemical determinations for glucagon have become readily available. Historically, this syndrome dates to the description by Becker *et al.* [73]. in 1942 of a patient who suffered from a distinctive chronic dermatitis and died from metastatic islet cell carcinoma. In 1966, McGavran *et al.* [74] demonstrated that the tumor associated with this syndrome is composed of glucagon-secreting α-cells. The distinctive dermatitis is now considered pathognomonic of the glucagonoma syndrome [75]. Mallinson *et al.* [71] noted that the dermatitis usually started and was most severe in the groin, perineum, lower abdomen, and between the thighs and buttocks but often became widespread to involve the face, hands, and feet.

Beginning as erythematous areas, the lesions progressed to superficial central bullous formations, rupturing to form crusts or a weeping surface with central healing and a sharply defined, spreading annular outline which healed in 1 to 2 weeks, with residual hyperpigmentation. Circumoral crusting was present in all patients and painful glossitis in most. The dermatitis usually preceded diagnosis of the pancreatic tumor by more than a year and in two cases by more than ten years. The lesions often become secondarily infected with bacteria or fungi and regress when the glucagon-secreting pancreatic tumor is completely resected [75] or when the associated marked depression of plasma amino acids is corrected by total parenteral nutrition [76].

Although the diabetes mellitus in most patients with the glucagonoma syndrome is usually mild and stable, patients have developed diabetic keto-acidosis [72] or have become insulin-resistant [77]. Although most patients with the glucagonoma syndrome have islet cell carcinoma with unresectable metastatic lesions [71], perhaps more widespread screening of appropriate diabetic patients with the radioimmunoassay for plasma glucagon will uncover a larger percentage of benign tumors or early resectable islet cell carcinoma [75]. Other paraneoplastic effects of glucagonoma appear to be diffuse neurologic involvement [78] and hypercalcemia with normal levels of plasma parathyroid hormone [77]. Like islet cell carcinomas secreting insulin, gastrin, or vasoactive intestinal peptide, those producing large amounts of glucagon or proglucagon may be responsive to chemotherapy with streptozotocin either alone [79] or in combination with 5-fluorouracil [78].

Somatostatin is a hypothalamic tetradecapeptide that inhibits the secretion of pituitary growth hormone [80]. Somatostatin has been demonstrated by immunofluorescence and electron micrographic techniques to be present in significant amounts in normal pancreatic and upper gastrointestinal tract D cells [81], and in both benign [82] and malignant [83] islet cell tumors. The clinical features of the somatostatinoma syndrome include diabetes mellitus, cholelithiasis, and steatorrhea. Recognition of these symptoms in a patient has permitted the preoperative diagnosis of somatostatinoma and the demonstration of an elevation of plasma somatostatin-like immunoactivity. The diabetic state has been observed to clear after complete resection of the pancreatic tumor [82]. Somatostatin-secreting pancreatic islet cell carcinomas also have been demonstrated to produce ectopic hormones, including calcitonin [83, 84] and corticotropin [85]. Ectopic Cushing's syndrome has been recognized to be associated with islet cell carcinoma [86], and in 17 collected instances of this association [87], most of the patients had intense generalized melanosis from ectopic production of melanocyte-stimulating hormone. Cure of a patient with acromegaly by resection of a large cystic β-cell adenoma of the pancreas containing substantial amounts of human growth hormone has recently been reported [88]. Ectopic production of chorionic gonadotropin and its subunits was found in 17 (63%) of 27 patients with functioning islet cell carcinomas by demonstration of both elevated plasma and tumor extract levels of human chorionic gonadotropin. In contrast, none of the 43 patients with islet cell adenoma or of the six patients with nonfunctioning islet cell carcinoma had elevated values of human chorionic gonadotropin. Thus, human chorionic gonadotropin and its subunits appear to be markers of malignant de-repression of the genome rather than simple hypersecretion by an aberrant 'cell rest' [89]. Other peptide substances localized in both the brain and the gut might be produced in excess by pancreatic or intestinal tumors in addition to somatostatin and vasoactive intestinal peptide [90]. Awareness of the potential clinical syndromes consistent with the known physiologic actions of neurotensin, enkephalins, substance P, or cholecystokinin could lead to identification of such an occurrence by application of available immunohistochemical and radioimmunoassy techniques.

O'Neal *et al.* [91] suggested that the polyhormonal secretory potential of islet cell carcinoma may on rare occasion include production of vasopressin (antidiuretic hormone).

Multiple endocrine neoplasia, type 1 (MEN, type 1), or Wermer's syndrome, is a rare, dominantly inherited genetic disorder that includes multicentric adenoma, carcinoma, or hyperplasia of pancreatic islet cells, as well as cells of the anterior pituitary and parathyroid glands and carcinoids of variable primary site [92]. Gastrinoma and insulinoma have been the most common islet cell syndromes [93]. MEN, type 2, or Sipple's syndrome, includes hyperparathyroidism plus pheochromocytoma and medullary thyroid carcinoma often associated with mucosal or cutaneous ganglioneuromatosis but not with islet cell tumors. Less common are the reports of MEN variants that combine tumors from MEN types 1 and 2, particularly pheochromocytoma and islet cell adenoma or carcinoma [92, 94], thus emphasizing the neuroendocrine origin of hyperplastic or neoplastic cells in MEN syndromes. These overlapping syndromes frequently occur in families with von Hippel-Lindau disease or neurofibromatosis.

4.2. Malignant Carcinoid Syndrome

The malignant carcinoid syndrome is most readily diagnosed when a patient presents with typical carcinoid cutaneous flushing involving the face, neck, and upper part of the chest associated with diarrhea and clinical evidence of advanced metastatic malignant disease, particularly hepatomegaly [95]. The urine commonly contains an increased amount of 5-hydroxyindoleacetic acid (5-HIAA), a metabolic breakdown product of 5-hydroxytryptamine (5-HT or serotonin), synthesized from tryptophan by these endocrine tumors. Blood levels of 5-HT may be elevated, but the level is technically much more difficult to determine than the readily available urinary 5-HIAA determination. While carcinoids can arise at any level in the gut, the vast majority of carcinoids giving rise to the malignant carcinoid syndrome are of midgut (small bowel or right colon) origin, most frequently the distal ileum, and excrete only 5-HIAA in the urine. The unusual carcinoids of foregut origin (gastric, pancreatic, or bronchial) may lack the ability to decarboxylate 5-hydroxytryptophan (5-HTP) to 5-HT and will excrete 5-HTP, 5-HT, and 5-HIAA [96].

Cutaneous flushing represents the classic clinical feature of malignant carcinoid syndrome. This visible episodic vasodilatation is extremely variable in frequency and severity but tends to be mild in most patients and to herald the presence of metastatic liver disease. Flushes characteristically last 2 to 5 minutes and are associated with a sensation of warmth spreading over the area of erythema. If the flushing is unusually severe, facial swelling, periorbital edema, conjunctival injection, and tachycardia or hypotensive symptoms may occur. Flushing that has been of long duration, particularly if frequent and severe, may lead to constant diffuse malar and facial purplish cyanotic erythema and telangiectasias. Precipitating factors tend to be those that produce vasomotor symptoms, such as emotion, exertion, imbibing alcoholic beverages, and postural changes. Eating, defecation, and hepatic palpation also precipitate flushing in many patients with malignant carcinoid syndrome. Because carcinoids are characteristically a very indolent nonaggressive cancer, many patients may harbor known metastatic disease for years before flushing becomes noticeable.

It was initially believed that release of serotonin by the tumor caused carcinoid flushes, but current thought incriminates kallikrein (bradykinin) as the usual mediator, with histamine and prostaglandins having a role in some [97]. While there is general correlation between the incidence of flushing and urinary 5-HIAA excretion, flushing is occasionally present with normal levels of 5-HIAA and, conversely, is absent with very high levels of 5-HIAA [95]. The so-called histamine flush is extremely rare, may last for hours and be intensely pruritic, and is considered characteristic of carcinoids of foregut origin. This type of carcinoid flush may respond to blockade with combined histamine H_1- and H_2-receptor antagonists [98]. Extreme variability in synthesis, storage, rate of release, platelet binding, and tissue inactivation of 5-HT may help explain the wide range of variability of symptoms as correlated with levels of serotonin or its metabolic products.

Diarrhea, like flushing, is seen in about two-thirds of patients with the malignant carcinoid syndrome. There is no constant relationship between diarrhea and flushing in individual patients. The diarrhea of the carcinoid syndrome is characteristically watery and varies greatly in frequency and severity. The major pathophysiologic mechanism contributing to carcinoid diarrhea is generally considered to be humoral stimulation of intestinal motility by an agent not clearly defined. 5-HT may have a role, as both p-chlorophenylalanine, an inhibitor of 5-HT synthesis, and methysergide, a 5-HT antagonist, may be effective in controlling the diarrhea of patients with malignant carcinoid syndrome. Both these agents have significant toxic potential and thus have not enjoyed wide clinical acceptance. Symptomatic control of diarrhea is often achieved with standard antidiarrheal agents such as codeine, tincture of opium, diphenoxylate, or loperamide. Other mechanisms that may be operational in the diarrhea of patients with carcinoid syndrome include partial intestinal obstruction due to kinking of the bowel wall by fibrosis about the tumor or mesenteric shortening and fibrosis. Steatorrhea may be due to diffuse mesenteric lymphatic obstruction from nodal metastases or fibrosis, to bowel ischemia from the compression of mesenteric arterial and venous vessels by intense fibrosis or internal elastic vascular sclerosis[99], or to chronic intestinal obstruction and stasis with bacterial overgrowth, or it may occur after ileal resection. Some patients may have choleretic or secretory diarrhea[100]. Multiple mechanisms seem to be operational in the genesis of diarrhea in some patients with malignant carcinoid syndrome.

Carcinoid heart disease is the most serious distant paraneoplastic effect of malignant carcinoid syndrome and may dominate the clinical course, frequently leading to progressive right heart failure and death[101]. This distinctive cardiopathy is caused by progressive fibrosis of the internal elastic lamina of the endocardium of the right heart, apparently secondary to prolonged exposure to high concentrations of an unknown humoral agent released by carcinoid hepatic metastatic lesions. The typical clinical findings are those of restrictive right heart disease dominated by tricuspid valve thickening and distortion with insufficiency and stenosis, usually with similar, less severe, pulmonary valve disease leading to pulmonary stenosis. A similar process may rarely involve the left heart in patients with bronchial carcinoid.

Pellagra is an additional paraneoplastic syndrome seen in patients with malignant carcinoid syndrome secondary to shunting of up to 60% of the dietary complement of the essential amino acid L-tryptophan into neoplastic synthesis of 5-HT, leading to reduced synthesis of nicotinic acid[102]. Significant clinical improvement may occur after treatment with nicotinic acid. Pellagra was noted in only two of the 91 patients with malignant carcinoid syndrome reviewed by Davis *et al.* [95], both of whom were in poor nutritional status due to advanced carcinomatosis. Other paraneoplastic effects seen in malignant carcinoid syndrome include retroperitoneal fibrosis [103], Peyronie's disease [104], arthropathy [105], and myopathy [106]. Reports of ectopic hormone secretion in the malignant carcinoid syndrome have included the ectopic corticotropin-melanocyte-stimulating syndrome (ACTH-MSH syndrome) and insulin production [97].

4.3. Ectopic Hormone Syndrome

In addition to the previously discussed ectopic hormone production by gastrointestinal endocrine carcinomas as a manifestation of the polyfunctional potential of cells of the APUD system, carcinomas of digestive tract origin originating in tissue not usually considered to have endocrine potential may also produce ectopic hormones and metabolic syndromes. By far the most commonly seen are those produced by primary liver cancers [107], including hypoglycemia and hypercalcemia with hepatocellular carcinoma and precocious puberty with hepatoblastoma. Less common paraneoplastic disorders observed with hepatocellular carcinoma include feminization, carcinoid syndrome [108], porphyria cutanea tarda [109], hyperlipemia [110], and osteoporosis [111]. Increased production of a number of proteins, in addition to the characteristic tumor marker α-fetoprotein, has been found in patients with hepatocellular carcinoma. These include dysfibrinogenemia [112], cryofibrinogenemia, polyclonal hypergammaglobulinemia [113], vitamin B_{12}-binding protein [114], and thyroxine-binding globulin [115].

Ectopic Cushing's syndrome (ectopic ACTH-MSH syndrome) is most frequently seen with small-cell lung cancer and malignant thymoma. This syndrome should be suspected when the patient is elderly and becomes rapidly and severely ill with signs and symptoms of adrenocortical hypersecretion. Loss of weight and muscle wasting and weakness rather than obesity are usually seen. Hypokalemia is frequently severe and often poorly responsive to potassium replacement. Severe mucocutaneous melanosis may occur secondary to ectopic production of melanocyte-stimulating hormone. Gastrointestinal carcinomas, other than islet cell tumors and carcinoids, which have been reported to lead to ectopic Cushing's syndrome, include those originating in the esophagus, stomach, and colon [116].

While the onset of hypercalcemia in patients with cancer most commonly is secondary to osseous metastasis, in a large number of these patients, bony metastases cannot be demonstrated. In most of these patients, the hypercalcemia is considered to be secondary to ectopic hyperparathyroidism, with secretion by the tumor of a substance identical or closely related to parathyroid hormone. These ectopic parathyroid hormone-like tumor products may on occasion differ immunologically from native parathyroid hormone and have less affinity for antibody to parathyroid hormone used in the parathyroid hormone radioimmunoassay, but they retain the usual physiologic actions of parathyroid hormone. Hypercalcemia of recent onset, with serum calcium levels of more than 14 mg/dl, especially if observed in a patient with anemia and loss of weight and without renal stones or evidence of bone resorption, is highly suggestive of ectopic hyperparathyroidism. While carcinoma of the lung and kidney produce most ectopic hyperparathyroidism, primary gastrointestinal carcinomas reported to be associated with the ectopic parathyroid hormone syndrome include those of esophageal [117], pancreatic, hepatic, and large bowel origin [118].

Extrapancreatic paraneoplastic hypoglycemia was caused by large mesenchymal abdominal or thoracic neoplasms in most (64%) of the series collected by Lipsett et al. [119]. Hepatoma made up 21%, whereas 6% were associated with carcinoma of other digestive tract origin, including stomach, bile duct, and cecum. Extrapancreatic tumors are believed to produce hypoglycemia by mechanisms other than elaboration of insulin [120], as ectopic extrapancreatic paraneoplastic insulin secretion has rarely been documented. Postulated neoplastic hypoglycemic mechanisms include marked consumption of glucose by large hypermetabolic tumors, secretion by the neoplastic cell of nucleic acids with insulin-like actions, and elaboration by tumors of tryptophan derivatives which are capable of inhibiting hepatic glyconeogenesis.

The syndrome of inappropriate antidiuretic hormone secretion (SIADH) has been reported in association with a wide range of clinical situations. These include central nervous system trauma, infection, neoplasm, or disease and thoracic disease represented by lung cancer, malignant thymoma, pulmonary tuberculosis, and pneumonia, as well as metabolic disorders such as acute intermittent porphyria [121]. Clinically, SIADH presents as water intoxication due to continued antidiuretic hormone (vasopressin) secretion in the presence of relatively hypo-osmolar serum and may progress to cerebral edema. The syndrome is characterized by renal sodium loss, hyponatremia, and abnormal or expanded extracellular fluid volume, all of which can be corrected by limiting intake of water. Levels of antidiuretic hormone can be measured in body fluid or tissue by radioimmunoassay or bioassay. Marks et al. [122] demonstrated, by both of these techniques, tissue levels of antidiuretic hormone which approximated those present in the human neurohypophysis in a pancreatic carcinoma from a patient with SIADH.

The functioning neoplasms that characteristically produce large amounts of gonadotropins are those of trophoblastic origin, such as choriocarcinoma and gonadal carcinomas that contain trophoblastic elements. As such, this gonadotropin production cannot be considered ectopic. Ectopic production of human chorionic gonadotropin and its subunits has been demonstrated by radioimmunoassay in a wide variety of nontrophoblastic malignant neoplasms [123], including hepatoma, hepatoblastoma, and other gastrointestinal cancers, notably gastric and pancreatic carcinoma. In male children with large, rapidly progressive hepatoblastoma, precocious puberty may result [124]. In men, ectopic paraneoplastic production of human chorionic gonadotropin is most commonly seen as a manifestation of lung cancer but also has been documented in primary hepatocellular carcinoma [125]. Feminization may occur in adolescents and gynecomastia alone in older men.

5. NEUROMUSCULAR MANIFESTATIONS

Primary neuromuscular disorders [126, 127] often present a combination of signs and symptoms that are not readily categorized into specific entities. Adding to this problem is the reverse situation, in which neuromuscular syndromes are secondary to malignant disease elsewhere in the body. Even more intriguing is evidence that these neuromuscular syndromes are not due to invasive metastatic disease but to some other remote mechanism. In a series [128] of 1,465 patients with carcinoma, 96 patients (6.6%) had an associated neuromyopathy. The incidence was significantly increased in patients with carcinoma of the lung (12 to 15%) and ovary (16%) but was considerably less frequent in patients with carcinoma of the prostate (6%), breast (4%), colon (3 to 5%), and rectum (less than 1%). Categorizing these carcinomatous neuromyopathies was difficult because of overlapping syndromes, but the most frequent symptoms were weakness and wasting of proximal muscles, occurring in 65% of the patients. Other syndromes delineated were myopathies, including myasthenia gravis, cerebellar degeneration, selective spinal cord motor neuron degeneration, and dementia. Unfortunately, the most consistent finding in carcinomatous neuromyopathy is its almost universally poor prognosis, with removal of the tumor having little or no effect.

6. RHEUMATOLOGIC MANIFESTATIONS

Acute and chronic nonspecific inflammatory reactions in the fibrous tissue around tendons and joints occur with some systemic diseases (e.g. viremia, collagen diseases). Similarly, such changes have been associated with malignant tumors. These include an atypical rheumatoid arthritis syndrome (carcinomatous polyarthritis) and hypertrophic osteoarthropathy (Marie-Bamberger syndrome) [129].

Rheumatoid arthritis-like joint symptoms in a patient more than 50 years old are suggestive of a systemic disorder, and an underlying malignancy

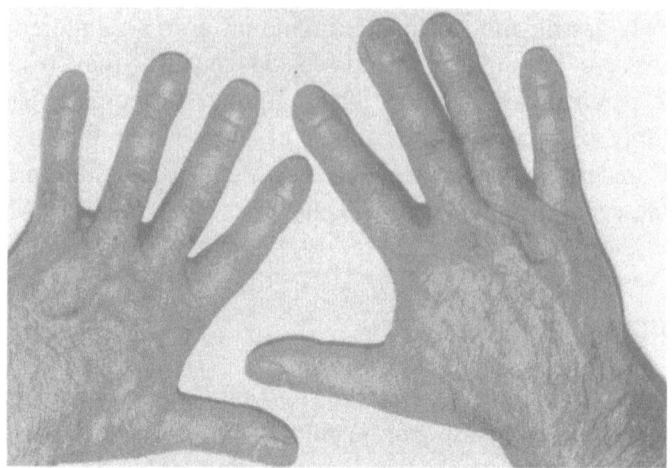

Figure 6. Hypertrophic pulmonary osteoarthropathy.

should be sought. Unusual features include an abrupt onset, asymmetric involvement of larger joints (less frequently seen in the usual form of rheumatoid arthritis) and the sparing of the commonly affected hand and wrist joints. Cancers manifesting these changes are found in the breast, bladder, bronchus, colon, and cervix.

Clinically, hypertrophic pulmonary osteoarthropathy may develop abruptly and consists of painful digital clubbing (Figure 6), with burning paresthesias and ossifying hypertrophic periostitis at the distal end of long bones, and synovitis. The condition is most commonly associated with intrathoracic disease, which may very from inflammation to primary or metastatic malignancy. In 50 patients with this syndrome, 19 had an underlying malignancy, with two having the origin of the lesion in the colon [129].

7. RENAL MANIFESTATIONS

All the common pathophysiologic syndromes of renal disease are occasionally seen as paraneoplastic vary;equences of gastrointestinal carcinoma. Renal failure can be precipitated either by hypercalcemia or, when disseminated intravascular coagulation eventuates in bilateral renal cortical necrosis, by extensive renal ischemia with infarction, or bilateral renal vein thrombosis. Deposition of tumor antigen–antibody complexes on glomerular basement membrane can result in paraneoplastic membranous glomerulopathy and the nephrotic syndrome. Presumptive evidence of soluble immune complex glomerulonephritis was demonstrated by Costanza and associates [130], who showed, by immunofluorescent staining, the presence of immunoglobulins and carcinoembryonic antigen on the glomerular basement membrane in a patient with the nephrotic syndrome and hepatic metastases secondary to carcinoma of the colon. A similar patient with the nephrotic syndrome and a resectable colon carcinoma has been described, in whom carcinoembryonic antigen could not be demonstrated on the glomerular basement membrane but in whom deposits of tumor antigen and antibody were detected by immunofluorescent techniques[131]. The patient improved after resection of the primary colon carcinoma, as did the patient reported by Cantrell[132] after resection of a gastric carcinoma.

Renal amyloidosis and renal vein thrombosis also may lead to the nephrotic syndrome. Tubular syndromes secondary to metastatic pancreatic carcinoma have been noted in isolated reports. These include the adult Fanconi syndrome of proximal tubular dysfunction[133] and renal failure secondary to tubular obstruction by proteinaceous casts in a patient with peritoneal carcinomatosis secondary to a mucoprotein-secreting adenocarcinoma[134]. The latter syndrome is most commonly a complication of multiple myeloma.

8. GASTROINTESTINAL MANIFESTATIONS

The common major constitutional paraneoplastic signs and symptoms of gastrointestinal cancer and the more rare and fascinating gastrointestinal genetic syndromes with dermatologic manifestations have been previously discussed in this chapter. Several other paraneoplastic effects of gut cancer deserve emphasis.

The patient with an otherwise asymptomatic gastric carcinoma may note dependent edema as an initial symptom secondary to pronounced hypoalbuminemia related to exudative protein-losing enteropathy. Waldmann et al. [135] demonstrated gastrointestinal protein loss in all seven patients with ulcerated gastric carcinomas whom they studied, as well as in patients with ulcerated colon and esophageal carcinomas. A more recent report[136] describes a patient with severe hypoalbuminemia and generalized edema from an ulcerated primary duodenal adenocarcinoma. The McKittrick-Wheelock syndrome represents a special variant of neoplastic protein-losing enteropathy and refers to the sometimes massive secretion of electrolytes and protein-rich mucus by soft, bulky villous tumors of the rectosigmoid. Patients with this syndrome may present with severe dehydration, potentially fatal shock, confusion, paralysis, and cardiac arrhythmias secondary to severe depletion of water, potassium, sodium, chloride, and serum proteins. The offending villous neoplasm may be so soft and jelly-like in consistency that detection by digital rectal examination may be very difficult[137]. The presence of firm areas, deep in the villous lesion, may betray the presence of an area of occult carcinoma and has been found in about 40% of these neoplasms. Deller *et al.* [138] found mild malabsorption and steatorrhea associated with minor atrophic changes in the mucosa of the small bowel of most of the 45 patients with cancer they studied, including two with rectal cancer. These findings suggest that mild paraneoplastic malabsorption may be a contributing factor to the loss of weight commonly experienced by patients with cancer. Lender [139] described patients who had systemic amyloidosis associated with carcinoma of the colon, stomach, and gallbladder. In a review of the literature, he found that only 7% of 944 patients with systemic amyloidosis had malignant neoplasms.

REFERENCES

1. Brown J, Winkelmann RK: Acanthosis nigricans: a study of 90 cases. Medicine (Baltimore) 47:33–51, 1968.
2. Curth HO, Hilberg AW, Machacek GF: The site and histology of the cancer associated with malignant acanthosis nigricans. Cancer 15:364–382, 1962.
3. Bartholomew LG, Schutt AJ: Systemic syndromes associated with neoplastic disease including cancer of the colon. Cancer 28:170–174, 1971.
4. Christianson HB, Brunsting LA, Perry HO: Dermatomyositis: unusual features, complications, and treatment. Arch Dermatol 74:581–589, 1956.
5. Williams RC Jr: Cited by Arundell FD, Wilkinson RD, Haserick JR: Dermatomyositis and malignant neoplasms in adults: a survey of twenty years' experience. Arch Dermatol 82:772–775, 1960.
6. MacMahon HE, Brown PA, Shen EM: Acinar cell carcinoma of the pancreas with subcutaneous fat necrosis. Gastroenterology 49:555–559, 1965.
7. Robertson JC, Eeles GH: Syndrome associated with pancreatic acinar cell carcinoma. Br Med J 2:708–709, 1970.
8. Howel-Evans W, McConnell RB, Clarke CA, Sheppard PM: Carcinoma of the oesophagus with keratosis palmaris et plantaris (tylosis). Q J Med 27:413–429, 1958.
9. Clarke CA, Howel Evans W, McConnell RB, Sheppard PM: Carcinoma of oesophagus in association with tylosis (letter to the editor). Br Med J 2:1100, 1959.
10. Shine I, Allison PR: Carcinoma of the oesophagus with tylosis (keratosis palmaris et plantaris). Lancet 1:951–953, 1966.
11. Hochberg FH, Dasilva AB, Galdabini J, Richardson EP Jr: Gastrointestinal involvement in von Recklinghausen's neurofibromatosis. Neurology 24:1144–1151, 1974.
12. Lukash WM, Morgan RI, Sennett CO, Nielson OF: Gastrointestinal neoplasms in von Recklinghausen's disease. Arch Surg 92:905–908, 1966.
13. Raszkowski HJ, Hufner RF: Neurofibromatosis of the colon: a unique manifestation of von Recklinghausen's disease. Cancer 27:134–142, 1971.
14. Hensley GT, Glynn KP: Hypertrichosis lanuginosa as a sign of internal malignancy. Cancer 24:1051–1056, 1969.
15. Hegedus SI, Schorr WF: Acquired hypertrichosis lanuginosa and malignancy: a clinical review and histopathologic evaluation with special attention to the 'mantle' hair of Pinkus. Arch Dermatol 106:84–88, 1972.
16. Gardner EJ: A genetic and clinical study of intestinal polyposis, a predisposing factor for carcinoma of the colon and rectum. Am J Hum Genet 3:167–176, 1951.

17. Gardner EJ, Plenk HP: Hereditary pattern for multiple osteomas in a family group. Am J Hum Genet 4:31–36, 1952.
18. Smith WG: Multiple polyposis, Gardner's syndrome and desmoid tumors. Dis Colon Rectum 1:323–332, 1958.
19. Schnur PL, David E, Brown PW Jr, Beahrs OH, ReMine WH, Harrison EG Jr: Adenocarcinoma of the duodenum and the Gardner syndrome JAMA 223:1229–1232, 1973.
20. Jeghers H, McKusick VA, Katz KH: Generalized intestinal polyposis and melanin spots of the oral mucosa, lips and digits: a syndrome of diagnostic significance. N Engl J Med 241:993–1005, 1949.
21. Bartholomew LG, Dahlin DC, Waugh JM: Intestinal polyposis associated with mucocutaneous melanin pigmentation (Peutz-Jeghers syndrome): review of literature and report of six cases with special reference to pathologic findings. Gastroenterology 32:434–451, 1957.
22. Bartholomew LG, Moore CE, Dahlin DC, Waugh JM: Intestinal polyposis associated with mucocutaneous pigmentation. Surg Gynecol Obstet 115:1–11, 1962.
23. Dozois RR, Judd ES, Dahlin DC, Bartholomew LG: The Peutz-Jeghers syndrome: is there a predisposition to the development of intestinal malignancy? Arch Surg 98:509–516, 1969.
24. Reid JD: Intestinal carcinoma in the Peutz-Jeghers syndrome. JAMA 229:833–834, 1974.
25. Dozois RR, Kempers RD, Dahlin DC, Bartholomew LG: Ovarian tumors associated with the Peutz-Jeghers syndrome. Ann Surg 172:233–238, 1970.
26. Christian CD: Ovarian tumors: an extension of the Peutz-Jeghers syndrome. Am J Obstet Gynecol 111:529–532, 1971.
27. Linos DA: Unpublished data.
28. Scully RE: Sex cord tumor with annular tubules: a distinctive ovarian tumor of the Peutz-Jeghers syndrome. Cancer 25:1107–1121, 1970.
29. Lieberman JS, Borrero J, Urdaneta E, Wright IS: Thrombophlebitis and cancer. JAMA 177:542–545, 1961.
30. Hawley PR, Johnston AW, Rankin JT: Association between digital ischaemia and malignant disease. Br Med J 3:208–212, 1967.
31. Andrasch RH, Bardana EJ Jr, Porter JM, Pirofsky B: Digital ischemia and gangrene preceding renal neoplasm: an association with sarcomatoid adenocarcinoma of the kidney. Arch Intern Med 136:486–488, 1976.
32. Van der Meulen J, The TH, Wouda AA: Le phénomène de Raynaud: un syndrome paranéoplastique? (letter to the editor). Nouv Presse Med 7:3935, 1978.
33. Spiral MA, Lynch EC: Autoimmune hemolytic anemia and carcinoma: an unusual association. Am J Med 67:753–758, 1979.
34. Miura AB, Shibata A, Akihama T, Endo Y, Sugawara M, Ono I, Watanuki T: Autoimmune hemolytic anemia associated with colon cancer. Cancer 33:111–114, 1974.
35. Lohrmann H-P, Adam W, Heymer B, Kubanek B: Microangiopathic hemolytic anemia in metastatic carcinoma: report of eight cases. Ann Intern Med 79:368–375, 1973.
36. Alpert LI, Benisch B: Hemangioendothelioma of the liver associated with microangiopathic hemolytic anemia: report of four cases. Am J Med 48:624–628, 1970.
37. Thorling EB: Paraneoplastic erythrocytosis and inappropriate erythropoietin production: a review. Scand J Haematol Suppl 17:1–166, 1972.
38. Hammond D, Winnick S: Paraneoplastic erythrocytosis and ectopic erythropoietins. Ann NY Acad Sci 230:219–227, 1974.
39. Robinson WA: Granulocytosis in neoplasia. Ann NY Acad Sci 230:212–218, 1974.
40. Isaacson NH, Rapoport P: Eosinophilia in malignant tumors: its significance. Ann Intern Med 25:893–902, 1946.

41. Ranke EJ: Eosinophilia and hepatocellular carcinoma: report of a case. Am J Dig Dis 10:548–553, 1965.
42. Bichel J: Lymphatic leukemia and lymphatic leukemoid states in cancer of the stomach. Blood 4:759–766, 1949.
43. Bowie EJW, Owen CA Jr: Introduction: symposium on the diagnosis and treatment of intravascular coagulation-fibrinolysis (ICF) syndrome, with special emphasis on this syndrome in patients with cancer. Mayo Clin Proc 49:635, 1974.
44. Sun NCJ, Bowie EJW, Kazmier FJ, Elveback LR: Blood coagulation studies in patients with cancer. Mayo Clin Proc 49:636–641, 1974.
45. Lurie BB, Bull DM, Zamcheck N, Steward AM, Helms RA: Diagnosis and prognosis in colon cancer based on a profile of immune reactivity. J Natl Cancer Inst 54:319–325, 1975.
46. Pearse AGE: The endocrine cells of the GI tract: origins, morphology and functional relationships in health and disease. Clin Gastroenterol 3:491–510, 1974.
47. Huizenga KA, Goodrick WIM, Summerskill WHJ: Peptic ulcer with islet cell tumor. Am J Med 37:564–577, 1964.
48. Marks V, Samols E: Insulinoma: natural history and diagnosis. Clin Gastroenterol 3:559–573, 1974.
49. Alsever RN, Roberts JP, Gerber JG, Mako ME, Rubenstein AH: Insulinoma with low circulating insulin levels: the diagnostic value of proinsulin measurements. Ann Intern Med 82:347–350, 1975.
50. Stefanini P, Carboni M, Patrassi N: Surgical treatment and prognosis of insulinoma. Clin Gastroenterol 3:697–709, 1974.
51. Regan PT, Malagelada J-R: A reappraisal of clinical, roentgenographic, and endoscopic features of the Zollinger-Ellison syndrome. Mayo Clin Proc 53:19–23, 1978.
52. Zollinger RM, Takeuchi O: Surgical treatment of gastrinoma and WDHA syndrome. Clin Gastroenterol 3:685–696, 1974.
53. Bonfils S, Bernades P: Zollinger-Ellison syndrome: natural history and diagnosis. Clin Gastroenterol 3:539–557, 1974.
54. Lamers CBH, Festen HPM, van Tongeren JHM: Long-term treatment with histamine H_2-receptor antagonists in Zollinger-Ellison syndrome. Am J Gastroenterol 70: 286–291, 1978.
55. Verner JV, Morrison AB: Islet cell tumor and a syndrome of refractory watery diarrhea and hypokalemia. Am J Med 25:374–380, 1958.
56. Verner JV, Morrison AB: Endocrine pancreatic islet disease with diarrhea: report of a case due to diffuse hyperplasia of nonbeta islet tissue with a review of 54 additional cases. Arch Intern Med 133:492–500, 1974.
57. McGill DB, Miller LJ, Carney JA, Phillips SF, Go VLW, Schutt AJ: Hormonal diarrhea due to pancreatic tumor. Gastroenterology 79:571–582, 1980.
58. Gardner JD: Plasma VIP in patients with watery diarrhea syndrome. Am J Dig Dis 23:370–373, 1978.
59. Rambaud J-C, Modigliani R, Matuchansky C, Bloom S, Said S, Pessayre D, Bernier J-J: Pancreatic cholera: studies on tumoral secretions and pathophysiology of diarrhea. Gastroenterology 69:110–122, 1975.
60. Chears WC Jr, Thompson JE, Hutcheson JB, Patterson CO: Pancreatic islet tumor with severe diarrhea. Am J Med 29:529–533, 1960.
61. Domschke S, Domschke W, Bloom SR, Mitznegg P, Mitchell SJ, Lux G, Strunz U: Vasoactive intestinal peptide in man: pharmacokinetics, metabolic and circulatory effects Gut 19:1049–1053, 1978.
62. Wacker WEC, Parisi AF: Magnesium metabolism. N Engl J Med 278:658–663, 1968.
63. Murray JS, Paton RR, Pope CE II: Pancreatic tumor associated with flushing and diarrhea:

report of a case. N Engl J Med 264:436–439, 1961.

64. Konturek SJ, Thor P, Dembínski A, Król R: Vasoactive intestinal peptide: comparison with secretin for potency and spectrum of physiologic action. In: Gastrointestinal hormones: a symposium. Thompson JC (ed). Austin: University of Texas Press, 1975, pp 611–633.

65. Welbourn RB, Polak JM, Bloom SR: Apudomas of the pancreas. In: Gut hormones, Bloom SR (ed). Edinburgh: Churchill Livingstone, 1978, pp 561–669.

66. Bloom SR: Vasoactive intestinal peptide, the major mediator of the WDHA (pancreatic cholera) syndrome: value of measurement in diagnosis and treatment. Am J Dig Dis 23:373–376, 1978.

67. Krejs GJ, Walsh JH, Morawski SG, Fordtran JS: Intractable diarrhea: intestinal perfusion studies and plasma VIP concentrations in patients with pancreatic cholera syndrome and surreptitious ingestion of laxatives and diuretics. Am J Dig Dis 22:280–292, 1977.

68. Jaffe BM: To be or not to VIP (editorial). Gastroenterology 76:417–420, 1979.

69. Jaffe BM, Kopen DF, DeSchryver-Kecskemeti K, Gingerich RL, Greider M: Indomethacin-responsive pancreatic cholera. N Engl J Med 297:817–821, 1977.

70. Pandol SJ, Korman LY, McCarthy DM, Gardner JD: Beneficial effect of oral lithium carbonate in the treatment of pancreatic cholera syndrome. N Engl J Med 302:1403–1404, 1980.

71. Mallinson CN, Bloom SR, Warin AP, Salmon PR, Cox B: A glucagonoma syndrome. Lancet 2:1–5, 1974.

72. Domen RE, Shaffer MB Jr, Finke J, Sterin WK, Hurst CB: The glucagonoma syndrome: report of a case. Arch Intern Med 140:262–263, 1980.

73. Becker SW, Kahn D, Rothman S: Cutaneous manifestations of internal malignant tumors. Arch Dermatol Syphilol 45:1069–1080, 1942.

74. McGavran MH, Unger RH, Recant L, Polk HC, Kilo C, Levin ME: A glucagon-secreting alpha-cell carcinoma of the pancreas. N Engl J Med 274:1408–1413, 1966.

75. Katz R, Fischmann AB, Galotto J, Guccio JG, Higgins GA, Ortega LG, West WH, Recant L: Necrolytic migratory erythema, presenting as candidiasis, due to a pancreatic glucagonoma. Cancer 44:558–563, 1979.

76. Norton JA, Kahn CR, Schiebinger R, Gorschboth C, Brennan MF: Amino acid deficiency and the skin rash associated with glucagonoma. Ann Intern Med 91:213–215, 1979.

77. Leichter SB, Pagliara AS, Greider MH, Pohl S, Rosai J, Kipnis DM: Uncontrolled diabetes mellitus and hyperglucagonemia associated with an islet cell carcinoma. Am J Med 58:285–293, 1975.

78. Khandekar JD, Oyer D, Miller HJ, Vick NA: Neurologic involvement in glucagonoma syndrome: response to combination chemotherapy with 5-fluorouracil and streptozotocin. Cancer 44:2014–2016, 1979.

79. Danforth DN Jr, Triche T, Doppman JL, Beazley RM, Perrino PV, Recant L: Elevated plasma proglucagon-like component with a glucagon-secreting tumor: effect of streptozotocin. N Engl J Med 295:242–245, 1976.

80. Brazeau P, Vale W, Burgus R, Butcher M, Rivier J, Guillemin R: Hypothalamic polypeptide that inhibits the secretion of immunoreactive pituitary growth hormone. Science 179:77–79, 1973.

81. Polak JM, Pearse AGE, Grimelius L, Bloom SR: Growth-hormone release-inhibiting hormone in gastrointestinal and pancreatic D cells. Lancet 1:1220–1222, 1975.

82. Ganda OP, Weir GC, Soeldner JS, Legg MA, Chick WL, Patel YC, Ebeid Am, Gabbay KH, Reichlin S: 'Somatostatinoma': a somatostatin-containing tumor of the endocrine pancreas. N Engl J Med 296:963–967, 1977.

83. Galmiche JP, Chayvialle JA, Dubois PM, Descos F, Paulin C, Ducastelle T, Colin R, Geffroy Y: Calcitonin-producing pancreatic somatostatinoma. Gastroenterology 78:

1577–1583, 1980.

84. Krejs GJ, Orci L, Conlon JM, Ravazzola M, Davis GR, Raskin P, Collins SM, McCarthy DM, Baetens D, Rubenstein A, Aldor TA, Unger RH: Somatostatinoma syndrome: biochemical, morphologic and clinical features. N Engl J Med 301:285–292, 1979.

85. Kovacs K, Horvath E, Ezrin C, Sepp H, Elkan I: Immunoreactive somatostatin in pancreatic islet-cell carcinoma accompanied by ectopic A.C.T.H. syndrome (letter to the editor). Lancet 1:1365–1366, 1977.

86. Riggs BL Jr, Sprague RG: Association of Cushing's syndrome and neoplastic disease: observations in 232 cases of Cushing's syndrome and review of literature. Arch Intern Med 108:841–849, 1961.

87. Schein PS, DeLellis RA, Kahn CR, Gordon P, Kraft AR: Islet cell tumors: current concepts and management. Ann Intern Med 79:239–257, 1973.

88. Caplan RH, Koob L, Abellera RM, Pagliara AS, Kovacs K, Randall RV: Cure of acromegaly by operative removal of an islet cell tumor of the pancreas. Am J Med 64: 874–882, 1978.

89. Kahn CR, Rosen SW, Weintraub BD, Fajans SS, Gorden P: Ectopic production of chorionic gonadotropin and its subunits by islet-cell tumors: a specific marker for malignancy. N Engl J Med 297:565–569, 1977.

90. Snyder SH, Uhl GR, Miller R: Brain peptides secreted by gut tumors (letter to the editor). N Engl J Med 298: 1259–1260, 1978.

91. O'Neal LW, Kipnis DM, Luse SA, Lacy PE, Jarett L: Secretion of various endocrine substances by ACTH-secreting tumors— gastrin, melanotropin, norepinephrine, serotonin, parathormone, vasopressin, glucagon. Cancer 21:1219–1232, 1968.

92. Tateishi R, Wada A, Ishiguro S, Ehara M, Sakamoto H, Miki T, Mori Y, Matsui Y, Ishikawa O: Coexistence of bilateral pheochromocytoma and pancreatic islet cell tumor: report of a case and review of the literature. Cancer 42:2928–2934, 1978.

93. Synder N III, Scurry MT, Deiss WP Jr: Five families with multiple endocrine adenomatosis. Ann Intern Med 76:53–58, 1972.

94. Carney JA, Go VLW, Gordon H, Northcutt RC, Pearse AGE, Sheps SG: Familial pheochromocytoma and islet cell tumor of the pancreas. Am J Med 68:515–521, 1980.

95. Davis Z, Moertel CG, McIlrath DC: The malignant carcinoid syndrome. Surg Gynecol Obstet 137:637–644, 1973.

96. Feldman JM: Serotonin metabolism in patients with carcinoid tumors: incidence of 5-hydroxytryptophan-secreting tumors. Gastroenterology 75:1109–1114, 1978.

97. Grahame-Smith DG: Natural history and diagnosis of the carcinoid syndrome. Clin Gastroenterol 3:575–594, 1973.

98. Roberts LJ II, Marney SR Jr, Oates JA: Blockade of the flush associated with metastatic gastric carcinoid by combined histamine H_1 and H_2 receptor antagonists: evidence of an important role of H_2 receptors in human vasculature. N Engl J Med 300:236–238, 1979.

99. Iozzo RV: Case 16-1979 — elastic vascular sclerosis and carcinoid tumors (letter to the editor). N Engl J Med 301:385–386, 1979.

100. Davis GR, Camp RC, Raskin P, Krejs GJ: Effect of somatostatin infusion on jejunal water and electrolyte transport in a patient with secretory diarrhea due to malignant carcinoid syndrome. Gastroenterology 78:346–349, 1980.

101. Trell E, Rausing A, Ripa J, Torp A, Waldenström J: Carcinoid heart disease: clinicopathologic findings and follow-up in 11 cases. Am J Med 54:433–444, 1973.

102. Swain CP, Tavill AS, Neale G: Studies of tryptophan and albumin metabolism in a patient with carcinoid syndrome, pellagra, and hypoproteinemia. Gastroenterology 71:484–489, 1976.

103. Morin LJ, Zuerner RT: Retroperitoneal fibrosis and carcinoid tumor (letter to the editor).

JAMA 216:1647–1648, 1971.

104. Bivens CH, Marecek RL, Feldman JM: Peyronie's disease: a presenting complaint of the carcinoid syndrome. N Engl J Med 289:844–845, 1973.

105. Plonk JW, Feldman JM: Carcinoid arthropathy. Arch Intern Med 134:651–654, 1974.

106. Berry EM, Maunder C, Wilson M: Carcinoid myopathy and treatment with cyproheptadine (Periactin). Gut 15:34–38, 1974.

107. Margolis S, Homcy C: Systemic manifestations of hepatoma. Medicine (Baltimore) 51:381–391, 1972.

108. Primack A, Wilson J, O'Connor GT, Engelman K, Hull E, Canellos GP: Hepatocellular carcinoma with the carcinoid syndrome. Cancer 27:1182–1189, 1971.

109. Thompson RPH, Nicholson DC, Farnan T, Whitmore DN, Williams R: Cutaneous porphyria due to a malignant primary hepatoma. Gastroenterology 59:779–783, 1970.

110. Santer MA Jr, Waldmann TA, Fallon HJ: Erythrocytosis and hyperlipemia as manifestations of hepatic carcinoma. Arch Intern Med 120:735–739, 1967.

111. Teng CT, Daeschner CW Jr, Singleton EB, Rosenberg HS, Cole VW, Hill LL, Brennan JC: Liver diseases and osteoporosis in children. I. Clinical observations. J Pediatr 59:684–702, 1961.

112. Gralnick HR, Givelber H, Abrams E: Dysfibrinogenemia associated with hepatoma: increased carbohydrate content of the fibrinogen molecule. N Engl J Med 299:221–226, 1978.

113. Fenoglio C, Ferenczy A, Isobe T, Osserman EF: Hepatoma associated with marked plasmacytosis and polyclonal hypergammaglobulinemia. Am J Med 55:111–115, 1973.

114. Kane SP, Murray-Lyon IM, Paradinas FJ, Johnson PJ, Williams R, Orr AH, Kohn J: Vitamin B_{12} binding protein as a tumour marker for hepatocellular carcinoma. Gut 19:1105–1109, 1978.

115. Nelson RB: Thyroxine-binding globulin in hepatoma (letter to the editor). Arch Intern Med 139:1063, 1979.

116. Balsam A, Bernstein G, Goldman J, Sachs BA, Rifkin H: Ectopic adrenocorticotropin syndrome associated with carcinoma of the colon. Gastroenterology 62:636–641, 1972.

117. Benrey J, Graham DY, Goyal RK: Hypercalcemia and carcinoma of the esophagus (letter to the editor). Ann Intern Med 80:415–416, 1974.

118. Lafferty FW: Pseudohyperparathyroidism. Medicine (Baltimore) 45:247–260, 1966.

119. Lipsett MB, Odell WD, Rosenberg LE, Waldmann TA: Humoral syndromes associated with nonendocrine tumors. Ann Intern Med 61:733–756, 1964.

120. Liddle GW, Ball JH: Manifestations of cancer mediated by ectopic hormones. In: Cancer medicine, Holland JF, Frei E III (eds). Philadelphia: Lea & Febiger, 1973, pp 1046–1057.

121. Baumann G, Lopez-Amor E, Dingman JF: Plasma arginine vasopressin in the syndrome of inappropriate antidiuretic hormone secretion. Am J Med 52:19–24, 1972.

122. Marks LJ, Berde B, Klein LA, Roth J, Goonan SR, Blumen D, Nabseth DC: Inappropriate vasopressin secretion and carcinoma of the pancreas. Am J Med 45:967–974, 1968.

123. Braunstein GD, Vaitukaitis JL, Carbone PP, Ross GT: Ectopic production of human chorionic gonadotrophin by neoplasms. Ann Intern Med 78:39–45, 1973.

124. McArthur JW, Toll GD, Russfield AB, Reiss AM, Quinby WC, Baker WH: Sexual precocity attributable to ectopic gonadotropin secretion by hepatoblastoma. Am J Med 54:390–403, 1973.

125. Kew MC, Kirschner MA, Abrahams GE, Katz M: Mechanism of feminization in primary liver cancer. N Engl J Med 296:1084–1088, 1977.

126. Rowland LP, Schneck SA: Neuromuscular disorders associated with malignant neoplastic disease. J Chronic Dis 16:777–795, 1963.

127. Richardson EP Jr: Neurologic effects of cancer. In: Cancer medicine, Holland JF, Frei E III

(eds). Philadelphia: Lea & Febiger, 1973, pp 1057–1067.

128. Croft PB, Wilkinson M: The incidence of carcinomatous neuromyopathy in patients with various types of carcinoma. Brain 88:427–434, 1965.

129. Mackenzie AH, Scherbel AI: Connective tissue syndromes associated with carcinoma. Geriatrics 18:745–753, 1963.

130. Costanza ME, Pinn V, Schwartz RS, Nathanson L: Carcinoembryonic antigen–antibody complexes in a patient with colonic carcinoma and nephrotic syndrome. N Engl J Med 289:520–522, 1973.

131. Couser WG, Wagonfeld JB, Spargo JB, Lewis EJ: Glomerular deposition of tumor antigen in membranous nephropathy associated with colonic carcinoma. Am J Med 57:962–970, 1974.

132. Cantrell EG: Nephrotic syndrome cured by removal of gastric carcinoma. Br Med J 2:739–740, 1969.

133. Myerson RM, Pastor BH: The Fanconi syndrome and its clinical variants. Am J Med Sci 228:378–387, 1954.

134. Hobbs JR, Evans DJ, Wrong OM: Renal tubular obstruction by mucoproteins from adeno-carcinoma of pancreas. Br Med J 2:87–89, 1974.

135. Waldmann TA, Broder S, Strober W: Protein-losing enteropathies in malignancy. Ann NY Acad Sci 230:306–317, 1974.

136. Mangla JC, Taylor E, Cristo C: Primary duodenal carcinoma with protein-losing enteropathy. Am J Gastroenterol 67:73–76, 1977.

137. Shamblin JR Jr, Huff JF, Waugh JM, Moertel CG: Villous adenocarcinoma of the colon with pronounced electrolyte disturbance. Ann Surg 156:318–326, 1962.

138. Deller DJ, Murrell TGC, Blowes R: Jejunal biopsy and malignant disease. Aust Ann Med 16:236–241, 1967.

139. Lender M: Amyloidosis associated with neoplastic diseases. S Afr Med J 48:1944–1946, 1974.

4. Epidemiology and Early Detection of Cancer of the Esophagus

PARVIZ SOROURI

1. INTRODUCTION

The esophagus functions as a conduit for passage of ingesta into the stomach, a relatively simple but vital function. Its proximity to many other essential organs, such as trachea, bronchi, aorta and other large vessels in the mediastinum, increases the possibility of carcinomatous involvement, both extrinsically and intrinsically. Surgical approach and removal is at best very difficult and is sometimes devastating. Unfortunately, the disease is usually beyond its early stages by the time the diagnosis of cancer of the esophagus is made in a symptomatic patient. Thus, any form of treatment would fall short of being curative. In recent years, a consensus of opinion has been formed that the diagnosis of early stages of cancer of the esophagus, particularly in subjects at high risk, is of utmost importance. The study of etiologic factors as well as the pattern of the disease in the geographic areas of high incidence are helpful in formulation of criteria for classification of high-risk populations as well as furnishing guidelines for early diagnosis and future preventive interventions.

2. INCIDENCE

Carcinoma of esophagus has been found more frequently in recent years, probably due partly to better diagnostic methods. The incidence varies considerably by geographical location, race and sex. Many different isolated and unrelated locations in the world have been reported to show high incidence for cancer of esophagus. The high incidence and the fatal outcome of this disease has been known for many years amongst the inhabitants of some of these high-incidence areas. For instance, the disease, its symptoms and its course, have been well known to the Turkoman tribes in the high-incidence area of Gonabad in the Caspian littoral of Iran for many generations and centuries[1]. The tribe has accepted it as a natural process of fate and thus resist any form of medical intervention.

Cancer of esophagus shows a marked variation of about 300-fold between the highest and lowest incidence rates in different countries[2]. The highest rates are reported in parts of Central Asia, in eastern and southern regions of Africa, and in Curaçao and parts of Brazil[2]. However, striking variations in the frequency of the disease have been found within relatively small areas. A belt of high incidence has been proposed. It runs from the Caspian littoral in Iran to Northern China with extremely high incidence rates reported from regions of Gonabad and Gorgan in Iran[3] and from the province of Honan in China[4]. The high rates in Turkmenia, Kazakhstan and Uzbekistan in the USSR[5] form the central portion of the belt. Many areas of high frequency are found in East and South Africa[6] especially Rhodesia[7] and parts of Transkei[8–10]. Rates are moderately elevated in France[11], particularly in the provinces of Brittany and Normandy[12], in India[7, 13], Japan, Puerto Rico[7, 14], in the black population of the U.S.[15], among the Chinese in Singapore[7, 16] and in southern Greenland[17].

In contrast to these areas of high and moderately elevated incidence, in most countries the incidence rates of esophageal cancer, age standardized to the world population, are below 10.0 per 100 000 for males and below 5.0 per 100 000 for females[7]. In the United States, the incidence for white males is about 4.7 per 100 000 and 1.6 per 100 000 for females and has remained stable for the past 40 years. However, the incidence in the black population in the U.S. has risen since 1940 and is now at 16.7 per 100 000 for black men and 4.8 per 100 000 for black women. Rates for Americans of Chinese and Japanese descent are somewhere in between and have not increased in recent years[18].

In India in the Greater Bombay study, the rate was reported to be 14.4 for males and 11.0 for females per 100 000[19]. In Northern Karnataka, cancer of esophagus constituted 14.1% of all malignancies seen and occurred in a slightly younger age population[20]. It is of interest to note that the moderately-high incidence of cancer of esophagus in the Indians persists even when they have immigrated to other countries. Of the 21 cases of the cancer of esophagus reported from Beersheba, Israel 43% occurred in Indian Jews who had immigrated to Israel about 1960. The incidence otherwise for the general population in Israel is 2.8 for males and 1.8 for females per 100 000[21].

A high incidence of cancer of esophagus had been reported in West Kenya in the past[22, 23]. Recently, a high incidence has also been reported from Central Kenya as compared to the low incidence in the Rift Valley and North Kenya[24].

In Saudi Arabia, cancer of esophagus comprises 5.9% of all cancers

Table 1. List of geographic locations with high incidence of cancer of the esophagus.

Location	Male per 100,000	Female per 100,000
Iran, Caspian littoral		
Gonabad region	93.1	110.0
Gorgan region	66.7	49.2
Gilan region	20.1	6.2
China, Linksien area	85.0	55.0
South Africa		
Transkei	70.4	33.3
Rhodesia		
Bulawayo	63.8	2.2
USSR		
Turkmenia	51.1	33.2
Kazakhstan	47.8	26.3
Uzbekistan	28.5	13.7
France		
Ille-et-Vilaine	29.4	1.2
Switzerland	20.0	4.0
Singapore		
Chinese	20.1	6.4
Cote D'Or		
Bourgogne	18.1	1.3
Greenland		
Greenlander	16.2	6.7
India		
Bombay	15.2	10.8
Puerto Rico	14.8	5.4
U.S. Blacks	13.9	3.3
Japan		
Miyagi	12.9	6.7

recorded there, the fifth most frequent cancer [25].

The incidence of cancer of esophagus in the Cote D'Or district of Bourgogne was found to be elevated at 18.1 for men and 1.3 for women per 100 000 [26]. The incidence rates are tabulated in Table 1.

3. SEX

Cancer of esophagus for world standard population is calculated to be 5.0 per 100 000 for males and 0.7 per 100 000 for females. The European standard records a rate of 7.1 per 100 000 for males and 1.0 per 100 000 for females. The risk of females developing esophageal cancer is very low, the average sex ratio being 5:1 (male:female). Reports from Poland, U.K., Denmark, Sweden, German Democratic Republic, Norway and the Federal Republic of Germany show that the incidence rate and sex ratio is about same [27]. Only in Brittany and Normandy in France is a very high incidence of 29.4 per 100 000 for males and 1.2 per 100 000 for females recorded, a ratio of 25:1 (male:female). In Finland, the incidence for males is 6.8 per 100 000 and for females 4.9 per 100 000, the ratio being 1.4:1 (male:female). In the Gonabad region of the Caspian littoral of Iran, the high incidence of 93.1 per 100 000 for males and 110.0 per 100 000 for females gives a sex ratio of 0.6:1 (male:female). However, in the Gorgan region, which is less than 200 km away from Gonabad, the incidence is 66.7 per 100 000 in males and 49.2 per 100 000 for females, the sex ratio being 1.4:1 (male:female). The same type of ratio is reported from the Transkei of South Africa.

Thus, it is generally accepted that carcinoma of the esophagus is more common in men with few geographic exceptions. A survey of 14 500 cases reported by various authors showed 72.25% in men and 27.75% in women [28]. In few areas such as the Gonabad region of the Caspian littoral in Iran [3], in Finland [29] and Indian Jews in Beersheba, Israel [21], the sex ratio is reversed and slightly more than one half are seen in females.

4. AGE

The majority of cases are found in the sixth and seventh decades. In most reported series, the average age is approximately 62 years. Cancer of esophagus generally occurs at a younger age in women [28]. In certain regions, particularly in the Caspian littoral in Iran, in India, in Transkei and Kenya, cancer of esophagus is found at approximately 5 to 15 years younger than the expected age of 62 years [3, 7–9, 13, 22–24].

5. RACE

It has been evident for many years from vital statistical reports in the U.S. that the incidence of cancer of esophagus per 100 000 population is highest in black males and less so in black females. No valid reason for this high incidence in the black population of the U.S. has been formulated. Some observers have implicated possible lower socioeconomic factors rather than racial factors [15].

In the high-incidence areas of the Caspian littoral in Iran, the people are of Turkic or Mongol origin. Ancient writings suggest that esophageal cancer has long been known in this part of he world. People of the same ethnic origin are also amongst the population of high-incidence areas in the USSR and

China. A genetic predisposition to esophageal cancer may be present in the Turkoman race. Study on the HLA profiles of the Turkomans has been initiated but results are not yet known [2].

6. ETIOLOGY

The cause of cancer of the esophagus is unknown. Attempts have been made to incriminate agents such as alcohol, hot food and liquids, smoking, and diseases such as syphilis, scleroderma, achalasia and oral sepsis, but no acceptable evidence for any single cause has been recorded. Epidemiological data amongst the high-incidence areas has been accumulating. In central Asia, the epidemiology of cancer of the esophagus is most fully documented in the Southern Caspian littoral in Iran which has the highest incidence of cancer of the esophagus localized in a small area. Joint Iran-International Agency for Research on Cancer Study Group has provided new and stimulating information about this area.

The study Group stratified the area into 15 regions and accumulated large quantities of information about the structure of the population and local agriculture, climate, vegetation, and geology. The people are of Turkic or Mongol origin. They lead a life dedicated to agriculture, either as semi-nomadic pastoralists or as settled-subsistence farmers. The crops are mainly wheat, barley and cotton. Sheep and goats are the principal livestock. Their mode of life has changed very little over many centuries.

Some important findings have been established. Alcohol and tobacco, two major factors in the etiology of cancer of the esophagus in many other regions, can be excluded in the Caspian cases. There is no evidence of use of local plants or herbs in the high-incidence areas, nor of unusual method of preserving or cooking. Clear regional variations in diet were, however, identified, with bread and tea emerging as the main staples in the high-incidence areas. It was also found that the people living in these regions had low calorie and total protein intake, and low intake of vitamin A, riboflavin and vitamin C. More hot tea is consumed in the high-incidence areas.

Measurements of morphine metabolites in urine indicated that addiction was widespread in the high-incidence areas, occurring in about 50% of the men and women aged 35 or more, despite poor verbal cooperation on interviews. Morphine is not only smoked in the form of opium in these areas, but also eaten as opium or in the form of a tarry residue scraped out of opium pipes called 'shireh.' Tests for known carcinogens in bread and tea such as aflatoxin, polycyclic aromatic hydrocarbons, and nitrosamines were all negative, but the grain is frequently contaminated in the field by fungi and foreign seeds, some of which, particularly the fungi, may elaborate carcinogenic toxins. Indeed potatoes from this high-incidence area were found to be infected with *Fusarium sulphurerum* Schlechtendal, which is capable of producing at least four different irritant trichothecenes [30].

The role of the diet is very important, not by what it contains but by what it lacks. The effects of chronic inadequate nutrition may both impair the normal structure and function of the esophagus and induce general effects on, for example, immune function extending back into infancy and early childhood [2]. An endoscopic survey was undertaken in Northern Iran on 430 persons in the high-incidence area [31]. This study revealed a chronic esophagitis, involving mainly the middle and lower thirds of the esophagus in 86% of the subjects and the frequency was very high even in the younger age groups. Also an incidence of 3.7% dysplasia and 2.6% invasive cancer of the esophagus was present in the people studied.

Clinically and histologically the esophagitis in this rural population was different from that observed in the low-risk areas of Europe and the United States where esophagitis is usually associated with reflux [32–37]. The low prevalence of incompetent cardias and hiatus hernias and absence of symptoms of heartburn in Iran suggested that the esophagitis is not of reflux origin. This was further supported by the frequent finding of a normal precardial mucosa in the presence of esophagitis. The absence of ulceration, even in the most severe cases of esophagitis is also noteworthy. The histological changes of the chronic esophagitis in this study is similar to the early changes seen before frank dysplasia and early cancer development in rats treated with N-M-N-nitrosaniline [38].

Little is known about precursor lesions of esophageal cancer in man. The changes in the mucosa surrounding the cancer are assumed to be of a precancerous nature [4, 39], but there is no information on the lesions preceding this dysplasia.

In follow-up studies in a high-risk population in China, 27% of obvious dysplasia progressed to cancer [42]. In another high-risk population in Central Asia, submucosal fibrosis has been incriminated as a precancerous condition [43].

A similar screening study was performed in the People's Republic of China on large numbers of persons in Linksien (Lin County, Honan Province) and nearby regions where mortality from esophageal cancer is reported to be approximately 100 per 100 000 per year [44]. In the Linksien area, 62 045 people over 30 years of age were examined by an exfoliative cytological technique between 1971 and 1975. The technique consisted of swallowing a gauze-covered balloon which was then inflated and withdrawn, carrying with it cells from the esophageal wall. Dysplasia was found in 2.2% and invasive or *in-situ* carcinoma in 1.2% of the cases examined. They reported that the technique used had very low false negative results. Among a series of 11 011 persons with normal cytology, only 13 were known to have developed cancer shortly afterwards. Preliminary study of patients with esophageal dysplasia who were followed up to 12 years revealed a high risk for esophageal cancer.

A vesiculo-papular oropharyngeal lesion called *Amaqhakuva* was reported in ten of 82 patiens with cancer of the esophagus in the Xhosa patients of the Transkei region [10]. In one of these patients, this lesion had preceded squamous cell carcinoma of the upper third of the esophagus by six months. Again, nutritional deficiencies leading to possible infection have been proposed as the cause of these lesions.

Plummer-Vinson syndrome (Paterson-Kelly, Sideropenic anemia with postcricoid dysphagia and the formation of webs or strictures in the upper part of the esophagus) has been considered a precancerous condition of esophageal cancer, which is otherwise rare at this site [45, 46]. The pathogenesis of this syndrome is not clear. Iron deficiency is important, but other nutritional deficiencies such as riboflavin, thiamine, pyridoxine and protein as well as genetic factors have been suggested (see Chapter 2). Pellagra was evident in 36 patients reported from the Scandinavian series of this syndrome [10]. Riboflavin has been shown to be essential for maintaining the integrity of the squamous epithelium of the esophagus [47]. Severe riboflavin deficiency in mouse and baboon caused atrophy and ulcerative lesions in the esophageal mucosa and some hyperplastic lesions were thought to be precancerous [48, 49].

Previous field studies have revealed a widespread riboflavin deficiency in Northern Iran, equally prevalent in the areas of both high and low-risk for cancer of the esophagus [50, 51]. The oral lesions associated with riboflavin deficiency regressed after 3–4 weeks of administration of riboflavin [50]. Endoscopic and histologic observations in the Caspian littoral suggested that a chain of events leading to cancer starts with chronic inflammation and some hyperplastic changes of the epithelium, evolving in some cases to dysplasia and finally cancer. This chronic inflammatory change has been found in patients 15 years of age indicating that the crucial injury may occur early in life [31].

Injury to the epithelium may be another factor involved. In Africa, traumatic insults include the eating of great quantities of farinaceous foods containing small particles of silica, wild spinach and stinging nettles. Kaffir beer, to which may be added various toxic substances, such as cleaning fluids, is also consumed, the overall diet being essentially deficient. In Iran, as well as in India, China and USSR and Scottish women, the drinking of hot tea may cause thermal injury on a weakened esophageal mucosa due to dietary deficiency [31]. The factor of thermal irritation has been felt to be the most constant predisposing factor by some [52].

The ratio of bread to rice in the Caspian littoral was found to have a tendency to rise with the incidence of esophageal cancer. The consumption of pulses, green vegetables and fresh fruit was lower among the high risk population as was the consumption of all types of animal protein. The diet in this area is restricted to little but home baked bread and tea[51]. The same restricted type of diet is reported from Northern Karnataka, India[20]. The diet is mostly restricted to '*Jowar Rotis*' taken with a paste of chillies and spices. The '*Rotis*' are often several days old, which may be contaminated with fungal growth or other toxins. The very hard nature of '*Rotis*' may also cause constant irritation to the esophageal mucosa. Ingestion of spiced foods is suggested as a factor in development of cancer of the esophagus in Saudi Arabia[25].

Various nitrosamine compounds have been found to be potent esophageal carcinogens in rodent models[59–65]. It has been demonstrated that methyl-alkyl-nitrosamines will specifically induce carcinomas of the esophagus regardless of their route of administration[53]. One of the more potent of these compounds, N-methyl-N-benzylnitrosamine (MBZN) produced papillomas in 100% of rats. Of the total number of neoplams, 66% were papillomas, 17% were pedunculated papillary carcinomas, and 17% were sessile carcinomas. Histologically, all of the neoplasms showed squamous differentiation[54]. As in the rats, squamous cell carcinoma is by far the most frequently observed type of human esophageal cancer[55]. The neoplasms are usually well differentiated, with varying degrees of keratinization, and are deeply invasive. Patterns of growth are also very similar to those found in the rat. Most of the cancers exhibit a fungating pattern with characteristic intra-luminal proliferation or an infiltrating pattern with extensive lateral sub-epithelial penetration. Ulceration is prominant in about 25% of the carcinomas. Although the predominant form of esophageal neoplasm in the rat, a papillary form, is rare in humans, a few cases have been reported[56].

In another study, methyl-n-amylnitrosamine (MNAN) was found to be not as specific a carcinogen for the esophagus as had been thought, since tracheal and nasal cavity tumors were also induced in rats. However, esophageal tumors might predominate more strongly if enhancers specific for the esophagus were administered in addition to MNAN[57]. This observation is interesting when the clinically high incidence of cancer of the esophagus is noted among the patients with primary head and neck tumors, suggesting MNAN as a possible etiologic factor[78].

Many reports have accumulated from various regions about nitrosamines being involved as carcinogenic factors in some of the high-incidence areas. Dimethylnitrosamine has been found in the fruit juice used by the Bantu to curdle milk which is their chief food for the first 20 years of life[58]. Nitrosamines are also found in larger amounts in certain foods in Greenland,

France and Iran.

In a study in the Transkei region of South Africa, the soil was found to be molybdenum-deficient in the areas with high incidence of esophageal cancer. This deficiency was felt to be possibly linked to accumulation of nitrates and nitrosamines in the food of cancer-prone natives [66].

A possible carcinogenicity of mycotoxins for esophageal cancer has been proposed because the toxic metabolities of *Fusarium* species have been shown to induce hyperkeratotic papillomatous growths in the squamous forestomach of rats and basal cell hyperplasia of the esophageal squamous epithelium in the rat.

The coordinating group for research on the etiology of esophageal cancer in North China has reported the presence of *Geotrichum candidum* link in the food of high-risk groups and advances some experimental evidence of cocarcinogenic properties of the fungus. Interestingly, chickens of this region share a high rate of esophageal neoplasm [17]. The role of food contaminated with fungi has already been mentioned in the study of the Caspian littoral [30].

The epidemic of alimentary toxic aleukia (ATA) which occurred in parts of the Soviet Union were almost certainly caused by similar trichothecenes and judging from various reports there seems to be some overlap of earlier ATA areas and current high esophageal cancer areas.

In Africa, there is a clear association between corn cultivation and occurrence of esophageal cancer [71]. Although this may largely be due to nutritional implications, the extreme frequency of *Fusarium* contamination of this crop in Africa [7] and elsewhere including the U.S. [8] raises the possibility of at least a carcinogenic effect of some irritant *Fusarium* metabolites which are known to cause lesions in the rat esophagus.

The highest known esophageal cancer rate in Africa occurs in southwestern districts of the Republic of Transkei whereas the incidence in the northeastern region of the country is relatively low [30]. Corn is the main dietary staple in the low as well as high-incidence areas. Earlier observations indicate that the extent of moldy corn consumption is not only a matter of expediency depending on the success of the crop, but that moldy ears are actually preferred by many Transkeians for beer making because of the allegedly improved flavor.

In one study, the data obtained are suggestive that higher levels of mycotoxins, deoxytrivalenol and zearalenone contamination occur in moldy kernels produced in a high- as compared to a low-incidence area of esophageal cancer in Transkei [30].

Many studies have shown that cigarette smoking increases the risk of carcinoma of the esophagus [9, 67–69]. In one report, multiple sections of the esophagus from 1202 autopsy specimens from men whose smoking history was known were examined. Atypical basal epithelial cells were found far more frequently in cigarette smokers, with a direct relationship between the amount of smoking and the frequency of atypical cells [70].

Several epidemiologic studies have found a correlation between carcinoma of the esophagus and alcohol consumption [11, 69, 71–74]. Alcohol may also promote the effect of tobacco. In a study in Ille-et-Vilaine in France, it was shown that the logarithmic risk of esophageal cancer in man was a linear function of the daily consumption of alcohol and tobacco, separately and also the effect was synergistic when taken together [69]. The consumption of any type of alcoholic beverages entails an increased risk of esophageal cancer. In addition, it has been found that the risk is greater for cider and digestives, particularly the distillate of apple cider. The additional risk is greater for strong beverages (digestives) than for lighter ones in France [73].

The mechanism of possible carcinogenicity of methanol is unknown. It may be possible that alcoholic beverages carry active carcinogens such as polycyclic hydrocarbons, nitrosamines, fusel oils and other still unknown substances.

Various additives to alcoholic beverages are reported from Jamaica, Puerto Rico, South of U.S., Transkei in Africa, India, Japan and Greenland and postulated as possible carcinogenic factors.

Various types of obstructive lesions have been associated with carcinoma of the esophagus. Lye strictures have been found to develop into cancer in 3.5–5.5% of patients, frequently at an unusually early age [76, 77]. In one study, the mean interval between lye ingestion and development of carcinoma was 43.5 years [78].

The incidence of carcinoma in achalasia has been variously reported from a fraction above 0 to 29% [78–100]. The true incidence is estimated to be approximately 3%. Malignant tumors arise at all levels, but the most common location has been found to be the middle third of the esophagus. Here, again, the average age at onset is earlier [48] as compared to spontaneously occurring tumors (average 62 years). The mean interval between diagnosis of achalasia and carcinoma has been reported to be approximately 18–28 years [78, 79]. Some authors believe chronic irritation plays an important role in its etiology. Early surgical treatment of achalasia to prevent esophageal dilatation has been advocated to help prevent subsequent development of carcinoma [80–86]. Carcinoma occurring after a clinically successful Heller procedure for achalasia has been reported [78]. If achalasia is treated without surgical repair, yearly esophagoscopy, esophagogram and cytologic examinations are recommended. In fact, in long-standing achalasia, biannual cytologic examination of washings has been suggested [79]. Almost 90% of cancer of the esophagus occurring in lye stricture and achalasia is squamous cell carcinoma.

Several retrospective studies and case reports have shown that there is an increased frequency of esophageal adenocarcinoma in patients with Barrett's epithelium [83-89]. The columnar cell-lined esophagus, called Barrett's epithelium, is a metaplasia of the distal esophagus which is associated with chronic reflux esophagitis. In a large study, 12 cases of adenocarcinoma was found among 140 patients with columnar lined esophagus [87]. Another retrospective review revealed that the tumor arose in Barrett's epithelium in 12 of 14 cases of primary esophageal adenocarcinoma [89]. Abnormal patterns of epithelial renewal have been associated with frank neoplasia or preneoplastic lesions elsewhere in the gastrointestinal tract [90-96] (see Chapter 1).

In a recent study, it was found that all three types of Barrett's epithelium (specialized columnar, junctional and fundic), when not associated with evidence for neoplasia, in general have proliferation kinetics which are typical of normal epithelia elsewhere in the gastrointestinal tract. However, a minority of patients who have Barrett's epithelium may have altered proliferation kinetics, such as expansion of the proliferative zone. Whether identification of an expanded proliferative zone will predict those individuals who are more likely to develop cancer is a subject which requires further investigation [97].

Although antireflux operations may prevent extension of the columnar epithelium within the esophagus, the columnar epithelium may persist for many years and retain its malignant potential [87]. Regression of Barrett esophagus or reversion to squamous lining after an antireflux procedure has been reported [98]. The reported incidence of carcinoma associated with Barrett esophagus varies from 8.5% to 26.3% [87, 98].

The most common roentgenographic findings in Barrett esophagus are hiatal hernia (85%), stricture (82%), mucosal abnormality (74%), reflux (62%) and ulcerations (54%) [99]. It has been suggested that this constellation of radiologic findings, particularly ulceration, may suggest a Barrett esophagus and thus identify the patient with an increased risk of esophageal cancer. One case is reported in whom adenocarcinoma from Barrett's epithelium simulated esophageal varices radiologically [111]. In another report, 4% of patients treated with dilatation for treatment of peptic esophageal stricture developed adenocarcinoma at the site of the stricture, raising the possibility that chronic irritation may have predisposed them to neoplastic change in addition to Barrett epithelium factor [100].

A relationship between diaphragmatic hiatal hernia and gastroesophageal carcinoma has also been suggested, particularly wih those hernias associated with a short esophagus [102-104]. In a study of 34 000 hiatal hernias, only in 0.2% were carcinomas detected [105]. Hiatus hernia seems to be more prevalent in Western Europe and the U.S. One report stated that 47% of patients with hiatus hernia were found to have erosive esophagitis [107]. In another survey, 25.7% of symptomatic patients with hiatus hernia were found to have erosive esophagitis [106].

Esophageal reflux is known to be a cause of esophagitis, stricture and ulceration. Histologically, basal cell hyperplasia as well as extension of the papillae close to the epithelial surface have been shown to have a good correlation with symptoms and with reflux studies [37].

Other studies have indicated that distal to an esophageal ulcer or stricture secondary to reflux, columnar epithelium may be found [108–110]. In another study of 1 225 patients with chronic reflux esophagitis, 140 patients were found to have columnar metaplasia of the distal esophagus. Adenocarcinoma of the distal esophagus developed in 8.5% of the 140 patients with metaplasia [87].

Carcinoma has been reported to occur in 0.31% of pharyngoesophageal diverticula [112].

Esophageal carcinoma is a common complication in sideropenic dysphagia (Plummer-Vinson syndrome) [107]. However, a more recent report has shown a marked decrease in esophageal carcinoma in younger women in Sweden [114].

Irradiation has been proposed as an etiologic factor in development of cancer of the esophagus in several patients [109]. Interestingly, a granular cell myeloblastoma of the esophagus is reported in a patient developing after irradiation for treatment of carcinoma of the esophagus [121].

Only six cases of carcinoma of the esophagus associated with scleroderma have been recorded so far [116–120].

Leukoplakia of the esophagus has been found in some reports to be a common pathologic condition, frequently associated with carcinoma, and possibly precancerous [122].

The esophageal mucosal changes in pellagra in man have been reported to consist of intense hyperemia, edema and multiple small ulcerations endoscopically responding promptly to therapy [123, 124]. Fourteen patients in a series of 700 cases of carcinoma of the esophagus gave a history of pellagra [28].

Carcinoma of the esophagus has been shown to exist in about 1.2% in the population of head and neck cancer patients, approximately ten times the incidence in a normal population [78]. In another study, the risk of developing a new primary carcinoma of the esophagus in patients with head and neck cancer, equaled the risk of metastatic disease from the initial head-neck tumor [125].

The association of head-neck carcinoma with esophageal carcinoma may be due in part to predisposing factors, such as heavy smoking and heavy alcohol consumption [126, 127], perhaps due to contaminating carcinogenic agents within the alcohol and tobacco [55].

7. HEREDITY

The role of influence of hereditary factors in carcinoma of the esophagus needs further investigation (see Chapter 2). In one study, it was found that 22.1% of 172 patients with carcinoma of the esophagus had a family history of carcinoma of the esophagus[128]. In keratosis palmaris et plantaris (tylosis), which is inherited as an autosomal dominant a high incidence of cancer of the esophagus is reported. In a study of 48 members of two families with tylosis, 18 developed cancer of the esophagus; an incidence rate of 37.5% [129]. Other reports later have described this association[130–132].

The hereditary factors in the Turkoman races in Northern Iran, USSR and China needs further evaluation. HLA studies are in progress in Northern Iran.

8. EARLY DETECTION

Two cases of microscopic carcinoma of the esophagus were diagnosed on endoscopic evaluation of the patients for hiatus hernia and reflux esophagitis. Carcinoma was not suspected at the time of endoscopy[132]. Few other cases of early carcinoma of the esophagus have been reported [86, 134, 135, 137–141, 143]. A large group of 28 cases of superficial squamous cell carcinomas diagnosed in early stages comes from Japan[135]. By far, the largest group reported is from China. Chinese report that use of a net-covered balloon for cytologic screening has lead to detection of early esophageal lesions and precancerous dysplasia. They detected 136 asymptomatic cases of esophageal cancer among 11 564 persons, and 70% of these patients were in an early stage. They claim that the overall resection rate has increased to 80%, and the overall five-year survival rate to 29%. However, in patients with early detection followed by early surgery, the five-year survival rate increases to about 90% in their series[42, 133, 142]. In the Mayo Clinic series of 1 657 patients, the five-year survival after resection for 31 middle esophageal lesions without nodal involvement was 41.9%. This contrasts to an overall five-year survival of 9%.

The detection of early cancer of the esophagus either fortuitously[132, 143] or through organized screening[42, 133, 135, 142], has resulted in early surgery with very encouraging five-year survival rates in recent years. An analogy may be drawn with carcinoma of the stomach in Japan where mass screening, early detection and treatment has given a 90%, five-year survival rate[144]. Possibly, similar efforts devoted to esophageal cancer may bring about a parallel success and break the traditional gloomy prognosis of this disease.

Any person with persistent progressive dysphagia must be evaluated thoroughly for the presence of cancer of the esophagus. However, dysphagia is also a common symptom for many of the associated conditions such as achalasia, lye stricture, Plummer-Vinson syndrome, Barrett esophagus, head and neck cancer, or stricture after surgery for head and neck cancer.

Usually by the time that the cancer of the esophagus produces dysphagia, the cancer is beyond its early stages. Thus, in order to detect early cancer of the esophagus, other criteria than clinical manifestations must be sought. The most important of these criteria would be cytological diagnostic measures. The high-risk group for cancer of the esophagus should be recognized and possibly followed by routine annual or biannual cytological diagnostic evaluation, regardless of lack of specific symptoms.

The high-risk groups are tabulated in Table 2.

Barium swallow should be used routinely in these high-risk patients to diagnose early and possibly resectable carcinomas. Double contrast roentgeno-

Table 2. High-risk group for development of cancer of the esophagus.

1. Long-standing malnutrition, particularly deficiency of vitamins A and C, riboflavin, proteins:
    1.1. – In certain geographic areas, such as Caspian littoral in Iran, Kenya, India, China, USSR
    1.2 – Untreated malabsorption of long-standing duration, particularly celiac sprue disease
    1.3 – Plummer-Vinson syndrome
2. Hereditary factors:
    2.1 – Turkoman or Mongol race in Iran, USSR and China
    2.2 – Black male population in U.S.
    2.3 – Tylosis
    2.4 – Celiac sprue
3. Achalasia
4. Benign stricture
    4.1 – Lye stricture
    4.2 – Stricture from peptic esophagitis
    4.3 – Post-surgical strictures
5. Barrett's esophagus
6. Hiatal hernia
7. Pulsion diverticulae
8. Carcinomas of other organs
    (most commonly head, neck and lung)
9. Heavy alcohol consumption
10. Heavy smoking
11. Long-standing history of intake of hot beverages and spiced foods
12. Reflux esophagitis:
    12.1 – Barrett's esophagus
    12.2 – Hiatal hernia
    12.3 – Post-gastric surgery

graphy of the esophagus seems to be the best method for detecting small lesions [78, 145].

Radioactive phosphorus for diagnosis [151], despite report of overall accuracy of 95% [152, 153], has not gained general application. It would also not be applicable for repeated annual screening.

Computerized tomography may be of benefit in demonstrating the extent of invasion outside the esophagus. No reports have been presented so far in regard to its application in early detection of cancer of the esophagus.

Cytological diagnosis by using washings, abrasive balloons, small sponges and different types of brushes introduced either blindly or under fluoroscopic control has been replaced by flexible endoscopy with sampling of the esophageal mucosa by direct brushing, washing or multiple biopsies in recent years. Endoscopic brushing of the esophagus has yielded the highest positive result ranging from 81.8 to 96.2% [146–150].

The following plan of screening is recommended for detection of early cancer of the esophagus developing in the high-risk population.
1. Endoscopic brush-washing cytology and multiple biopsies every 6 months.
2. Double contrast esophagogram yearly.
3. Both double contrast esophagogram and endoscopic brush cytology and biopsy at any time when dysphagia or changes in symptom complex occurs.

9. PREVENTION

Most of the factors cited as playing an etiologic role in cancer of the esophagus, such as nitrosamines, alcohol, cigarettes, and deficient nutrition have had their effects over a long period of time. Thus, correction of these factors may not decrease the risk in the present generation, but it may reduce the risk in the future generations. However, early detection of reflux esophagitis and its correction may decrease the risk of development of the cancer of the esophagus in each individual patient.

REFERENCES

1. Dowlatshahi K, Daneshbod A, Mobarhan S: Early detection of cancer of esophagus along Caspian littoral. Lancet 1:125–126, 1978.
2. Anonymous: Esophageal cancer on the Caspian littoral. Lancet 1:641–642, 1978.
3. Mahboubi E, Kmet J, Cook PJ, Day NE, Ghadirian P, Salmasizadeh S, Esophageal cancer studies in the Caspian littoral of Iran. The Caspian Cancer Registry. Br J Cancer 28:197–208, 1973.

4. Coordinating group for research on etiology of esophageal cancer in North China: The epidemiology and etiology of esophageal cancer in North China. A preliminary report. Chin Med J 1:167–183, 1975.

5. Tuyns AJ: Cancer morbidity and mortality data in USSR. In: Medicina, Moscow (1970. International technical report 70/003 Serenko ÁF, Romenski AA (eds). Lyon: International Agency for Research on Cancer, 1970.

6. Cook PJ, Burkitt DP: Cancer in Africa. Br Med Bull 27:14–20, 1971.

7. Waterhouse J, Muir C, Correa P, Powell J (eds): Cancer incidence in five continents, 1st edn. Vol 3, pp 492–495. Lyon: International Agency for Research on Cancer, 1976.

8. Rose ER: Esophageal cancer in the Transkei, 1955–1969. J Natl Cancer Inst 51:7–16, 1973.

9. Warwick CP, Harrington JS: Some aspects of the epidemiology and etiology of esophageal cancer with particular emphasis on the Transkei, South Africa. Adv Cancer Res 17:81–229, 1973.

10. Mannell A, Plant M: The first symptoms of carcinoma of the esophagus, with particular reference to Amaghakuva. A report from the Republic of Transkei. S Afr Med J 55:803–6, 1979.

11. Audigier JC, Tuyns AJ, Lambert R: Epidemiology of esophageal cancer in France. Digestion 13:209–219, 1975.

12. Tuyns AF, Masse G: Cancer of the esophagus in Brittany: an incidence study in Ille-et-Vilaine. Int J Epidemiol 4:55–59, 1975.

13. Gangadharan P: Epidemiology of cancer of the esophagus in India. Ind J Surg 36:293–298, 1974.

14. Martinez I: Factors associated with cancer of the esophagus, mouth and pharynx in Puerto Rico. J Natl Cancer Inst 42:1069–1094, 1969.

15. Third National Cancer Survey: Incidence data. National Cancer Institute Monograph 41, Bethesda, 1975.

16. deJong UW, Breslow N, Goh Ewe Hong J, Sridharan M, Shanmugaratnam K: Etiological factors in esophageal cancer in Singapore Chinese. Int J Cancer 13:291–303, 1974.

17. Nielsen NH, Mikkelsen F, Hansen JPH: Esophageal Cancer in Greenland; selected epidemiological and clinical aspects. J Cancer Res Clin Oncol 94:69–80, 1979.

18. Cutler SF, Young JLJr: Third National Cancer Survey: Incidence Data. National Cancer Institute Monograph 41, 1975.

19. Paymaster JC, Sanghivi LD, Gandharan P: Cancer in the gastrointestinal tract in western India. Cancer 21:279–288, 1968.

20. Deka BC, Deka AC, Patil RB, Joshi SG: Carcinoma of the esophagus in northern Karnataka; an observation on 161 cases. Indian J Cancer 15:23–27, 1978.

21. Odes HS, Krawiec J: Carcinoma of the esophagus in Indian Jews in Beersheba, Israel. Front Gastroint Res 4:96–100. Basel: Karger, 1979.

22. Ahmed N: Geographical Incidence of Esophageal Cancer in West Kenya. E African Med J 43:235–240, 1966.

23. Ahmed N, Cook P: The incidence of cancer of the esophagus in West Kenya. Brit J Cancer 23:302–312, 1969.

24. Gatei DG, Odhiambo PA, Orinda DAO, Muruka FJ, Wassuna A: Retrospective study of carcinoma of the esophagus in Kenya. Cancer Research 38:303–307, 1978.

25. Stirling G, Khalil AM, Nada GM, Saad AA, Raheem MA: Malignant neoplasms in Saudi Arabia. Cancer 44:1543–1548, 1979.

26. Legoux JL, Faivre J, Martin F, Michiels R, Cabanne F, Klepping C: Incidence of cancer of the esophagus in the Department of the Cote D'Or. Rev Fr Gastroenterol 149:41–45, 1979.

27. Kayser K, Burkhardt Hu: The incidence of gastro-intestinal cancer in North Baden (West Germany) 1971-1977. J Cancer Res Clin Oncol 93:301-321, 1979.
28. Postlethwait RW, Sealy WC: Surgery of the esophagus. New York: Appleton-Century-Croft, 1979.
29. Kirivanta UK: Carcinoma of the esophagus, its incidence, age and sex distribution, and prognosis in Finland. Acta Octolaryngol 42:73-80, 1952.
30. Marasas WFO, van Rensburg SJ, Mirocha CJ: Incidence of Fusarium species and the mycotoxins, deoxynivalenol and zearalenone in corn produced in esophageal cancer areas in Transkei. J Agric Food Chem 27:1108-1112, 1979.
31. Crespi M, Grassi A, Amiri G, Munoz N, Aramesh B, Mojtabai A: Esophageal lesions in northern Iran: a premalignant condition? Lancet 2:217-221, 1979.
32. Savary M, Guignand G: Adenocarcinogenesis of the lower esophagus. Acta Endoscop Radiocin 7:217-230, 1977.
33. Rasmussen CW: A new endoscopic classification of chronic esophagitis. Am J Gastroenterol 65:409-415, 1976.
34. Clemençon G: Inflammatory stenosis of the esophagus following non-gastric surgery. Acta Endoscop Radiocin 7:323-328, 1977.
35. Kobayashi S, Kasugai T: Endoscopical biopsy criteria for the diagnosis of esophagitis with a fiberoptic esophagoscope. Digest Dis 19:345-352, 1974.
36. Hattori K, Winans CS, Archer F, Kirsner JB: Endoscopic diagnosis of esophageal inflammation. Gastroint Endosc 20:102-104, 1974.
37. Ismail-Beigi F, Horton P, Pope CE: Histological consequences of gastroesophageal reflux in man. Gastroenterology 58:163-174, 1970).
38. Napoleon NW, Pozharisk K: Morphogenesis of experimental tumors of the esophagus. J Nat Cancer Inst 42:922-940, 1969.
39. Postlethwait RW, Wendell Musser A: Changes in the esophagus in 1000 autopsy specimens. J Thorac Cardiovasc Surg 68:953-956, 1974.
40. Mukada T, Sato E, Sasono N: Comparative studies on dysplasia of esophageal epithelium in four prefectures of Japan (Miyagi, Nara, Wakayama and Amori) with reference to risk of carcinoma. Tohoku J Exp Med 119:51-63, 1976.
41. Mandard AM, Chasle J, Marnay J: Cancer of the esophagus and dysplasia (preliminary results). Eur J Cancer (Suppl): 15-26, 1978.
42. Coordinating Group for the Research of Esophageal Carcinoma, Chinese Academy of Medical Sciences and Honan Province. Studies on the relationship between epithelial dysplasia and carcinoma of the esophagus. Chin Med J 11:674-690, 1974.
43. Kolysheva VJ: Data on the epidemiology and morphology of precancerous changes and of cancér of the esophagus in Kazakhstan, USSR. Thesis, Alma Ata, 1974.
44. Li FP, Shiang El: Screening for esophageal cancer in 62,000 Chinese. Lancet 2:804, 1979.
45. Larsson LG, Sandstrom A, Westling P: Relationship of Plummer-Vinson to cancer of the upper alimentary tract in Sweden. Cancer Res 35:3308-16, 1975.
46. Entwistle CC, Jacobs A: Histological findings in the Pattersen-Kelly Syndrome. J Clin Pathol 18:403-413, 1965.
47. Foy H, Mbaya V: Riboflavin. Prof Fd Nutr Sci 3:357-394, 1977.
48. Wynder EL, Klein UE: The possible role of riboflavin deficiency in epithelial neoplasia. Cancer 18:167-180, 1965.
49. Foy H, Gilman T, Kondi A: Histological changes in the skin of baboons deprived of riboflavin. in: Medical primatology. Goldsmith EI, Moor-Janowski J (eds). Basel: Karger, 1972, pp 159-168.
50. Kmet J, McLaren DS, Siassi F: Epidemiology of esophageal cancer with special reference to

nutritional studies among the Turkoman of Iran. In: Advances in modern human nutrition (in press).

51. Joint Iran/Irac Study Group: Esophageal cancer studies in the Caspian littoral of Iran: results of population studies in a prodrome. J Nat Cancer Inst 59:1127–1138, 1977.

52. Watson WL, Goodner JT: Carcinoma of the esophagus. Amer J Surg 93:259–270, 1957.

53. Druckrey H: Organospecific carcinogenesis in the digestive tract. In: Topics in chemical carcinogenesis. Nakahara W, Takayama S, Sugimura T (eds). Baltimore: University Park Press, 1972, pp 73–103.

54. Stinson SF: Animal model: esophageal carcinoma in the rat induced with methyl-alkyl-nitrosamines. Tumor Pathology Branch, National Cancer Institute, National Institutes of Health, Bethesda, MD 20014.

55. Ming SC: Tumors of the esophagus and stomach. In: Atlas of tumor pathology, 2 series: Fascicle 7. Washington, DC: Armed forces Institute of Pathology, 1973, pp 1–8.

56. Minielly JA, Harrison EGJr, Fontana RS, Payne WS: Verrucous squamous cell carcinoma of the esophagus. Cancer 20:2078–2087, 1967.

57. Bulay O, Mirvish SS: Carcinogenesis in rat esophagus by intraperitoneal injection of different doses of methyl-n-amylnitrosamine. Cancer Research 39:3644–3646, 1979.

58. DuPlessis LS, Nunn JR, Roach WA: Carcinogen in a Transkeian Bantu Food additive. Nature 222:1198–1207, 1969.

59. Napalkov NP, Pozharisski KM: Morphogenesis of experimental tumors of the esophagus. J Natl Cancer Inst 42:927–936, 1969.

60. Nakamura T, Matsuyama M, Kishimoto H: Tumors of the esophagus and duodenum induced in mice by oral administration of n-ethyl-n'-nitro-n-nitrosoguanidine. J Natl Cancer Inst 52:519–525, 1974.

61. Deyasi SK, Aikat BK, Sehgal S: Nitrosamine-induced carcinoma of the esophagus. Ind J Pathol Bacteriol 17:180–186, 1974.

62. Baker JR, Mason MM, Yerganian G, Weisburger EK, Weisburger JH: Induction of tumors of the stomach and esophagus in inbred Chinese hamsters by oral diethylnitrosamine. Proc Soc Exp Biol Med 146:291–298, 1974.

63. Reuber MD: Carcinomas of the esophagus in rats ingesting diethylnitrosamine. Eur J Cancer 11:97–106, 1975.

64. Lijinsky W, Taylor HW: Increased carcinogenicity of 2,6-dimethylnitrosomorpholine compared with nitrosomorpholine in rats. Cancer Res 35:2123–2138, 1975.

65. Schmahl D: Investigations on esophageal carcinogenicity by methylphenyl-nitrosamine and ethyl alcohol in rats. Cancer Lett 1:215–218, 1976.

66. Esophageal cancer (leading articles). Brit Med J 2:718–728, 1966.

67. Bradshaw E, Schowland M: Smoking, drinking, and esophageal cancer in African males of Johannesburg, South Africa. Brit J Cancer 30:157–166, 1974.

68. Weir JM, Dunn JE: Smoking and mortality: a prospective study. Cancer 25:105–110, 1970.

69. Tuyns AJ, Pequignot G, Jensen DM: Role of diet, alcohol and tobacco in esophageal cancer, as illustrated by two contrasting high-incidence areas in the north of Iran and west of France. Front Gastrointest Res 4:101–110. Basel: Karger, 1979.

70. Averbach O, Stout AP, Hammond EC, Garfinkel L: Histologic changes in esophagus in relation to smoking habits. Arch Environ Health 11:4–17, 1965.

71. Cook P: Cancer of the esophagus in Africa. A summary and evaluation of the evidence for the frequency of occurrence, and a preliminary indication of the possible association with the concumption of alcoholic drinks made from maize. Br J Cancer 25:853–861, 1971.

72. Hakulinen T, Lehtimaki L, Lehtonen M, Teppo L: Cancer morbidity among two male cohorts with increased alcohol consumption in Finland. J Natl Cancer Inst 52:1711–1722,

1974.

73. Tuyns, AJ, Pequignot G, Aggatucci JS: Esophageal cancer and alcohol consumption: importance of type of beverage Int J Cancer 23:443–447, 1979.

74. Jensen OM, Tuyns AJ, Pequignot G: Usefulness of population controls in retrospective studies of alcohol consumption. J Studies Alcohol 39:175–182, 1978.

75. Tuyns AJ, Pequignot G, Hensen OM: Le cancer de l'esophage en Ille-et-Vilaine en fonction des niveaux de consommation d'alcool et de tabac. Des risques qui se multiplient. Bull Cancer 64:45–60, 1977a.

76. Benedict EB: Carcinoma of the esophagus developing in a benign stricture. New Eng J Med 224:408–411, 1941.

77. Bigger JA, Vinson PP: Carcinoma secondary to burn of the esophagus from ingestion of lye. Surgery 28:887–890, 1950.

78. Norton GA, Postlethwait RW, Thompson WM: Esophageal carcinoma: a survey of population at risk. Southern Med J 73:25–27, 1980.

79. Just-Viera JO, Haight C: Achalasia and Carcinoma of the esophagus. Surg Gynec Obstet 128:1081–1084, 1969.

80. Carter R, Brewer LA: Achalasia and esophageal carcinoma studies in early diagnosis for improved surgical management. Am J Surg 130:114–120, 1975.

81. Wychulis AR, Woodam GL, Anderson HA et al: Achalasia and carcinoma of the esophagus. JAMA 215:1638–1641, 1971.

82. Pierce WS, MacVaugh H, Johnson J: Carcinoma of the esophagus arising in patients with achalasia of the cardia. J Thorac Cardiovasc Surg 59:335–339, 1970.

83. Carrie A: Adenocarcinoma of the upper end of the esophagus arising from ectopic gastric epithelium. Brit J Surg 37:474–481, 1950.

84. Hawe A, Payne WS, Weiland LH, Fontana RS: Adenocarcinoma in the columnar epithelial lined lower (Barrett) esophagus. Thorax 28:511–514, 1973.

85. Hankins JR, Cole FN, Attar S, Frost JL, McLaughlin JS: Adenocarcinoma involving the esophagus. J Thorac Cardiovasc Surg 68:148–158, 1974.

86. Belladonna JA, Hajdu SI, Bains MS, Winawer SF: Adenocarcinoma in-situ of Barrett's esophagus diagnosed by endoscopic cytology. New Eng J Med 291:895–896, 1974.

87. Naef AP, Savary M, Ozello L: Columnar-lined lower esophagus: an acquired lesion with malignant predisposition. J Thorac Cardiovasc Surg 70:826–835, 1975.

88. McDonald GB, Brand DL, Thorning DR: Multiple adenomatous neoplasma arising in columnar-lined (Barrett's) esophagus. Gastroenterology 72:1317–1321, 1977.

89. Haggitt RC, Tryzelaar J, Ellis FH, Colcher H: Adenocarcinoma complicating columnar epithelium-lined (Barrett's) esophagus. Amer J Clin Pathol 70:15, 1978.

90. Cole JW, McKalen A: Studies on the morphogenesis of adenomatous polyps in the human colon. Cancer 16:998–1002, 1963.

91. Deschner EE, Lipkin M, Solomon G: Study of human rectal epithelial cells *in vitro*. II. H3-thymidine incorporation into polyps and adjacent mucosa. J Natl Cancer Inst 36:849–855, 1966.

92. Lieb LM, Lisco H: *In vitro* uptake of titrated thymidine by carcinoma of the human colon. Cancer Res 26:733–740, 1966.

93. Winawer S, Lipkin M: Cell Proliferation kinetics in the gastrointestinal tract of man, IV. Cell renewal in the intestinalized gastric mucosa. J Natl Cancer Inst 42:9–17, 1969.

94. Bleiberg H, Mainguet P, Galand P, Chretien J, DuPont, Mairesse N: Cell renewal in the human rectum. *In vitro* autoradiographic study on active ulcerative colitis. Gastroenterology 58:851–855, 1970.

95. Bleiberg H, Mainguet P, Galand P: Cell renewal in familial polyposis; comparison between polyps and adjacent healthy mucosa. Gastroenterology 63:240–245, 1972.

96. Eastwood GL, Trier JS: Epithelial cell renewal in cultures rectal biopsies in ulcerative colitis, Gastroenterology 64:383–390, 1973.
97. Pellish LF, Hermos JA, Eastwood GL: Cell proliferation in three types of Barrett's epithelium. Gut 21:26–31, 1980.
98. Radigan LR, Glover JL, Shipley FE et al.: Barrett esophagus. Arch Surg 112:486–491, 1977.
99. Robbins AH, Vincent ME, Saini M et al.: Revised radiologic concepts of the Barrett esophagus. Gastrointest Radiol 3:377–381, 1978.
100. Ogilvie AL, Ferguson R, Atkinson M: Outlook with conservative treatment of peptic esophageal stricture. Gut 21:23–25, 1980.
101. Kirivanta UK: Corrosion carcinoma of the esophagus; 381 cases of corrosion and 9 cases of corrosion carcinoma. Acta Otolaryngol (Stockh) 42:89–95, 1952.
102. Adler RH, Rodriquez J: The association of hiatus hernia and gastroesophageal malignancy. J Thorac Surg 3:553–559, 1959.
103. Resano H, Malenchini M, Barain JC, Barg S: Esophage court et cancer. Ann Otol (Paris) 74:150–161, 1957.
104. Tager IL: Hernia of the esophageal opening and Cardio-esophageal cancer. Acta Un Int Cancrum 19:1263–1266, 1963.
105. Michel JC, Arthur MO, Dockerty MB: The association of diaphragmatic hiatal hernia and gastroesophageal carcinoma. Surg Gynec Obstet 124:583–589, 1967.
106. Palmer ED: Therapy of hiatal hernia. In: The esophagogastric junction, Katz D, Hoffman F (eds). Amsterdam: Excerpta Medica, 1971, p 143.
107. Cronstedt J, Carling L, Vestergaard P, Berglund J: Esophageal disease revealed by endoscopy in 1000 patients referred principally for gastroscopy. Acta Med Scand 204:413–416, 1978.
108. Abrams I, Heath D: Lower esophagus lines with intestinal and gastric epithelia. Thorax 20:66–72, 1965.
109. Heitmann P, Strauszer T, Sapunar J: Lower esophagus lined with columnar epithelium: Morphological and physiological correlation. Gastroenterology 53:611–624, 1967.
110. Burgess JN, Payne WS, Andersen HA et al.: Barrett esophagus: the columnar epithelial lined lower esophagus. Mayo Clinic proc 46:728–734, 1971.
111. Nelson AM, Grayer DI: Adenocarcinoma from Barrett's epithelium simulating esophageal varices. Connecticut Med 43:553–554, 1979.
112. Wychulis AR, Gunnlugsson GH, Clagett OT: Carcinoma occurring in pharyngo-esophageal diverticulum: report of three cases. Surg 66:976–979, 1969.
113. Lindvall N: Hypolaryngeal carcinoma in sideropenic dysphagia. Acta Radiol 39:17–20, 1953.
114. Larson LG, Sanstrom A, Westling P: Relationship of Plummer-Vinson disease to cancer of the upper alimentary tract in Sweden. Cancer Res 35:3308–3316, 1975.
115. Chudecki B: Radiation cancer of the thoracic esophagus. Br J Radiol 45:303–309, 1972.
116. Johnson BB, Monroe LS: Carcinoma of the esophagus developing in progressive systemic sclerosis. Gastrointest Endosc 19:181–191, 1973.
117. Kilton L, Gottlieb JA: Scleroderma and carcinoma of the esophagus (letter to the editor). Lancet 2:707, 1971.
118. Matzner MF, Trachtman B, Medelbaum RA: Co-existent carcinoma and scleroderma of the esophagus. Am J Gastroenterol 39:31–42, 1963.
119. Wittaker JA, Bishop R: Scleroderma with carcinoma of the esophagus. Am J Gastroenterol 71: 496–500, 1979.
120. Mattingly PC, Mowat AG: Rapidly progressive scleroderma associated with carcinoma of the esophagus. Ann Rheum Dis 38:177–178, 1979.

121. Domen RE, Tang P, Harshman KV: Granular cell myeloblastoma of the esophagus after irradiation for carcinoma. Southern Med J 72:1207–1209, 1979.
122. Schaer H: Systematic examination of the occurrence of prestages of cancer in the human esophagus. Z Krebsforsch 31:217–228, 1930.
123. Fisher GE: The esophagical manifestations of pellagra. South Med J 37:446–458, 1944.
124. Fisher GE: The esophageal manifestation of pellagra. Trans Am Acad Ophthalmol Otolaryngol 48:175–188, 1944.
125. Sugarbaker EV, Jesse RH: Second primary carcinoma of the 'foregut'; high risk of head and neck patients. Cancer (in press).
126. Wynder EL, Mushinski MH, Spivak JC: Tobacco and alcohol consumption in relation to the development of multiple primary cancers. Cancer 40:1872–1878, 1977.
127. Jayant K, Balakrishnan V, Sanghvi LD et al.: Quantification of the role of smoking and chewing tobacco in oral, Pharyngeal and esophageal cancers. Br J Cancer 35:232–235, 1977.
128. Wuyk, Loucks HH: Carcinoma of the esophagus or cardia of the stomach. An Analysis of 172 cases with 81 resections. Ann Surg 134:946–952, 1961.
129. Howel-Evans W, McConnel RB, Clarke CA, Sheppard PM: Carcinoma of the esophagus with keratosis palmaris et plantaris (Tylosis). Q J Med 27:413–421, 1958.
130. Shine I, Allison PR: Carcinoma of the esophagus with tylosis (keratosis palmaris et plantaris). Lancet 1:951–960, 1966.
131. Schwindt WD, Bernhardt LC, Johnson S: Tylosis and intrathoracic neoplasms. Chest 57:590–598, 1970.
132. Ritter SB, Petersen G: Esophageal cancer, hyperkeratosis and oral leukoplakia: follow-up family study. JAMA 237:1844–1862, 1976 (letter).
133. British Medical Journal. Editorial: cancer of the esophagus. Brit Med J 21:135–136, 1976.
134. Burke EL, Strum J, Williamson D: The diagnosis of microscopic carcinoma of the esophagus. Digestive Dis 23:148–151, 1978.
135. Nabeya K: Early carcinoma of the esophagus. Stomach and Intestine (Tokyo) 5:1205–1213, 1970.
136. Gunnlaugsson GH, Wychulis AR et al.: Analysis of the records of 1657 patients with carcinoma of the esophagus and cardia of the stomach. Surg Gynec Obstet (June 1970): 997–1005, 1970.
137. Moulinier B, deOliveira C, Lambert R, Ruet D, Lesbros F, Brault A: Early carcinoma of the esophagus: report of a case. Arch Fr Mal App Dig 62:489–494, 1973.
138. Suzuki H, Kobayashi S, Endo M, Nakayama K: Diagnosis of early esophageal cancer. Surgery 71:99–103, 1972.
139. Ilzuka T, Hirata K, Mitomi T et al.: Intraepithelial carcinoma of the esophagus. JPN J Clin Oncol 12:105–112, 1973.
140. Ushigone S, Spjut HJ, Noon GP: Extensive dysplasia and carcinoma in situ of esophageal epithelium. Cancer 20:1023–1029, 1967.
141. Kakuta NH, Fujushima M, Chiba K et al.: A case of early esophageal carcinoma. Jpn J Cancer Clin 19:1190–1192, 1973.
142. Coordinating Group for Research on Esophageal Cancer. Chin Med J 2:113–121, 1976.
143. Ferlic RM: Superficial esophageal cancinoma diagnosed solely by endoscopy. Nebraska MJ (June 1978): 184–186, 1978.
144. Shida S: Early detection of cancer of stomach. Gann Monogr Cancer Research 11:207–216, 1971.
145. Laufer I: Double contrast gastrointestinal radiology with endoscopic correlation. Philadelphia: WB Saunders, 1979, pp 79–80.

146. Villardel F: Cytological diagnosis of digestive cancer. Amer J Gastroenterol 70:357–364, 1978.
147. Winawer SJ, Sherlock P, Belladonna JA, Melamed M, Beattie EJ Jr: Endoscopic brush cytology in esophageal cancer. JAMA 232:1358–1368, 1975.
148. Bemvennuti GA, Hattori K, Levin R et al.: Endoscopic sampling for tissue diagnosis in gastrointestinal malignancy. Gastroint Endosc 21:159–161, 1975.
149. Halter F, Witzel L, Gretillat PA et al.: Diagnostic value of biopsy guided lavage and brush cytology in esophagogastroscopy. Am J Dig Dis 22:129–131, 1977.
150. Prolla JC, Reilly RW, Kirsner JB et al.: Direct vision endoscopic cytology and biopsy in the diagnosis of esophageal and gastric tumors. Acta Cytol 21:339–402, 1977.
151. Nakayama K, Hirota K: Experiences of about 3000 cases with cancer of the esophagus and the cardia. Aust NZ J Surg 31:222–236, 1962.
152. Nelson RS, Dewey WC, Rose RG: The use of radioactive phosphorus P32 and a miniature Geiger tube to detect malignant neoplasia of the gastrointestinal tract. Gastroenterology 46:8–16, 1964.
153. Nelson RS, Lanza FL: Radioisotope evaluation of the esophagus. JAMA 204:216–224, 1968.

5. Epidemiology of Gastric Cancer and its Precursor Lesions

PELAYO CORREA

1. INTRODUCTION

Our understanding of the epidemiology of gastric cancer has been characterized by alternating periods of progress and stagnation, generally matching technologic developments that have facilitated its study. For many years the information available was based on mortality statistics, which called attention to the fact that there were marked intercountry contrasts in the frequency of the disease [1]. Studies of relative frequency complemented mortality statistics and indicated that interpopulation contrasts were also found within several countries [2]. Studies of migrant populations became available around the 1960 decade and revealed drastic changes in both incidence and mortality associated with migration, generating the notion of previously unsuspected dynamic changes in the epidemiology of the disease [3]. The same studies suggested that forces at play in the premigration period, most probably in the first decades of life, were responsible for the high risks observed after migration to low-risk countries.

The histopathology of gastric cancer was then correlated with demographic parameters and it was reported that one histologic type, the so-called intestinal type, predominated in high-risk populations [4]. The same histologic type was accompanied by atrophic and metaplastic changes in the surrounding gastric mucosa [5]. These nontumoral changes were found to be very prevalent in autopsy material of high-risk populations, both providing an indicator of such risk and suggesting a possible explanation for the prolonged latency period found in migrant populations [6]. Fiberoptic endoscopy became available and facilitated the study of patients with precursor lesions.

A long search for experimental models became fruitful when some N-nitroso compounds were found active, and these experiments contributed to the present interest in the role of this family of chemical compounds as human carcinogens [7]. Although it has been suspected for a long time that dietary patterns are responsible for the interpopulation variability in gastric cancer, extensive search for carcinogens in dietary items led to no clear conclusions. The discovery that carcinogens can be formed intragastrically in experimental animals by simultaneous feeding of nitrite and secondary amines has deemphasized the search for complete carcinogens in the diet and strengthened work on the hypothesis of in situ synthesis of carcinogens, especially N-nitroso compounds [8].

We will summarize separately the most relevant factors related to the epidemiology of gastric cancer and its precursor lesions.

2. GASTRIC CARCINOMA

2.1. Geographic Distribution

It has long been known that some countries have very high mortality and morbidity rates for stomach cancer. Japan has always been at the top of the list. The average annual incidence rate in Miyagi males, adjusted to the world population from 1968 to 1971, was 94.6 per 100 000 [9]. Andean populations in Latin America have generally high risks. Costa Rica and Chile have displayed high rates, although not as high as those of Japan. In 1974, the mortality rate in males from Chile was 50.8 and in Costa Rica 49.5 per 100 000 [10]. Some Nordic countries have also displayed high risks, although there has been a marked decrease in recent years. Age-adjusted incidence rates for 1968 to 1972 were 24.6 per 100 000 in Norway, 37.5 per 100 000 in Finland and 43.0 per 100 000 in Iceland. Unites States whites and Australia–New Zealand have been at the other end of the risk spectrum in most intercountry comparisons. The age-adjusted incidence rate for the state of Connecticut in 1968–1972 was 13.5 per 100 000; the comparable rate for New Zealand (non Maori) was 15.3 per 100 000 [9].

2.2. Sex Ratio

There is a predominance of male rates in all countries but the magnitude of the excess varies with age. The male:female ratio is close to unity at ages under 35, after that age it rises until it reaches a peak of about 2:1 around age 55 and, thereafter, declines to about 1.3:1 at the oldest age [11].

2.3. Time Trends

There has been a consistent decline in mortality and incidence rates of gastric cancer first noticed in the United States and later in most other countries [12]. The decline is seen in both sexes and all age groups, especially younger cohorts.

2.4. Migrant Studies

Observations in immigrants to the United States who were born in countries at high risk for stomach cancer revealed that they continued to experience the risk characteristic to the population of origin [13]. This pattern was observed for the first generation of immigrants only. Their United States-born offspring displayed rates similar to those of the adopted country. Similar observations have been made in Australia and the intracountry migratory populations of Colombia [6].

2.5. Histopathology

Observations made about 30 years ago reported that most gastric carcinomas reproduced well-formed glandular elements lined by mucus-secreting cells similar to those found in intestinal tumors. They frequently arose from

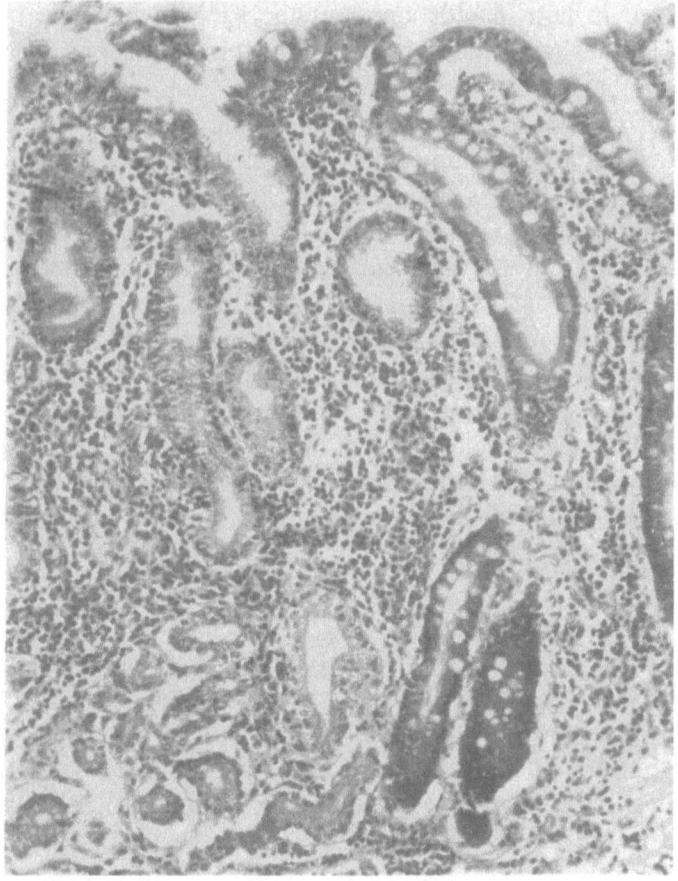

Figure 1. Gastric mucosa showing loss of glands, marked inflammatory infiltrate in the lamina propria and intestinal metaplasia. The metaplastic glands (right side) have numerous mucous goblets similar to those found in the intestine.

gastric mucosa that had previously been transformed to intestinal-like muco-sa [5]. For those reasons, tumors with these histologic patterns were called 'intestinal type.' Other tumors did not show the cohesiveness needed to form glandular structures and invaded the gastric wall in a diffuse fashion, which has resulted in the name 'diffuse type' being applied to them. It was noted that males had a higher proportion of the intestinal type than females and there was a tendency for an increased proportion of such tumors to occur with advanced age in both sexes [4].

Studies of the histology of gastric tumors in Japanese populations in their native land and in Hawaii led to the following conclusions: 1) The age-specific incidence rate for diffuse carcinoma remained little changed among Japanese migrants; the decrease in intestinal type accounted for most of the decline in the total gastric cancer incidence in Hawaii. 2) The predominance of the diffuse type in the young and of the intestinal type in older persons has been preserved in both populations, but the age at which the transition in type occurs has changed; the transitional age comes earlier in Japan, where a high risk for stomach cancer still prevails [14].

Histological classification of gastric carcinoma in Latin America showed that the intestinal type accounted for most of the excess incidence in high-risk populations and it was, therefore, labeled the 'epidemic type' [6]. This type was found less frequently in populations at low risk. It was later found that the intestinal type accounted for most of the declining rates observed in recent decades in several countries [15]. The diffuse type displayed less inter-country variation in rates and has been associated with a lesser decline in rates in the United States and European populations [16, 17]. Further evidence of the independency of the intestinal and diffuse carcinomas was provided by the age-specific incidence rates for each histologic type in native Japanese and in Japanese migrants to Hawaii. The slope of the intestinal-type curve was much steeper than that of the diffuse type and only the former type showed any decline with migration [14].

2.6. Blood Groups

A small excess in blood group A distribution in gastric cancer patients has been noted for a long time. When blood group types were correlated with histology it was found that the group A excess was restricted to the diffuse histologic type in populations of different ethnic groups (Colombia, Norway, Hawaiian Japanese), apparently suggesting some kind of genetic susceptibili-ty [14, 18] (see Chapter 2).

2.7. Socioeconomic Class

A marked inverse socioeconomic gradient in risk has been noted in many countries with the lower classes having approximately 2.5 times the risk of the upper classes. This has not been accompanied by a consistent pattern of excess risk in specific occupations although miners, fishermen and agricultural workers have been considered at higher risk than other occupations [19]. An urban–rural gradient is described in some studies but is not a constant feature of the epidemiology of the disease. In general, urbanization is associated with lower-risk. Urban–rural differences, however, may be determined by migration patterns. In some countries a high risk has been observed in some rural areas but not in others. Since first generation migrants maintain their original risk, the risk of the population of any given city will be equivalent to a weighted average of the risks of the native and migrant populations. A city with heavy migration from high-risk rural areas may, therefore, display a risk much greater than expected on the basis of the native population alone. If, on the other hand, migration is predominantly from low-risk rural areas, the risk of the city will tend to be low. In populations with heavy immigration a strong correlation can be found between the gastric cancer risk of the immigrants and that of their place of birth [6].

2.8. Geochemistry

There have been suggestions that gastric cancer is related to occupations involving close contact with the soil. Acidic soils are generally found in areas of high risk for stomach cancer. Deficiencies of trace elements have been suggested but no consistent pattern has emerged [20]. An association between high nitrate content of the drinking water and cancer risk has been suspected in England and in Colombia [21].

2.9. Diet

The marked interpopulation differences in gastric cancer risk and in dietary habits, as well as the fact that the gastric mucosa sustains prolonged contact with food, were the basis for etiologic hypotheses pointing to dietary habits. It has been speculated that diet may have a carcinogenic role in a number of ways: a) food items may be carcinogenic; b) they may be vehicles for carcinogens; c) they may be converted to carcinogens in the food preparation process; d) they may contain promoters of carcinogens; and, e) they may lack inhibitors of carcinogens. It is also recognized that the above characteristics are not mutually exclusive and that there may still be other unknown ways in which diet may influence carcinogenesis [19].

Descriptions of dietary habits of populations at high risk have led to suspected associations between cancer and a variety of food items: rice in Japan, fried foods in Wales, potatoes in Slovenia, grain products in Finland, spices in Java, and smoked fish in Iceland. In many descriptive studies starchy foods were the most frequently implicated items [22]. In the United States it has been observed that the decline in cancer mortality coincided with

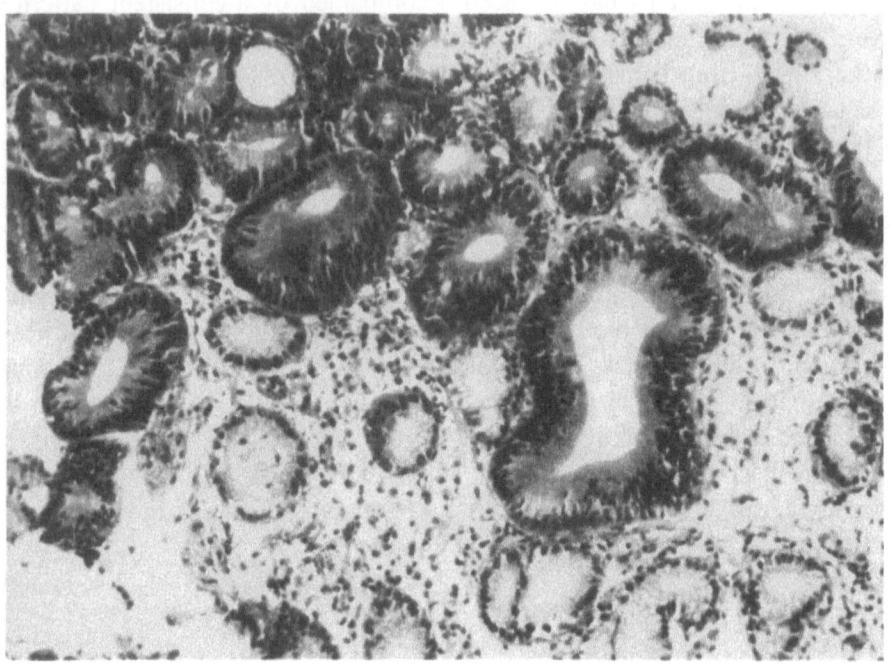

Figure 2. Metaplastic gastric antral mucosa with adenomatous dysplasia. The metaplastic gland (upper part) shows decreased mucous secretion and elongated hyperchromatic nuclei with pseudostratification.

a decrease in the consumption of cabbage and an increase in the consumption of lettuce and citric foods [12]. A considerable number of case-control studies have focused on dietary items in several parts of the world. Wynder *et al.* [23] found no noteworthy differences between cases and controls in Iceland, Slovenia and the United States. Meinsma reported a higher frequency of bacon and a lower frequency of citric fruits in cases than in controls in Holland [24]. Acheson and Doll found no significant case-control differences in England [22]. Higginson reported a more frequent use of fried foods by cases in Kansas City [25]. Graham *et al.* in Buffalo found a smaller porportion of cases who use raw vegetables (lettuce, tomatoes, cole slaw) [26]. Hirayama reported that cases in Japan consume less milk and more salted foods than controls [27].

Although no unanimity can be found to implicate any food as positively associated with gastric cancer risk, a number or studies have reported that green leafy vegetables such as lettuce, as well as citric fruits, are associated with lower risk. Bjelke has interpreted his findings in Norway and the United States as showing an independent protective effect of a vitamin C index [28]. There is speculation, therefore, that vitamin C may play an inhibitory role in gastric carcinogenesis. Bjelke has pointed out that some items such as salted fish and vitamin C index may interact with respect to histologic expression of the carcinoma. It thus appears that the effect of any specific item might be dependent on the presence of other items and that a very complex interaction of a variety of food items may determine whether potential dietary carcinogens are expressed or remain inactive.

2.10. Pernicious Anemia

It has been well established for many years that patients with pernicious anemia carry an increased risk of gastric cancer. It has also been known that pernicious anemia patients develop progressive atrophy of the mucosa of the corpus and fundus of the stomach, probably related to antiparietal cell antibodies, and that gastric carcinoma in such patients arises in the same topographic area of the stomach showing the atrophy. The atrophic area is also the site of extensive transformation of the normal mucosal glands into intestinal-type glands, so-called intestinal metaplasia. However, the great majority of gastric cancer patients, especially outside Scandinavian countries, do not have a history of pernicious anemia.

3. PRECURSOR LESIONS

3.1. Historic Aspects

The concept of gastric cancer precursors has evolved from a series of observations of the pathology and epidemiology of the disease. Its origins date back to 1883 when Kupfer described in the gastric mucosa islets of intestinal glands [29]. According to the prevailing concepts of pathogenesis at that time, they were interpreted as misplaced embryonal rests and duly labeled 'heterotopias.' Little consideration was given to the possibility that these heterotopias may have pathologic significance until Bonne et al. in 1938 described Chinese immigrants who had a high frequency of both gastric carcinoma and atrophic gastritis with 'goblet cell metaplasia,' which is equivalent to the so-called heterotopias [30]. By contrast, the native Malays had a low frequency of carcinoma and a low prevalence of metaplasia. Jarvi and Lauren in 1951 described carcinomas resembling those of the intestine originating in such areas of 'heterotopia' [31]. The true nature of these heterotopias began to be reevaluated and the idea that they may not be really embryonic rests but rather a change from the gastric to intestinal mucosa, 'metaplasia,' began to find some supporters. In 1955 Morson described small gastric carcinomas originating in areas of intestinal metaplasia [32]. Siurala repeatedly biopsied individuals followed over a period of years and described progression from atrophic gastritis to gastric carcinoma [33]. Figure 1 illustrates the metaplastic changes.

3.2. Interpopulation Correlations

Recently the epidemiology of precursor lesions has been studied in Colombia where a cancer registry in the city of Cali reported that the immigrants from the Andean mountains of Nariño had a very high incidence of gastric carcinoma, especially of the intestinal type [6]. A systematic search for intestinal metaplasia in autopsy material from six groups of immigrants, as well as from the local natives, revealed a positive correlation between the incidence of gastric cancer, especially of the intestinal type, and the frequency of metaplasia [6]. Imai *et al.* reported a similar positive correlation between metaplasia and carcinoma in a comparison of Japanese and U.S. populations [34]. The association with metaplasia is largely limited to intestial-type carcinoma. In surgical specimens, carcinomas of the intestinal type are usually surrounded by severe intestinal metaplasia. The presence of intestinal metaplasia in specimens with diffuse carcinoma was found with about the same prevalence as that of the population under study [15]. In low-risk populations, diffuse carcinomas are usually surrounded by normally appearing mucosa.

3.3. Histologic Characteristics

From detailed studies of the gastric mucosa in high-risk populations, a series of lesions have been described that apparently represent a continuum of change from normal to carcinoma [35]. The complete process is believed to take a long time: 16 to 24 years in cell kinetics studies [36].

The mildest and, therefore, probably earliest lesion observed is superficial gastritis, characterized by infiltration of lymphocytes, plasma cells and polymorphonuclear leukocytes in the superficial portion of the lamina propria. Superficial gastritis is usually accompanied by necrosis of epithelial cells and regenerative changes in the glandular neck region. It is widely believed that this type of gastritis can be produced by a variety of injuries and that it may be repaired ad-integrum. The lesion considered to be next in the severity scale is chronic atrophic gastritis, characterized by loss of glands as determined by the visualization of areas of lamina propria devoid of glands and occupied only by connective tissue and white blood cells. There are varying degrees of severity of atrophy. On this atrophic background the process of intestinal metaplasia sets in with the appearance of glands lined by cells normally present only in the intestine: absorptive cells, goblet cells, argentaffin cells and Paneth's cells. These cells are distinguished by their morphologic characteristics, as well as by the abnormal set of enzymes they contain: alkaline phosphatase, leucine aminopeptidase and sucrase. When all of the morphologic and enzymatic characteristics expressed in the phenotype of these cells correspond to those of the normal intestine, the metaplasia is usually labeled mature and, as long as it remains mature, the transformation to neoplastic cells appears remote.

In some patients, however, there are metaplastic cells which appear less mature and do not show the complete set of intestinal enzymes, suggesting that they lose that phenotypic expression and that their intestinalization, as judged by this set of enzymes, is incomplete. In specimens with gastric carcinomas surrounded by metaplasia, the set of intestinal enzymes is frequently incomplete [37]. These same metaplastic cells show abnormalities of nuclear morphology characterized by increased size, hyperchromatism and irregular shape. In pathology terminology these changes are known as 'dysplasia,' which also implies distortion of the glandular architecture. These architectural changes have been divided in two groups: when they resemble hormonally-induced proliferations of glandular tissue they are called 'hyperplastic dysplasia,' and when they resemble a benign proliferation of tubular glands they are called 'adenomatous' or 'villous' dysplasia [38]. Dysplasia is believed to carry an increased risk of transformation into invasive carcinoma. Figure 2 illustrates adenomatous dysplasia.

3.4. Distribution by Sex and Age

Although gastric cancer is more frequent in males than in females, studies in Finland and Colombia have found equal prevalence of atrophic gastritis in both sexes. Dysplastic changes, on the other hand, are more common in men, apparently indicating that the promotional stages of the carcinogenic process are expressed more strongly in men. Atrophic gastritis and intestinal metaplasia increase with age in both sexes, not only in prevalence but also in surface area covered by the lesion. Detailed studies of the dynamics and especially of the rate of conversion from one stage of the precursor lesions to the next, reveal that the proportion of individuals in a given community who enter into the precursor lesion cycle, is achieved rather early. After the third decade of life, the porportion of individuals with some of the precursor lesions remains constant. This apparently indicates that the selection of the members of the community who will (or will not) enter the cycle of precursor lesions is achieved before the end of the third decade. The later stages, characterized by increase in the surface area covered by metaplasia and by dysplasia, show a constant increment with age [35].

3.5. Diet

Few studies of diet in patients with atrophic gastritis have been done. Since the prevalence of precursors is probably high in areas at high risk for stomach cancer, it may be assumed that the same dietary patterns described for stomach cancer are applicable to its precursors.

Studies conducted in the high-risk area of Nariño, Colombia, show an excessive consumption of corn, wheat and cabbage [39]. An inverse relationship (less use of these items in the high-risk area) was found for lettuce and other green leafy vegetables. Individuals with atrophic gastritis reported a higher consumption of corn and lima beans and a lower consumption of lettuce and other green leafy vegetables than the controls. The data suggested a peculiar interaction of food items: lettuce seemed to prevent the association between atrophic gastritis and corn consumption only when the amount of corn eaten was not excessive. Concerning food preparation, salting of food for preservation was generally more common in high risk areas.

3.6. Nitrate Intake

Nitrate is present in the water supply of some populations at high gastric cancer risk such as Colombia, England, Chile, Israel and Newfoundland [40]. In Nariño, Colombia, the content of nitrate in the water was found to be higher in towns where cancer and precursor lesions were more frequent. A significantly higher concentration of nitrates was found in the urine of persons living in high-risk villages. In the same villages, a greater proportion of the population obtained their drinking water from dug wells and it was precisely in the water from such wells that high-risk levels of nitrate were found [21].

4. CONCLUSIONS

The epidemiology of gastric cancer and its precursors, as summarized above, has given rise to speculations about the etiology of the disease, as summarized in the following quote [8]:

'It is postulated that one major subtype of gastric carcinoma ("intestinal type") is the end result of a series of mutations and cell transformations begun in the first decade of life. The mutagen could be a nitroso compound synthesized in the upper gastrointestinal tract by the action of nitrite (i.e., from food or saliva) on naturally occurring nitrogen compounds. Under normal conditions these nitroso compounds do not reach the gastric epithelial cell, presumably because their synthesis is inhibited by antioxidants present in food or because of their inability to pass the mucosal barrier. The barrier may be overcome by abrasives or irritants such as hard grains, food with high sodium chloride concentration, or surfactants.

Once the first mutation occurs, the glandular gastric epithelium is gradually changed to intestinal-type epithelium, the mucous barrier altered and the pH elevated. Under these conditions, bacteria proliferate in the gastric cavity and facilitate the conversion of nitrates to nitrites, thereby increasing the nitrite pool and the probability of formation of mutagenic-carcinogenic nitroso compounds. This process of gastric atrophy and intestinal metaplasia goes on for 30 to 50 years until some of the individuals affected have the final mutation or cell transformation which allows the cell to become autonomous and invade other tissues.'

Work on this hypothesis continues in several countries. Although it cannot be said that the hypothesis has been proven correct, so far all further explorations of it have been consistent with the main theme. No other alternative hypotheses have been proposed in recent times.

REFERENCES

1. Barrett MK: Avenues of approach to gastric-cancer problem. J Natl Cancer Inst 7:127–157, 1946.
2. Dunham LJ: World maps of cancer mortality rates and frequency ratios. J Natl Cancer Inst 41:155–203, 1968.
3. Haenszel W, Kurihara M, Segi M, Lee RKC: Stomach cancer among Japanese in Hawaii. J Natl Cancer Inst 49:969–988, 1972.
4. Lauren P: The two histological main types of gastric carcinoma: diffuse and so-called intestinal-type carcinoma. An attempt at a histo-clinical classification. Acta Pathol Microbiol Scand 64:31–49, 1965.
5. Jarvi O: A review of the part played by gastrointestinal heterotopias in neoplasmogenesis. Proc Finnish Acad Sci, pp 151–187, 1962.
6. Correa P, Cuello C, Duque E: Carcinoma and intestinal metaplasia of the stomach in Colombian migrants. J Natl Cancer Inst 44:297–306, 1970.
7. Sugimura T, Fujimura S, Baha T: Tumor production in the glandular stomach and alimentary tract of the rat by N-methyl-N'-nitro-N-nitrosoguanidine. Cancer Res 30:455–465, 1970.
8. Correa P, Haenszel W, Cuello C, Archer M, Tannenbaum S: A model for gastric cancer epidemiology. Lancet 2:58–60, 1975.
9. Waterhouse J, Muir C, Correa P, Powell J (eds): Cancer Incidence in five continents, vol III, Scientific Publication No. 15. Lyon: International Agency for Research on Cancer, 1976.
10. Segi M: Age-adjusted death rates for cancer for selected sites in 51 countries in 1974. Nagoya: Segi Institute of Cancer Epidemiology, 1979.
11. Griffith FW: The sex ratio in gastric cancer and hypothetical considerations relative to aetiology. Brit J Cancer 22:163–172, 1968.
12. Haenszel W: Variation in incidence of and mortality from stomach cancer, with particular reference to the United States. J Natl Cancer Inst 21:213–262, 1958.
13. Haenszel Wb: Cancer mortality among the foreign-born in the United States. J Natl Cancer Inst 26:37–132, 1961.
14. Correa P, Sasano N, Stemmermann GN, Haenszel W: Pathology of gastric carcinoma in Japanese populations: comparisons between Miyagi Prefecture, Japan, and Hawaii. J Natl Cancer Inst 51:1449–1459, 1973.
15. Muñoz N, Correa P, Cuello C, Duque E: Histologic types of gastric carcinoma in high- and low-risk areas. Intern J Cancer 3:809–818, 1968.
16. Muñoz N, Asvall J: Time trends of intestinal and diffuse types of gastric cancer in Norway. Intern J Cancer 8:144–157, 1971.
17. Muñoz N, Connelly R: Time trends of intestinal and diffuse types of gastric cancer in the United States. Intern J Cancer 8:158–164, 1971.
18. Correa P: IAP Maude Abbott Lecture. Geographic pathology of cancer in Colombia. Intern Pathol 11:16–22, 1970.

19. Haenszel W, Correa P: Developments in the epidemiology of stomach cancer over the past decade. Cancer Res 35:3452–3459, 1975.

20. Stocks P, Davies RI: Epidemiological evidence from chemical and spectrographical analysis that soil is concerned in the causation of cancer. Brit J Cancer 14:8–22, 1960.

21. Cuello C, Correa P, Haenszel W, Gordillo G, Brown C, Archer M, Tannenbaum S: Gastric cancer in Colombia. I. Cancer risk and suspect environmental agents. J Natl Cancer Inst 57:1015–1020, 1976.

22. Acheson ED, Doll R: Dietary factors in carcinoma of the stomach: a study of 100 cases and 200 controls. Gut 5:126–131, 1964.

23. Wynder EL, Kmet J, Dungal N, Segi M: An epidemiological investigation of gastric cancer. Cancer 16:1461–1496, 1963.

24. Meinsma L: Voeding en Kanker. Voeding 25:357–365, 1964.

25. Higginson J: Etiological factors in gastro-intestinal cancer in man. J Natl Cancer Inst 37:527–545, 1966.

26. Graham S, Schotz W, Martino P: Alimentary factors in the epidemiology of gastric cancer. Cancer 30:927–938, 1972.

27. Hirayama T: The epidemiology of cancer of the stomach in Japan with special reference to the role of diet. Unio Intern Contre Cancrum Monograph Ser 10:37–48, 1967.

28. Bjelke E: Epidemiologic studies of cancer of the stomach, colon and rectum; with special emphasis on the role of diet. Scand J Gastroenterol 9 (Suppl. 31) 1:253, 1974.

29. Kupfer C: Fetschrift. Arz Verein Munch, P 7, 1883.

30. Bonne C, Hartz Ph H, Klerks JV, Postuma JH, Radsma W, Tjokronegoro S: Morphology of the stomach and gastric secretion in Malays and Chinese and the different incidence of gastric ulcer and cancer in these races. Amer J Cancer 33:265–279, 1938.

31. Jarvi O, Lauren P: On the role of heterotopias of the intestinal epithelium in the pathogenesis of gastric cancer. Acta Pathol Microbiol Scand 29:26–44, 1951.

32. Morson B: Carcinoma arising from areas of intestinal metaplasia in the gastric mucosa. Br J Cancer 9:377–385, 1955.

33. Siurala M, Varis K, Wiljasalo M: Studies of patients with atrophic gastritis: a 10–15 year follow-up. Scand J Gastroenterol 1:40–48, 1966.

34. Imai T, Kubo T, Watanabe H: Chronic gastritis in Japanese with reference to high incidence of gastric carcinoma. J Natl Cancer Inst 47:179–195, 1971.

35. Correa P, Cuello C, Duque E, Burbano L, García FT, Bolaños O, Brown C, Haenszel W: Gastric cancer in Colombia. III. Natural history of precursor lesions. J. Natl Cancer Inst 57:1027–1035, 1976.

36. Fujita S, Takanori H: Cell Proliferation, differentiation and migration in the gastric mucosa: a study of the background of carcinogenesis. In: Pathophysiology of carcinogenesis in digestive organs, Farber E et al. (eds). University of Tokyo Press, 1977, pp 21–36.

37. Matsukura N: Personal communication, 1980.

38. Cuello C, Correa P, Zarama G, López J, Murray J, Gordillo G: Histopathology of gastric dysplasias. Correlations with gastric juice chemistry. Am J Surg Pathol 3:491–500, 1979.

39. Haenszel W, Correa P, Cuello C, Guzmán N, Burbano L, Lores H, Muñoz J: Gastric cancer in Colombia. II. Case-control epidemiologic study of precursor lesions. J Natl Cancer Inst 57:1021–1026, 1976.

40. Fraser P, Chilvers C, Beral V, Hill M: Nitrate and human cancer: a review of the evidence. Int J Epidemiol 9:3–11, 1980.

6. Early Detection of Gastric Cancer

SEIBI KOBAYASHI

1. PREFACE

What does early detection of gastric cancer mean? It probably means the detection of a curable cancer which is not necessarily an asymptomatic lesion. A scirrhous lesion of gastric cancer can become advanced even when it is still asymptomatic and can be already inoperable when it becomes symptomatic.

On the other hand, a symptomatic lesion is not necessarily incurable. In most cases, even a curable lesion will cause some sort of symptoms, but such a lesion will be asymptomatic in much earlier period.

What will a curable cancer mean substantially? It would be a lesion that can be radically resected together with involved or uninvolved regional lymph nodes. The most curable is a lesion that is localized in the stomach without lymph node involvement. Since Ewing's publication in 1936[1], several authors[2–4] have referred to curable or early gastric cancer, but detection of such lesion has been extremely difficult.

Gastric cancer has been a national disease among the Japanese for a long time. From long-term studies on gastric cancer in Japan, the depth of cancerous invasion within the gastric wall seems most valuable to assess the curability of a lesion. Early recognition of gastric cancer has been greatly improved by recent progress in X-ray and endoscopic examination mainly in Japan. It is now evident that the features of a carcinomatous lesion are very different roentgenologically and endoscopically depending upon the presence or absence of involvement of the propria muscle by carcinomatous tissues.

Based on this idea, the definition and classification of early gastric carcinoma were proposed by the Japanese Gastroenterological Endoscopy Society in 1962[5]. Early gastric carcinoma is defined as that in which the tumor is still confined to the mucosa or/and the submucosa regardless of lymph node involvement. A five year survival rate of such tumors can exceed 90% after radical operation[6, 7]. Being familiar with the gross features of such tumors,

J. J. DeCosse and P. Sherlock (eds.), Gastrointestinal cancer 1, 131-164. All rights reserved.
Copyright © 1981 Martinus Nijhoff Publishers, The Hague/Boston/London.

one can facilitate early recognition of gastric cancer on X-ray and endoscopic examination.

However, the early detection of gastric cancer is still very insufficient on an out-patient basis even in Japan, unless patients with such a tumor visit an experienced doctor chronologically earlier. Therefore, a mass screening method using double contrast X-ray technique was devised in Japan approximately 20 years ago. In addition, further progress in fiberoptic endoscopy combined with cytology and biopsy has contributed substantially to early detection of gastric cancer not only in Japan, but also throughout the world.

2. DEFINITION AND CLASSIFICATION OF EARLY GASTRIC CANCER

The definition and classification of early carcinoma of the stomach were proposed in 1962 to the Japanese Gastroenterological Endoscopy Society [5] and in 1963 to the Japanese Research Society for Gastric Cancer. Early carcinoma of the stomach was defined as carcinoma in which cancerous invasion was confined to the mucosa or/and the submucosa regardless of lymph node involvement.

Early gastric carcinoma, in the experience of Japanese workers, can be macroscopically classified as one of three basic types: type I, protruded type; type II, superficial type; subtype IIa, elevated; subtype IIb, flat; subtype IIc, depressed; type III, excavated type (Figure 1).

2.1. Type I: Protruded Type
A protrusion into the gastric lumen is very prominent. It sometimes resembles a benign semipedunculated or sessile polyp. A malignant lesion, in general, presents an irregular contour, unevenness of the surface, and bleeding with or without definite ulcerations on the surface. Redness, lobulation,

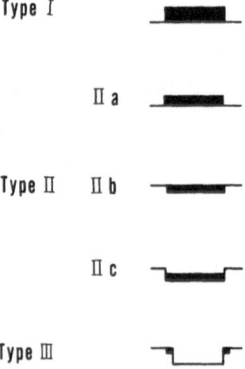

Figure 1. Macroscopic classification of early gastric carcinoma.

and erosion of the surface are not always observed in malignant lesions. Lesions greater than 2 cm in diameter must be considered likely to be malignant.

2.2. Type II: Superficial Type

The unevenness of the gastric surface is relatively inconspicuous. This type is classified into three subtypes.

2.2.1. Type IIa (Elevated). This type is characterized by sessile mucosal elevation of plateau-like or flower bed pattern. The height of elevation is less than two times that of the surrounding mucosa. This elevation commonly surrounds an area of central depression and then is designated as type IIa + IIc.

2.2.2. Type IIb (Flat). This type shows neither elevation nor depression of the gastric surface and may be recognized only because of discoloration of the mucosa. These lesions may be very small. The diagnosis of the pure IIb is considered very difficult.

2.2.3. Type IIc (Depressed). This type is a slightly depressed lesion and sometimes has a dirty appearance with adherent mucus or exudate. The margins of the depressed area are irregular and may be hemorrhagic. Island-like residues of intact mucosa may be observed in the depressed area. The mucosal folds are disrupted and clubbed. Tumors of this type are frequently seen in association with the deeper type III lesions and are then called type IIc + III. This type and its combinations (IIc + III, IIa + IIc) are the most commonly observed types in early gastric cancer.

These lesions probably correspond to the 'superficial erosive carcinoma' of Ewing[1] and many instances of the superficial spreading carcinoma of Gutman *et al.* [2] and Stout [4].

2.3. Type III: Excavated Type

This type appears as an ulcer, quite similar by inspection or radiologic examination to a benign peptic ulcer, except when there is invasion of the surrounding mucosa, creating a superficial depression around the ulcer, then called type III + IIc. When the depressed area is more prominent, the case is classified as IIc + III.

3. CONTROVERSY ABOUT THE TERM 'EARLY GASTRIC CANCER'

A question will be raised why we do not use the term 'superficial carcioma' or 'superficial spreading carcinoma.' The carcinoma is superficial histologically, but the term 'superficial carcinoma' might be misconstrued to mean that the tumor exists only in the mucosa, and is not capable of invading the muscularis mucosae.

Our present definition of 'early gastric cancer' was established by agreement among internists, surgeons, and pathologists in Japan over 15 years ago. In the discussion on terminology between Murakami[8] and Prolla[9], Prolla stated that insofar as the definition is based on morphologic features and the histological depth of cancerous invasion, this type of carcinoma should be called 'superficial gastric carcinoma'. He did not agree to the term 'superficial spreading carcinoma' as used by Stout[4] because it is not certain that all of these tumors have spread superficially, at the time and in the place they are observed.

An ulcerated lesion such as the type IIc+III or III+IIc, according to the Japanese classification seems to exist for many years without spreading through the gastric mucosa, and occasionally shows temporary healing.

By our definition, 'early gastric cancer' can include even prominent polypoid (type I) and deeply ulcerated (type III) lesions that still are relatively localized in the gastric wall.

We decided to reserve the term 'superficial type' for the relatively flat lesions that may be slightly elevated (type IIa), flush with the mucosal surface (type IIb), or slightly depressed (type IIc). Therefore, the adjective 'superficial' cannot encompass all of the different types of early gastric cancer.

As Murakami stressed[8], 'early' was important to emphasize the benefit of prompt detection of gastric cancer. It is well known that gastric cancer has been an enormous, nationwide problem in Japan. Early detection by radiographic and endoscopic techniques is essential for a chance of curative resection. In this light, the term employed should appeal to the mass communication media and to the public, emphasizing that early detection is an important means of solving this national problem.

It is true that 'early gastric cancer,' by our definition, can progress to lymphatic involvement and even to distant metastases in rare instances, but the usual reported prognosis is excellent, the 5-year survival rate being over 95% [7]. For this reason, we think that the term 'early gastric cancer' is more appropriate than 'superficial carcinoma' or 'superficial spreading carcinoma.'

4. INCIDENCE OF EARLY GASTRIC CANCER

At our hospital (AACH), the incidence of an early lesion among all gastric carcinoma is shown in Table 1, accounting for a mean of 13.1% from 1964 to 1977. The incidence has not shown a significant increase since 1967. Takagi

Table 1. Incidence of early gastric carcinoma (Aichi Cancer Center Hospital).

Year	No. with gastric cancer	No. early gastric cancer resected radically	% early cancer
1964	5	2	40.0
1965	303	20	6.6
1966	295	24	8.0
1967	256	27	10.5
1968	271	51	18.8
1969	282	33	11.7
1970	280	38	13.6
1971	260	37	14.2
1972	266	36	13.5
1973	270	35	13.0
1974	254	41	16.1
1975	279	31	11.1
1976	293	51	17.4
1977	266	43	16.2
Total	3580	469	13.1

et al. [10] reported that a ratio of early cancers to all gastric cancers operated on had shown a significant increase during past decades. The rate was 2.1% during the period from 1946 to 1955, 9.7% from 1956 to 1965, and 28.1% from 1966 to 1975, respectively. In the United States, Ito *et al.* [11] reported that the rate of early gastric cancer was 8.3% in the series of the University of Chicago.

5. RADIOLOGICAL DIAGNOSIS

Radiological diagnosis of early gastric cancer stems from Gutmann's pioneer work over 40 years ago [2]. A significant improvement was made by Shirakabe *et al.* [12], who established a double contrast radiologic method.

5.1. Method of Examination

The patient is premedicated intramuscularly with an antispasmodic 5 to 10 minutes before the examination to lessen gastric motility and to avoid rapid flow of barium into the duodenum. For constipated patients, laxatives or a cleansing enema should be given to eliminate colonic gas and feces.

To provide good visualization, it is necessary to give a patient a sufficient amount of barium and air. The volume of barium given is usually more than 200 ml. With less barium the entire gastric mucosa cannot be coated evenly to obtain good double contrast images. The volume of air to insufflate the

Table 2. Pick-up rate by X-ray and endoscopic examination.

Period	X-ray	Endoscopy
1959–1962	66.7%	94.4%
1963–1967	86.3%	95.0%
1969–1971	86.7%	95.0%

Shirakabe *et al.* [14].

stomach adequately is also important. According to Maruyama, at least 300 ml of air is required for this purpose [13].

5.2. Results

A pick-up rate of abnormalities in the stomach by double contrast X-ray examination was reported by Shirakabe *et al.* (Table 2) and compared with that by endoscopic examination [14].

During the period 1959 to 1963, the detection rate was low, showing 66.7% by X-ray examination, and endoscopy was superior to X-ray examination in detection of abnormalities. During the period 1969–1971, X-ray examination was improved, and the detection rate improved to 86.7%. Endoscopy did not impact on this improvement.

Diagnostic accuracy for detection of malignancy is shown by Shirakabe *et al.* [14] (Table 3). During the period 1959–1962, X-ray and endoscopic examination demonstrated diagnostic accuracies of 66.7% and 66.1% respectively. During the period 1963–1967, the rates were elevated up to 82.5% and 83.8%, respectively. During the last period 1969–1971, a further significant improvement was attained up to 95.0% and 93.4%, respectively.

5.3. Radiologic Findings of Early Gastric Cancer
5.3.1. Produced Types (Type I and IIa)

Barium filling study. Protruded types of early gastric cancer are generally small and flat, usually without ulceration or scar formation. Therefore, barium-filled roentgenograms of the stomach may not disclose a typical filling

Table 3. Diagnostic accuracy of gastric malignancy.

Period	X-ray	Endoscopy
1959–1962	66.7%	66.1%
1963–1967	82.5%	83.8%
1969–1971	95.0%	93.4%

Shirakabe *et al.* [14].

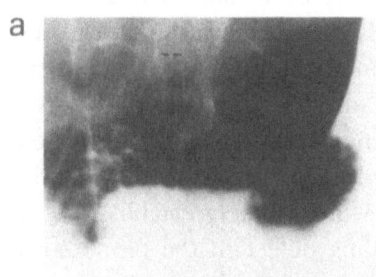

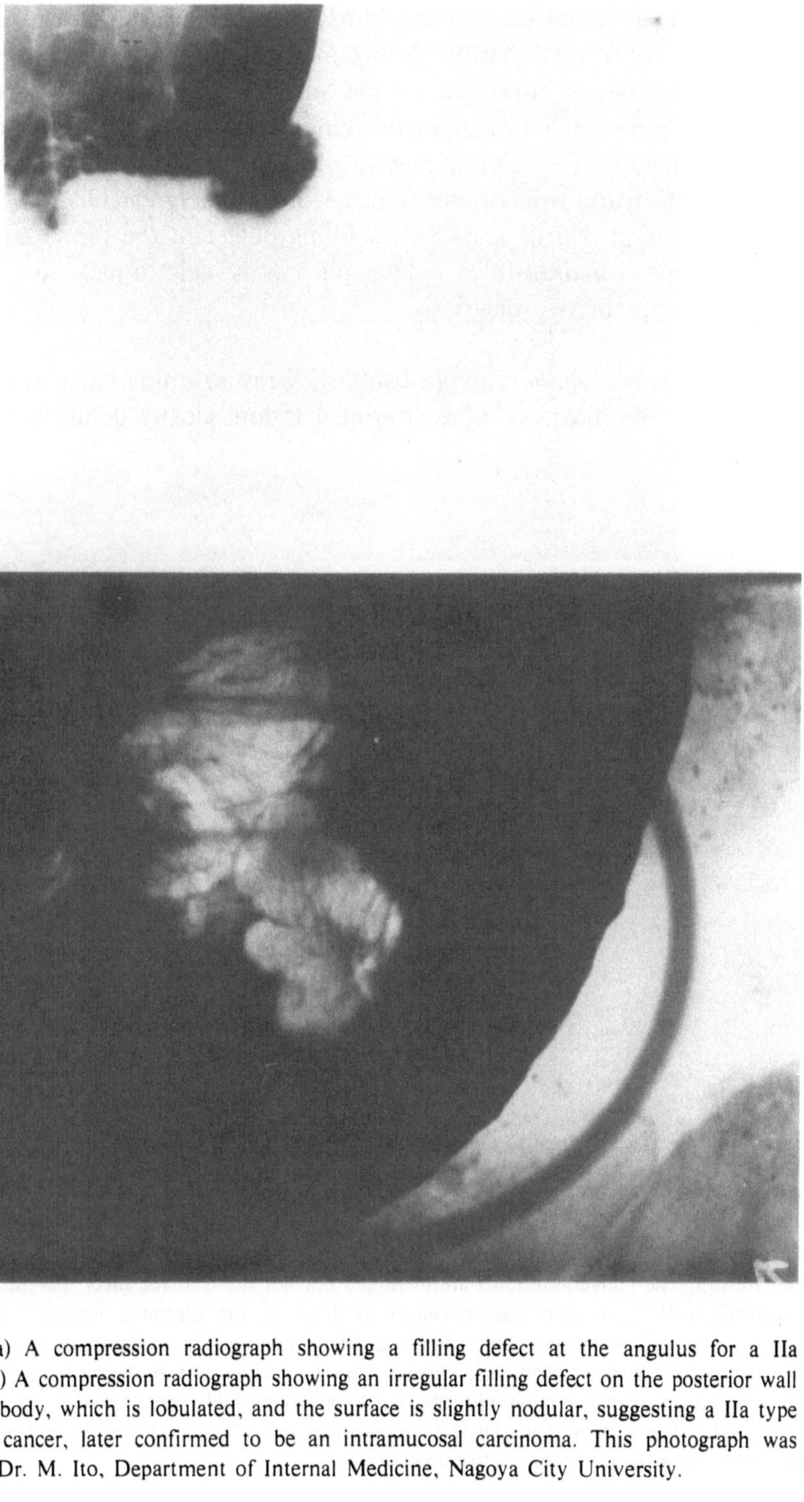

Figure 2. (a) A compression radiograph showing a filling defect at the angulus for a IIa carcinoma. (b) A compression radiograph showing an irregular filling defect on the posterior wall of the lower body, which is lobulated, and the surface is slightly nodular, suggesting a IIa type early gastric cancer, later confirmed to be an intramucosal carcinoma. This photograph was provided by Dr. M. Ito, Department of Internal Medicine, Nagoya City University.

defect or even an indirect finding suggestive of a lesion. Unless at least a part of the lesion is delineated on the films, the diagnosis of an elevated cancer will not be made by a barium filling method. If a lesion is present on the lesser or the greater curvature, or the adjacent area, the diagnosis could be made with barium filled radiographs demonstrating a small filling defect or an irregular contour. If a lesion is present on the anterior or the posterior wall of the stomach, barium-filled radiography will not likely establish the diagnosis. An antral lesion will be shown as a filling defect in the prone position of a patient. Thus, a barium-filled radiograph may be able to pick up a lesion, but not make a qualitative diagnosis.

Double contrast study. Double contrast X-ray examination plays an important role in the diagnosis of a protruded lesion, clearly delineating its confi-

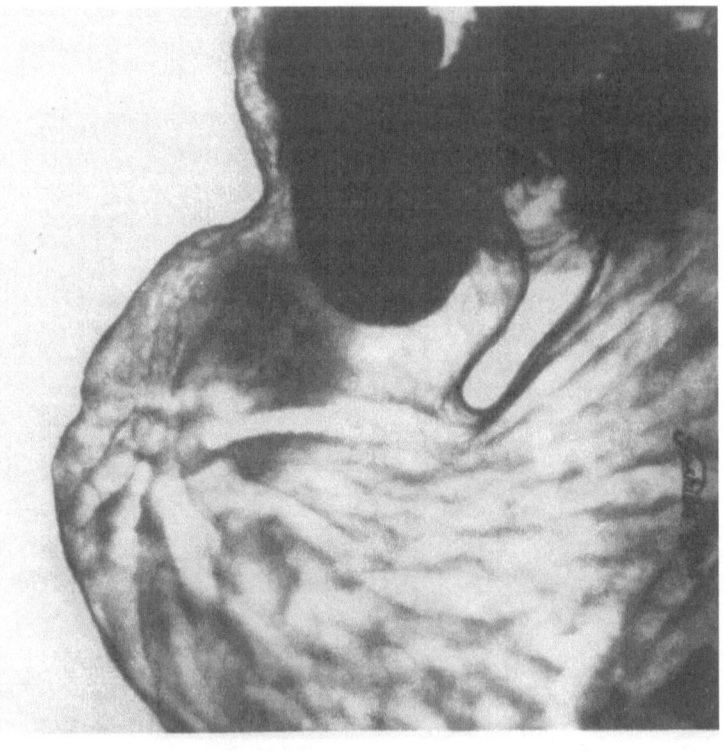

a

Figure 3. (a) A double contrast radiograph showing an irregular ulceration with a granular base in the antrum. The converging folds are disrupted but not fused at the ulcer margin. This finding suggested a IIc type early gastric cancer localized in the ulcerated region, later confirmed histologically to be intramucosal carcinoma. This photograph was provided by Dr. M. Ito, Department of Internal Medicine, Nagoya City University. (b) A double contract radiograph showing an irregular ulceration with thickened converging folds which are clubbed, disrupted but not fused at the ulcer margin. There findings suggested a IIc type early gastric cancer involving the submucosa, later confirmed histologically.

guration, size and features of the surface, but does not well delineate the presence or absence of a stalk or the margins of the tumor, which are better demonstrated by a compression study. the presence or absence of a stalk on a protruded lesion is a key point to determine the diagnosis. A lesion in the fundus or the upper body of the stomach cannot be effectively demonstrated by compression. Such lesions will be better delineated in a semi-upright, left oblique position on double contrast X-ray examination.

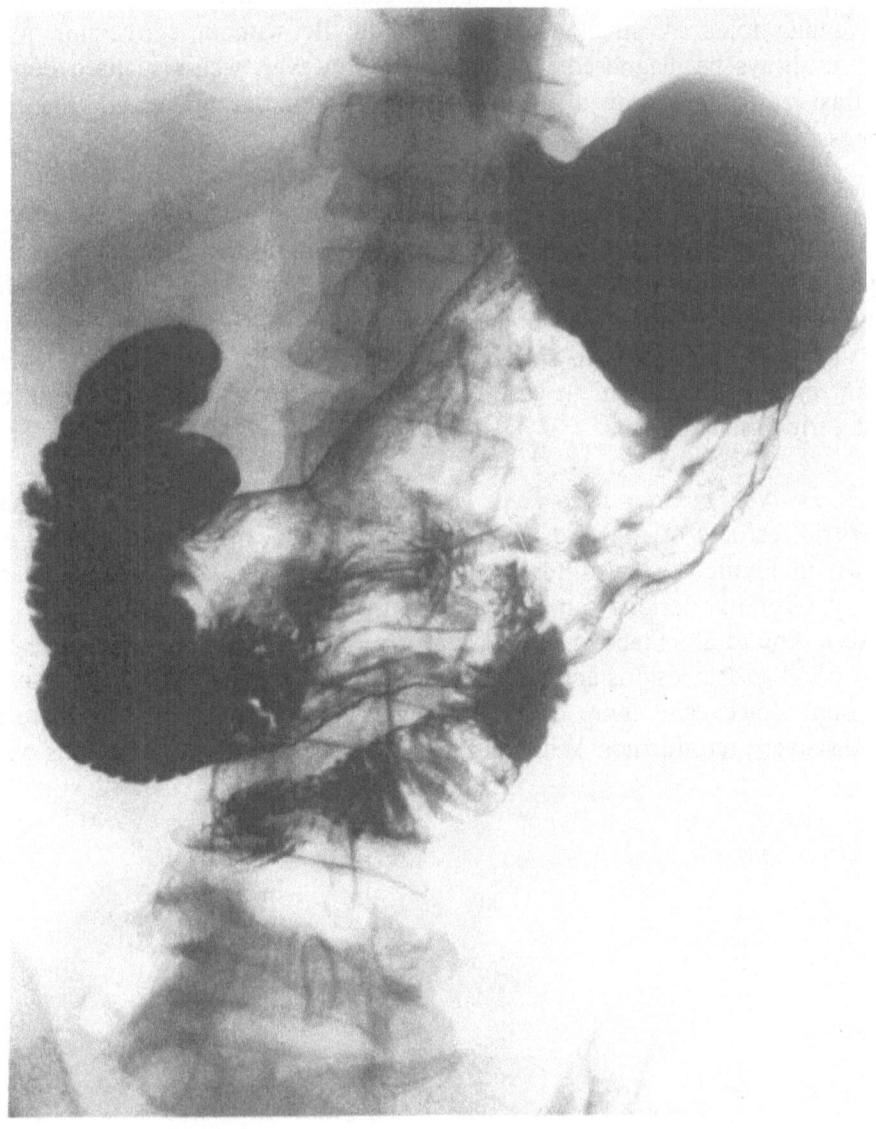

b

Compression study. A compression study plays an important role in the diagnosis of protruded early gastric cancers. The configuration, size and surface features are well demonstrated by compression, especially in a lesion of the lower body or the antrum of the stomach. Furthermore, a compression study can reveal the presence or absence of a stalk and the border of a tumor. A successful compression study can, therefore, make a diagnosis of a protruded early gastric cancer (Figure 2).

5.3.2. Depressed Types

Types IIc and IIc+III. The characteristic features of these types are irregular margins, a depressed base, and thinning, clubbing and fusion of the tips of converging folds. A small and very shallow IIc without converging folds cannot always be diagnosed with certainty. However, well-visualized double contrast radiographs show a barium fleck on a IIc appearing area and a deeper depression represents III (Figure 3).

Types III, III+IIc and benign peptic ulcer. To identify a III+ IIc cancer and to distinguish it from a benign peptic ulcer, one should be alert to the adjacent mucosa of a benign appearing ulcer niche on X-ray films. A IIc area may be identified during a healing process of an ulcer with medical treatment. An ulcer niche decreases in size. This phenomenon has been called a 'malignant cycle of ulceration' in gastric cancers and is commonly seen in ulcerated early gastric cancers.

5.3.3. Features of Converging Folds in Depressed Early Gastric Cancers.
Characteristic features of the folds related to depressed early gastric cancers are shown in Figure 4. The differential diagnosis between early malignant and benign ulcerative lesions can be made on the basis of these features.

According to Shirakabe *et al.* [14], a routine radiologic examination revealed 86% of all gastric lesions and subsequent endoscopy added 9% to the discovery rate. However, a more detailed radiologic examination did not increase the discovery rate further. With routine X-ray series, 32% of all lesions were

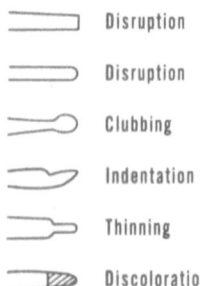

Figure 4. Features of folds in early gastric carcinoma.

interpreted as malignant, 30% as suspicious and 25% as benign. Subsequent endoscopic examination reduced the rates of suspicious and benign radiologic findings to 19% and 17% respectively. At a detailed X-ray series, 68% were interpreted as malignant, 8% suspicious and 18% as benign. With detailed radiologic and endoscopic examination, 86% were diagnosed as malignant, 8% as suspicious and 6% as benign. Shirakabe *et al.* concluded that biopsy procedure would be needed in the diagnosis of 14% of the lesions [14].

Finally, the authors conclude that double contrast radiography plays an important role in detecting early gastric cancers. Continuing correlative studies with endoscopic findings and gross appearances of the resected specimens would be required for a more detailed understanding of the radiologic findings of early gastric cancers.

6. ENDOSCOPIC DIAGNOSIS

A total of 476 patients with 496 early gastric cancers, found at the Gastrointestinal Endoscopy Unit, the Aichi Cancer Center Hospital during the period 1965 to 1977 were classified by the Japanese Classification (Table 4). The endoscopic diagnosis of the cases was evaluated at the following three different stages: (1) the initial endoscopic examination; (2) before positive biopsy or cytology; and, (3) after review of gastroscopic photographs following positive biopsy or cytology.

Table 4. Macroscopic classification of 476 cases of early gastric cancer.

Type	1965–1977	
	No. lesions	%
I	43	8.7
I + IIc	5	
IIa	35	7.1
IIa + IIb	2	
IIa + IIc	52	10.5
IIc + IIa	13	2.6
IIc + IIb	5	
IIc	238	48.0
IIc + III	86	17.3
III + IIc	16	3.2
III	1	
Total	496	100.0

Table 5. Initial endoscopic diagnosis of early gastric cancer.

	1965–1977	
Endoscopic diagnosis	No. cases	%
Malignant		
early cancer	246	51.7
advanced cancer	98	20.6
total cancer	344	72.3
Nonmalignant or inconclusive		
ulcer or ulcer scar	87	18.3
polyps	16	3.4
gastritis	20	4.2
atypical epithelium	3	
submucosal tumor	2	
others	4	
total	132	27.7
Total	476	100.0

6.1. Initial Endoscopic Diagnosis (Table 5)

At the inital gastroscopy, 246 (51.7%) of 475 cases of early gastric cancer were correctly diagnosed and 98 (20.6%) were interpreted as advanced cancer. A total of 344 cases (72.3%) were, therefore, correctly read as cancer on the films taken at the initial gastroscopy. On the other hand, 132 (27.7%) were regarded as non-malignant or inconclusive with the following diagnosis: benign ulcer or ulcer scar, 87 (18.3%); polyps, 16; gastritis of various types, 20; submucosal tumor, 2; atypical epithelium (dysplasia), 3; and others, 4.

6.2. Endoscopic Diagnosis Before Biopsy or Cytology, (Table 6)

Before biopsy or cytology, repeat gastroscopy was performed in some cases to improve diagnostic accuracy or to observe varied changes during a follow-up period. A correct interpretation was made in 305 cases (64.1%) of early malignancy and 106 (22.3%) of the total 476 cases were again read as advanced cancer. However, 411 cases (86.4%) were correctly interpreted as malignant lesion at this stage. Conversely, the number of the cases regarded as benign were significantly reduced to 65 (13.6%) by repeat gastroscopic examinations.

6.3. Final Endoscopic Diagnosis (Table 7)

Gastroscopic films of all but one of the cases were carefully reviewed after malignancy had been confirmed by cytology or biopsy procedures. Either

Table 6. Endoscopic diagnosis prior to biopsy and cytology.

	1965–1977	
Endoscopic diagnosis	No. cases	%
Malignant		
early cancer	305	64.1
advanced cancer	106	22.3
total cancers	411	86.4
Nonmalignant or inconclusive		
ulcer or ulcer scar	50	10.5
polyps	10	2.1
atypical epithelium	3	
submucosal tumor	1	
other	1	
total	65	13.6
Total	476	100.0

cytology or biopsy, or both done under direct vision with a fibergastroscope were positive for malignancy in all of the 475 cases examined.

The diagnosis of early gastric cancer was successfuly made in 387 cases (81.3%). However, the remaining 88 cases (18.5%) were still regarded as advanced cancer in endoscopic appearance. Endoscopic criteria based upon the Japanese classification of early gastric carcinoma were helpful in differentiating early carcinoma from advanced cancer in the majority of the cases, but one should realize the limits of endoscopy as long as macroscopic criteria alone are applied.

Table 7. Final endoscopic diagnosis of early gastric cancer.

	1965–1977	
Endoscopic diagnosis	No. cases	%
Early cancer	387	81.3
Advanced cancer	88	18.5
Gastric ulcer*	1	0.2
Total	476	100.0

* Biopsy or cytology not done before surgery.

Table 8. Endoscopic misdiagnosis in relation to macroscopic type of early gastric cancer.

Type	A No. lesions	B Those erroneously diagnosed as benign or inconclusive	B/A (%)
I	43	10	23.3
I + IIc	5	0	0
IIa	35	7	20.0
IIa + IIb	2	1	50.0
IIa + IIc	52	2	3.8
IIc + IIa	13	0	0
IIc + IIb	5	1	20.0
IIc	238	33	13.9
IIc + III	86	12	14.0
III + IIc	16	7	43.8
III	1	1	100.0
Total	496	74	14.9

6.4. *Endoscopic Misdiagnosis in Relation to Macroscopic Type of Early Gastric Cancer* (Table 8)

Before biopsy or cytology, 65 cases (13.6%) were still diagnosed as benign or inconclusive by endoscopic observation or film interpretation. The 65 cases included 50 interpreted on endoscopic examination as benign ulcer or ulcer scar, 10 as a polyp, 3 as a typical epithelium (dysplasia) and 2 as others (Table 8).

Type I and IIa were occasionally diagnosed as gastric polyps. Type III + IIc were often interpreted as a benign gastric ulcer because the IIc component can be easily overlooked. Type IIc + III and IIc were less frequently misdiagnosed. Thus, we found that the endoscopic differentiation between benign and malignant lesions is difficult in some cases of early gastric cancer [16].

6.5. *Role of Endoscopic Biopsy*

Endoscopic biopsy plays an important role in establishing the correct diagnosis of malignancy and in determining the extent of the cancer, mainly its upper margin and rarely, the lower margin [16]. The sites of biopsy are important.

In an ulcer that appears benign, at least four biopsy specimens are taken, one from each of the four sectors of the ulcer margin (Figure 5). If the ulcer is malignant, at least one specimen can be expected to be positive. From a lesion having the type IIc configuration, at least three specimens are obtained from a suspicious area to establish the diagnosis, and an additional

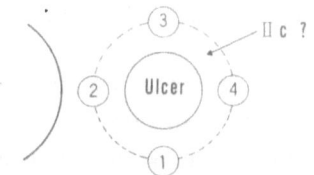

Biopsy is taken from four corners of the ulcer
margins to make a differential diagnosis.

Figure 5. Site of biopsy in benign appearing ulcer.

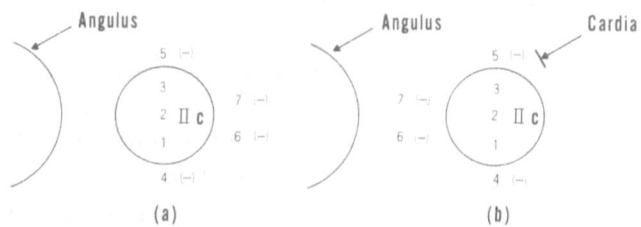

(a) Distal gastrectomy will be done.
(b) Proximal gastrectomy will be considered.

Figure 6. Site of biopsy in IIc appearing lesion.

four biopsies are taken from the surrounding margins to delineate the extent
of cancer (Figure 6). This information can help the surgeon in designing the
extent of resection and deciding whether a distal or proximal gastrectomy will
be required.

In our experience biopsy provides an accurate diagnosis in 94.6% of cases
at the first examination. Thus, cytologic examination is usually unnecessary
in the diagnosis of early gastric cancer (Table 9). We now utilize brush
cytology selectively in cases with negative biopsy or stenosis proximal to the
tumor, and more often in cancer of the cardiac area of the stomach [17, 18].

Table 9. Results of endoscopic biopsy in 464 patients with early gastric cancer — 1965-1977.

Sequence of endoscopic procedures	No. yielding positive results	Cumulative diagnostic accuracy
First	439	94.6%
Second	18	98.5%
Third	2	98.9%

6.6. Endoscopic Differential Diagnosis of Early Gastric Cancer and Benign Peptic Ulcer [16]

Considerable number of gastric cancers resemble a benign peptic ulcer. Endoscopic recognition of a IIc area surrounding a deper benign appearing ulcer is most important to avoid a delay in diagnosis. A IIc area usually appears so red that the differentiation between a IIc cancer and regenerating tissues at the margins of a benign peptic ulcer is sometimes difficult. Therefore, an appropriate biopsy method is imperative for differentiation.

The authors [19] collected 16 cases of early gastric cancer from a surgical series at the University of Chicago during the period from 1955 to 1969. Of the 13 cases examined endoscopically, 4 were regarded as benign peptic ulcers.

Evans et al. [20] commented that, while the early detection of gastric cancer has been facilitated by endoscopy and endoscopic biopsy, endoscopic diagnosis by observation alone was correct in only four of nine cases of early gastric cancer; the remaining five cases were interpreted as benign peptic ulcers. Biopsy was positive in six patients. In most cases misdiagnosed by endoscopic inspection, a small IIc area surrounding a deeper peptic ulceration (III) was overlooked. As Ito et al. [11] pointed out, a lesion may be seen only tangentially and then incompletely with a forward-viewing instrument, so that important features of early gastric cancer such as disruption and clubbing of the folds and irregular depression of the ulcer margin may be poorly demonstrated. With a side-viewing instrument with gastrocamera, it is usually possible to photograph the lesion, en face and to scrutinize more details of the folds and ulcer margin.

In our experience, intragastric photography using a side-viewing instrument, such as the Olympus GTF, has been very helpful in detecting small IIc areas on film and has aided in guiding subsequent endoscopic biopsy.

The following are typical samples of depressed types of early gastric cancer. Figure 7 shows a discolored area with converging folds representing IIc. Figure 8 shows a discolored area with converging folds representing a IIc cancer surrounding a deeper central ulceration, making IIc+III. Figure 9 shows a close view of an ulcer demonstrating an apparently benign ulcer. However, a more distant view (Figure 10) demonstrates a shallow depression surrounding the benign-appearing ulcer, suggesting this lesion to be malignant, namely III+IIc-type of early gastric cancer.

6.7. Illustrative Cases

6.7.1. Case 1. A 28-year-old man presented with mild fasting epigastric pain. Gastroscopy revealed a punched-out ulcer at the angulus (Figure 11). Our endoscopic impression was that the ulcer was undoubtedly benign. However, biopsy from the area of erythema on the anterior aspect of the ulcer

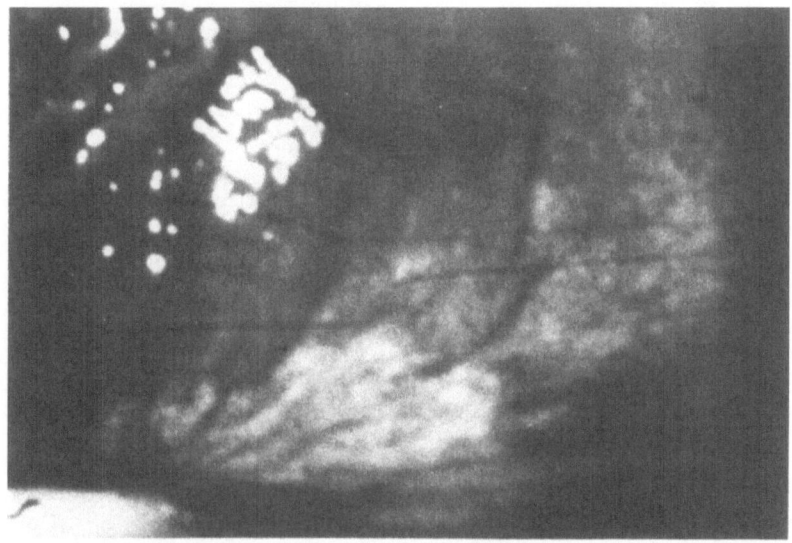

Figure 7. Gastroscopy revealed a discolored area representing IIc..

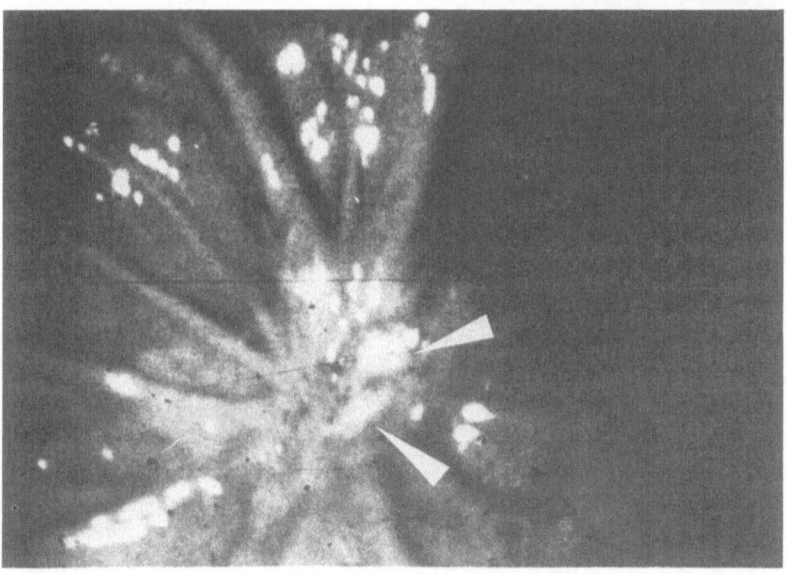

Figure 8. Gastroscopy revealed a discolored area with converging folds representing a IIc surrounding a deeper central ulceration (arrows), making IIc + III.

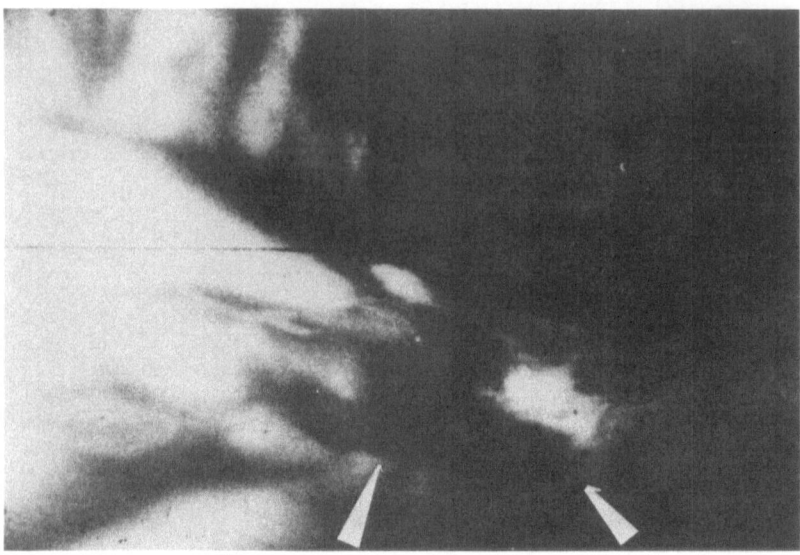

Figure 9. Gastroscopy revealed a close view of an ulcer (arrows) demonstrating an apparently benign ulcer.

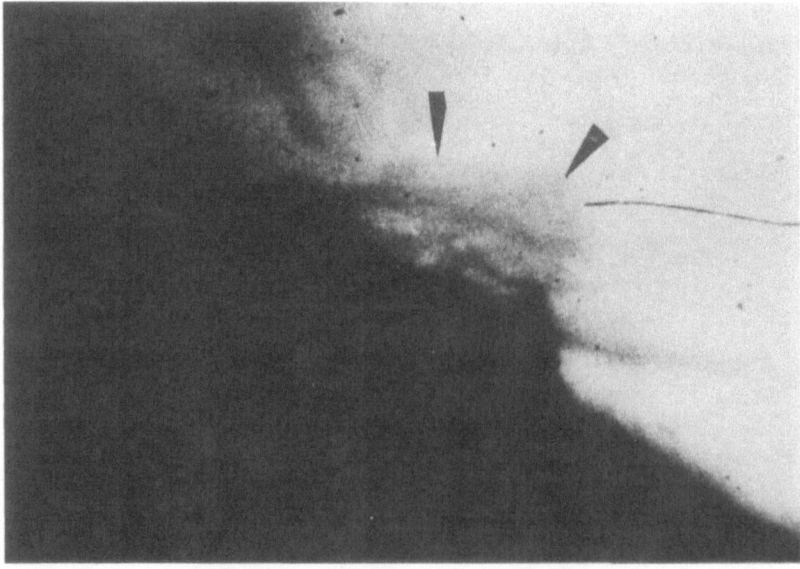

Figure 10. A more distant view of the ulcer in Figure 9 demonstrating a shallow depression (arrows) surrounding the benign appearing ulcer, suggesting the lesion to be malignant, namely III + IIc type of early gastric cancer.

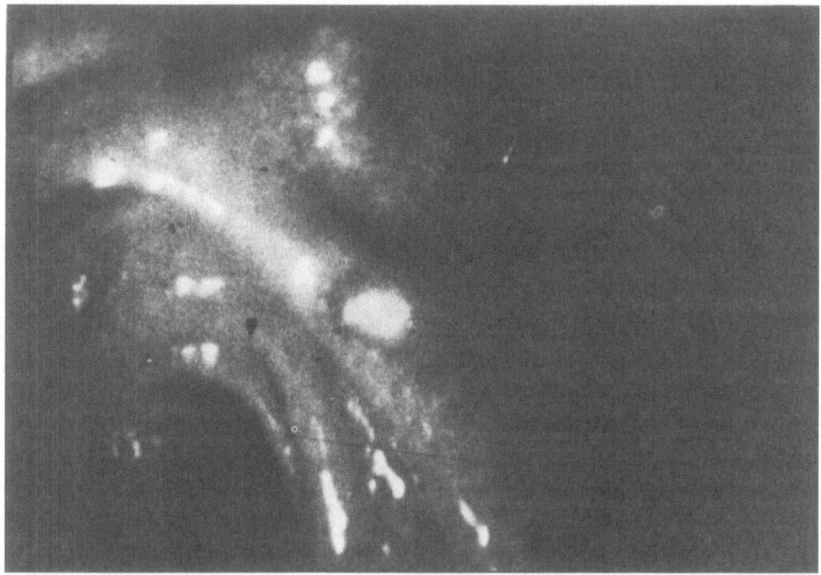

Figure 11. Gastroscopy revealed a punched-out ulcer at the angulus.

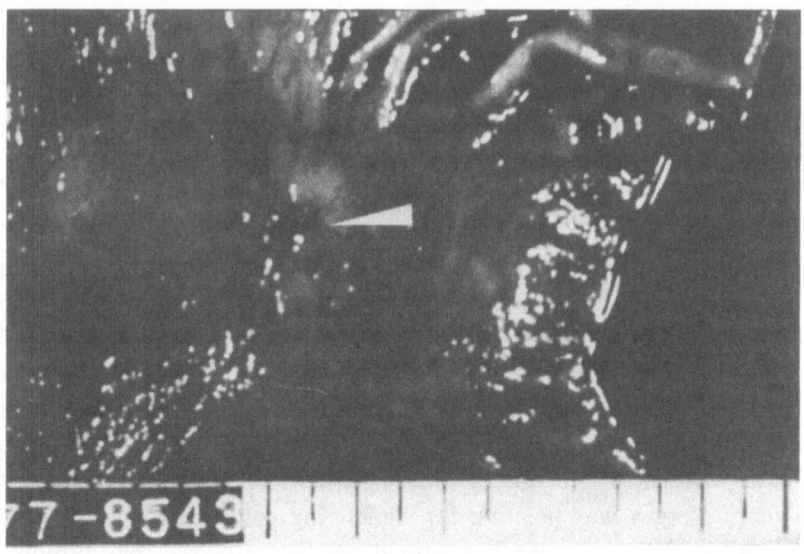

Figure 12. The gross specimen showing the ulcer almost healed (arrow).

revealed signet-ring cells. In the resected specimen the ulcer was almost healed (Figure 12). Histologically, cancer cells were limited to the mucosa (Figure 13). This was our most difficult case in distinguishing a small type IIc area at the margin of a deeper ulcer crater that appeared benign.

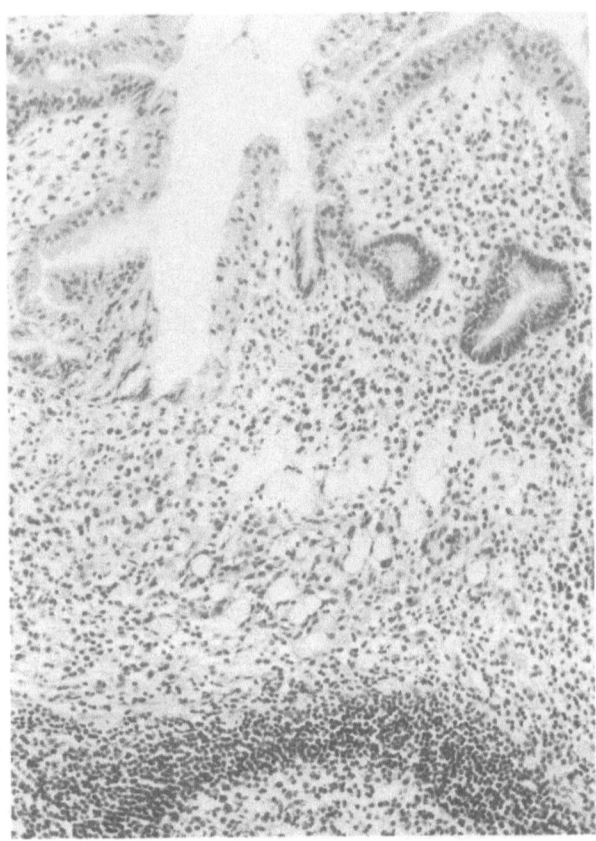

Figure 13. Cancer cells of signet-ring and presignet-ring types are limited to the lamina propria.
HE × 137.

6.7.2. Case 2. A 49-year-old man who had had a long history of gastric
ulcer presented with a recurrent fasting epigastric pain in August 1979.
Gastroscopy on admission revealed a peptic ulcer at the angulus. After 6
weeks of cimetidine treatment the ulcer showed almost healing. Two months
after discharge gastroscopy showed relapsing of the ulcer with an irregular
upper margin (Figure 14). A III + IIc early cancer was suspected. Endoscopic
biopsy was performed and one of four specimens taken from the four sectors
of the ulcer margin was positive for signet-ring cells. Gastrectomy was performed and cancer cells were confined to the mucosa. No lymph node
involvement was found.

The author would like to emphasize the importance of identifying a IIc area
at the margins of a deeper ulcer to distinguish a depressed type of early
gastric cancer from a benign peptic ulcer. In addition, it is important that
biopsy be performed earlier during the period of follow-up of even benign-
appearing lesions in order to avoid delay in appropriate treatment.

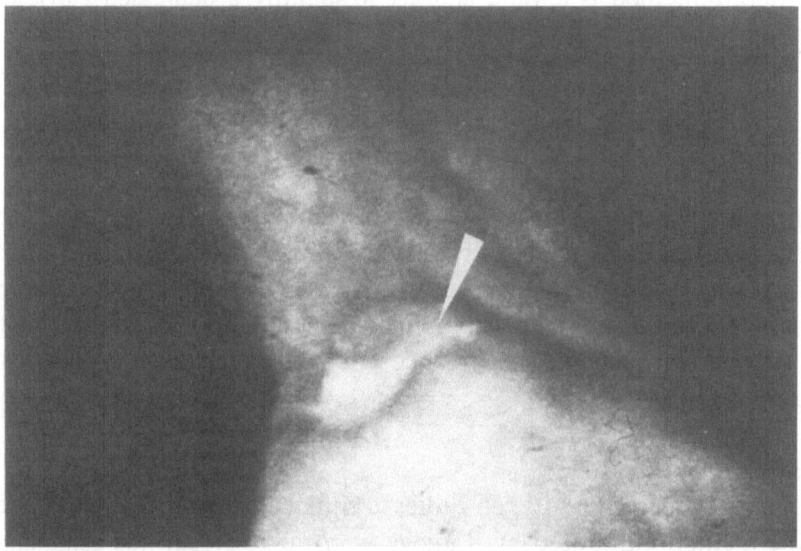

Figure 14. Gastroscopy revealed relapsing of ulcer with an irregular upper margin (arrow), suggesting a suspicion of III+IIc type early cancer.

6.8. Endoscopic Dye-Scattering Method

A small malignant gastric cancer may be overlooked by ordinary endoscopic examination. In an attempt to make such lesions conspicuous, a dye-scattering method with methylene blue was introduced by Yamakawa *et al.* in 1966 [21].

To obtain adequate staining, a proteolytic enzyme solution is initially given orally to the patient to remove gastric mucus covering the surface of the stomach. Then a small amount of 0.5% methylene blue is given orally or through a nasogastric tube. The patient is required to move frequently to spread the dye solution evenly throughout the stomach. Then the gastroscope is introduced into the stomach. Dark blue staining is observed in cancer and intestinal metaplasia. Normal gastric mucosa, peptic ulcer or scar, erosion, benign polyp and gastritis without intestinal metaplasia do not stain. In a depressed type of early gastric cancer such as IIc, this method is very helpful to delineate the contour of a lesion by staining the depression with methylene blue. This helps not only to identify a depressed lesion but also to determine the extent of cancer. Biopsy should be performed on both the inside and outside of the depression.

Suzuki *et al.* [22] reported that of 36 gastric cancers, 33 (92%) were successfully stained and demonstrated that methylene blue is clearly visible in the superficial cells of cancerous lesions and intestinal metaplasia. Thus, a dye-scattering method is a valid adjunct to identify a depressed early gastric cancer and its extent.

7. CYTODIAGNOSIS

As mentioned earlier, biopsy is accurate in the diagnosis of gastric cancer at the first examination. Therefore. cytologic approaches became less important. When a lesion is visualized endoscopically, biopsy is the method of choice for diagnosis. Those lesions with a proximal stricture through which the fiber-scope cannot reach should be brushed to make a cytological diagnosis of gastric cancer [17].

7.1. Brushing Technique

Because of the complexity of earlier technique, a gastric lavage cytology brushing method introduced by Kameya *et al.* in 1964 [23] was established at the Gastrointestinal Endoscopy and Cytology Laboratories, University of Chicago in August 1968 [24]. After a lesion has been brought into the center of a visual field on gastroscopy, a nylon brush is introduced through a biopsy channel and advanced to the lesion. Bleeding is usually seen at the site or in the vicinity of the lesion after successful brushing. The material is smeared on glass slides immediately after withdrawing the brush. Fixation, staining and reading are subsequently made.

Since June 1970 we have been employing a brushing technique through fiberoptic instruments in the following circumstances [25, 26]: (1) cases with negative biopsy results; and (2) the presence of a marked stenosis which does not allow the biopsy forceps to reach the site of the tumor itself under direct vision. Thus, brushing cytology plays a supplementary role to biopsy in many cases. This technique is particularly useful for the diagnosis of carcinoma of the cardia of the stomach with a marked stricture [18]. A combined use of biopsy and brushing made a correct diagnosis in 121 (90%) of 135 patients with carcinoma of the cardia (Table 10).

Although the presence of malignancy is quite probable in cases with a marked stenosis in the esophagus or the cardia, the possibility of a benign stricture should first be excluded. A definitive histological diagnosis should be made to facilitate the choice of appropriate treatment on the basis of the cellular type. Therefore, it is especially important to obtain a positive brushing result in cases with negative biopsy in order to initiate an appropriate therapeutic approach for a juxtacardial lesion suggestive of malignancy. Cytology is more accurate than biopsy in gastric cancer involving the cardia and also is more reliable in stenosing tumors as reported by us [18, 26] and by Witzel *et al.* [27]. A combined use of biopsy and brushing raised diagnostic

Table 10. Results of brushing cytology in 135 patients with carcinoma of the cardia — June 1970 to Dec. 1976.

Brushing	Biopsy	No. patients
Positive	Positive	81
Positive	Negative	23
Positive	Not done	2
Negative	Positive	15
Negative	Negative	14

Brushing positive	106/135 (78%)
Biopsy positive	96/133 (72%)
Brushing and/or biopsy positive	121/135 (90%)

accuracy approximately 20% in gastric cancer involving the cardia or the lower esophagus in cases showing a mucosal elevation, thick folds or a tight cardia stenosis on esophagoscopic examination [18]. Therefore, the brushing technique is especially recommended for use on such occasions.

8. HEALING OF ULCERATION IN GASTRIC CANCER

There has been controversy on the malignant transformation of a benign peptic ulcer of the stomach. In 1940, Mallory [1] reported four cases of ulcer cancer which had shown a healing tendency. In 1944, Palmer and Humphreys [28] also reported the role of peptic digestion in ulceration in preexisting carcinoma that could heal completely with medical treatment.

In 1960, Murakami [29] pointed out that there seems a life cycle of ulceration, healing and recurrent ulceration for malignant ulcers, especially in early gastric cancer and later termed the course as 'malignant cycle.'

From December 1964 to December 1974, 13 patients with gastric cancer were followed up for more than 6 months with the initial diagnosis of a benign gastric ulcer [30]. Nine of the 13 lesions demonstrated the so-called 'malignant cycle' during the follow-up period (Table 11). With regard to the depth of these lesions, three were intramucosal cancers, two invaded the submucosa and four were advanced cancers with involvement of the propria muscle. It is also interesting that all of the signet-ring cell carcinomas and all poorly-differentiated adenocarcinomas showed a malignant cycle. These lesions are very similar to benign peptic ulcers in clinical symptoms, gross type and location. A peptic etiology for the ulceration is suggested by the presence of acid secretion in all the six patients examined in our series. Sakita

Table 11. Malignant cycle.

Number of cases	9 (13)
Depth of cancer	
m·	3 (6)
sm	2 (3)
pm	4 (4)
Histologic type	
signet ring cell	3 (3)
poorly diff.	3 (3)
well diff.	3 (3)
mod. diff.	0 (2)

( ) Total number.

et al. also noted that all their patients showing a malignant cycle of ulceration demonstrated acid secretion [31]. With the progress in biopsy technique, a delay in the diagnosis of such malignant ulcers showing a healing tendency has been reduced.

8.1.1. Case. A 59-year-old man presenting with epigastric pain followed by hematemesis was treated as a benign peptic ulcer for three months in 1963. In may 1969, the patient developed epigastric pain and upper gastrointestinal series revealed a niche on the lesser curvature of the lower body which was thought to be benign (Figure 15). Gastroscopy demonstrated an ulcer with whitish exudate, also appearing benign (Figure 16). Four months later in September 1969, The ulcer almost healed with converging folds. Gastroscopy demonstrated a tiny ulcer at that time (Figure 17). In January 1970, the ulcer recurred on the lesser curvature of the lower body (Figure 18), again appearing benign, and healed in three months. In May 1970, the ulcer recurred, appearing irregular in shape with disrupted converging folds (Figure 19). The ulcer base was smooth but the margins were irregular and slightly depressed in the vicinity of a whitish base. A III+IIc type early gastric cancer was suspected. Biopsy was positive for signet-ring cells. Gastrectomy was performed but it was still difficult to make a diagnosis of gastric cancer, even from the gross specimen, which did not show characteristic features of malignancy. Histologically, signet-ring cell carcinoma was found.

As shown in this case, complete or considerable healing is not a criterion for benignity of an ulcerated lesion, which phenomenon has also been described in the western literature [32].

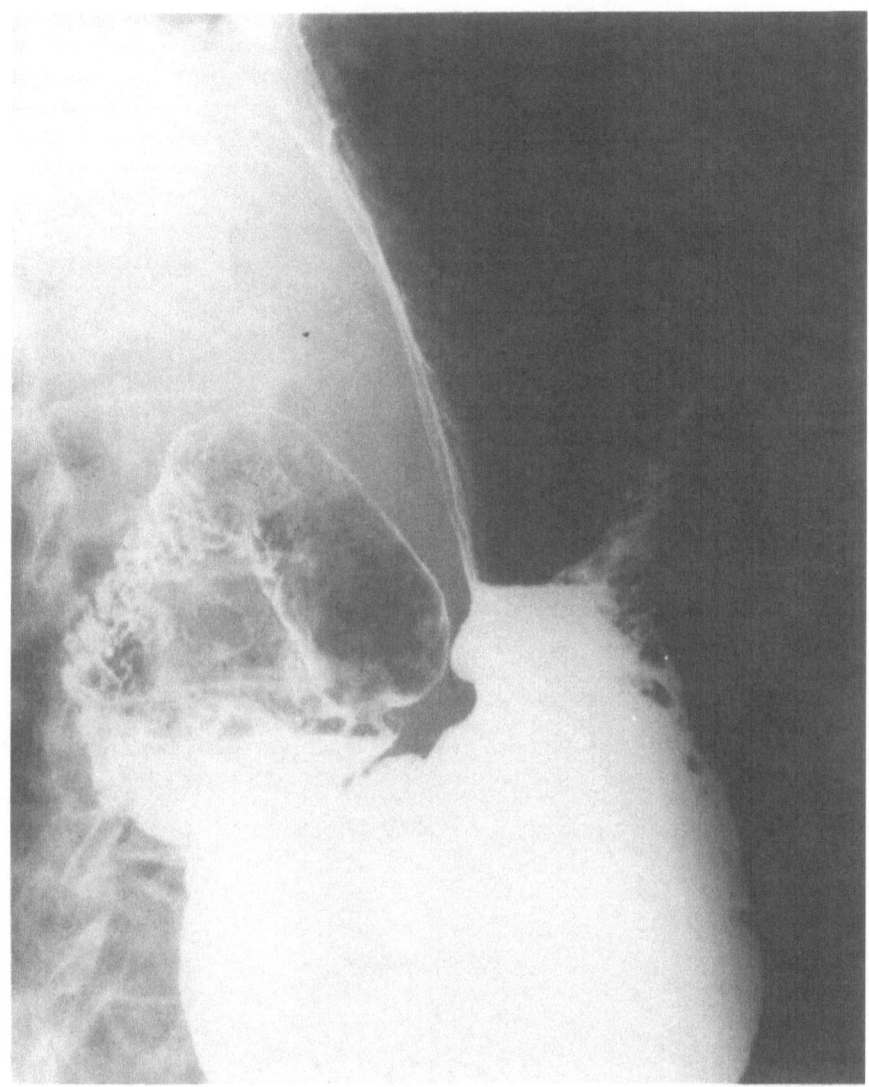

Figure 15. UGI series revealed a niche on the lesser curvature of the lower body which was thought to be benign.

9. SMALL CANCER OF THE STOMACH

A recent advance has been in detection of small gastric cancers, the so-called 'microcarcinoma.' A small lesion is likely to ˙be an early cancer, although even a large lesion can still be early on rare occasions. Our current efforts center on improving detection of 'microcarcinoma.'

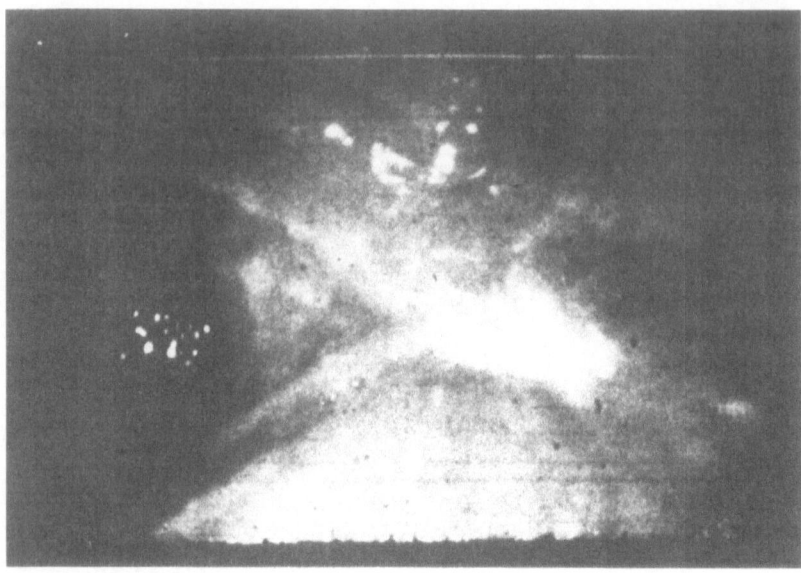

Figure 16. Gastroscopy demonstrated an ulcer with whitish exudates, appearing benign.

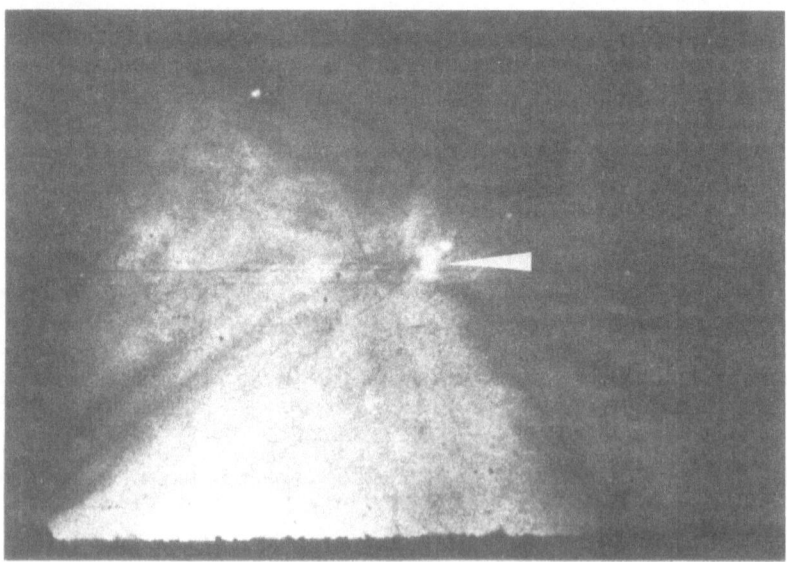

Figure 17. Gastroscopy demonstrated an almost healed ulcer (arrow).

During a 12-year period from 1965 to 1977, 'microcarcinoma' of the stomach less than 1 cm in size on the gross specimen was found in 19 (3.9%) of 484 patients with early gastric carcinoma operated on at the Aichi Cancer Center Hospital [33].

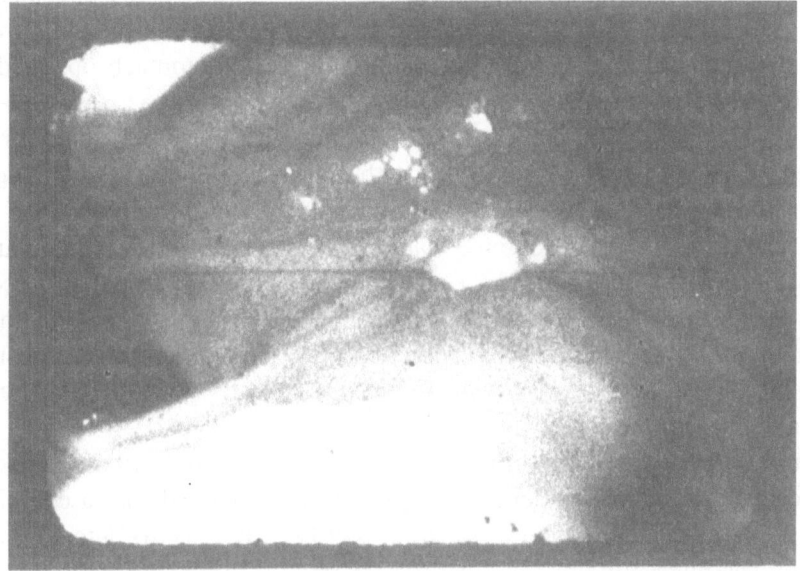

Figure 18. Gastroscopy revealed the ulcer recurred, still appearing benign.

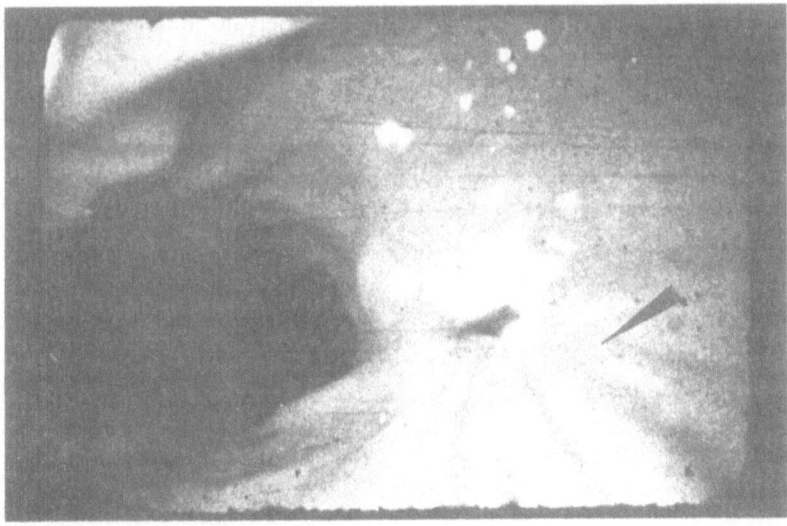

Figure 19. The recurred ulcer was irregular in shape and the converging folds appeared disrupted (arrow).

Three asymptomatic patients were suspected to have a small lesion by mass screening X-ray examination of the stomach. Three asymptomatic and six symptomatic patients came to the outpatient clinic to undergo a thorough examination of the upper gastrointestinal tract. Three were thought as follow-up to have a benign lesion (polyp or peptic ulcer). Two patients developed a second lesion during the follow-up of a benign disease. In the remaining two, a second tumor was incidentally found on the resected stomach operated on for early gastric carcinoma.

There were 13 symptomatic and 6 asymptomatic patients. The former included 10 with epigastric pain and 3 with epigastric fullness. X-ray diagnosis was correct in only three (16%), probably benign in nine (47%) and normal in seven (37%). Endoscopic diagnosis was correct in six (32%), suspicious of malignancy in eight (42%) and benign in five (26%). An endoscopic biopsy established a diagnosis of cancer in 15 of 17 patients on the initial examination. A repeat biopsy was required in two patients to make a positive diagnosis. Regarding the gross type, IIc was seen in ten (53%), IIa in seven (73%) and IIa+IIc in two.

Roentgen diagnosis was less reliable than endoscopy, which could pick up an abnormality in all the patients. It is, therefore, concluded that a combined use of X-ray and endoscopic examination will be necessary to detect a small lesion of gastric carcinoma and early performance of biopsy will make a definitive diagnosis.

A representative case is presented. A 56-year-old man presented with epigastric pain. Upper gastrointestinal series revealed no abnormality. However, gastroscopy revealed a small irregular depression on the greater curvature of the antrum, which was thought to be a IIc lesion (Figure 20). Biopsy was

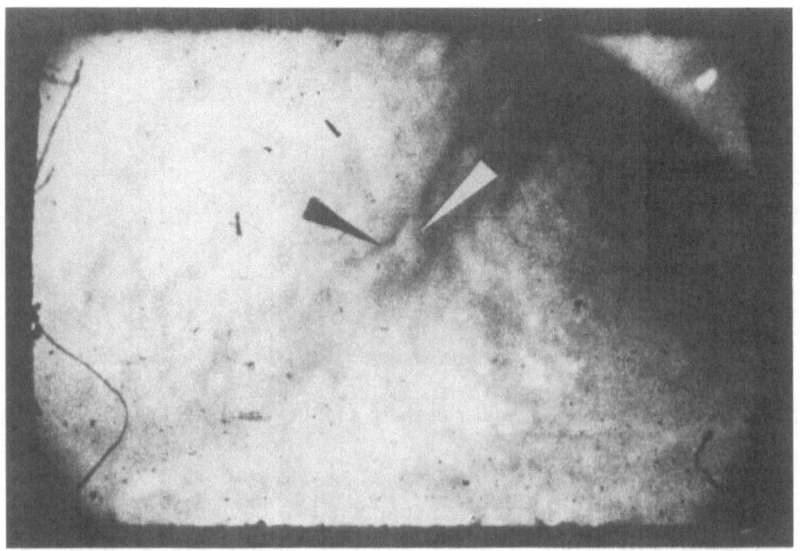

Figure 20. Gastroscopy revealed a small irregular depression (arrows) on the greater curvature of the antrum, which was thought to be a IIc lesion.

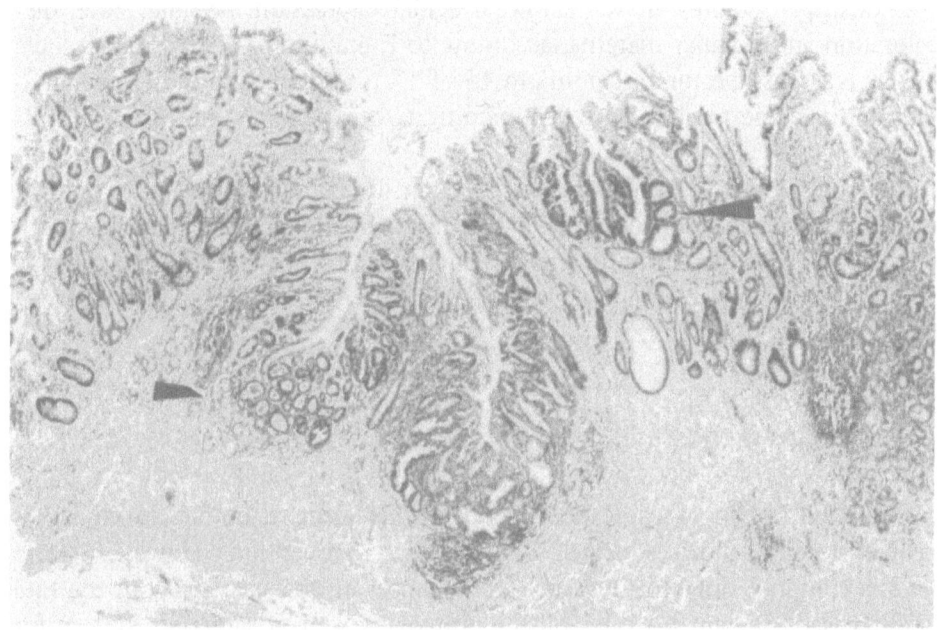

Figure 21. Microscopic photograph revealed a minute focus (arrows) of well differentiated adeno-carcinoma without invasion to the muscularis mucosae. HE×30.

positive for well-differentiated adenocarcinoma. The patient underwent a distal hemigastrectomy and the gross specimen showed a 3×3 mm shallow depression. Histologically, it was a well-differentiated adenocarcinoma without invasion of the muscularis mucosae (figure 21).

The frequency of 'microcarcinoma' less than 1 cm in size was reported to be 3–13% in a collective review in 1969[34]. It is very important that advanced cancer was seen in 1.5% of such small cancers, which makes efforts to detect such small lesions extremely valuable.

Such a small cancer is sometimes misdiagnosed as a benign disease or is occasionally found as the second lesion during follow-up of a preexisting benign lesion. Even a benign lesion should be followed up very carefully to avoid a misdiagnosis, especially in patients at high risk for gastric cancer, namely patients over the age of 40 or with a family history of gastric cancer, or members of a race with high incidence. In our series, six of 19 patients (30%) were asymptomatic. Thus, a smaller lesion has more chance to be asymptomatic.

Endoscopy was superior to radiologic examination as a diagnostic method for detecting a small cancer because it could indicate some abnormalities in all the lesions in our series. A differential diagnosis from benign disease was not very easy even by endoscopic examination. A correct interpretation was made in only 30% of the cases in our series.

Endoscopic features are a shallow, irregular depression, irregular base, discoloration and nodular margins, according to Fukutomi *et al.* [35]. Endoscopic biopsy was positive for carcinoma in 15 of 17 patients at the initial examination and became positive in the remaining two patients at the repeat examination.

Although endoscopic biopsy is decisive, an ill-planned biopsy may result in inadequate visualization because of bleeding: to establish the diagnosis with one biopsy specimen. Improvements of biopsy techniques with magnifying observation or dye-scattering techniques emphasizing the surface features can be expected in the future.

10. MASS SCREENING FOR GASTRIC CANCER

Detection of early gstric cancer has been increasing at outpatient clinics as people become more educated about cancer prevention. However, early lesions comprise only 15–20% of gastric cancer at present. How can the rate be increased? In Japan, we have been employing a mass screening system for detection of gastric cancer mainly in asymptomatic populations since 1960, using a bus equipped with an X-ray machine for an indirect barium meal study.

Mass screening by a radiologic method was first attempted in the United States a long time ago [36–38] but did not last long due to both financial reasons and rapid decline in the incidence of gastric cancer in the United States. A similar idea occurred later to the Japanese, who have had a very high incidence of gastric cancer in the past 30 years. Mass screening employing X-ray methods has rapidly expanded throughout the country and is currently contributing greatly to early detection of gastric cancer in Japan. In 1975, 3,000,000 people underwent gastric mass screening and of these, 3022 were found to have gastric cancer, including 934 with early cancer [39].

10.1. Method

The branch of Japanese anticancer society in each prefecture has its own bus equipped with X-ray instruments. Each morning a bus can deal with 50–60 subjects for X-ray examination of the stomach in a certain factory or town.

250 ml of barium and gas-producing agent are given to take double contrast X-ray films. Each examination finishes in 3–4 minutes after taking six films of the following:
1. Mucosal folds in supine position.
2. Mucosal folds in prone position.
3. Double contrast method in supine position.

4. Barium filling in prone position.
5. Barium filling in upright position.
6. Barium filling in right oblique, upright position.

Presently, these six exposures are thought to be appropriate to cover the entire stomach after detailed assessment.

10.2. Results

Ten to fifteen per cent of the subjects examined are recalled for further evaluation. The method for the second check is based on the finding on mass screening X-ray films and is usually endoscopic examination. At the same time, endoscopic biopsy is done for a suspicious lesion. X-ray examination is not often employed as a detailed procedure of evaluation.

Gastric cancer is detected in an average of 0.5% of all examinees in this mass screening method. In 1975, early cancer accounted for 31% of all gastric cancer in an overall series throughout the country [39]. However, the frequency of early cancer is only 13% among all the gastric cancers treated at the Aichi Cancer Center Hospital, Nagoya, Japan.

According to Kaneko et al. [40], the five-year survival rate for gastric cancer was 53.4% in patients from mass screening and 27% in patients found at the clinics. In advanced gastric cancer, the five-year survival rate was 29% in mass screened patients compared to 24% in hospitalized patients. The rate of early cancer reported by Kaneko et al. was 42.6% in mass screening group and 22.7% in hospitalized patients with gastric cancer [40]. At the ACCH, the rate was less than 10% in the initial period (1965–1966) but was raised more than 10% after 1967, the highest being 18.8% in 1968. The mean value was 13.1% during the period 1965–1977 (Table 1).

To increase the finding of early gastric cancer in the future, screening to bring such patients to the hospital should be expanded or the rate will never go up to 20%. Once such patients visit the hospital, early cancer will be readily recognized by currently available diagnostic procedures such as double contrast X-ray examination, endoscopy, cytology and biopsy.

The age at the diagnosis of gastric cancer is generally younger in the mass screening group than in hospitalized patients [41]. This suggested that if those patients detected in mass screening did not take a mass screening examination, they would develop subjective symptoms within a certain period and visit a clinic some years later.

10.3. Problems to be Resolved in Mass Screening

In Japan, a mass screening program for detection of gastric cancer has been supported by the Japanese government as a public health policy. Nevertheless, the population undergoing the survey is not over 10% of those over the age of 40. It is evident that this policy cannot be nationwide even for the Japanese people, who suffer from a high incidence of gastric cancer.

This method can deal with a number of subjects for a short time, but causes a considerably high false-positive rate. Those examined undergo a psychological burden until the final diagnosis has been made.

The next is a financial problem. Ten to fifteen per cent of subjects examined are sent for further evaluation, which costs $15,000 to detect a gastric cancer and $40,000 to detect an early cancer [42]. Yearly X-ray examination for mass screening may raise a problem of radiation injury in the future.

However, Ichikawa [43] stated that a yearly check-up will give far more benefit than losses from radiation injury in a high-risk population. Hirayama [44] reported that although no increased incidence of leukemia has been observed in the screened group compared to the general population, a careful follow-up would be needed to investigate this problem further.

From the above, it seems very difficult to expand this screening program for many reasons. However, there seems no better way of mass screening than the simple X-ray method currently being done. It will be mandatory to establish a mode of epidemiologic prevention in the near future.

REFERENCES

1. Ewing J: The beginnings of gastric cancer. Am J Surg 31:204–206, 1936.
2. Gutmann RA, Bertrand I, Péristany Th J: Le Cancer de l'estomac au début. Paris: Gaston Doin & Cie 1939.
3. Mallony TB: Carcinoma in situ of the stomach and its bearing on the histogenesis of malignant ulcers. Arch Pathol 30:348–362, 1940.
4. Stout AP: Superficial spreading type of carcinoma of the stomach. Arch Surg 44:651–657, 1942.
5. Tasaka T: Statistics of early gastric cancer in Japan. Gastroenterol Endosc (Tokyo) 4:4–14, 1962.
6. Hayashida T, Kidokoro T: End results of early gstric cancer collected from 22 institutions. Stomach Intestine (Tokyo) 4:1077–1085, 1969.
7. Yamada E, Nakazato H, Koike A, Suzuki K, Kato K, Kito T: Surgical results for early gastric cancer. Intl Surg 59:7–14, 1974.
8. Murakami T: On 'considerations about superficial and early gastric carcinoma'. Stomach Intestine (Tokyo) 4:1186–1188, 1969.
9. Prolla JC: Considerations about superficial and 'early' gastric carcinoma. Stomach Intestine (Tokyo) 4:1183–1185, 1969.
10. Takagi K, Ohashi I, Ohta T, Tokuda H, Kamija J, Nakagoshi T, Maedea M, Motohara T: Historical transfiguration in gastric cancer. Stomach Intestine (Tokyo) 15:11, 1980.
11. Ito Y, Blackstone MO, Riddell RH, Kirsner JB: The endoscopic diagnosis of early gastric cancer. Gastrointest Endosc 25:96–101, 1979.
12. Shirakabe H, Ichikawa H, Kumakura K, Nishizawa M, Higurashi K, Hayakawa H, Murakami T: Atlas of X-ray diagnosis of early gastric cancer. Philadelphia: J. B. Lippincott, 1966.
13. Maruyama M: Early gastric cancer. In: double contrast gastrointestinal radiology with Endoscopic correlation, Laufer I (ed.), Philadelphia: W. B. Saunders, 1979, pp 241–287.

14. Shirakabe H, Nishizawa M, Hayakawa H, Yoshikawa Y, Kurihara M: Clinical diagnosis of early gastric cancer during this thirteen years. Stomach Intestine (Tokyo) 7:295–300, 1972.
15. Kobayashi S, Sugiura H, Kasugai T: Reliability of endoscopic observation in diagnosis of early carcinoma of the stomach Endoscopy 4:61–65, 1972.
16. Kobayashi S, Kasugai T, Yamazaki H: Endoscopic differentiation of early gastric cancer from benign peptic ulcer. Gastrointest Endosc 25:55–57, 1979.
17. Kobayashi S. Yoshii Y. Kasugai T: Selective use of brushing cytology in gastrointestinal strictures. Gastrointest Endosc 19:77–78, 1972.
18. Kobayashi S, Kasugai T: Brushing cytology for the diagnosis of gastric cancer involving the cardia or the lower esophagus. Acta Cytol 22:155–157, 1978.
19. Kobayashi S, Prolla JC, Kirsner JB: Statistics of early gastric carcinoma at an institution in the United States. Stomach Intestine (Tokyo) 6:1337–1341, 1971.
20. Evans DMD, Craven JL, Murphy F, Clesary BK: Comparison of early gastric cancer in Britain and Japan. Gut 19:1–9, 1978.
21. Yamakawa K, Naito S, Kanai T, Tsuda Y, Aoki S: Superficial staining of gastric lesions by fibergastricscope. Proc First Intl Soc Endosc, Tokyo, 1966, pp 586–590.
22. Suzuki Sh, Suzuki H, Endo M, Takemoto T, Kondo T, Nakayama K: Endoscopic dyeing method for diagnosis of early cancer and intestinal metaplasia of the stomach. Endoscopy 5:124–129, 1973.
23. Kameya S, Nakamura S, Mizutani K, Hayakawa H, Higashiyama S, Kutsuna K: Gastrofiberscope for biopsy. Gastroenterol Endosc (Tokyo) 6:36–40, 1964.
24. Kobayashi S, Prolla JC, Kirsner JB: Brushing cytology of the esophagus and stomach under direct vision by fiberscope. Acta Cytol 14:219–223, 1970.
25. Kasugai T, Kobayashi S: Evaluation of biopsy and cytology in the diagnosis of gastric cancer. Am J Gastroenterol 60:199–205, 1974.
26. Kobayashi S, Yoshii Y, Kasugai T: Biopsy and cytology in the diagnosis of early gastric cancer. 10-year experience with direct vision techniques at a Japanese institution. Endoscopy 8:53–58, 1976.
27. Witzel L, Halter F, Gretillat PA, Scheurer U, Keller M: Evaluation of specific value of endoscopic biopsies and brush cytology for malignancies of the esophagus and stomach. Gut 17:375–377, 1976.
28. Palmer WL, Humphreys EM: Gastric carcinoma: observations on peptic ulceration and healing. Gastroenterology 3:257–274, 1944.
29. Murakami T, Urushihara H, Nakamura A, Miyashita H: Gastric ulcer and cancer. Treatment (Tokyo) 42:261–266, 1960.
30. Kobayashi S, Mizuno H, Kasugai T: Gastric cancer detected during follow-up of benign appearing ulcer. Jap J Cancer Clin (Tokyo) 23:951–956, 1977.
31. Sakita T, Oguro Y, Takasu S, Fukutomi H, Yoshimori M: Observation on the healing of ulcerations in early gastric cancer: the life cycle of the malignant ulcer. Gastroenterology 60:835–844, 1971.
32. Stadelman O, Miederer SE, Loffler A, Muller R, Kaufer O, Elster K: So-called early gastric cancer and its detection. Endoscopy 5:70–76, 1973.
33. Sugiura H, Kobayashi S, Kasugai T: Present status in the diagnosis of minute carcinoma of the stomach. Gastroenterol Endosc (Tokyo) 21:717–720, 1979.
34. Takagi K: Macroscopic diagnosis of minute gastric cancer. Stomach Intestine (Tokyo) 5 939–949, 1970.
35. Fukutomi H, Takezawa H: Endoscopic diagnosis of gastric carcinoma less than 1 cm in diameter. Stomach Intestine (Tokyo) 5:961–970, 1970.
36. Roach JF, Sloan RD, Morgan RH: The detection of gastric carcinoma by photofluorographic

methods. Part I. Introduction. Am J Roentgenol 61:183–194, 1949.

37. Roach JF, Sloan RD, Morgan RH: The detection of gastric carcinoma by photofluorographic methods. Part III. Findings. Am J Roentgenol 67:68–75, 1952.

38. Russell W, Swenson PC: Photofluorography for the detection of unsuspected gastric neoplasms. Am J Roentgenol 69:242–267, 1953.

39. Hirayama T: A collective review of gastric mass screening in 1975. Gastric Cancer (Tokyo) 38:8–31, 1977.

40. Kaneko E, Nakamura T, Umeda N, Fujino A, Niwa H: Outcome of gastric carcinoma detected by gastric mass survey in Japan. Gut 68:626–630, 1977.

41. Yamaguchi M, Koshi S: Comparison of gastric cancer cases between those discovered in gastric mass survey and in outpatient clinic and their prognoses. Stomach intestine (Tokyo) 6:751–758, 1971.

42. Hattori K, Suzuki T, Kato Y, Kato H, Nishikawa H: Appraisal of gastric mass screening with reference to cost benefit. Gastric Cancer (Tokyo) 38:71–77, 1977.

43. Ichikawa H: Mass screening for stomach cancer in Japan UICC Technical Report Series 40, 'Screening in Cancer', Miller AB (ed.). Geneva: International Union Against Cancer, 1978, pp 279–299.

44. Hirayama T: Outline of stomach cancer screening in Japan. UICC Technical Report Series 40 'Screening in Cancer', Miller AB (ed.). Geneva: International Union Against Cancer, 1978, pp 264–278.

7. Cancer of the Gastric Stump

KLAUS DAHM

Cancer of the gastric stump in patients previously operated on for benign disease was first mentioned by Balfour[1] in 1922 and was subsequently described after gastroenterostomy by several authors[2, 3]. Today, cancer of the gastric stump is no longer the great rarity it was once considered to be. By 1972, Morgenstern[4] had found more than 1100 cases and, by 1979, about 3000 cases had been published[5]. Although the etiology is not yet known completely, the possible development of cancer within the gastric stump has influenced trends of modern gastric surgery toward more conservative procedures such as vagotomy in the treatment of peptic ulcer. Our present knowledge of carcinoma of the gastric stump is the result of a close collaboration among gastroenterologists, surgeons and pathologists. The facts collected from all these sources have contributed substantially to the pathogenesis of this malignancy.

1. DEFINITION

Cancer of the gastric stump comprises a carcinoma developing after either partial gastrectomy or after gastroenterostomy. Cancer is rarely observed today after gastroenterostomy, because gastroenterostomy as the only procedure has been abandoned in the treatment of ulcer disease.

When defining a cancer of the gastric stump, two criteria should be fulfilled: 1. The previous operation (partial gastrectomy or gastroenterostomy) should have been carried out for benign disease; and 2. To rule out the presence of an occult carcinoma at the time of the first operation, a time interval of at least five years should have elapsed since the original gastric resection.

2. INTERVAL BETWEEN RESECTION FOR ULCER AND MANIFESTATION OF GASTRIC STUMP CANCER

The average interval from the first operation (resection for ulcer) and the time of the diagnosis of the stump carcinoma varied between from 23 to 27 years [6–8]. The mean interval calculated from our patients treated at the University Hospital of Hamburg was 24 years (Figure 1). Several authors have pointed out the increasing risk that threatens the patient with partial gastrectomy from the tenth year onwards [9–11]. The relative risk from gastric stump cancer is very low before the tenth year; it rises to six to eight times as much between the 15th and the 30th year after the intitial operation [12]. Similar results were found using endoscopy as a screening method [13]. According to these findings, one can expect that, after a latency of 20 years or more following partial gastrectomy every fifth patient may develop a cancer of the gastric stump. Several authors noted that the interval was greater for those who underwent surgery at a younger age [10, 14–16].

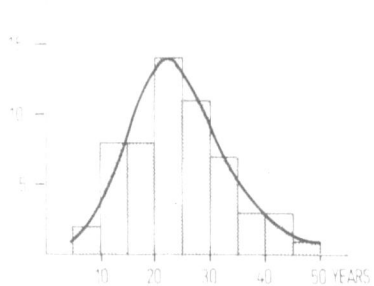

Figure 1. Mean interval between resection for ulcer disease and manifestation of cancer of the gastric stump (*n* = 58; University Hospital of Hamburg).

3. EPIDEMIOLOGY

The frequency of cancer of the gastric stump varies considerably in different parts of the western hemisphere. Cancer of the gastric stump has been reported to occur often in Central Europe [7, 10, 17], especially in the regions of the Alps [13, 18–20] as well as in certain parts of Scandinavia [8, 12, 21, 22]. Contrary to these findings, this special form of malignancy seems to be observed seldom in Great Britain and in the United States [3, 4, 23–27]. Only a few reports, describing individual cases, have been published in France and in Italy [28–30]. In Japan, where gastric cancer is six times more frequent than in the United States, cancer of the gastric stump is not observed more often than common gastric cancer [31]. The epidemiology is influenced not only by the eating habits or possible contact with noxious substances but also by the type of partial gastrectomy employed for ulcer treatment in the respective medical centers. Also, the interest of the gastroenterologists to look for special sequelae such as gastric stump carcinoma in gastrectomized patients fluctuates considerably and may, therefore, alter the true picture.

The age distribution of patients with a gastric stump carcinoma does not differ from that of patients with common gastric cancer. There is a mean age peak of 64 ± 4 years [6, 16, 18, 19]. The mean age of patients treated or seen for common gastric cancer at the University Hospital of Hamburg was 66 years.

Cancer of the gastric stump is much more common in men than in women. The figures reported so far vary between 3.5:1 (male to female) and 10:1 [4, 18, 21, 25, 32, 33]. According to Saegesser [34], the sex ratio is 17:1. The ratio for the common gastric cancer amounts to 1.76:1 in Central Europe [35]. The predominance of the gastric stump carcinoma in the male sex may be explained by the fact that the underlying ulcer disease leading to partial gastrectomy has a higher incidence in men than in women. It is unknown whether estrogen hormones are able to stimulate cytoprotective agents such as prostaglandins in the stomach mucosa of patients subjected to partial gastrectomy.

Blood group A is seen more often in association with gastric cancer than in the general population, and the same is found in patients with carcinoma of the gastric stump [16, 36].

4. OCCURRENCE

4.1. Autopsy Studies

A strictly controlled retrospective study, based on autopsy material, was performed in Oslo 1971 [11]. Among 630 cases of gastric cancer submitted to necropsy, the frequency of previous gastric surgery for ulcer was increased to about six times the frequency among matched controls for those patients operated on 25 years and more before death. The difference was statistically significant ($p < 0.005$). A similar study was made in Helsinki [37]. Of 464 patients dying with gastric cancer, nine had previously undergone a partial gastrectomy, while the respective number among the controls was five. The difference between the two groups was not statistically significant and, therefore, a conclusive answer to the question whether partial gastrectomy implies an increased risk for carcinoma cannot be given from this report.

Two statistical studies based on a large amount of autopsy material have been published in Austria. Among 50 000 autopsies at the University Hospital of Vienna, 363 cases of gastric cancer were observed to have had a partial gastrectomy either according to Billroth II, or to Billroth I or a simple gastroenterostomy [19]. Forty of them showed a cancer of the gastric stump (11%). The respective figure of common gastric cancer in the rest of the 49 637 cases was 5.3%. This ratio demonstrated that gastric cancer was twice as frequent in partially gastrectomized subjects as cancer in the population not operated on. In Innsbruck, similar results were found from a smaller number of autopsies ($n = 9857$) [38]. In this study, the proportion with cancer of the gastric stump was 8.2%, whereas the incidence of gastric cancer in intact controls amounted to 5.4%.

4.2. Follow-up Studies

Retrospective long term follow-up studies of patients after partial gastrectomy were performed in Norway as well as in Sweden [8, 22]. In Oslo, Helsingen and Hillestad [8] drew attention to the fact that it was not the proportion of stump cancer in itself that is deciding but one must compare the observed incidence with the total expected incidence in the whole population. These authors divided the observation period into ten-year segments with men and women considered separately. The incidence of cancer among those whose stomach was partially resected for *gastric* ulcer was three times higher than expected, while in those operated on for duodenal ulcer, the figure was of the order expected. In Sweden, Krause [22] followed up the fate of 362 patients with partial gastrectomy operated on between 1905 and 1933. Of the total, 212 had succumbed, 28 from cancer of the gastric stump (7.7%). In southern Germany, Griesser and Schmidt [7] examined 580 patients several decades after partial gastrectomy for *gastric* ulcer; these authors found a gastric stump carcinoma in 77 (13.3%).

Similar results were obtained by different authors using endoscopic screening methods to follow up patients with partial gastrectomy. Schmid et al. [10] evaluated 24 000 gastroscopies and found 609 patients with a gastrojejunostomy (Billroth II procedure). Of the 609, 39 showed a cancer of the gastric stump (6.4%). The increased incidence of cancer of the gastric stump, compared to the incidence of cancer in the normal population, has been confirmed by other endoscopists [9, 13, 39]. In Switzerland, 6341 patients with partial gastrectomy were analyzed in different centers of endoscopy [13] after a postoperative interval of ten years or more. The overall incidence of cancer of the gastric stump was 15.1%, whereas the incidence among patients not operated on ($n = 29\,361$) was 0.95%. Based on endoscopy, Domellöf and coworkers [9] reported the expected and observed number of stump carcinomas in patients operated on according to Billroth I or Billroth II. They noted that an increased risk is found only in male patients 12 years and more after operation (Figure 2).

In summarizing the results reported in the literature, most authors agree to

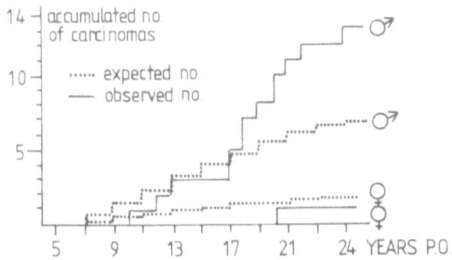

Figure 2. The expected and observed accumulated numbers of stump carcinomas in male and female patients operated on for benign disease (according to [39]).

a causal relationship of partial gastrectomy and increased risk of development of cancer in the gastric remnant. However, some investigators did not observe in their material a higher frequency of stump carcinomas than expected in the normal population with intact stomach [37, 40, 41]. Therefore, the question whether gastric resection for ulcer disease implies an increased risk for subsequent cancer remains a matter of dispute. It seems justified, however, to make the following remarks.

1. Prospective controlled analyses covering 5 to 40 years do not exist. On ethical as well as practical grounds, it seems impossible to accomplish such studies in the future.

2. Autopsy studies as well as endoscopic studies may be involved with the error of a positive selection of the patients.

3. Clinical follow-up studies supplying dates about a possible cancer risk reflect the situation at the point of examination. They show a momentary view and, as all survivors might still be able to develop a stump cancer, published values are the least possible figures.

4. In about 75% of the cases , common gastric cancer is localized to the antrum and corpus regions. When this portion of the stomach is removed because of ulcer disease, the expected frequency in later cancer development should amount to about 25%. However, the opposite seems to occur.

5. ETIOLOGY

5.1.. Duodenogastric Reflux and the Development of Gastric Stump Cancer

Clinical as well as experimental observations have pointed to the important role of duodenogastric reflux occurring in the gastric remnant from certain types of gastroenteric anastomosis. Bile, the main component of the duodenogastric reflux, is known to act as a detergent, thereby damaging the mucosal barrier of the stomach [42]. Atrophic gastritis, intestinal metaplasia, and cystification of the mucosal glands are the alterations typically occurring in

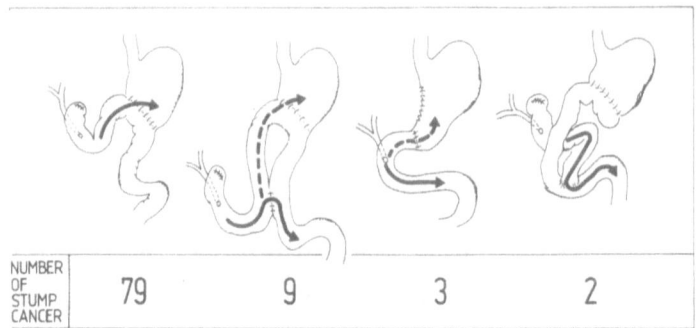

Figure 3. Development of gastric stump carcinoma following different types of partial gastrectomy. Polya type B II resection undergoes unavoidable reflux, Roux's GE undergoes no reflux (*n* = 93; cases were collected from various hospitals of Hamburg).

the vicinity of a gastroenteric anastomosis[4, 39]. Atrophic gastritis is thought to be the main risk factor for the development of gastric carcinoma[43, 44].

Analysis of the different gastroenteric anastomosis, close to which the malignant growth often is observed, has shed some light on the effect of duodenogastric reflux on the development of a gastric stump carcinoma. In the majority of cases, gastric stump carcinoma arises in patients operated on decades earlier according to the Billroth II procedure – Polya-type[45]. When a Polya-type Billroth II procedure is performed, reflux of bile and duodenal secretions regularly pass through the gastric stump, whereas other gastroenteric anastomosis such as Braun's type GE or the Billroth I procedure effect only a partial reflux into the gastric remnant (Figure 3). The high incidence of stump cancer, following a Polya type Billroth II resection, is due not only to the relative frequency of this type of gastric resection but also to the unavoidable reflux after this procedure. Therefore, it seems probable that cancer of the gastric stump develops as the consequence of an unintentional 'experiment' taking several decades to manifest itself.

In animal models, cancer of the gastric stump develops preferentially in the gastric mucosa underlying a continuous duodenogastric reflux[46, 47].

5.2. Development of N-nitroso-compounds in the Gastric Stump

Increasing attention has been paid to the influence of gastric surgery on bacterial flora of the gastric juice[48–50]. Metabolically active bacteria capable of generating nitrite from nitrate and of catalyzing nitrosation may occur in the gastric juice under certain circumstances such as hypochlorhydria or achlorhydria[49]. On the premiss of a high ingested concentration of nitrite the formation of carcinogenic nitrosamines is possible[48]. In a recent study, the concentration of nitrite and N-nitroso-compounds was examined in the fasting gastric juices of 44 patients operated on for ulcer disease [51]. Two and a half years had elapsed since operation. A significant increase of nitrite concentration was found in the gastric juices of subjects undergoing partial gastrectomy according to Billroth I as well as to Billroth II. However, N-nitroso-compounds were elevated only in patients operated on according to the Billroth II procedure as compared to healthy controls. The results of this study demonstrated that the Billroth II type gastroenteric anastomosis creates conditions leading to the formation of potent carcinogens.

5.3. Relationship of Type of Ulcer Disease and Gastric Stump Cancer

The question whether the underlying ulcer disease, i.e. gastric ulcer or duodenal ulcer, affects the late prognosis of patients with partial gastrectomy is still a matter of dispute. The study of Helsingen and Hillestad [8] demonstrated that, in the group of patients operated on for gastric ulcer, the observed frequency of stump cancer was three times higher than expected ($p < 0.001$). In the group operated on for duodenal ulcer, observed and expected frequencies were practically identical. Griesser and Schmidt [7] found among 580 cases who had a stomach resection because of gastric ulcer 77 patients (13.3%) suffering from a stump carcinoma decades later. When the indication for stomach resection was a duodenal ulcer, only 6.25% of the patients developed a cancer. On the other hand, cancer also appeared later in patients with gastric ulcer treated conservatively, the percentage being 10.7%.

Therefore, the possibility has to be considered that gastric ulcer *per se,* apart from any changes caused by the operation, might be a factor in cancer pathogenesis. In other investigations, no difference was shown in the incidence of cancer of the gastric stump as related to the primary ulcer site [11, 32]. Hammar [21], reporting on 56 cases with cancer of the gastric stump, observed a predominance of duodenal ulcer.

6. DIAGNOSIS AND THERAPY

6.1. Clinical and Diagnostic Symptoms

The physician runs the risk of attributing the symptoms of a developing cancer of the gastric stump to a benign disorder of the remaining stomach. Therefore, special attention must be paid to patients who have undergone gastric resection ten years or more earlier and who, after remaining in good health, suddenly develop epigastric disorders, accompanied with a deterioration of the general state of health.

Symptoms are as follows (Figure 4): 1. Loss of weight, pain or feeling of epigastric heaviness, loss of appetite, and fatigue. These symptoms do not differ from those seen in gastric cancer in general. 2. Vomiting of gastric

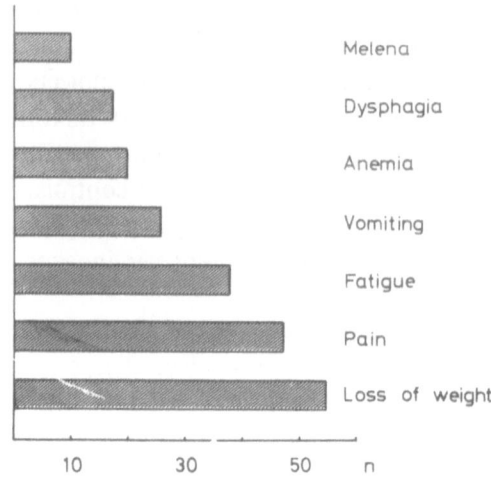

Figure 4. Clinical symptoms in 58 patients with cancer of the gastric stump (University Hospital of Hamburg).

contents suggests malignant obstruction of the anastomosis. When the cancer occupies the proximal part of the stomach as well as the distal esophagus, patients complain of regurgitation, dysphagia and sialorrhea. 3. Anemia is a common symptom whereas massive gastrointestinal hemorrhage with hematemesis and melena is seldom observed. The average duration of these symptoms is 8 months [34].

6.2. Endoscopy

Endoscopic observation of the postoperative stomach is adequately performed by the modern forward-viewing fiberoptic gastroscopes. Gastroscopy not only provides an accurate localization of malignancy (Figure 5) but also offers the definite histological diagnosis by biopsy or by cytology. Due to gastroscopy, an increasing number of cancers of the gastric stump have been detected [9, 10, 26, 41]. Several authors conclude that a higher number of gastric stump carcinomas may be detected at an early stage [10, 41, 52] and that endoscopy of the whole gastric stump, with multiple biopsies and brush cytology from the gastrojejunal anastomosis, is of crucial importance to improve the prognosis of these patients.

6.3. Radiologic Examination

Cancer of the gastric stump is not as easy to recognize for the radiologist as is cancer of the intact stomach. The literature contains numerous references to the limitations of X-ray examination in the diagnosis of cancer in the gastric remnant. Most of the interpretations by X-ray were marginal ulcer or recurrent duodenal ulcer with complications [53–55]. Conventional radiologic

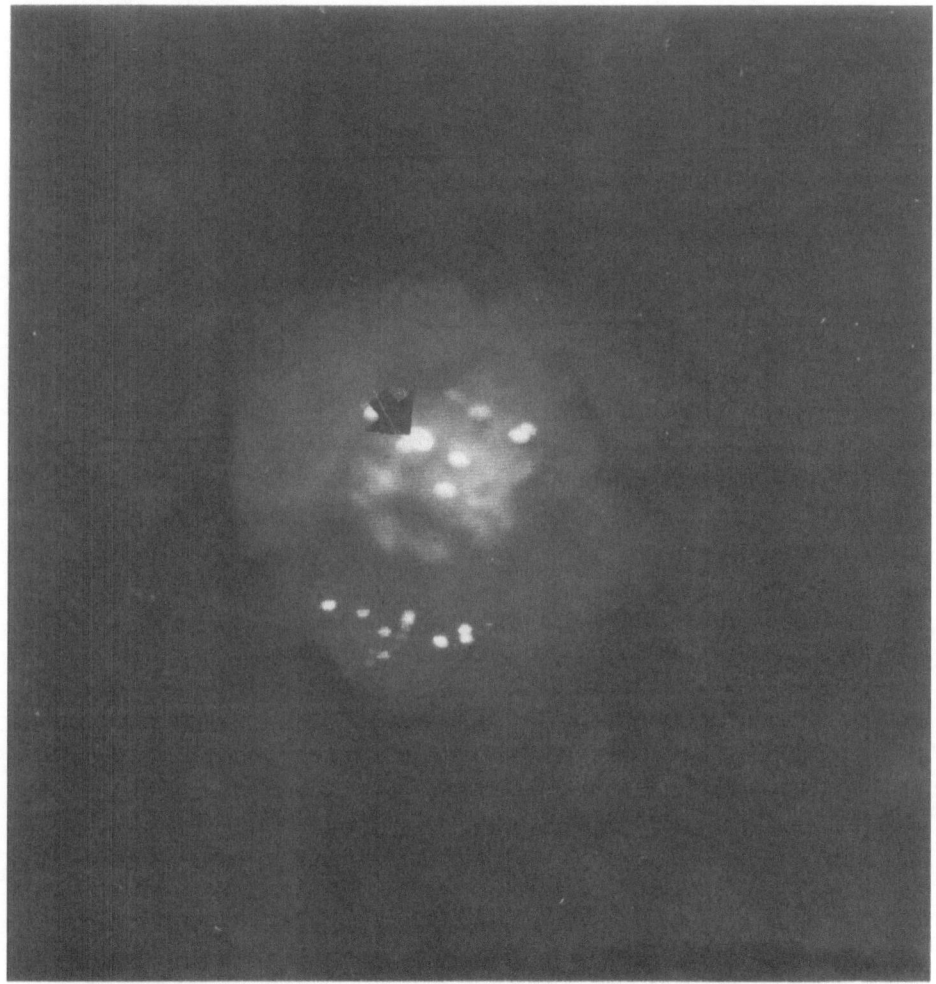

Figure 5. View through fibergastroscope to a tumour (arrow) arising from a gastrojejunal anasto-mosis of a patient with partial gastrectomy (Billroth II).

examination can not confirm the diagnosis in more than 50% of cases [55]. However, the double contrast Roentgen method has been emphasized as helpful in the early diagnosis of cancer of the gastric stump [56]. One of the radiological problems is to know with certainty what operation was in fact originally performed. The malignant lesions are capable of imitating various morphological alterations effected by the previous surgical procedures. In the advanced state, the hourglass stomach is a common feature of cancer of the gastric stump (Figure 6). However, a funnel-shaped rigidity of the wall of the gastric remnant is not at all a definite sign of cancer (Figure 7). In order to

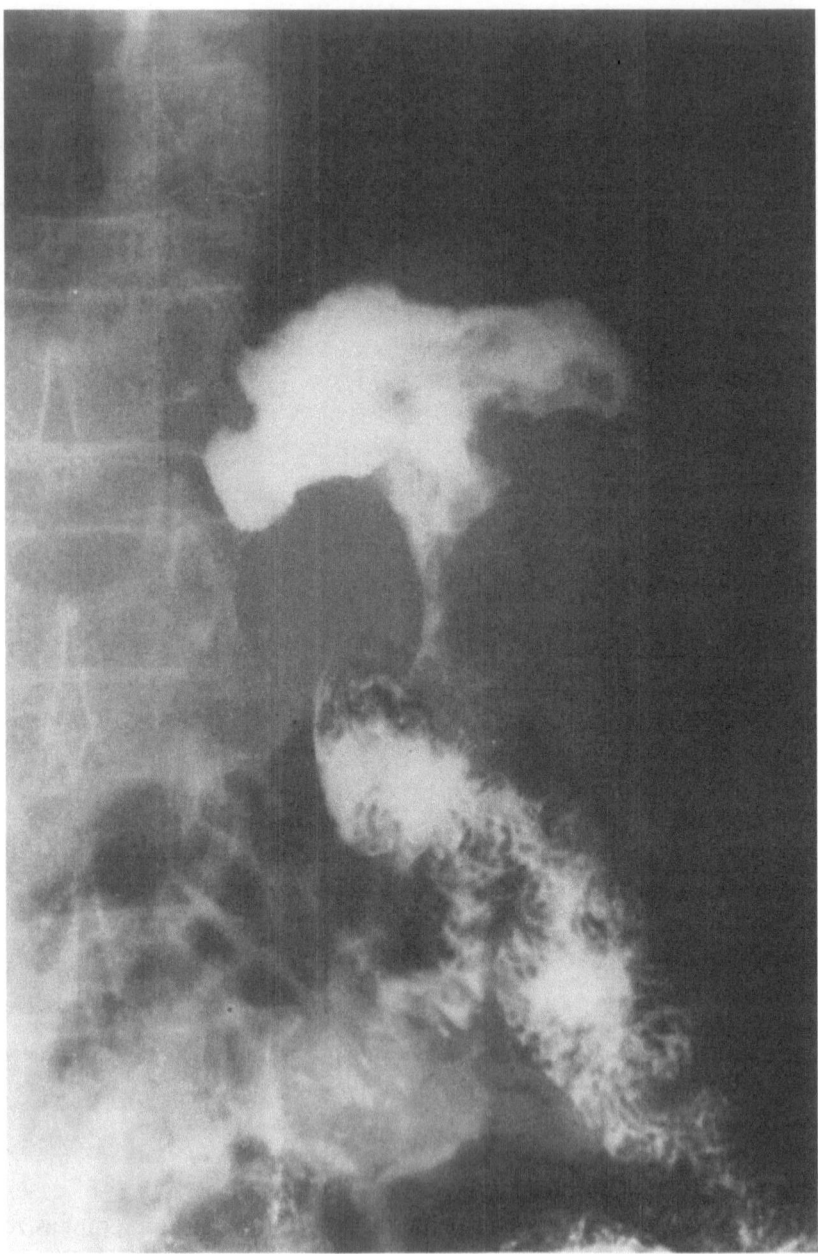

Figure 6. X-ray examination of a gastric stump showing irregular constriction due to a narrowing cancer in the advanced stage.

exclude or to prove a stump carcinoma, we combine radiological examination with subsequent gastroscopy.

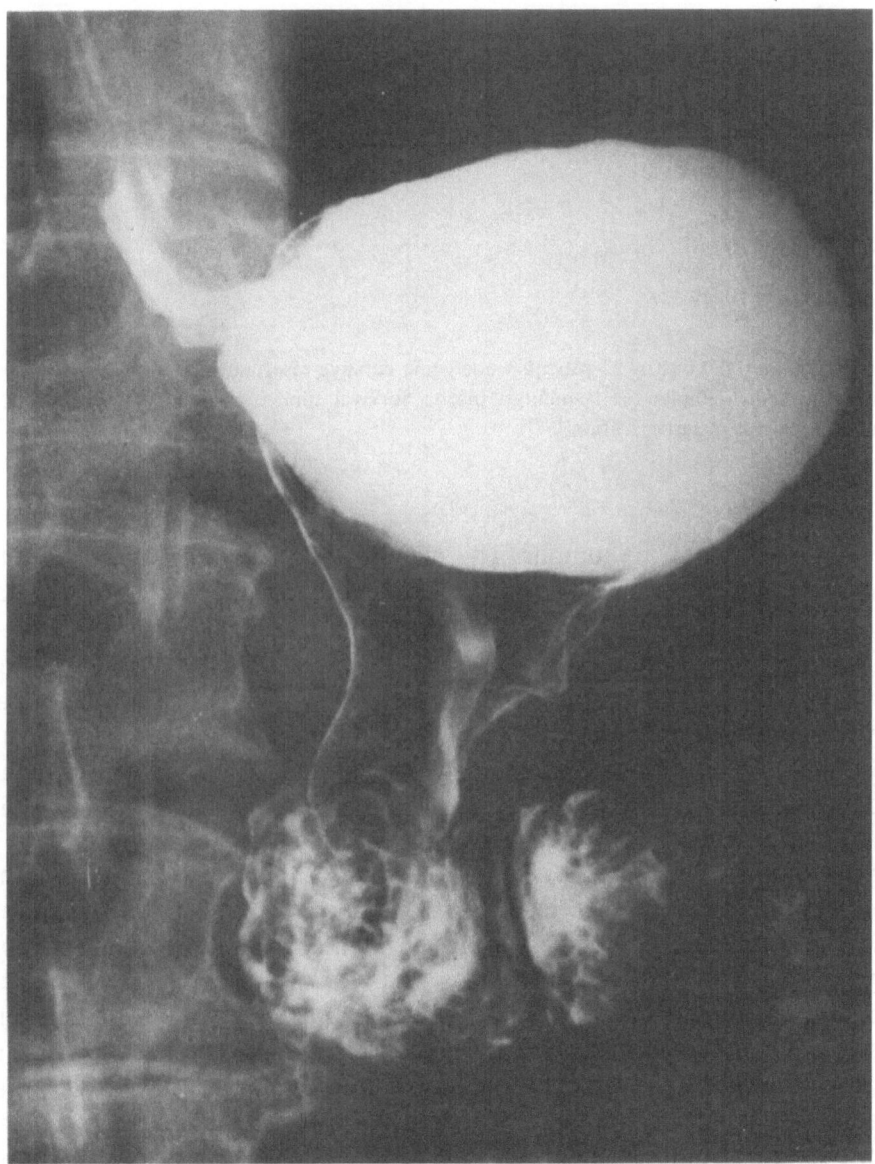

Figure 7. X-ray examination of a gastric stump, 28 years after partial gastrectomy (Polya type B II resection). No tumour was found at laparotomy. The funnel-shaped rigidity of the distal part of the stomach was due to adhesions.

6.4. Surgical Therapy

A considerable number of patients suffering from cancer of the gastric stump are inoperable by the time they come to surgery. Only 22 of 58 patients treated at the University Hospital of Hamburg were eligible for

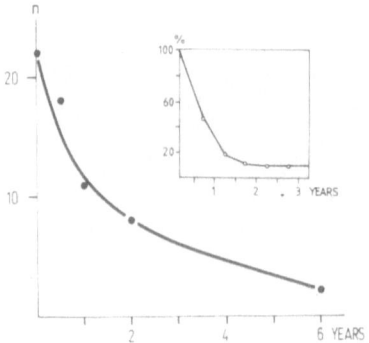

Figure 8. Time of survival of 22 patients undergoing curative resection for cancer of the gastric stump (University Hospital of Hamburg). Insert: Survival time of patients not operated on because of general metastasis (from [57]).

curative resection of the tumour. The majority of cases with a gastric stump cancer are no longer curable due to the existence of visceral or general metastasis, but some can benefit from palliative measures.

The prognosis for cure is poor [4, 16, 24, 57]. Sporadic cases of long time survivors rarely appear in the literature [36, 54, 57]. Figure 8 shows the duration of survival of our patients undergoing curative resection as compared to those not subjected to surgical therapy. Among the 22 of our patients who underwent resection for cure, three are living, apparently free of tumour, six years after extirpation of the cancer of the gastric stump.

Apart from general metastasis, surgical interventions are limited by the advanced age of the patients. Due to the invasive growth of the gastric stump cancer, resection for cure can be achieved in the majority of cases only by removing parts of the adjacent organs such as the pancreas, liver or large intestine. In our patients, a variety of surgical procedures have been performed: Subtotal gastrectomy, 12; total gastrectomy, 10; splenectomy, 5; partial pancreatectomy, 3; resection of the left lobe of the liver, 2; and, partial resection of the large bowel, 5. The continuity of the digestive tract was reconstructed by different methods such as Roux en Y-esophagojejunostomy, interposition of an isolated jejunal loop between esophagus and duodenum, gastroduodenostomy or gastrojejunostomy.

7. PATHOLOGY

7.1. Macroscopic Findings

Carcinoma of the gastric stump is either exophytic or appears as an ulcer. Exophytic tumours are more common. Because of the late onset of symp-

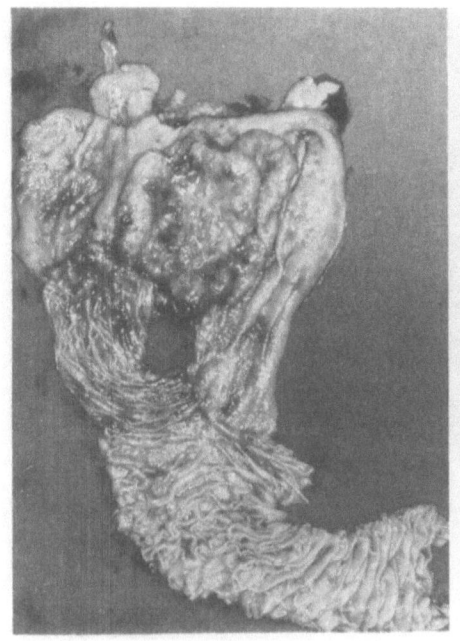
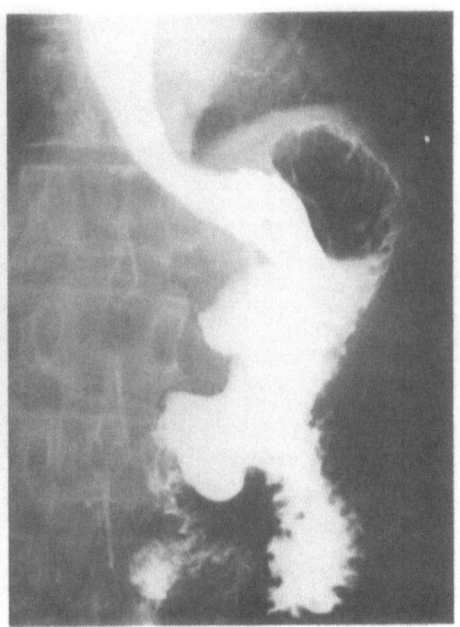

A   B

Figure 9. A. Operation specimen of a huge carcinoma covering the whole gastric stump of a 68-year-old man, 19 years after partial gastrectomy for ulcer. B. X-ray examination of the tumour.

toms, the surgeon often finds huge carcinomas encompassing nearly the entire gastric stump (Figure 9). The direction of the malignant growth is mainly along the minor site of the gastric remnant from distal to proximal. At an early stage, adjacent organs such as pancreas, liver, and colon are infiltrated by tumour. Several authors have focused attention on the resistance of small intestine to invasion by the stump carcinoma [4, 34].

7.2. Localization

Studies concerning the localization of cancer of the gastric stump have pointed to the gastroenteric stoma as a specific area that seems to be particular liable to cancerous changes [4, 22, 26, 33, 46, 57]. Early cancer of the gastric stump arises often at or near the anastomosis [41, 52]. In the University Hospital of Hamburg, seven patients were gastrectomized because of early cancer of the gastric stump. In all but one, early gastric cancer developed near the anastomosis of a Billroth II partial gastrectomy (Polya type) (Figure 10). Hammar studied 65 autopsy specimens and provided strong evidence for a typical site of cancer growth within the Billroth II stoma, the tumour extending towards the posterior wall near the efferent loop [21].

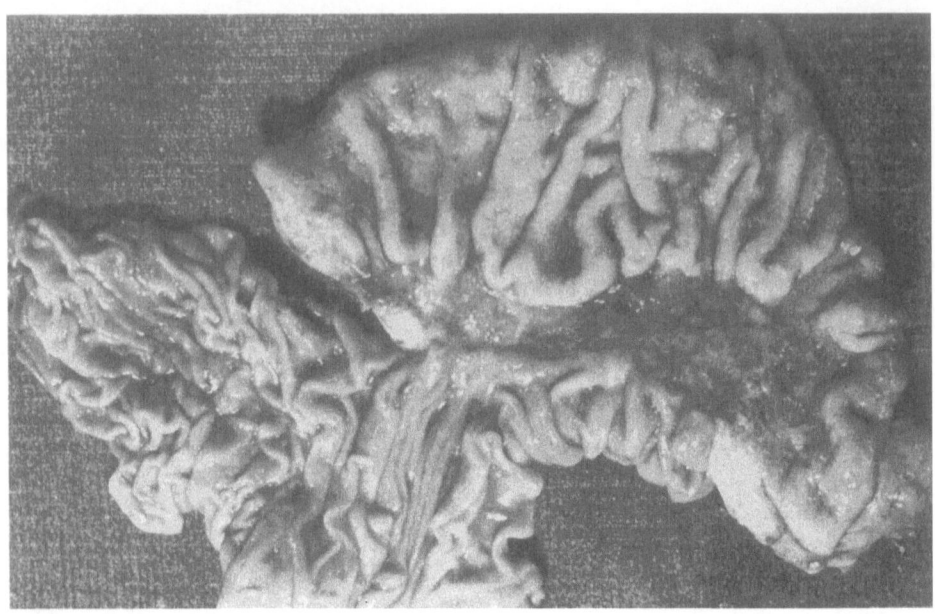

Figure 10. IIc-type of the Japanese classification of early gastric cancer developing in a gastroenteric anastomosis.

7.3. Microscopic Findings

The histology shows all forms of gastric carcinoma. According to our experience, adenocarcinoms form the major group. Beside these, solid as well as anaplastic forms are observed. The new classification of gastric cancer according to Laurèn [58], used more often in recent years, has not shown new findings [59].

7.3.1. Polyps.
More interesting are those changes that might point to an increased risk of cancer development or are reactions accompanied with a gastric stump carcinoma. Polyps are more frequent in the residual gastric remnant than in the intact one [60]. In any case, suspect polypoid findings should be removed by the endoscopist using snare biopsy. Histological examination often shows reactive or regenerative changes of the anastomosis or of the gastric remnant described as foveolar hyperplasia [27, 61], gastritis cystica pseudopolyposa (Figure 11) [4, 62, 63] or regenerative polyps [64]. Malignant transformation has not been demonstrated in these alterations. In contrast to regenerative polyps, adenomatous polyps occurring also in the gastric stump should be regarded as premalignant [65].

7.3.2. Intestinalization.
Another morphologic change, often observed near a gastroenterostomy, is the intestinalization of the gastric mucosa (Figure

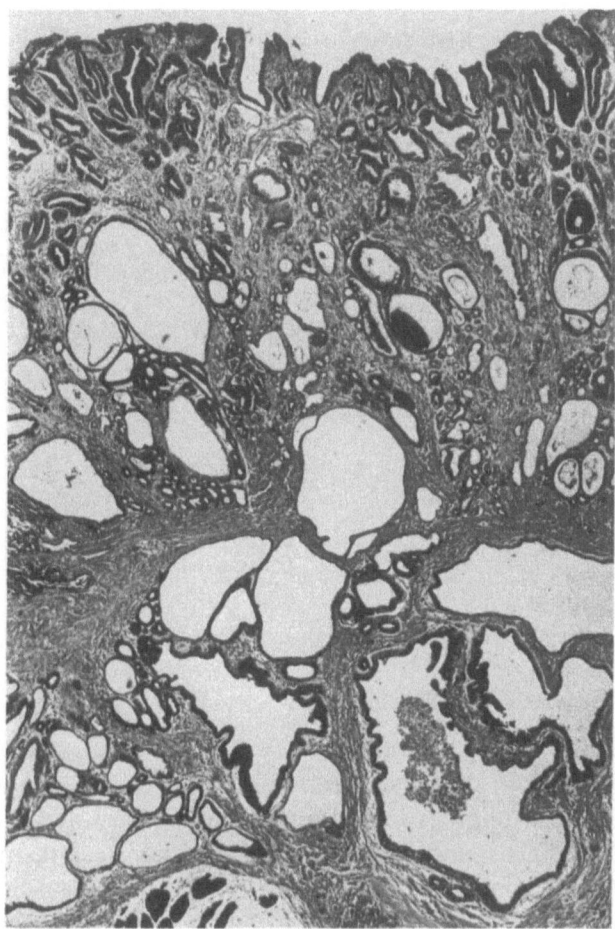

Figure 11. Gastritis cystica polyposa occurring in a gastroenteric anastomosis. Note dilated glands partially dislocated into the submucosa (hematoxylin–eosin, ×40 (from [80]).

12) [4, 64, 66]. Intestinal metaplasia is more frequent following a gastroduodenostomy (Billroth I) than it is after gastrojejunostomy (Billroth II) [64]. Some authors have suggested that intestinal metaplasia bears an increased risk of cancer [67], whereas other point to the fact that goblet cells and Paneth cells are highly differentiated and that carcinoma and intestinal metaplasia are not necessarily correlated [68] (see Chapter 5).

7.3.3. Lipid Islands. Lipid islands, visible as small white or yellow-white patches in the gastric mucosa, are frequently observed in postoperative patients [69]. Histologically, these patches consist of foam cells beneath the surface epithelium. The occurrence of single or multiple islands increases with

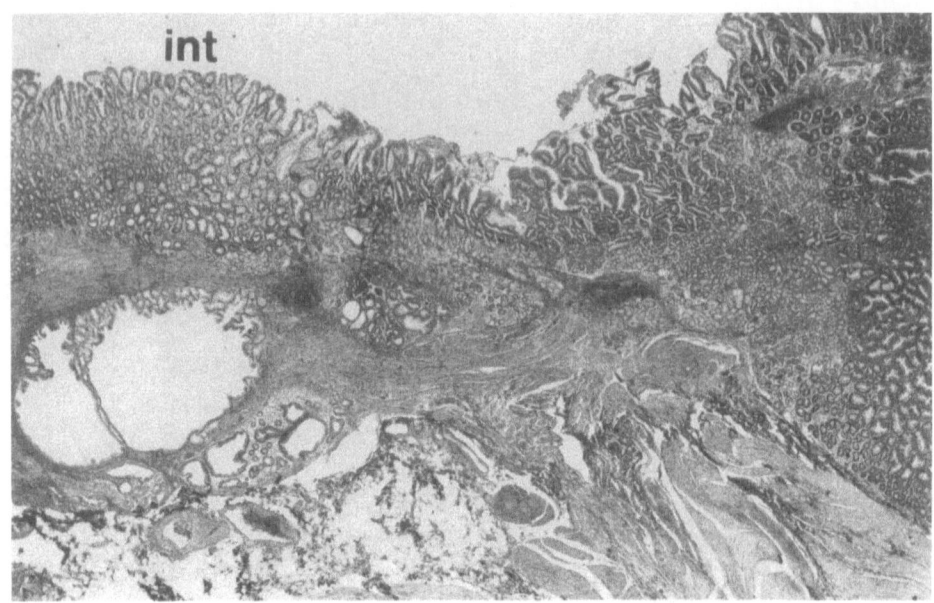

Figure 12. Gastric mucosa showing intestinalization (int), 44 years after gastroenterostomy (hematoxylin–eosin, ×16 (from [80]).

time after operation, independently of the original ulcer disease or the type of operation performed. In diagnosing early gastric carcinoma at gastroscopy in the stomach operated on, it is important for the clinician and the pathologist to be aware of the lipid islands because these alterations can be mistaken for a signet ring cell carcinoma [70].

7.3.4. Dysplasia. Some possible precancerous lesions found in the gastric mucosa are defined as dysplasias (Figure 13) (see Chapters 1 and 5). Dysplasia of the gastric glands is characterized on the basis of cytological as well as structural abnormalities [71]. These are divided into three degrees of mild, moderate and severe dyplasia. Dysplasias are often observed in the neighbourhood of early gastric cancer as well as in the mucosa of a gastric remnant decades after partial gastrectomy [72]. In some cases, they are situated either immediately bordering early gastric cancer or showing transitions to the latter. According to our present knowledge, severe dysplasia of the mucosa of the gastric remnant should be regarded as a possible precancerous lesion. No indication exists for surgical intervention in patients exhibiting severe dysplasia only. However, supervision by gastroscopy is mandatory.

7.3.5. Atrophic Gastritis. Since the extensive studies of G.E. Konjetzny [73, 74], it has been known that chronic atrophic gastritis is a premalignant

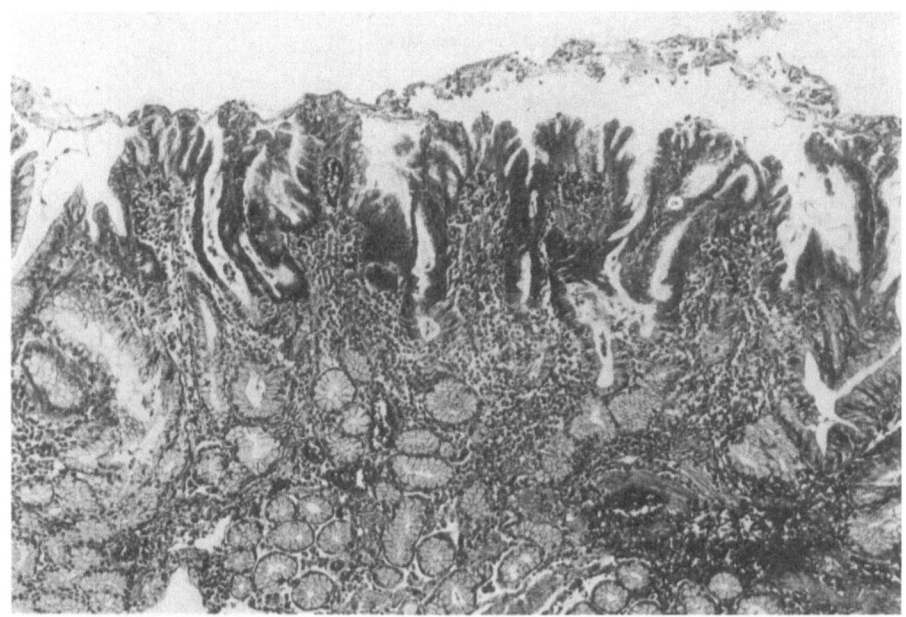

Figure 13. Moderate dysplasia of the foveolar glands in a gastric remnant, 26 years after partial gastrectomy. Note metaplasia of pseudopyloric glands (hematoxylin–eosin, ×100).

condition prone to transform in time into gastric cancer. Partially gastrectomized patients show atrophic gastritis at a higher frequency and to a more severe degree than age-matched controls with intact stomachs [7, 60, 75, 76]. In long-term follow-up studies, patients with chronic atrophic gastritis have a higher incidence of gastric carcinoma than the general population [43, 44]. Although atrophic gastritis is supposed to have an increased risk of cancer development, some authors hesitate to regard it as a precancerous condition leading unavoidably to cancer of the gastric stump [78].

8. EXPERIMENTAL CANCER OF THE GASTRIC STUMP

Many questions concerning the pathogenesis of the gastric stump carcinoma have not been answered by clinical research. Therefore, we looked for an experimental model in order to resolve the following problems: First, is the gastric remnant really more susceptible to cancer development than the intact one? Second, is there any influence of chronic duodenogastric reflux on cancer development?

In the first series of experiments, 66 male Wistar rats were subjected to partial gastrectomy according to either the Billroth I or the Billroth II procedure. These rats, as well as control animals, were fed the carcinogen N-methyl-N'-nitro-N-nitrosoguanidine (MNNG). Of 66 rats, 25 developed carci-

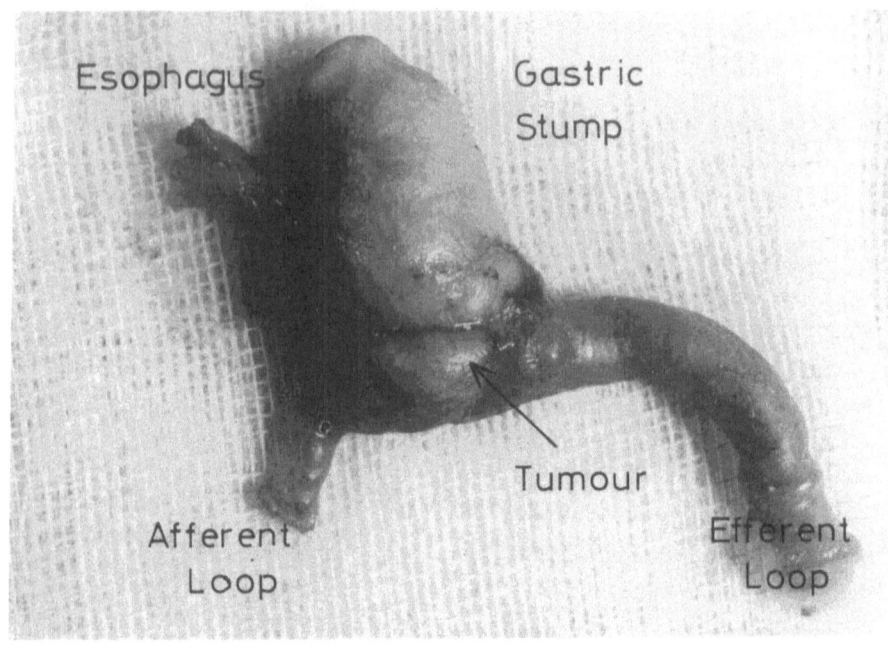

Figure 14. Carcinoma of the gastric stump arising from the gastrojejunal anastomosis of a rat, 31 weeks after daily oral administration of MNNG (from [46]).

noma in the gastric remnant. The tumours were characterized histologically as adenocarcinoma. Mostly, the carcinomas were localized near the gastroenteric anastomosis (Figure 14). The process of tumour development in the partially resected stomach of the rat was completed within 17 to 31 weeks on continuous feeding of MNNG in a concentration of 120 mg/l in the drinking water. Control animals, either with intact stomachs treated with the carcinogen or operated on and kept under normal diet and tap water, showed no development of cancer up to the 31st week. In contrast to these findings, the formation of cancer in the intact stomachs required on average 41 weeks under the same experimental conditions. With regard to the incidence of malignant changes, no significant difference was observed between animals undergoing the Billroth I procedure and those undergoing the Billroth II procedure. The results suggested that the partially resected stomach of the rat is more susceptible to induction of cancer than the intact one. Exposure of the resected stomach to an oral carcinogen (MNNG) induced carcinogenesis predominantly in the anastomotic region [46].

In a second series of experiments, we tried to answer the question whether the duodenogastric reflux has any influence on the malignant cell growth in the gastric stump, especially at the anastomosis. Seventy-two male Wistar rats were subjected to partial stomach resection. A gastroenteric anastomosis (GE) was performed either as short loop anastomosis (Polya type Billroth II; $n = 39$), thus providing a continuous duodenogastric reflux, or as Y-shaped GE (according to Roux; $n = 33$). By the latter technique, bile and pancreatic juices were diverted into the jejunum without coming into contact with the gastric remnant. All animals, including a control group with intact stomachs, were fed MNNG in the drinking water. At autopsy, most of the tumours were found in the animal group subjected to chronic duodenogastric reflux (Polya–Billroth II group). The incidence of carcinomas of the gastric stump was significantly lower in rats without reflux (Roux group or intact control group). The results of these experiments demonstrated that, in rats, the duodenogastric reflux contributed substantially to the development of cancer of the gastric stump[47].

REFERENCES

1. Balfour DC: Factors influencing the life expectancy of patients operated on for gastric ulcer. Ann Surg 76:405–408, 1922.
2. Beatson GT: Carcinoma of the stomach after gastrojejunostomy. Br Med J 1:15, 1926.
3. Nicholls JC: Carcinoma of the stomach following partial gastrectomy for benign gastroduodenal lesions. Br J Surg 61:244–249, 1974.
4. Morgenstern L, Yamakawa T, Seltzer D: Carcinoma of the gastric stump. Am J Surg 125:29–37, 1973.
5. Peitsch W, Becker HD: Was ist gesichert in der Pathogenese und Häufigkeit des primären Carcinoms im operierten Magen? Chirurgica 50:33–38, 1979.
6. Gerstenberg E, Albrecht A, Krentz K, Voth H: Das Magenstumpfkarzinom: eine Spätkomplikation des operierten Magens? Dtsch Med. Wschr. 90:2185–2190, 1965.
7. Grüsser G, Schmidt H: Statistische Erhebungen über die Häufigkeit des Karzinoms nach Magenoperation wegen eines Geschwürsleidens. Med Welt 2:1836–1840, 1964.
8. Helsingen N. Hillestad L: Cancer development in the gastric stump after partial gastrectomy for ulcer. Ann Surg 143:173–179, 1956.
9. Domellöf L, Januger K-G: The risk for gastric carcinoma after partial gastrectomy. Am J Surg 134:581–584, 1977.
10. Schmid E, Vollmer R, Adlung J, Blaich E, Goebell H, Heinkel K, Kimmig J-M, Probst M: Zur endoskopischen Diagnostik des Karzinoms im operierten Magen. Z Gastroent 14:521–530, 1976.
11. Stalsberg H, Taksdal S: Stomach cancer following gastric surgery for benign conditions. Lancet II:1175–1177, 1971.
12. Stalsberg H: Reply of the author. Selected summaries Gastroenterology 62:1276,1972.
13. Clemencon G, Baumgartner R, Leuthold E, Miller G, Neiger A: Das Karzinom des operierten Magens. Dtsch med Wschr 101:1015–1020, 1976.
14. Kivelitz H, Müller E, Kleinschmidt F, Loose D: Das Magenstumpfkarzinom nach Ulkusresektion. Bruns Beitr Klin Chir 220:253–258, 1973.
15. Lüders K, Radomsky J, Ungeheuer E: Magenstumpfkarzinom. Med Klinik 74:91–100, 1979.
16. Terjesen T, Erichsen HG: Carcinoma of the gastric stump after operation for benign gastroduodenal ulcer. Acta Chir Scand 142:256–260, 1976.

17. Dahm K, Werner B: Das Karzinom Im operierten Magen. Dtsch Med Wschr 100:1973-1078, 1975.

18. Kronberger L, Hafner H: Über das primäre Stumpfcarcinom nach Ulcusresektion. Chirurg 39:118-122, 1968.

19. Kühlmayer R, Rokitansky O: Das Magenstumpfcarcinom als Spätproblem der Ulcuschirurgie. Langenbecks Arch Klin Chir 278:361-373, 1954.

20. Schwamberger K, Reissigl H, Troyer E: Diagnose und Therapie des Magenstumpfcarcinoms: Eigene Ergenbnisse. Akt. Gastrologie 5:375-380, 1976.

21. Hammar E: The localization of precancerous changes and carcinoma after previous gastric operation for benign condition. Acta Path Microbiol Scand Sect A 84:495-507, 1976.

22. Krause U: Late prognosis after partial gastrectomy for ulcer. A follow-up study of 361 patients operated upon from 1905 to 1933. Acta Chir Scand 114:341-354, 1957.

23. Eberlein TJ, Lorenzo FV, Webster MW: Gastric carcinoma following operation for peptic ulcer disease. Ann Surg 187:251-256, 1978.

24. Goldenkranz R, Thorbjarnarson B: Carcinoma of the stomach following previous peptic ulcer surgery. New York St J Med 78:733-735, 1978.

25. Klarfeld J, Resnick G: Gastric remnant carcinoma. Cancer 44:1129-1133, 1979.

26. Kobayashi S, Prolla JC, Kirsner JB: Late gastric carcinoma developing after surgery for benign conditions. Endoscopic and histologic studies of the anastomosis and diagnostic problems Dig Dis 15:905-912, 1970.

27. Mitschke H: Pathologisch-anatomische Grundlagen der Krebsrisikoerkrankungen und des Frühcarcinoms des Magens. Chirurgica 49:465-472, 1978.

28. Breger PR, Kerneis JP, Badel Y: Cancer primitif du moignon gastrique après gastrectomie pour ulcère. Ann Chir (Paris) 14:303-309, 1960.

29. Giacosa A, Molinari F, Perasso A, Cheli R: Endoscopic experience in the diagnosis of gastric stump cancer. Front. Gastrointest. Res 5:160-163, 1979.

30. Hivet M, Lagadec B, Gutman R: Cancer d'une ancienne gastro-enterostomie. Sem Hop Paris 48:1265-1267, 1972.

31. Sugimura T: Personal communication.

32. Freedman MA, Berne CJ: Gastric carcinoma of gastrojejunal stoma. Gastroenterology 27:210-217, 1954.

33. Schönleben K, Langhans P, Schlake W, Kautz G, Bünte H: Gastric stump carcinoma — carcinogenic factors and possible preventive measures. Acta Hepato-Gastroent 26:239-247, 1979.

34. Saegesser F, Jämes D: Cancer of the gastric stump after partial gastrectomy (Billroth II principle) for ulcer. Cancer 29:1150-1159, 1972.

35. Frentzel-Beyme R, Leutner R, Wagner G, Wiebelt H: Cancer atlas of the Federal Republic of Germany. Berlin: Springer, 1979, pp 12-13.

36. Saegesser F, Waridel D: Primary cancers of the gastric stump. In: Current problems in surgery, vol 14. Baltimore: Williams & Wilkins, 1970, pp 613-636.

37. Kivilaakso E, Hakkiluoto A, Kalima TV, Sipponen P: Relative risk of stump cancer following partial gastrectomy. Br J Surg 64:336-338, 1977.

38. Hilbe G, Salzer GM, Hussl H, Kutschera H: Die Carcinomgefährdung des Resektionsmagens. Langenbecks Arch Klin Chir 323:142-153, 1968.

39. Januger K-G, Domellöf L, Eriksson S: The development of mucosal changes after gastric surgery for ulcer disease. Scand J Gastroent 13:217-223, 1978.

40. Liavaag K: Cancer development in gastric stump after partial gastrectomy for peptic ulcer. Ann. Surg. 155:103-106, 1962.

41. Osnes M, Løtveit T, Myren J, Serck-Hansen A: Early gastric carcinoma in patients with a Billroth II partial gastrectomy. Endoscopy 9:45-49, 1977.

42. Davenport HW: Destruction of the gastric mucosal barrier by detergents and urea. Gastroenterology 54:175–181, 1968.

43. Siurala M, Varis K, Wiljasalo M: Studies of patients with atrophic gastritis; a 10–15 year follow-up. Scand J Gastroent 1:40–48, 1966.

44. Walker IR, Strickland RG, Ungar B, Mackay IR: Simple atrophic gastritis and gastric carcinoma. Gut 12:906–911, 1971.

45. Dahm K, deHeer K: Cancer risk of the stomach resected for ulcer: The role of duodeno-gastric reflux. Z. Krebsforsch. 87:343–344, 1976.

46. Dahm K, Werner B: Experimentelles Anastomosencarcinom. Ein Beitrag zur Pathogenese des Magenstumpfcarcinoms. Langenbecks Arch Chir 333:211–236, 1973.

47. Dahm K, Eichen R, Mitschke H: Das Krebsrisiko im Resektionsmagen. Zur Bedeutung des duodenogastrischen Refluxes bei verschiedenen gastroenteralen Anastomosen. Langenbecks Arch Chir 344:71–82, 1977.

48. Hawksworth GM, Hill MJ: Bacteria and the N-nitrosation of secondary amines. Br J Cancer 25:520–526, 1971.

49. Ruddell WSJ, Bone ES, Hill MJ, Walters CL: Gastric juice nitrite. Lancet 13:1037–1039, 1976.

50. Schlag P, Böckler R, Meyer H, Belohlavek D: Nitrite and N-nitroso-compounds in the operated stomach. In: Gastric cancer, Herfarth C, Schlag P (eds). Berlin: Springer, 1979, pp 120–128.

51. Schlag P, Böckler R, Ulrich H, Peter M, Merkle P, Herfarth C: Are nitrite and N-nitroso compounds in gastric juice risk factors for carcinoma in the operated stomach? Lancet i: 727-729, 1980.

52. Rehner M, Soehendra N, Eichfuss HP, Dahm K, Eckert P, Mitschke H: Frühkarzinome im (Billroth II)-Resektionsmagen. Dtsch Med Wschr 99:533–534, 1974.

53. Berkowitz D, Cooney P, Bralow SP: Carcinoma of the stomach appearing after previous gastric surgery for benign ulcer disease. Gastroenterology 36:691–697, 1959.

54. Pack GT, Banner RL: The late development of gastric cancer after gastroenterostomy and gastrectomy for peptic ulcer and benign pyloric stenosis. Surgery 44:1024–1033, 1958.

55. Pygott F, Shah VL: Gastric cancer associated with gastroenterostomy and partial gastrectomy. Gut 9:117–124, 1968.

56. Fridman EG: Cancer of a resected stomach: analysis of 194 cases. Acta Un Int Cancer 19:1257-1260, 1963.

57. Boeckl O, Lill H: Über das Magenstumpfkarzinom. Münch Med Wschr 105:615–618, 1963.

58. Laurèn P: The two histological main types of gastric carcinoma: Diffuse and so-called intestinal-type carcinoma. An attempt at a histo-clinical classification. Acta Path Microbiol scand 64:31–49, 1965.

59 Taksdal S, Stalsberg H: Histology of gastric carcinoma occurring after gastric surgery for benign conditions. Cancer 32:162–166, 1973.

60. Domellöf L, Eriksson S, Januger K-G: Carcinoma and possible precancerous changes of the gastric stump after Billroth II resection. Gastroenterology 73:462–468, 1977.

61. Stemmermann GN: Intestinal metaplasia of the gastric mucosa: A gross and microscopic study of its distribution in various disease states. J Nat Cancer Inst 41:627–633, 1968.

62. Griffel B, Englebert M, Reiss R, Saba K: Multiple polypoid cystic gastritis in old gastroenteric stoma. Arch. Path. 97:316–318, 1974.

63. Littler ER, Gleibermann E: Gastritis cystica polyposa. Cancer 29: 205–209, 1972.

64. Domellöf L, Eriksson S, Januger K-G: Late precancerous changes and carcinoma of the gastric stump after Billroth I resection. Am J Surg 132:26–31, 1976.

65. Ming SC, Goldman H: Gastric polyps. A histogenetic classification and its relation to carcinoma. Cancer 18:721–726, 1965.

66. Schrumpf E, Stadaas J, Myren J, Serck-Hansen A, Aune S, Osnes M: Mucosal changes in the gastric stump 20–25 years after partial gastrectomy. Lancet II:467–469, 1977.
67. Morson BC: Carcinoma arising from areas of intestinal metaplasia in the gastric mucosa. Br J Cancer 9:377–385, 1955.
68. Stemmermann GN, Hayashi T: Hyperplastic polyps of the gastric mucosa adjacent to gastroenterostomy stomas. Am J Clin Pathol 71:341–345, 1979.
69. Domellöf L, Eriksson S, Helander HF, Januger K-G: Lipid islands in the gastric mucosa after resection for benign ulcer disease. Gastroenterology 72:14–18, 1977.
70. Heilmann K: Lipid islands in gastric mucosa. Beitr. Path. 149:411–419, 1973.
71. Oehlert W, Keller P, Henke M, Strauch M: Die Dysplasien der Magenschleimhaut. Das Problem ihrer klinischen Bedeutung. Dtsch. Med Wschr 100:1950–1956, 1975.
72. Grundmann E, Schlake W: Histology of possible precancerous stages in the stomach. In: Gastric cancer, Herfarth C, Schlag P (eds.). Berlin: Springer, 1979, pp 72–82.
73. Konjetzny GE: Der Magenkrebs. Stuttgart: Enke 1938, p 108.
74. Konjetzny GE: Die Beziehung zwischen Gastritis und Magenkrebsentwicklung. Langenbecks Arch Klin Chir 204:4–63, 1943.
75. Siurala M, Isokoski M, Varis K, Kekki M: Prevalence of gastritis in a rural population. Scand J Gastroent 3:211–223, 1968.
76. Werner B, Leppin A, Seiler I, Mitschke H, Soehendra N, Farthmann E, Rehner M, Dahm K: Duodenaler Reflux und Gastritis im Billroth-I-Magen. Dtsch Med Wschr 100:2385–2388, 1975.
77. Burn JI, Welbourn RB: Cancer of the stomach. In: Gastric surgery, Smith R (ed.). London: Butterworths, 1975, pp 121–148.
78. Mitschke H, Dahm K: Definition, Häufigkeit, Pathogenese, Pathologische Anatomie. In: Das Karzinom im operierten Magen, Dahm K, Rehner M (eds). Stuttgart: Thieme, 1975, p 6.
79. Böttcher H, Hantschmann N: Das Magenstumpfkarzinom. Med Klin 68:175–179, 1973.
80. Vitek J, Vrubel F, Zejda V: Primäre Magenstumpfkarzinome an Ulcusreseziertern. Zbl. Chir. 88:246–253, 1963.

8. Metabolic Epidemiology of Large Bowel Cancer

M. J. HILL

1. INTRODUCTION

Large bowel cancer is one of the major neoplasms in western countries and is the major site of carcinogenesis in the United States[1]; the prognosis is relatively good (compared with, for example, cancer of the stomach, lung or pancreas) so that lung cancer remains the major cause of death from malignancy with colorectal cancer second to lung cancer in men, to breast cancer in women and to lung cancer when both sexes are combined.

Because bowel cancer appears to be related to life style it is potentially preventable; consequently, during the last 23 years (since the key paper by Wynder and Shigematsu[2]) there has been great interest in determining the etiology of the disease. In this paper I shall describe the epidemiology of the disease and the predisposing and associated diseases. The possible causative agents will then be described followed by a summary of the evidence for a role for the bile acids as co-carcinogens. These results of the metabolic epidemiology will then be discussed in terms of the results of the histopathology of the disease and the adenoma-carcinoma sequence.

2. EPIDEMIOLOGY OF COLORECTAL CANCER

There have been many previous in-depth studies of the epidemiology of colorectal cancer; examples include these by Wynder[3], Correa and Haenszel[4], Hill[5], Berg and Howell[6] and Burkitt[7]. The reader is referred to these for a detailed treatment of the subject; here I will give a summary of the types of observation that have been made together with some of the more recent findings.

J. J. DeCosse and P. Sherlock (eds.), Gastrointestinal cancer 1, 187-226. All rights reserved.
Copyright © 1981 Martinus Nijhoff Publishers, The Hague/Boston/London.

2.1. Geographical Distribution

There have been a number of studies comparing the incidence of colorectal cancer in various countries based on the data compiled by cancer registries. These include the regular compilations by Segi[8], and by the International Agency for Research in Cancer[9, 10]; in addition, publications have included estimates from less reliable sources to give a wider coverage of Asia and Africa[11]. The clear indications from these are that the disease is common in North-West Europe, North America and Australasia and, relatively rare in Africa, Asia, Central and South America and Eastern Europe (Table 1). In South America there are areas of high incidence in Uruguay and Northern Argentina (the River Plata area) adjacent to areas of low incidence. In Europe the incidence is lower in the south and east than in the north and west. At a

Table 1. The incidence of colon and rectal cancer in various countries (data from ref. [11] for men, age adjusted 35–64 years per 100,000 per annum).

	Colon	Rectum
Asia		
India	6.6	8.0
Japan, Miyagi	5.0	8.1
Singapore	4.6	8.5
Africa		
Nigeria	2.8	3.1
S. Africa – white	17.9	10.8
– coloured	13.7	5.6
– Indian	2.5	5.1
– African	6.6	4.5
Mozambique	5.3	0.1
S. America		
Colombia	5.7	3.9
Chile	5.8	6.0
Venezuela	7.3	4.4
N. America		
USA – white	26.6	15.6
– black	25.6	16.0
Canada – Alberta	20.3	12.4
Europe		
England and Wales – Birmingham	17.4	20.7
Denmark	17.1	20.8
France	20.2	16.8
Bulgaria	7.8	13.2
Italy	16.0	11.6
Poland	8.2	7.5

cursory glance the distribution of the disease indicates a genetic predisposition to the disease in populations of Anglo-Saxon or Scandinavian origin.

2.2. Migrant Studies

The study of migrants is a powerful tool in the investigation of the relative importance of genetic and environmental factors in the causation of disease. Migrants from Europe to the United States and to Australia, and from Japan to the United States have been investigated in great depth; in all of these studies it is clear that persons moving from an area with a low risk of colorectal cancer to the United States or Australia, both of which have a high risk of the disease, rapidly achieve an incidence of the disease similar to that of their new homeland and very much higher than that of their country of origin [12, 13]. From these studies it is apparent that genetic factors are of only minor importance compared with environmental factors in determining the risk of the disease in populations. This does not imply that genetic factors are unimportant *per se*; indeed in individuals it is likely that they are very important. However, the full genetic predisposition to the disease may only be expressed under certain environmental conditions.

2.3. Colon Cancer Incidence within a Country

Within a country, the risk of a cancer may vary between regions, between sexes, between socioeconomic groups, between races, and between areas of different population density. It may also vary with time. These will be discussed in turn.

2.3.1. Variation between Regions. Such variations have been noted in many countries. In the United Kingdom there is an increasing incidence from south to north and from east to west (Table 2). Similarly there is a variation between the Canadian provinces (Table 2). Within the United States the incidence is highest in the north and east and lowest in the south and west [14]. Within the Sudan, the incidence is much higher in the north than in the south [15], this may be due to differences in social class.

2.3.2. Variations between the Sexes. Large bowel cancer is one of the few cancers that are as common in women as in men (Table 3), the ratio being between 0.8 and 1.2 in most countries. This apparent uniformity in incidence hides some differences; the incidence of colon cancer is greater in women than men below the age of 60–70 but is higher in men in the older age groups and is higher in men at all ages for rectal cancer.

2.3.3. Variations between Socioeconomic Groups. In the high risk populations of the western world there is little difference in the incidence of

Table 2. Variation in the incidence of cancer of the colon and rectum by region in the United Kingdom and in Canada (data from ref. [11] and from Doll (personal communication).).

	Incidence of colon cancer		Incidence of rectal cancer	
	Males	Females	Males	Females
Scotland	28.2	34.2	23.3	17.3
England — Liverpool	24.1	25.8	15.4	10.5
— Birmingham	17.4	20.9	20.7	12.9
— S. Metropolitan	15.8	20.5	16.2	10.9
— S. West	17.2	18.2	16.6	10.3
Northern Ireland	21.9	33.7	18.7	16.0
Canada — Alberta	20.3	26.0	12.4	9.0
— Saskatchewan	18.0	25.4	18.8	14.2
— Manitoba	29.8	33.0	15.2	15.1
— New Brunswick	24.1	38.0	16.8	17.1
— Newfoundland	24.9	25.5	5.5	9.4

Table 3. Ratio of age adjusted incidence rates in males: females for colon cancer (for details see ref. [5]).

	<0.8	0.8–1.0	1.0–1.2	>1.2
Africa	Uganda	S. Africa—white	Nigeria	S. Africa—black
Asia		Israel	Japan	Taiwan India
S. America	Venezuela Jamaica	Chile	Colombia	Uruguay
Europe	England	Belgium Germany	France Bulgaria	Yugoslavia Czechoslovakia

colorectal cancer between various socioeconomic groups. In England and Wales the standardised mortality rates for colon cancer for the professional and managerial (class I), for the partly skilled (class IV) and unskilled (class V) workers are 120, 92 and 109 respectively [16]. For rectal cancer there is a somewhat higher incidence in the lower social groups than in class I persons, but the difference is not great. In contrast, there is a clear correlation between social class and the incidence of large bowel cancer in low incidence countries such as Colombia, Japan and Hong Kong. The analysis has been most detailed in Cali, Colombia, where Haenszel *et al.* [17] observed that when the population was divided into four classes (upper (I), middle (II), low (III) and very low (IV) there was an overall gradient in standard incidence rate from

Table 4. Standardised incidence rates for large bowel cancer by subsite of the cancer and by sex and socioeconomic class of the patient for Cali, Colombia (data from ref. [17]).

Site of the cancer	Both sexes		Males		Females	
	Class I & II	Class III	Class I & II	Class III	Class I & II	Class III
All large bowel cancers	145	92	145	96	145	88
Caecum	105	119	89	119	122	119
Ascending and transverse	198	72	209	65	185	80
Descending, sigmoid and rectosigmoid	165	81	242	47	119	104
Rectum	113	100	106	119	118	82

140 (class I) to 29 (class IV); there was no gradient for cancer of the caecum or rectum, the excess for classes I and II being confined to the segment from the ascending to the rectosigmoid colon. The gradient was more marked for men than for women (Table 4). A similar gradient has been noted in Hong Kong [18] and in Japan [19].

2.3.4. Variations between Races and Religions. The existence of interracial differences in incidence of large bowel cancer is dependent on parallel differences in life style. Thus in South Africa the white, black, coloured and Indian populations have widely different incidences in large bowel cancer, as do the different religious groups in Bombay (Table 5); these are related to differences in cultural environment. Similar differences in incidence of large bowel cancer have been noted between the various races in Hawaii (Japanese, Chinese, White American and indigenous) and between the various sub-groups of Chinese in Singapore. In all of these examples, the various racial groups share

Table 5. Large bowel cancer in various religious groups in Bombay (data from ref. [20]).

Religious group	Colorectal carcinomas as a percentage of all gastrointestinal neoplasms	
	Males	Females
Hindus — Maharashtra	11.5	9.7
— Gujarat	8.0	9.9
Moslems	9.3	7.2
Christians	14.5	14.8
Parsees	28.6	27.6

the same physical environment (e.g. climate, air pollution, latitude) but have greatly different life styles, particularly dietary.

A similar separation of the effects of physical and cultural environment can be obtained by studying various religious groups. In this respect, the various religious groups in Bombay (Table 5), all of whom share the same physical environment, have interesting differences in incidence of colorectal cancer with the meat-eating religions having a higher incidence than the vegetarians [20]. Similarly, in the United States the vegetarian 7th Day Adventists have an incidence of the disease below the national average [21], as do the Mormons [22].

2.3.5. Variation with Population Density. In general, urban dwellers are more likely to develop carcinoma than are rural persons, because of the very much higher level of environmental carcinogens (air pollution, industrial exposure, etc.) in the urban areas. In England and Wales the ratio in incidence of colon cancer between urban and rural persons is about 1.1 [16], a small excess compared with that for lung cancer, for example (Table 6). In the United States the ratio is somewhat higher than in England and Wales; urban–rural differences have been reported from a number of other countries.

2.3.6. Temporal Variations. There has been a general upward trend in incidence of colorectal cancer around the world although there have been a few exceptions. In the United States, although the mortality has remained constant between 1935 and 1970 this was due to improved treatment and masked a 50% increase in incidence. In Japan the incidence, which has traditionally been very low, has been increasing rapidly since 1950 [23]. In West Germany the incidence of large bowel cancer has also been increasing steadily during the last thirty years (since registration began). In contrast, in England and Wales the pattern has been more complex. Overall, the incidence has changed little during this century; this masks a steady increase to a

Table 6. The incidence of colon and rectal cancer in urban areas compared with rural areas.

Country	Population	Sex	Cancer site	Incidence in urban areas / rural areas
United States	White	Male	Colon	1.4
	Non-white		Colon	1.5
	White		Rectum	1.4
	Non-white		Rectum	1.7
England and Wales	All	Male	Colon & rectum	1.1
		Female	Colon & rectum	1.1

maximum in 1935–1940 followed by a steady decrease at the rate of about 2% per year [23]. In general, the incidence is increasing rapidly in the newly developing countries and is more static in the more socially stable populations of North-West Europe.

2.4. Subsite Distribution

Until recently there has been little detailed data about the subsite distribution of colorectal cancers. However this aspect of the disease has received a lot of recent attention. Haenszel and Correa [24] used data from seven countries to investigate the reported relative excess of right sided tumours in low incidence countries; the tumours were classified into caecum and ascending colon, transverse and descending colon, sigmoid colon and rectum and their conclusions were that the incidence of cancer of the caecum plus ascending colon and of the rectum varied little and that the geographical variation in incidence of the disease was due to the variation in incidence of tumours of the sigmoid colon. A similar conclusion was drawn by Haenszel et al. [17] from the socioeconomic differences in incidence in Cali, Colombia; the excess in social class I being entirely due to tumours in the ascending to sigmoid colon, in particular the sigmoid colon.

In contrast, De Jong et al. [25] studied data from 12 countries, including high incidence (North America, New Zealand), low incidence (Eastern Asia) and intermediate (Scandinavia, England) countries, and found that the proportional subsite distribution was similar in all countries and increased from the caecum to the sigmoid colon. Powell [26] has carried out a more detailed study which gave a different picture from that described by the other groups; she divided the large bowel into caecum, ascending colon, hepatic flexure, transverse colon, splenic flexure, descending colon, sigmoid colon and rectum and found the incidence to be high in the caecum, sigmoid colon and rectum, low at the flexures and intermediate at the other subsites. She could only analyse data from Birmingham, England, cancer registry since only there were the data recorded in sufficient detail.

The question as to whether the incidence of carcinoma in the ascending, transverse and descending colon is the same (as shown by Powell) or increases sequentially (as shown by De Jong et al.) may prove difficult to resolve in the light of the observation by Rhodes et al. [27] that the subsite distribution is changing; they noted that in a large midwestern United States hospital the proportion of rectal and sigmoid tumours has progressively decreased during the last 30 years whilst the proportion of proximal tumours (caecum and ascending colon) has increased. Thus the results obtained by Powell could be explained as being due to the use of more recent data.

The subsite distribution is important in evaluating the relative importance of various etiologies of colorectal cancer and will be discussed later.

2.5. Relation of the Cultural Environment

There have been a number of case-control studies of large bowel cancer indicating that there is no role for smoking, alcohol consumption (except beer, to be discussed later), use of drugs and laxatives, bowel habits, etc. The major factor in the cultural environment to be incriminated has been diet, although there is little agreement on the dietary item implicated.

Studies of diet take various forms. Many groups have studied the mean intake of dietary items by various populations (usually taken from tables of food consumption prepared by the Food and Agriculture Organisation) compared with the large bowel cancer incidence in these populations. By this method, Gregor et al. [28] showed a strong correlation with dietary animal protein, Drasar and Irving [29] showed a strong correlation with animal protein and with fat, especially bound fat, whilst Armstrong and Doll [30] showed strong correlations with meat and with fat. These studies suffer from the drawback that the data used for food intake are not reliable (for example, they take no account of home grown vegetables). In the study by Gregor et al., current diet was more strongly correlated than was the diet consumed 15–20 years previously [28], indicating that diet is more likely to have a tumour promoting role than to cause tumour initiation. In contrast, Liu et al., who studied data from 20 countries showed that, when the incidence of colon cancer was related to the diet 10–15 years previously, the strongest correlation was with cholesterol rather than total fat or meat [31]. Clearly the picture is not clear and, in view of the quality of the available data on diet, is unlikely to become more so.

There have been many case-control studies relating diet to bowel cancer; in these, patients with bowel cancer and suitable controls are quizzed about their diet. Clearly the current diet of a person with gastrointestinal disease bears no relation to what it was when they were healthy, and so the investigator has to rely on dietary recall, usually back to at least a few years ago. A quick survey of friends and aquaintances will reveal that people are unaware of having changed their diet and, whereas this may be true of the healthy controls it is certainly not true, of the cases. In consequence, it is not surprising that these studies either reveal no correlation [e.g. 32, 33] or give a wide range of results implicating fat [19, 34], vitamins A and C [35], fibre as a protective agent [36] or in the form of string beans as a causative agent [37], meat [37] and so on.

These two approaches have been combined in studies of the diet of representives of populations within an area which have widely different incidences of bowel cancer. Such studies have been carried out on Japanese migrants to Hawaii compared with those born there (correlation with intake of meat and beans) [37], on three socioeconomic groups in Hong Kong (correlation with meat, fat and fibre) [38] and on two populations in Scandinavia (correlation with beer consumption and inverse correlation with milk and fibre) [60].

Table 7. The relation between diet and the incidence of large bowel cancer.

Dietary item	Type of study	Reference
Meat	International study of 23 countries	30
	Case control study	37
Animal protein	International study of 23 countries	30
	International study of 28 countries	28
	International study of 37 countries	29
Fat	International study of 28 countries	28
	International study of 37 countries	29
	International study of 23 countries	30
	Case control study	2
	Case control study	34
Fibre (protective)	Qualitative comparison of Africa and UK	7
	Case control study	36
	International study of 2 countries	60
Fibre (causative)	Case control study	37
	Study of 3 populations in Hong Kong	38
Beer	International study of 47 countries	61
	International study of 2 countries	60
Vitamins A and C (protective)	Case control study in 2 countries	35
Milk (protective)	International study of 2 countries	60

The data relating diet to bowel cancer is summarised in Table 7. The conclusion to be drawn is that no simple relationship exists between a single item of the diet and bowel carcinogenesis; however there is good evidence for a role for dietary meat or fat from all three types of study. Any hypothesis on the etiology of bowel cancer, whilst allowing a role for a wide variety of dietary components, must be able to explain this apparent primary role for dietary meat or fat.

3. PREDISPOSING AND ASSOCIATED DISEASES

Diseases that predispose to colorectal cancer are often confused with those which are merely associated with this malignancy. The distinction is important because the former are presumably causally related whilst some of the latter may be coincidental relationships.

3.1. Predisposing Diseases

The diseases that clearly predispose to colorectal carcinogenesis are inflammatory bowel disease, adenomatosis coli, 'cancer family' syndrome and carriage of villous adenomas.

3.1.1. Inflammatory Bowel Disease. In 1928 Bargen first suggested there was a link between ulcerative colitis and bowel cancer [39] and since that time there have been many studies confirming that ulcerative colitis predisposes to colorectal carcinogenesis [40–42]. There is a consensus about characteristics of the carcinogenesis in these patients. The most important is the latency of the process; there is no increased risk of malignancy during the first ten years of colitis, and the mean interval between the onset of colitis and the diagnosis of cancer is 15 to 20 years. The risk is greatest if the symptoms of colitis are chronic and continuous rather than the acute relapsing type of disease. As the age of onset of colitis is reduced, so the risk of malignancy is increased; MacDougall [43] showed that in persons whose symptoms had lasted for more than ten years the risk of malignancy in persons whose age of onset of colitis was less than 25 years was $2\frac{1}{2}$ times greater than that in other persons. Only those with total involvement of the colon are greatly at risk of carcinogenesis whilst in those with only distal involvement the risk of malignancy is negligible. In his review of cancer in colitis, MacDougall [44] concluded that patients with total colonic involvement for more than ten years had 30 times the normal risk of colon cancer whilst those with subtotal involvement had no excess risk regardless of the other characteristics of the disease. The development of cancer is preceded by dysplastic changes over an area sufficiently extensive to be recognised by rectal biopsy [41, 45], the dysplasia progressing from mild through moderate to severe and finally becoming malignant. The current status of the precancer lesion in ulcerative colitis has recently been reviewed by Dobbins [46].

Until relatively recently Crohn's disease (regional ileitis) was thought to be limited to the small bowel. However, involvement of the colon is now recognised as a common manifestation of the disease and Weedon *et al.* [47] have shown that persons with Crohn's disease of the colon may have the same risk as colitics of developing a malignancy.

3.1.2. Adenomatosis Coli. Adenomatosis coli (familial polyposis coli) is a genetically determined disease. Its familial nature was first reported by Cripps in 1882 [48] and its association with colorectal cancer was reported only eight years later by Handford [49]. It was described and characterised by Dukes [50] and has recently been reviewed by Bussey [51]. It is caused by an autosomal dominant gene and is defined as a disease in which large numbers of adenomatous polyps (never fewer than 100, by definition) develop from the colorectal mucosa. The polyps are fairly evenly distributed throughout the large bowel and normally appear when the affected person is in the late teens; the average age of patients presenting with symptoms is 33 and the average age at which they present with cancer is 40 years. The mean interval between detection of adenomas and the detection of carcinomas is ten years; the adenomas in patients with adenomatosis are indistinguishable from the discrete adenomas carried by a high percentage of normal people at postmortem, and their progression to malignancy appears to be identical to that in 'normal' discrete adenomas.

There are a number of extra-colonic manifestations of adenomatosis which may be present. In its severe form there are osteomas detectable in all bones (particularly in the mandibles) and carcinoid lesions at a range of possible sites; the disease is then classified as Gardner's syndrome. Recently there have been many reports of gastric polyps (particularly in Japan where apparently more than 40% of adenomatosis patients have such lesions) and of tumours in the duodenum [52].

Morson [53] has suggested that, although the development of adenomatosis is genetically determined, the progression to carcinoma is due to environmental factors; although multiple colorectal carcinomas are common it is clear that only a tiny proportion of the polyps become malignant. The cancer in these patients has normally progressed so far at diagnosis that the prognosis is poor, but follow-up of the children, with regular annual sigmoidoscopy from the age of 15 years enables the disease to be detected early (it will, of course, affect about 50% of the children since it is determined by an autosomal dominant gene) and treated by total colectomy. Thus, in this group true cancer prevention is practised.

3.1.3. Cancer Family Syndrome. 'Cancer families' have been described in which a high proportion of first degree relatives of an index case develop large bowel cancer. The disease was described by Lynch and Krush [54] and is characterised by its early onset and by the fact that it is not preceded by the development of large numbers of adenomas (indeed adenomas are rarely detected at the time of tumour resection). Large bowel cancer in the female members of cancer families is strongly associated with additional cancer of the endometrium.

Cancer family syndrome in the extreme form described by Lynch and Krush is rare, but may be an extreme form of the genetic predisposition of first degree relatives to develop large bowel cancer [55, 56].

3.1.4. Colorectal Adenomas. It is now well established that the vast majority, if not all, colorectal carcinomas arise in pre-existing adenomas. The evidence for this has been summarised by Morson [53, 57] and by Enterline [58]. A high proportion of adenomas more than 2 cm in diameter already contain areas of focal carcinoma (Table 8) indicating that carcinoma can arise in adenomas. When the histopathology of colorectal carcinomas is examined, a high proportion of Dukes'A carcinomas contain an area of adenomatous tissue; a smaller proportion of Dukes'B and only a tiny proportion of

Table 8. The proportion of adenomas containing a malignant component and of carcinomas containing a non-malignant component.

Adenoma characteristic	Percentage containing a malignant component
Adenomas less than 0.5 cm diameter*	0
less than 1.0 cm diameter	1.3
between 1 and 2 cm diameter	9.5
greater that 2 cm	46.0
Tubular adenomas	4.8
Villous adenomas	40.7
Tubulovillous	22.5

* Data from ref. [59]; other data from ref. [57].

Dukes'C tumours contain a non-malignant component and this is compatible with the thesis that carcinomas arise in non-malignant adenomas and, as the malignant area grows, progressively replace the non-malignant remnant.

There has been a growth of interest recently in the causation of colorectal adenomas. This has been hampered by the lack of reliable data; there are registries of carcinomas and there are many centres from which reliable incidence data on colorectal carcinomas are available, but most large bowel adenomas are undiagnosed and are only detected at post-mortem. There are few areas of the world where a high proportion of persons undergo post-mortem examination and even in such areas the large bowel is not necessarily opened and examined by hand-lens. Nevertheless, some data are available and have been reviewed by Correa [62]. The general conclusions that can be drawn are that:

(a) In areas where large bowel cancer is rare, such as Colombia, Nigeria, Iran, Japan and in Black South Africans, colorectal adenomas are also rare. Where large bowel cancer is common, as in the United States, colorectal adenomas are also common. Where the incidence of colorectal cancer is intermediate (e.g. Sao Paulo, Sweden, Britain) the incidence of adenomas is also intermediate (Table 9).

(b) When Japanese migrate to the United States their incidence of colorectal adenomas and of colorectal carcinomas increases to a level similar to that of native Americans (Table 10).

(c) Despite this apparent correlation between the incidence of adenomas and of carcinomas, countries with a common low incidence of colorectal carcinoma have a wide range in incidence of colorectal adenomas (Table 8).

(d) In general, adenomas arise earlier than carcinomas by approximately 5–10 years.

(e) Whereas colorectal carcinomas are much more common in the left colon than in the right, adenomas detected at autopsy are evenly distributed along the length of the large bowel (Table 11). Large adenomas, however have the same distribution as carcinomas. There is considerable debate

Table 9. Relation between the incidence of colorectal adenoma and carcinomas in various countries.

Population	Colon cancer frequency	Prevalence rate of adenomas (men aged 40–50) (%)	Reference
Hawaiian Japanese	Very high	69	62
New Orleans — white	High	39	62
— black	High	26	62
Brazil — Sao Paulo	Intermediate	14	62
Sweden — Malmo	Intermediate	13	69
Japan — Miyagi	Low	9	62
Costa Rica — San Jose	Low	6	62
Colombia — Cali	Low	7	62
Iran	Low	1	64
Nigeria	Low	<1	65
Bolivia	Low	<1	66

Table 10. Prevalence of adenomas in Japanese living in Hawaii, analysed by place of birth (data from ref. [67]).

	Prevalence of adenomas in Japanese		
	Living in Japan (Akita)	Born in Japan	Born in Hawaii
Age 0–49		0	46%
50–79		59%	67%
All ages	35%	61%	63%

Table 11. The distribution of adenomas and carcinomas by subsite within the large bowel.

Subsite	Sweden		Colombia		U.S.A.	
	ad	ca	ad	ca	ad	ca
Caecum and ascending colon	24%	20%	18	30%	24	16%
Transverse and descending colon	30%	14%	41	13%	35	18%
Sigmoid colon	30%	41%	20	9%	22	25%
Rectum	16%	24%	21	48%	19	42%
Reference	69	69	68	70	68	70

concerning the subsite distribution of adenomas, with hospital and colonoscopy series showing a distribution similar to that of colorectal carci-
nomes. This may be because the very small adenomas that are found in
the right colon at autopsy are not seen at colonoscopy or by X-ray.
From the geographical epidemiology of colorectal adenomas and from the
studies of migrants, it is apparent that adenomas are caused by environmental
factors associated with the western life style. The even distribution of adenomas along the large bowel suggests that the environmental factor either enters
the caecum preformed or else is readily activated.

In addition to these studies of the role of environmental factors, there have
been studies of the role of familial and genetic factors, summarised by
Veale [71], which led to the conclusion that the predisposition to develop
adenomas is determined by a recessive autosomal gene (p); a person who is
pp is prone to develop adenomas when exposed to the relevent environmental
factors whilst presons who are np or nn (where n is the normal variant of p)
will not develop adenomas regardless of how much environmental factor the
person is exposed to. This hypothesis is very difficult to test; since adenomas
are normally asymptomatic there are no published records concerning the
familial carriage of adenomas.

The histopathology and the causation of the progression from adenoma to
carcinoma will be discussed at length later in section 6.

3.2. Associated Diseases

A number of diseases have been associated with colorectal cancer, including a range of cancers of other sites, the so-called 'diseases of fibre depletion', and a number of other miscellaneous diseases.

3.2.2. Associated Cancers.
The cancers associated with colorectal cancers
are the hormone-dependent ones such as cancer of the breast, ovary, endometrium and prostate, together with cancers of the digestive system such as the
pancreas and kidney. Cancer of the large bowel, breast, endometrium, ovary
and prostate all associated geographically, being more common in western
countries than in Africa, Asia and South America; migrants from low incidence countries to high incidence areas such as the United States experience
an increased incidence of all five cancers reaching that of the new homeland
by the next generation. All are associated with each other in patients with
multiple primary carcinomas. The female members of 'cancer families' are
highly likely to develop endometrial as well as colorectal cancer. All are
associated with a western-type diet rich in fat and meat (Table 12), and in all
steroid hormones or bile acids have been implicated in the etiology. Oestrogens have been implicated in breast carcinogenesis by many groups, and the
causation of breast cancer has been reviewed by McMahon et al. [72]. The

Table 12. The association between various cancers.

	Large bowel	Breast	Ovary	Endometrium	Prostate
Incidence in western countries	High	High	High	High	High
Incidence in Asia, Africa and South America	Low	Low	Low	Low	Low
Social class gradient	None	None	None	None	None
Association in 2nd primaries	Breast Endometrium	Large bowel Endometrium Ovary	Breast Endometrium	Colon Breast Ovary	None
Postulated role of steroid hormones	None	+ +	+ +	+ +	+ +
Dietary associations	Fat Meat	Fat	Fat	Fat	Fat
Abnormal urinary steroids	?	+ +	?	?	+ +

etiology of endometrial cancer has been reviewed by Armstrong [73] who has postulated a major role for oestrogen and for dietary fat. The role of steroid hormones in the causation of cancer of the prostate has been deduced from the beneficial effect of the removal of androgen sources by orchidectomy or by the reversal of androgen action by oestrogen therapy [74]. The etiology of ovarian cancer has been reviewed by Lingeman [75], who has discussed the role of oestrogens in carcinogenesis.

Thus in all of the associated cancers there is a key role for steroid hormones and all are associated with a high intake of dietary fat. Because of the strength of the association it is likely that the relationship is not coincidental but indicates a common component in their causation. The associations have been discussed in detail by Hill [5].

3.2.2. Diseases of Fibre Depletion. A number of ' diseases of fibre depletion ' have been described by Burkitt [7] and by Cleave [77] based on observations of the prevalence of the diseases in Africa compared with the United States or the United Kingdom (Table 13). It has been suggested [78] that an ' association of a number of effects of unknown causation suggests that they are due wholly or in part to some cause common to each ' and that the ' common cause ' is fibre depletion. The ' associated diseases ' described included constipation, diverticular disease, appendicitis, hiatus hernia, polyps and colon cancer, and dietary supplementation with 2−6 g dietary fibre per day was advo-

Table 13. The association between large bowel cancer and the 'diseases of fibre depletion'

Disease	Suggestion for association	Evidence for association	
		fibre depletion	large bowel cancer
Constipation	76, 78	Treatable with bran	No association [2]
Appendicitis	76, 78	?	No association [79]
Diverticular disease	76, 78	Treatable with bran in short term	No association [80]
Polyps	78	?	Adenomas progress to carcinoma [57]
Hiatus hernia	78	?	?
Gallstones	7	?	Not associated [80]
Coronary heart disease	7, 76	?	Not associated [81]
Ulcerative colitis	7	?	Predisposes to bowel cancer [40]
Diabetes	7	?	?

cated to correct the depletion. If this really is the answer then there should be quite a strong association. To date little information regarding these correlations has been presented; the little evidence available does not indicate such an association. Castleden [80] has studied the relationship between gallstones and large bowel cancer and has shown that there is none. Fredrick *et al.* [81] have used the Oxford Record Linkage data to check an association between large bowel cancer and coronary heart disease, appendicitis and diverticulitis and have found none. Moertal *et al.* [79] studied prospectively the association between appendicitis and large bowel cancer and found none. Wynder and Shigematsu [2] studied the relationship between obesity and large bowel cancer and found none. To date, apart from adenomas and ulcerative colitis, which have been discussed already in section 3.1.1 and 3.1.4, none of the suggested associations has survived scrutiny.

3.2.3. Other Associated Diseases. In a study of the geographical epidemiology of multiple sclerosis, Wolfgram [82] studied a wide range of diseases of which only colon cancer had a similar geographical distribution. No hypothesis has been suggested to explain the association.

4. POSSIBLE CAUSATIVE AGENTS

In discussing the agents that might be implicated in large bowel carcinogenesis, we must turn to the epidemiology of the disease for leads. This implicated the cultural environment, which includes smoking, alcohol, diet, etc. Factors associated with the physical environment appear to be unimportant. Although the causative agent might be exogenous (e.g. U.V. light, air pollutants, water pollutants, cigarette smoke, hair dyes, food colours) or endogenous (e.g. steroid hormones, metabolites produced by gut bacteria, etc.) it must be related to the cultural environment in some way. The various factors implicated in carcinogenesis in general may be divided into the following broad classes:

(a) physical factors;

(b) radiation (both natural and therapeutic);

(c) immunological factors;

(d) virological factors;

(e) environmental agents;

(f) endogenous agents;

(g) nutrition; and

(h) genetic factors.

4.1. Stress and Physical Factors

Stress was the first factor to be implicated in carcinogenesis when Imhotep, in 3000 BC, stated that cancer resulted from injury [83]. There have been many reports of large bowel cancers arising at suture lines following bowel resection but there is little support for a role of physical factors, either stress or physical irritation, in the causation of large bowel cancer (although irritation was implicated in the causation of cancer of the scrotum [84] by Percival Pott in 1775).

4.2. Radiation

Radiation is known to be important in the causation of skin cancer and many leukemias. There is unlikely to be a role for solar radiation in large bowel carcinogenesis – populations exposed to the highest levels of sunlight tend to have low incidences of the disease – and large bowel cancer was not associated with exposure to the radiation following the atomic bombs in Japan. There has been continuing interest in a possible role for therapeutic radiation, but there have been few indications that this is a risk factor in colorectal carcinogenesis.

4.3. Immunological Factors

Although immunological studies account for a large part of the overall budget for large bowel cancer research, the main thrust of these studies is into the early detection of the disease rather than to its causation and management.

There is a widely held view that immune surveillance plays an important part in the normal host defence against cancer and that, when cancer becomes manifest, this represents a failure in the immune surveillance mechanism. In support of this, it has been widely noted that persons with immunological deficiency or who are on immunosuppressive therapy are more likely than 'normal' persons to develop cancer [85]. The excess cancers reported in these persons, however, tend to be lymphomas and leukemias and do not include colorectal neoplasms.

Berlinger *et al.* [86] reported defective recognitive immunity in 44% of cancer-free individuals from colon cancer families. These individuals had no other pre-cancerous symptoms but the immune defect is similar to that noted by many others in persons with established malignancies. It has been reported that cellular immunity plays an important role in controlling the rate of growth of tumours, and Bone *et al.* [87, 88] have produced data to support this in colorectal cancer patients. However, the reduced delayed hypersensitivity responses in the patients with fast growing tumours may be the result of the general debility of those patients rather than the cause of the rapid growth.

Using animal models, the effect of stimulating the delayed hypersensitivity response by injecting BCG appears not to protect the animals; indeed in some reports [89] there is evidence of tumour promotion.

In summary, there is little clear evidence that immune factors play a major part in the causation of large bowel cancer.

4.4. Virological Factors

To date, no reasonable evidence has been produced to indicate a role for viruses in human colorectal carcinogenesis; indeed, there is little evidence for such a role in the causation of cancer at any other site in humans.

4.5. Environmental Agents

Under this heading I include all preformed chemical carcinogens to which persons are exposed. In contrast to the situation with lung and bladder cancer, very few potential colorectal carcinogens have been detected in the environment [90, 91].

It has been reported that asbestos workers in the United States have an increased risk of colorectal cancer [92]; although similar results have not been obtained in the U.K [93]. Asbestos dust is known to have an irritant effect on the lung and, in combination with smoking, gives rise to very high incidences of lung cancer; the dust particles caught in the nasal or oral passages and swallowed might have a similar irritant effect in the colon. However, even if it is shown to cause colorectal cancers, the amount of asbestos to which the normal population is exposed is very small and it is unlikely that it plays a major part in the causation of colorectal cancer.

It has been noted that the incidence of the disease is higher in urban than in rural populations, suggesting a role for industrial exposures or atmospheric

Table 14. The role of dietary carcinogens in human carcinogenesis.

Carcinogen	Reference	Populations studied	Suggested target	Incidence of colorectal cancer in the same population
Aflatoxin	94	Thailand	Liver	Very low
	95	Africa	Liver	Very low
P.A.H.s	96	Iceland	Stomach	Very low
N-nitroso compounds	97	Transkei	Oesophagus	Very low

pollutants. To date, studies of groups working with known carcinogens (e.g. diazo dyes, aromatic amines, N-nitroso compounds, etc.) have revealed no excess risk of colorectal cancer. Although polycyclic aromatic hydrocarbons (PAHs) are present in the atmosphere as a result of combustion of fuels, motor exhaust fumes, etc., our main exposure to this group of known carcinogens is through the inhalation of cigarette smoke; Wynder and Shigematsu [2] found no correlation between cigarette smoking and colorectal cancer.

A wide range of carcinogens are known to be present in food, including aflatoxins, N-nitroso compounds, PAHs, the products of pyrolysis of protein (e.g. harman, nor-harman) etc., but none of these has been implicated in colorectal carcinogenesis and the populations exposed to high levels of them tend to have a low level of colorectal cancer (Table 14).

4.6. Endogenous Agents

A range of endogenous compounds or products of bacterial metabolism of endogenous compounds have been claimed to be carcinogenic or co-carcinogens and are known to reach the colon. In only a few cases have their tumor initiating or promoting actions been tested in the colon and so this section contains rather more hypothesis than fact. The compounds to be studied include cholesterol, bile acids, steroid oestrogens, tryptopan metabolites, tyrosine metabolites, N-nitroso compounds and other compounds.

The group of compounds contains three classes of steroids; interest in the steroids as possible endogenous carcinogens began following the early work of Cook [98], who had noted the structural similarity between steroids and the PAHs. He suggested that endogenous steroids produced as a result of abnormal steroid metabolism might be the cause of spontaneous neoplasms – a hypothesis that lives on in various theories on the causation of breast, endometrial and colorectal cancer. Fieser [99], as a result of early studies on structure–activity relationships thought that, if this were so, then the main candidates would be the aromatic or partially aromatic steroids. More recently Yang et al. [100] went so far as to suggest that PAHs are carcinogenic *because* of their structural similarity to steroid hormones, which would enable them to block binding sites etc. The steroid carcinogens have been reviewed by Bischoff[101].

The evidence implicating these various endogenous compounds in human colorectal carcinogenesis has been reviewed elsewhere [5, 102–104] and will be summarised briefly here.

4.6.1. Cholesterol. In a series of studies summarised in 1958, Hieger demonstrated that when cholesterol is injected subcutaneously in mice as an oily solution it is weakly carcinogenic [105]. These experiments were repeated by various groups with equivocal results, but Bischoff[101] in his review has presented evidence that the original results are due to solid state carcinogenesis and not due to any carcinogenic properties of cholesterol itself. In studies in which animals are treated with solutions of compounds by rectal instillation, Reddy *et al.* [106] have shown that neither cholesterol, its epoxide or cholestriol is carcinogenic for the rat large bowel and neither were they co-carcinogenic in rats treated in the same way after first being treated with the tumour initiator dimethylhydrazine (which in rodents is organ-specific for the large bowel).

In contrast, Cruse *et al.* [107] showed that rats fed a soluble defined diet developed fewer colorectal tumours than those animals fed the same diet but supplemented with cholesterol, both groups having been treated with dimethylhydrazine. From this they concluded that cholesterol is co-carcinogenic in the rat colon.

4.6.2. Bile Acids. Bile acids have been shown to be co-carcinogenic in skin painting studies, in rectal instillation experiments, in mutagenesis assays in bacteria and in *Drosophila* (Table 15); deoxycholic acid has been found to be

Table 15. Evidence that bile acids have tumour promoting or initiating properties.

Bile acid studied	Reference	Test system	
Deoxycholic acid	108 109	Painting in oily vehicle on rat skin	Co-carcinogen
Deoxycholic acid Lithocholic acid	110	Rectal instillation	Co-carcinogen
Deoxycholic acid Lithocholic acid	111	Salmonella mutagenesis	Co-carcinogen
Deoxycholic acid	112	Drosophila	Mutagen
Lithocholic acid	113	Cell transformation assay	Mutagen
Total bile acids	114, 115	Bile diversion studies	Co-carcinogen

Table 16. The effect of diet on faecal bile acid concentration and on the incidence of tumours in rats treated with dimethylhydrazine.

Dietary changes	Effect on FBA concentrations	Effect on tumour incidence
Added fat	Increase	Increase
Added meat	Increase	Increase
Added pectin	Increase	Increase
Added bran	Decrease	Decrease
Added lactulose	Decreased metabolism	Decrease
Change to Vivonex diet	Decrease	Decrease

For references, see ref. [104].

co-carcinogenic in all of these systems whilst lithocholic acid and a range of other bile acids have proved to be positive in a number of test systems.

In bile diversion studies, where the concentration of bile acid in the large bowel of rats treated with dimethylhydrazine was increased by surgical treatment, by the use of dietary changes or treatment with sequestrants, bile acids were again shown to be co-carcinogenic. Table 16 lists studies in which dietary or other treatment has changed the faecal bile acid concentration and has similarly changed the incidence of colorectal tumours. The animal models of large bowel carcinogenesis have been reviewed by LaMont and O'Gorman [116].

Thus there is a considerable body of evidence that bile acids can act as co-carcinogens in the rat large bowel. Similar evidence from studies of humans will be discussed later.

4.6.3. Steroid Oestrogens. The evidence that steroid oestrogens can act as tumour initiators or promoters in animals has been discussed by Bischoff [101] and is summarised in Table 17. The role of oestrogens in human carcinogen-

Table 17. Evidence from animal studies that steroid oestrogens can act as tumour initiators or promotors (for references, see ref. [101]).

Tumour site	Animal	Route of administration
Breast	Rat	S.C. implant of estradiol
Endometrium	Mouse	
	Rabbit	S.C. implant of estradiol
	Rat	Oestrogen dependence in castrates
	Mouse	
Adrenal cortex	Rat	Estrone implant
Kidney	Hamster	S.C. implant of estradiol

Table 18. Tryptophan metabolites shown to be carcinogenic or co-carcinogenic in various test systems (for references, see ref. [59]).

Tryptophan metabolite	Test system
Indole Indoleacetic acid	} A.A.F. treated rats
3-Hydroxykynurenine 3-Hydroxyanthranilic acid 8-Hydroxyquinaldic acid Xanthenuric acid Quinaldic acid	} Bladder implantation
3-Hydroxykynurenine 3-Hydroxyanthranilic acid	} Mutagenicity in cultured mammalian tissue cells

esis has been reviewed by McMahon [107], but to date there is no evidence that oestrogen can cause bowel cancer in animals or in humans, although it is clear that quite large amounts of estradiol, estriol and estrone reach the colon and are excreted in faeces [118].

4.6.4. Tryptophan Metabolites. A number of tryptophan metabolites have been claimed to be carcinogens or tumour promotors (Table 18) although most of the data are open to criticism. In particular, the bladder implantation method used by Bryan *et al.* [119] appears to be as likely to depend on the solid state carcinogenesis by the cholesterol carrier as on the test compound. All of the metabolites of tryptophan listed on Table 18 have been shown to be produced by bacteria and so it is possible that they are produced in the human colon by bacterial action on dietary trystophan.

4.6.5. Tyrosine Metabolism. Tyrosine is metabolised by the gut bacteria to phenol and p-cresol, both of which are excreted in large amounts in normal

Table 19. The factors affecting the production of phenol and p-cresol in the human intestine (these phenols are excreted in the urine after absorption from the colon).

	Effect on urinary volatile phenols excreted
Small bowel overgrowth	Increase total U.V.P.; increase phenol = p-cresol ratio
Total colectomy or removal of gut flora by pre-operative bowel preparation	Great decrease in U.V.P./day
Increase dietary protein	Increase U.V.P./day
Increase dietary fibre	Decrease U.V.P./day

human urine together with small amounts of a number of other urinary volatile phenols (U.V.P.s). The factors affecting the normal amounts of U.V.P. are shown in Table 19.

A range of volatile phenols including phenol and p-cresol have been shown to be co-carcinogenic in skin painting studies in rats treated with a tumour initiating dose of dimethylbenzanthracene. They have yet to be tested as tumour promotors in the rat colon.

4.6.6. N-nitroso Compounds. N-nitroso compounds are formed by the action of nitrite on a suitable nitrogen compound at acid pH or, when mediated by bacterial action, at neutral pH: the receptor molecule maybe a secondary, tertiary or quaternary amine (giving a dialkylnitrosamine), an amide (giving an N-nitrosamide) or an alkylurea (giving N-nitrosourea). The N-nitroso compounds are a group of very potent carcinogens active in all animals in which they have been tested to date, and there is no reason to believe that humans are uniquely resistant to their carcinogenic action (although there is, as yet, no unambiguous evidence that N-nitroso compounds cause human cancers).

Although N-nitrosamides and N-nitrosoureas are direct-acting carcinogens giving rise to tumours at the site of application, N-nitrosamines need activation to give a proximate carcinogen and so give rise to tumours at a site distant from the site of application. This activation appears to take place in specific organs since the N-nitrosamines are target organ specific, the target organ varying from animal to animal and from nitrosamine to nitrosamine (Table 20). The carcinogenicity of the N-nitroso compounds has been reviewed by Magee and Barnes[120] and their possible role in human carcinogenesis has been summarised by Hill[121].

Although there has been little work on the mechanism, it appears that the mixed bacterial populations found in the human gastrointestinal tract may be able to activate N-nitroso compounds making N-nitrosamines relevant to local carcinogenesis. Volatile N-nitrosamines have been detected in human

Table 20. Target organ of N-nitrosamines in various animal species[120]).

Target organ	N-nitrosamine	Test animal
Kidney	Dimethylnitrosamine, single dose i.p.	Rat
Liver	Dimethylnitrosamine, divided doses i.p.	Rat
Oesophagus	N-nitrosopiperidine	Rat
Lung	N-nitrosomorpholine	Rat
Bladder	Dibutylnitrosomine	Rat
Liver	N-nitrosopiperidine	Hamster
Oesophagus	N-nitrosomorpholine	Hamster

faeces [122] and in the urine/faeces of patients with ureterosigmoid anastamosis [121].

4.6.7. Other Endogenous Carcinogens/Mutagens. Several groups of workers have described the presence of mutagens in human faeces [e.g. 123–125]. Since ileostomy effluent contains no mutagens, the mutagens in faeces were presumably formed during transit through the colon. These mutagens have yet to be identified and their relevance to human colorectal carcinogenesis is the subject of much speculation.

Commoner *et al.* [126] have described the formation of mutagens in beef and beef extract during cooking, and there have been many other reports of dietary carcinogens but these are unlikely to be related to the faecal mutagens; they are all lipid-soluble and so would be readily absorbed from the upper small intestine and would not, therefore, reach the colon. The absence of mutagens in ileal effluent confirms this.

4.7. Nutrition

The possible role of various components of diet has already been referred to in section 2.5 where the studies correlating dietary components with the risk of large bowel cancer were described. There have been a number of studies in animals indicating that the nutritional status of the animal is an important factor in carcinogenesis. Tannenbaum and Silverstone in a series of studies showed that rats fed diets rich in protein had a higher incidence of spontaneous liver tumours [127], whilst Tucker [128] showed that animals fed a low calorie diet lived much longer and had a much lower incidence of spontaneous tumours.

4.8. Genetic Factors

Although the studies of migrants indicate that environmental factors are the major determinants of the incidence of colorectal cancer in a population, there are indications from other work that genetic factors should not be ignored.

Cancer family syndrome and familial polyposis coli, both of which are determined by autosomal dominant genes account for only a small proportion of the total incidence of colorectal cancer. However, Lovett [55] in a study of relatives of 209 bowel cancer cases showed that first order relatives (parents, siblings and offspring) had an excess risk varying from 3-fold (for parents) to 5.5-fold (for siblings); when segregated by sex the male relatives had a 5-fold excess and the female relatives a 3-fold excess risk of colorectal cancer. In addition, the relatives had an excess risk of the associated cancers (cancer of the prostate × 2 in males, cancer of the uterus × 1.4 and of the breast × 1.8 in females); they also had an excess risk of stomach cancer (×1.8 in males and ×2.5 in females). An association between cancer of the large bowel and cancer of the stomach has not been reported before.

The adenoma–carcinoma sequence has already been described in section 3.1.4; the genetic component of bowel carcinogenesis might be due to a role in adenoma formation or progression to carcinoma. Veale [71] has suggested that large bowel adenomas show an inherited tendency and postulated a recessive autosomal gene that makes the affected person adenoma-prone. In support of this, Kirsner *et al.* [129] showed that of 421 patients who had an adenoma removed from the large bowel, 41% developed further adenomas within 11 years. It is difficult to dissociate genetic from environmental factors in interpreting the findings of Lovett or of Kirsner *et al.*, but if the hypothesis of a genetic factor in adenoma formation is substantiated then it would indicate that environmental factors determine the overall incidence of adenomas in a population whilst genetic factors determine which persons within a uniformly exposed population will actually develop the disease. It would also provide a valuable lead in cancer prevention, since it would strongly indicate that relatives of colorectal cancer or colorectal adenoma patients should be followed up rigorously whilst those with no family history of the disease would be unlikely to develop a large bowel malignancy.

5. ROLE OF BILE ACID METABOLITES

5.1. Role of Bile Acids as Tumour Promotors on the Human Large Bowel

Since the first suggestion by Aries *et al.* [130] that large bowel cancer might be caused by a metabolite produced by gut bacterial action on the bile acids, much effort has been expanded by many groups in trying to validate (or otherwise) and to clarify the role of bile acids in colorectal carcinogenesis. The current position is not clear.

There have been a number of studies showing that populations with a high incidence of colorectal cancer have a higher faecal bile acid (FBA) concentration than do populations with a low incidence of the disease (Table 21). Hill *et al.* [131] studied nine populations in eight countries and found a good correlation between FBA concentration and bowel cancer incidence and similar results were obtained in studies of various racial groups recently migrated to New York [132], of three socioeconomic groups in Hong Kong [18] and of four Scandinavian populations (urban and rural Finns compared with urban and rural Danes) – this being an extension of a previous study [134], which found no difference in FBA concentration between urban Danes and another group of rural Finns. In addition, a study of two populations in South Africa, which set out to relate faecal steroids to diet, coincidentally showed that, when eating their normal diet, White South Africans have a higher FBA concentra-

Table 21. Faecal bile acid (FBA) concentration in populations with a high incidence of colorectal (CR) cancer compared with that in populations with a low incidence of the disease.

Populations studied	Observation	Reference
1) 6 populations in various parts of the world	FBA concentrations correlated with CR cancer	131
2) 5 populations in New York	FBA concentrations correlated with CR cancer	132
3) 3 populations in Hong Kong	FBA concentrations correlated with CR cancer	18
4) Black and white South Africans	FBA concentrations correlated with CR cancer	136
5) Finland and Denmark	No relation	60
6) Finland (2 populations) and Denmark (2 populations)	FBA concentrations correlated with CR cancer	134
7) Finland and New York	FBA concentrations correlated with CR cancer	135

tion than do Black South Africans (and also have a higher incidence of colorectal cancer). A study comparing two groups of Japanese with greatly different incidences of bowel cancer found no differences in faecal bile acid concentration [133].

Case-control studies have been less favourable to the bile acid hypothesis. Those by Hill *et al.* [137] and by Reddy and Wynder [138] found that bowel cancer patients had a higher FBA concentration than did control persons, but Blackwood *et al.* [139], Mudd *et al.* [140] and Moskvitch *et al.* [141] found no difference; the latter provided a possible explanation for the discrepancy by noting that those patients with other cancers but with liver metastases had low FBA concentrations (so reducing the mean value); they presumably had too few colorectal cancer cases to justify separation in those with and those without liver metastases but Hill [104] has done so (Table 22); if those cases with Dukes'A tumours are removed then the difference between cases and controls becomes small, and disappears if right-sided tumours are considered.

Prospective studies are in progress in high risk populations and in a population of 8000 normal persons aged 45–75; these have been described by Hill [103] and should provide good evidence on the role of bile acids in human colorectal carcinogenesis.

Studies of animals have been much less ambiguous, possibly because of the nature of the animal model used and possibly because the experimental conditions are much 'cleaner'. The model involves the treatment of rats with a dose of dimethylhydrazine or azoxymethane, both of which are organ-

Table 22. FBA concentration in large bowel cancer cases (analysed by subsite and by Dukes' classification) and control person (data from ref. [104]).

Type of colorectal carcinoma	Number of patients	Mean FBA concentration (mg/g dry weight)
All large bowel cancers	84	10.1
colon cancers	30	10.6
caecum & ascending & transverse	10	9.0
descending & sigmoid	20	11.4
rectal cancers	38	10.3
upper third	13	10.3
mid third	12	10.8
lower third	13	10.0
Dukes' A	17	10.6
Dukes' B	36	10.7
Dukes' C	25	9.6
Dukes' C-2	6	7.7
Wealthy control persons*		7.8

* Persons living in South Wales aged 45-75 who formed a random sample from our prospective study population in that area.

specific carcinogens for the large bowel. The dose is one which gives a low incidence of colorectal tumours and then the diet etc. is modified to change the FBA concentration. The results have already been discussed (Table 16) and appear to indicate unambiguously that *in this model* bile acids act as tumour promoters. The question remaining is the relevence of this model, which is an excellent one for the studies of the histopathology of the adenoma–carcinoma sequence, to studies of colorectal carcinogenesis in humans.

The bile acids have been postulated to be implicated in the causation of large bowel cancer by dietary fat or meat and in the prevention of bowel carcinogenesis by dietary fibre. The faecal bile acid concentration is increased with increasing dietary fat [142, 143] and it has been postulated that dietary fat causes an increase in the amount of bile acid substrate for the production of tumour promotors in the large bowel [5]. In this respect, the less readily digestible bound fat would be expected to have a greater effect than free fat, in agreement with the observations of Drasar and Irving [29]. Dietary meat would be effective on this mechanism because of its bound fat component; since meat is the major source of dietary bound fat, the observation by Armstrong and Doll [30] that meat is more strongly correlated with bowel cancer than is total fat would be entirely reasonable.

Burkitt [7] has suggested that dietary fibre increases faecal bulk, thereby diluting the faecal carcinogens, and speeds transit, thereby giving the carcinogens less time to be formed and to act. It has been pointed out that the argument relating speed of transit to the ability of carcinogens to act is fallacious [144], but in any case in the only epidemiological studies in which fibre has been inversely related to bowel cancer incidence [60, 134], there was no difference in transit time between the populations. In the many studies relating FBA concentration to fibre intake, summarised in refs. [145] and [104], only cereal fibres cause a dilution of the faecal steroids whilst pectin ('fruit fibre') and lignin either increase the FBA concentration or have no effect, in accordance with the data of Irving and Drasar [146] that only cereal fibre is inversely related to bowel carcinogenesis whilst fruit fibres positively correlated with the disease.

In addition, it is known that beer drinking increases FBA loss. Vitamin C, which is a general scavenger of electrophiles, could act by removing the mutagens or promotors produced from the bile acids as they are formed and before they are able to act. Thus, the bile acids are good potential substrates for colon carcinogen production and could offer a rationalisation of many of the observed correlations with diet. If co-carcinogens *are* produced from bile acids and if these *are* the cause of large bowel cancer then we would not necessarily expect a clear-cut correlation with a single dietary item and the complex relationship observed between diet and bowel cancer incidence is entirely reasonable.

5.2. Bacterial Metabolism of Bile Acids

The bacterial metabolism of bile acids in the human gut has been summarised by Hill [147]. The principle reactions (Table 23) include deconjugation of

Table 23. Metabolism of bile acids by human gut bacteria.

Reaction	Enzyme	Organisms carrying out the reaction
1) Deconjugation of bile salts	Cholylglycine hydrolase	*Bacteroides* spp., *Clostridium* spp. *Bifidobacterium* spp.
2) Hydroxysteroid dehydrogenation at the C-3, C-7 and C-12 hydroxyl groups	3-Hydroxysteroid dehydrogenase 7 HSDH 12 HSDH	*Eubacterium lentum* *Esch. coli* *Clostridium* spp
3) 7-Dehydroxylation	7-Cholyldehydroxylase	*Bacteroides* spp. *Clostridium* spp. *Bifidobacterium* spp.
4) 4–5 Dehydrogenation of the bile acid nucleus	3-Oxo-Δ4-dehydrogenase	*Cl. paraputrificum* *Cl. tertium*

the amino acid conjugates, hydroxysteroid oxidoreductase action at the C-3, C-7 and C-12 position, and dehydroxylation at the C-7 position. In addition to these reactions on the substituents on the cholanoyl nucleus, there are a number of reactions involving the steroid nucleus itself, including the 3-oxo-Δ^4-dehydrogenase, which produces steroids with a 4-en-3-one configuration from the saturated bile acids. In addition to these enzymic activities, a range of additional reactions have been described by the group led by Dr. R. Bilton and Dr. A. Mason [148, 149], when organisms were incubated with bile acids as sole carbon source for prolonged periods. These include side-chain cleavage and ring-opening reactions.

Of these many enzymic activities, two have been incriminated in large bowel carcinogenesis; these are the Δ^4-dehydrogenase and the 7-dehydroxylase. The evidence in favour of a role for Δ^4-dehydrogenase comes from studies of the carriage of the organisms able to carry out the reaction. In a very detailed survey of gut organisms by Goddard et al. [150], only certain clostridia referred to as NDC (for nuclear dehydrogenating clostridia to distinguish them from those only able to dehydrogenate the hydroxyl substituents and from those unable to carry out either reaction) were able to produce unsaturated bile acids from those found in the normal human gut. These NDC were found to be carried by 30–40% of persons living in England, a higher proportion in Americans but none of the Japanese, Indians or Ugandans tested [151]. Similar results to those found in England have been obtained in Scotland [139], Denmark and Finland [60]. In case-control studies, a much higher proportion of bowel cancer cases than control persons carried NDC [137, 139].

The evidence for a role for 7-dehydroxylase comes from two sources:
(a) Studies of the faecal bile acids of various populations showed that the faecal concentration of deoxycholic acid correlated better with bowel cancer than did the total FBA concentration [131]; deoxycholic acid is the product of 7α-dehydroxylase action on the biliary bile acid cholic acid;
(b) The activity of 7α-dehydroxylase is very much higher in faeces from bowel cancer cases than in faeces from control persons [152].

Animal studies indicate a role for bacterial metabolites since, in the dimethylhydrazine model, the incidence of tumours in germ-free animals was very much lower than that in conventional animals. This is unlikely to be due to the release of enterohepatically circulated carcinogens by β-glucuronidase, as suggested by Renwick and Drasar [153], since there is no difference in faecal activity of β-glucuronidase between bowel cancer cases, patients with high risk diseases (adenomatous polyps or colitis) and control persons [152] and is more likely to be related to bile acid degrading enzymes. In humans the combination of high FBA concentration with carriage of NDC described more than 70% of bowel cancer cases compared with less than 10% of con-

Table 24. The proportion of persons with high FBA and carrying NDC in persons with large bowel cancer (analysed by subsite and by Dukes' classification) and in control persons.

Patient group	Number of persons	% with high FBA/NDC*
Normal healthy persons	100	8
Large bowel cancer cases	84	48
caecum and ascending colon	10	30
sigmoid and rectum	58	57
Dukes' A	17	77
Dukes' B	36	52
Dukes' C	25	32
Dukes' C-2	6	0

* 'High FBA' is defined as above the level of the 80th percentile in a normal healthy British population, and is currently 9.9 mg/g dry weight.

trols[137]. This FBA/NDC discriminant described a high proportion of persons whose tumour was in the rectum or left colon but only a small proportion of persons whose tumour was on the right side (Table 24); Haenszel and Correa[24] have already produced evidence from epidemiology that the causation of right-sided colon cancer differs from that of cancer of the left colon and rectum.

In summary, from studies in germ-free compared with conventional animals, it is apparent that the presence of bacteria in the colon increases the rate of carcinogenesis; from studies in humans the metabolic reactions that are of importance are 7-dehydroxylation and Δ^4-dehydrogenation and a 3-oxo-4, 6-chaladien-24-oic acid has been postulated[147] as the possible causative agent. This compound has been tested and shown to be mutagenic in the salmonella mutagenesis assay system (Bilton, personal communication).

6.   ETIOLOGY OF THE ADENOMA–CARCINOMA SEQUENCE

6.1. Description of the Adenoma–Carcinoma Sequence

In section 3.1.4, I have described briefly the etiology of colorectal adenomas, and summarised the evidence for the adenoma–carcinoma sequence. In summary, the prevalence of adenomas in a population appears to be related to the cultural environment, probably the diet, whilst the persons who actually develop adenomas amongst a population evenly exposed to the etiological agent are determined by genetic factors. I will now consider the evidence on the progression from adenoma to carcinoma. This has been reviewed and summarised by Morson[57], and by Correa[62].

Although almost all (if not all) carcinomas arise in performed adenomas, most adenomas do not progress to malignancy. This is clear from the prevalence rates of colorectal adenomas and carcinomas in various countries (Table 9); even in the populations with the highest colorectal cancer rates, less than 5% of the population will develop the disease during their lifetime, whereas more than 25% of the men aged 60 years in high risk countries carry one or more colorectal adenomas. It is clear that the risk of an adenoma becoming malignant depends on the size of the adenoma (Table 8), on whether it is villous or tubular (Table 8) and on the degree of dysplasia in the adenoma. The distribution of adenomas along the large bowel is fairly even in autopsy studies whilst carcinomas tend to be much more likely to arise in the left colon and rectum (Table 11); most large adenomas are found in the left colon, their distribution being similar to that of carcinomas. Similarly, adenomas in the left colon are more likely than those in the right colon to exhibit advanced dysplasia [62].

Thus, the adenoma–carcinoma sequence can be described as a series of steps (Figure 1):

(1) There is an autosomal recessive gene p, which confers adenoma-proneness on a person. Since it is recessive this will only be expressed in persons who are pp; those who are pn (where n is the normal variant of p) or nn will not be adenoma-prone.

(2) When a population is exposed to an environmental agent (termed E-1) those people who are pp will be prone to develop adenomas whilst persons who are pn or nn will be resistant to the action of E-1 and will develop adenomas only rarely; these latter persons will therefore play no further role in the adenoma–carcinoma sequence.

(3) Most adenomas in persons living in countries with a low risk of large bowel cancer remain small and have a low malignant potential but in persons living in high risk (of carcinoma) countries a higher proportion of adenomas grow to a large size with a high malignant potential (Table 25). These large adenomas are more common in Japanese living in Hawaii than in Japanese living in Japan; this and other evidence indicates that a

Table 25. The size distribution of adenomas in various countries (data from ref. [154]).

Population	Risk of large bowel cancer	% of adenomas greater than 10 mm diameter
Colombia	Low	2
Japan	Low	5
Sweden	High	27
England	High	39

Table 26. The relation between malignant potential and adenoma volume.

Mean diameter of adenoma	Mean volume of adenoma*	Malignant potential	Malignant potential per unit volume
<0.5 cm	0.05	0	0
0.5–1 cm	1.3	1.3	1
1-2 cm	10.5	9.5	1
>2 cm	49.5	46.0	1

* Volume calculated on the assumption that the polyp is a sphere, with a mean diameter midway in the range (i.e. 0.25 for those <0.5 cm, 0.75 for those 0.5 –1 cm, 1.5 for those 1–2 cm and 2.5 for those >2 cm).

factor related to the cultural environment (termed E-2) causes small adenomas to grow to a large size.

(4) Large adenomas are more common in the left colon and rectum than in the right colon whilst small adenomas are evenly distributed throughout the large bowel.

(5) A further factor C causes adenomas to become dysplastic and eventually malignant. This factor is much more active on large adenomas than on small adenomas, but this may be related simply to the number of adenomatous cells for C to act on, since the malignant potential is related to the volume of the adenoma (Table 26). The malignant potential of adenomas greater than 2 cm diameter is the same in Japan, Britain and Sweden, indicating that C is not related to the environment. It may represent the 'chance' of mutation in adenoma cells.

The postulated mechanism of the adenoma–carcinoma sequence as described above is illustrated diagramatically in Figure 1 and has been reviewed by Hill [154].

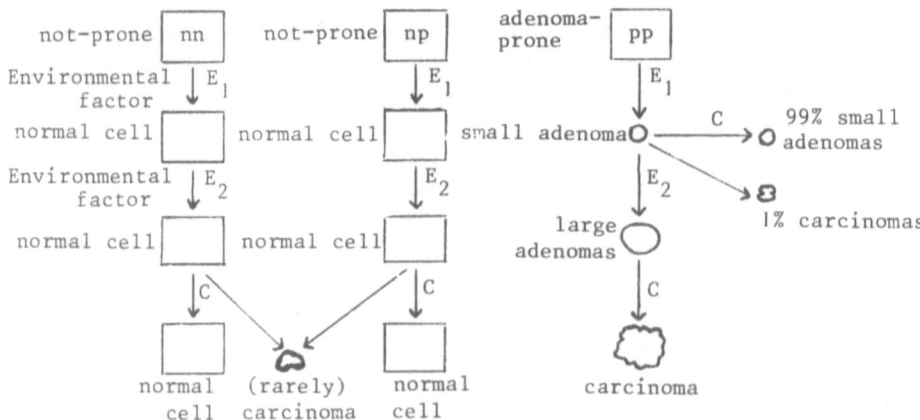

Figure 1. A proposed mechanism for the adenoma-carcinoma sequence.

Table 27. The relation between mean FBA concentration and carriage rate of NDC and adenoma size.

	Mean FBA concentration	% carrying NDC
Normal persons	7.8	35
All patients with polyps	8.1	36
those with non-adenomatous polyps	6.8	31
adenomas 0–5 mm diameter	6.6	20
adenomas 5–10 mm diameter	7.4	28
adenomas 10–20 mm diameter	8.7	54
adenomas >20 mm diameter	10.1	67

6.2. Identification of E-1, E-2 and C

If the postulated mechanism of the adenoma–carcinoma sequence is correct, then certain deductions can be made. The first is that in most countries the incidence of adenomas is very much higher than the incidence of carcinomas. Thus the rate-limiting step in colorectal carcinogenesis is not the rate of adenoma formation but the rate of adenoma growth and the characteristics of the epidemiology of colorectal carcinomas are those of E-2. In Africa, however, where colorectal adenomas are very rare it is likely that the rate of adenoma formation is the rate-limiting step.

It can be concluded, then, that the amount of E-2 to which a person is exposed is related to diet, particularly to dietary fat and meat. The concentration of E-2 is greater in the distal large bowel than in the proximal colon. It is greater in urban than in rural persons. From the case-control studies it is likely that the environmental factor E-2 causing adenomas to grow is the bile acid metabolite produced by the NDC described in section 5.2. In support of this, it has been demonstrated in a study of 102 patients with colorectal adenomas that:

(1) Patients with adenomas have the same mean FBA concentration and carriage rate of NDC as persons with no adenomas (Table 27), indicating that the bile acid metabolite is not related to E-1.
(2) The mean FBA concentration and carriage rate of NDC increases with adenoma size, supporting the hypothesis that the FBA/NDC discriminant is related to E-2.
(3) There was no relation between FBA concentration or NDC carriage and degree of dysplasia in the adenomas, indicating that the FBA/NDC discriminant is not related to C.

We know little about the environmental agent causing adenomas to be formed, E-1, because we have little detailed data on the causation of adenomas. The results of studies of populations living in various countries and of migrants indicate that E-1 is related to the cultural environment, probably to diet. The subsite distribution of adenomas indicates that E-1 enters the caecum pre-formed or is readily released (as, for example, the glucuronide conjugate of an enterohepatically circulated carcinogen), and is not continuously generated or released during transit through the large bowel.

Colorectal adenomas are more likely to arise in men than in women [62], the sex-ratio being similar to that for carcinomas in the rectum and in the stomach. This indicates that hormonal factors may play a promoting role in the action of E-2 or C, since the proportion of adenomas progressing to carcinomas must be much higher in women than in men in order to give the observed sex-ratio of colorectal carcinomas. Oestrogen receptors have been observed in the human colon, and a role for oestrogens would explain the association between colon cancer and cancers of the breast, ovary and endometrium; it might also explain the change in sex-ratio of colorectal cancer with age.

Persons with adenomatosis coli readily develop large numbers of adenomas. This would represent an extreme form of adenoma-proneness (or extreme sensitivity to factor E-1) so that even the limited exposure to E-1 of, for example, Japanese persons, is sufficient to give rise to very large numbers of adenomas. In cancer families, in contrast, there must be a very high proportion of adenomas progressing to carcinomas and so, on our postulated mechanism, this would be explained as extreme sensitivity of adenomas to E-2. In ulcerative colitis, where there appears to be no mediating adenoma, the 'normal' mucosa has apparently been rendered sensitive to the direct action of C by the long-term inflammation and, perhaps, the loss of the normal proctective mucin barrier.

7. CONCLUSIONS

In this presentation I have described the epidemiology of large bowel cancer and offered a unified hypothesis of the etiology of the adenoma-carcinoma sequence in which at least three factors together with genetic predisposition are involved. This provides the flexibility necessary to explain the very complex epidemiology of the disease. Whether or not it is correct remains to be demonstrated.

REFERENCES

1. Cutler SJ, Young JI: In: Persons at high risk of cancer, Fraumeni J (ed.). New York: Academic Press, 1975, pp 307–342.

2. Wynder EL, Shegematsu T: Environmental factors in cancer of the colon and rectum. Cancer 20:1520–1561, 1967.
3. Wynder EL: The epidemiology of large bowel cancer. Cancer Res 35:3388–3394, 1975.
4. Correa P, Haenszel W: The epidemiology of large bowel cancer. Adv Cancer Res 26:1–141, 1978.
5. Hill MJ: The etiology of colon cancer. Crit Rev Toxicol 4:31–82, 1975.
6. Berg J, Howell MA: The geographic pathology of large bowel cancer. Cancer 134:807–814, 1974.
7. Burkitt DP: Relationship as a clue to causation. Lancet ii:1237–1240, 1970.
8. Segi M, Kurihara M: Cancer mortality for selected sites in 24 countries, No 4: Sendai, Japan: Dept. of Public Health, Tokohu Univ. School of Medicine, 1966.
9. Doll R, Muir CS, Waterhouse JAH (eds): Cancer incidence in five continents, vol 2. Geneva: U.I.C.C., 1970.
10. Waterhouse J, Muir C, Correa P, Powell J (eds): Cancer incidence in five continents, vol 3. Lyon: IARC Sci. Publication No. 15, 1976.
11. Doll R: The geographical distribution of cancer. Br J Cancer 23:1–8, 1969.
12. Haenszel W: Cancer among foreign born in the United States. J Natl Cancer Inst 26:37–132, 1961.
13. Haenszel W, Kurihara M: Studies of Japaneses migrants. 1. Mortality from cancer and other diseases among Japanese in the United States. J Natl Cancer Inst 40:43–68, 1968.
14. Haenszel W, Dawson EA: A note on the mortality from cancer of the colon and rectum in the united States. Cancer 18:265–272, 1965.
15. Elmasri SH, Boulos PB: Carcinoma of the large bowel in the Sudan. Br J Surg 62:284–286, 1975.
16. Registrar General's Statistical Review of England and Wales. London: HMSO.
17. Haenszel W, Correa P, Cuello C: Social class differences in large bowel cancer in Cali, Colombia. J Natl Cancer Inst 54:1031–1035, 1975.
18. Crowther JS, Drasar BS, Hill MJ, MacLennan R, Magnin D, Peach S, Teoh-Chan CH: Faecal steroids and bacteria and large bowel cancer in Hong Kong by socio-economic groups. Br J Cancer 34:191–198, 1976.
19. Wynder EL, Kajitani T, Ishikawa, S, Dodo H, Takano A: Environmental factors of cancer of the colon and rectum. II. Japanese epidemiological data. Cancer 23:1210–1220, 1969.
20. Paymaster JC, Sanghri LD, GangadharanP: Cancer in the gastrointestinal tract in Western India. Cancer 21:279–288, 1968.
21. Phillips RL: Role of life-style and dietary habits in risk of cancer among Seventh-day Adventists. Cancer Res 35:3513–3522, 1975.
22. Lyon JL, Klauber MR, Gardner JW, Smart CR: Cancer incidence in Mormons and non-Mormons in Utah, 1966–1970. New Eng. J Med 294:129–133, 1976.
23. Lee JAH: Recent trends of large bowel cancer in Japan compared to United States and England and Wales. Int J Epidemiol 5:187–194, 1976.
24. Haenszel W, Correa P: Cancer of the large intestine. Epidemiological findings. Dis Colon Rectum 16:371–377, 1971.
25. De Jong UW, Day NE, Muir CS et al.: Sub-site distribution of colorectal cancer. Int J Cancer 10:463–477, 1972.
26. Powell J: Malignancy in the large bowel, the interrelationship of sex, age and subsites. Br J Cancer 32:249, 1975.
27. Rhodes JB, Holmes FF, Clark GM: Changing distribution of primary cancers in the large bowel. J.A.M.A. 238:1641–1643, 1977.
28. Gregor O, Toman R, Prusova F: Gastrointestinal cancer and nutrition. Gut 10:1031–1034, 1969.

29. Drasar BS, Irving D: Environmental factors and cancer of the colon and breast. Br J Cancer 27:167–172, 1973.
30. Armstrong B, Doll R: Environmental factors and cancer incidence and mortality in different countries, with special reference to dietary practices. Int J Cancer 15:617–631, 1975.
31. Lice K, Stamler J, Moss D, Garside D, Persky V, Soltero I: Dietary cholesterol, fat and fibre and colon cancer mortality. Lancet ii:782–785, 1979.
32. Higginson J: Etiological factors in gastrointestinal cancer in man. J Natl Cancer Inst 37:527–545, 1966.
33. Haenszel W, Locke FB, Segi SegiM: A case-control study of large-bowel cancer in Japan. J Natl Cancer Inst 64:17–22, 1980.
34. Pernu J: An epidemiological study on cancer of the digestive organs and respiratory system. Ann Med Intern Fenn 49:1–117, 1960.
35. Bjelke E. Epidemiologic studies of cancer of the stomach, colon and rectum, with special emphasis on diet. Scand J Gastro 9:(supplement 31), 1974.
36. Modan B, Barell V, Lubin F, Modan M, Greenberg R and Graham S: Low fibre intake as an etiologic factor in cancer of the colon. J Natl Cancer Inst 55:15–18, 1975.
37. Haenszel W, Berg JW, Segi M, Kwihara, M, Locke FB: Large bowel cancer in Hawaiian Japanese. J Natl Cancer Inst 51:1765–1779, 1973.
38. Hill, MJ, MacLennan R, Newcombe K: Diet and large bowel cancer in three socioeconomic groups in Hong Kong. Lancet i:436, 1979.
39. Bargen JA: Chronic ulcerative colitis associated with malignant disease. Arch Surg 17:561–576, 1928.
40. Goldgraber MB, Kirsner JB: Carcinoma of the colon in ulcerative colitis. Cancer 17:657–665, 1964.
41. Cook, MG, Goligher JC: Carcinoma and epithelial displasia complicating ulcerative colitis. Gastroenterology 68:1127–1136, 1975.
42. Greensten AJ, Sachar DB, Smith H, Pucillo A, Papatestas AE, Kreel I, Geller SA, Janowitz HD, Aufses AH: Cancer in universal and left-sided ulcerative colitis: factors determining risk. Gastroenterology 77:290–294, 1979.
43. MacDougall IPM: Clinical identification of those cases of ulcerative colitis most likely to develop cancer of the bowel. Dis Col & Rect 7:447–450, 1964.
44. MacDougall IPM: In: The prevention of cancer, Raven RW, Roe FJC (eds). London: Butterworths, 1967.
45. Morson BC, Pang LSC: Rectal biopsy as an aid to cancer control in ulcerative colitis. Gut 8:423–434, 1967.
46. Dobbins WO: Current status of the pre-cancer lesion in ulcerative colitis. Gastroenterology 73:1431–1433, 1977.
47. Weedon DD, Shorter RC, Ilstriep DM et al.: Crohn's disease and cancer. N Eng J Med 289:1099–1103, 1974.
48. Crips WH: Two cases of disseminated polyposis of the rectum. Trans Pathol Soc (London) 33:165, 1882.
49. Handford H: Disseminated polypi of the large intestine becoming malignant strictures (malignant adenoma) of the rectum and splenic flexure. Trans Pathol Soc (London 41:133, 1890.
50. Dukes, CE: Familial intestinal polyposis. Ann Eugen 17:1–29, 1952.
51. Bussey HJR: Familial polyposis coli. Baltimore: Johns Hopkins Univ Press, 1975.
52. Yao T, Lida M, Ohsato K, Watanabe H, Omae T: Duodenal lesions in familial polyposis of the colon. Gastroenterology 73:1086–1092, 1977.
53. Morson BC: Evolution of cancer of the colon and rectum. Cancer 34:845–849, 1974.
54. Lynch HT, Krusch AJ: Heredity and adenocarcinoma of the colon. Gastroenterology 53:517–527, 1967.

55. Lovett E: Familial factors in the etiology of carcinoma of the large bowel. Proc Roy Soc Med 67:751–752, 1974.
56. Peltokallio P, Peltokallio V: Relationship of familial factors to carcinoma of the colon. Dis Colon Rectum 9:367–370, 1966.
57. Morson BC: The polyp–cancer sequence in the large bowel. Proc R Soc Med 67:451–457, 1974.
58. Enterline, HT: Significance of adenomatous polyps in colon carcinogenesis. In: Colon cancer, Grundmann E (ed.). Stuttgart: Fischer Verlag, 1978, pp 57–66.
59. Granqvist D, Gabrielsson N, Sundelin, P: Diminutive colonic polyps — clinical significance and management. Endoscopy 11:36–42, 1979.
60. I.A.R.C. Intestinal Microecology Group. Dietary fibre, transit time, fecal bacteria, steroids and colon cancer in two Scandinavian populations. Lancet ii:207–211, 1977.
61. Enstrom JE: Colrectal cancer and beer drinking. Br J Cancer 35:674–683, 1977.
62. Correa P: Epidemiology of polyps and cancer. In: The pathogenesis of colorectal cancer, Morson BC (ed.). London: Saunders, 1978, pp 126–152.
63. Barge T, Ekelund G, Mellner C, Pihl B, Wenckert A: Carcinoma of the colon and rectum in a defined population. Acta Chir Scand Suppl 438, 1973.
64. Haghighi P, Nasr K, Mohallattee E, Ghassemi H, Sadri S, Nabizadeh I, Sheikholaslami M, Nostafavi N: Colorectal polyps and carcinoma in southern Iran. Cancer 39:274–278, 1977.
65. Williams AO, Chung EB, Aghata A, Jackson MA: Intestinal polyps in American negros and Nigerian Africans. Br J Cancer 31:485–491, 1975.
66. Rios-Dalenz J, Smith LB, Thompson TF: Diseases of the colon and rectum in Bolivia. Am J Surg 129:661–664, 1975.
67. Stemmermann GN, Yatani R: Diverticulosis and polyps of the large intestine. Cancer 31:1260–1270, 1973.
68. Hill MJ: Etiology of the adenoma-carcinoma sequence. In: The pathogenesis of colorectal cancer, Morson BC (ed.). London: Saunders, 1978, pp 153–162.
69. Ekelund G: On cancer and polyps of the colon and rectum. Acta Pathol Microbiol Scand. 59:165–170, 1963.
70. Correa P, Dugue E, Cuello C, Haenszel W: Polyps of the colon and rectum in Cali, Colombia. Br J Cancer 9:86–92, 1972.
71. Veale AMP: Intestinal polyposis. London: Eugenics Lab. Memoirs, Ser. 40, Cambridge Univ. Press, 1965.
72. McMahon B, Cole P, Brown J: Etiology of human breast cancer: a review. J Natl Cancer Inst 50:21–42, 1973.
73. Armstrong BK: The role of diet in human carcinogenesis with special reference to endometrial cancer. In: Origins of human cancer, Hiatt H, Watson J, Winsten J (eds.). New York: Cold Spring Harbour Lab. Press, 1977, pp 557–566.
74. Wynder EL, Mabuchi K, Whitmore WF: Epidemiology of cancer of the prostate. Cancer 28:344 360, 1971.
75. Lingeman CH: Etiology of cancer of the human ovary: a review. J Natl. Cancer Inst 53:1603–1618, 1974.
76. Burkitt DP: Epidemiology of cancer of the colon and rectum. Cancer 28:3–13, 1971.
77. Cleave, TL: The saccharine diseases. Bristol: Wright, 1974.
78. Burkitt DP: An epidemiological approach to cancer of the large intestine: the significance of disease relationship. Dis. Colon Rectum 17:456–461, 1974.
79. Moertal CG, Nobrega FT, Elveback LR, et al.: A prospective study of appendicectomy and predisposition to cancer. Surg Gynecol Obstet 138:549–553, 1974.
80. Castleden WR, Doouss TW, Jennings KP, Leighton M: Gallstones, Carcinoma of the colon and diverticular disease. Clin Oncol 4:139–144, 1978.

81. Frederick J: Personal communication.
82. Wolfgram F: Similar geographical distribution of multiple sclerosis and cancer of the colon. Acta Neurol Scand 52:294–302, 1975.
83. Imhotep. In: The Edwin Smith surgical papyrus. Chicago: Chicago Univ. Press, 1930.
84. Pott, P: In: Works of Pott, vol 2: Dublin: James Williams, 1775, p 403.
85. Hoover R: Effect of drugs — immunosuppression. In: Origins of human cancer, Hiatt H, Watson J, Winsten J (eds.). New York: Cold Spring Harbour Lab. Press, 1978, pp 369–380.
86. Berlinger NT, Lopez C, Lipkin M, Vogel JE, Good RA: Defective recognitive immunity in family aggregates of colon carcinoma. J Clin Invest 59:761–769, 1977.
87. Bone G, Appleton DR, Lauder I: Cutaneous delayed hypersensitivity responses to 2, 4-dinitrobenzene. A prognostic guide in malignant disease. Br J Surg 60:906–913, 1973.
88. Bone G, Lauder I: Cellular immunity, peripheral blood lymphocyte count and pathological staging of tumours in the gastrointestinal tract. Br J Cancer 30:215–221, 1974.
89. Martin MS, Martin F, Justabo E, Michel MF, Lagneau A: Effet de l'immunotherapie par le BCG sur la cinétique de croissance de 5 lignées de cancers colique chimio-induits chez le rat. Gastroenterol Clin Biol 3:247–253, 1979.
90. Clayson DB: Chemical carcinogenesis. London: Churchill, 1962.
91. Hueper WC, Conway WD: Chemical carcinogenesis and cancers. Springfield: Thomas, 1964.
92. Selikoff A: Cancer risk and asbestos exposure. In: Origins of human cancer, Hiatt, H, Watson J, Winsten J (eds.). New York: Cold Spring Harbour Lab. Press, 1978, pp 1765–1784.
93. Doll R: Mortality from lung cancer in asbestos workers. Br J Ind Med 12:81–86,.1955.
94. Wogan GN: Dietary factors and special epidemiological situation of liver cancer in Thailand and Africa. Cancer Res 35:3499–3502, 1975.
95. Peers FG, Linsell CA: Dietary aflatoxin and liver cancer: a population based study in Kenya. Br J Cancer 27:473–484, 1973.
96. Dungal N: Stomach cancer in Iceland. Can Cancer Conf 6:441–450, 1966.
97. Roach WA: The possible presence of nitrosamines in Transkei foodstuffs. In: N-nitroso compounds: analysis and formation, Bogovski P, Preussman R, Walker EA (eds). Lyon: I.A.R.C., 1972, pp 74–78.
98. Cook JW: Discussion on experimental production of malignant tumours. Proc Roy Soc B 113:273–285, 1933.
99. Fieser LF: Bicentenary Conference. Philadelphia: Univ. of Pennsylvania, 1941.
100. Yang NC, Castro AJ, Lewis M et al.: Polynuclear aromatic hydrocarbons, steroids and carcinogenesis. Science 134:386–387, 1961.
101. Bischoff F: Carcinogenic effects of steroids. Adv Lipid Res 7:165–244, 1969.
102. Hill MJ: Bacterial metabolism. In: Topics in gastroenterology No. 5, Truelove S, Lee E (eds). Oxford: Blackwell, 1977, pp 45–64.
103. Hill MJ: In: Origins of human cancer, Hiatt H, Watson J, Winsten J (eds). New York: Cold Spring Harbour Lab. Press, 1978, 1627–1640.
104. Hill MJ: The etiology of colorectal cancer. In: Recent advances in gastrointestinal pathology, Wright R (ed). London: Saunders, 1980, pp 297–310.
105. Hieger I: Cholesterol carcinogenesis. Br Med Bull 14:159–160, 1958.
106. Reddy BS, Watanabe, K: Effect of cholesterol metabolites and promoting effect of lithocholic acid in colon carcinogenesis in germ-free and conventional F344 rats. Cancer Res 39:1521–1524, 1979.
107. Cruse JP, Lewin MR, Ferulano GP Clark CG: Co-carcinogenic effects of dietary cholesterol in experimental colon cancer. Nature 276:822–824, 1978.

108. Cook JW, Kennaway EL, Kennaway NM: Production of tumours in mice by deoxycholic acid. Nature 145:627, 1940.

109. Salaman MH, Roe FJC: Further tests for tumour initiating activity: N, N-di-(2-chloroethyl)-p-aminophenylbutyric acid (CB 1348) as initiator of skin tumour formation in the mouse. Br J Cancer 10:363–378, 1956.

110. Narisawa T, Magadia NE, Weisburger JH, Wynder EL: Promoting effect of bile acid on colon carcinogenesis after intrarectal instillation of M.N.N.G. in rats. J Natl Cancer Inst 53:1093–1097, 1974.

111. Silverman SJ, Andrews AW: Bile acids: co-mutagenic activity in the Salmonella–mammalian–microsome mutagenicity test. Brief communication. J Natl Cancer Inst 59:1557–1559, 1977.

112. Demerec M: Mutations induced by carcinogens. Br J Cancer 2:114–117, 1948.

113. Kelsey MI, Pienta RJ: Transformation of hamster embryo cells by cholesterol-x-epoxide and lithocholic acid. Cancer Lett 6:143–149, 1979.

114. Chomchai C, Bhadrachan N, Nigro ND: The effect of bile on the induction of experimental intestinal tumours in rats. Dis. Colon Rectum, 17:310–312, 1974.

115. Nigro N, Singh DV, Campbell RL, Pak MS: Effects of dietary beef fat on intestinal tumour formation by azoxymethane in rats. J Natl Cancer Inst 54:439–442, 1975.

116. LaMont JT, O'Gorman, TA: Experimental colon cancer. Gastroenterology, 75:1157–1169, 1978.

117. McMahon B, Cole P: Endocrinology and epidemiology of breast cancer. Cancer 24:1146–1150, 1969.

118. Goldin BR, Adlercreutz H, Dwyer JT, Swenson L, Warren JH, Gorbach SL: The effect of diet on excretion of oestrogens in pre- and post-menopausal women. Cancer Res. (in press).

119. Bryan GT: Pellet implantation studies of carcinogenic compounds. J Natl Cancer Inst 43:255–261, 1969.

120. Magee, PN, Barnes JM: Carcinogenic citrose compounds. Adv Cancer Res 16:163–246, 1967.

121. Hill MJ: Bacterial metabolism and human carcinogenesis. Br Med Bull 36:89–94, 1980.

122. Wang T, Kazikoe T, Dion P, Furrer R, Varghese AJ, Bruce WR: Volatile nitrosamines in normal human faeces. Nature 276:280–282, 1978.

123. Bruce WR, Varghese AJ, Wang S, Dion, P: In: Naturally occurring carcinogens — mutagens and modulators of carcinogenesis, Miller EC et al. (eds). Baltimore: Japan Sci Soc Press, 1979, pp 221–228.

124. Mower H: Personal communication cited in ref. [123].

125. Ehrich M, Aswell J, Van Tassell R, Wilkins T, Walker ARP, Richardson N: Mutagens in the feces of 3 South African populations at different levels of risk of colon cancer. Mutation Res 65:231–240, 1979.

126. Commoner B, Vithayathil A, Dolaro P, Nair S, Madyastha P, Cuca G: Formation of mutagens in beef and beef extract during cooking. Science 201:913–916, 1978.

127. Tannenbaum A, Silverstone H: Genesis and growth of tumours; effect of varying the proportion of protein (casein) in the diet. Cancer Res. 9:162–173, 1949.

128. Tucker MJ: The effect of long term food restriction on tumours in rodents. Int J Cancer 23:803–807, 1979.

129. Kirsner JB, Rider JA, Moeller HC et al.: Polyps of the colon and rectum: Statistical analysis of a long-term follow-up study. Gastroenterology 39:178–182, 1960.

130. Aries VC, Crowther JS, Drasar BS, Hill MJ, Williams REO: Bacteria and the aetiology of cancer of the large bowel. Gut 10:334–335, 1969.

131. Hill MJ, Drasar BS, Aries VC, Crowther JS, Hawksworth GM, Williams REO: Bacteria and the etiology of large bowel cancer. Lancet i:95–100, 1971.

132. Reddy BS, Wynder EL: Large bowel carcinogenesis: fecal constituents of populations with diverse incidence rates of colon cancer. J Natl Cancer Inst 50:1437–1442, 1973.

133. Mower HF, Ray RM, Shoff R *et al.*: Fecal bile acids in two Japanese populations with different colon cancer risks. Cancer Res 39:328–331, 1979.

134. Hill M, Taylor A, Thompson M, Wait R: Fecal steroids and urinary volatile phenols in four Scandinavian populations. Nutrition and Cancer (in press).

135. Reddy BS, Hedges A, Laakso K, Wynder EL: Fecal constituents of a high risk North American and a low risk Finnish population for the development of large bowel cancer. Cancer Letters 4:217–222, 1978.

136. Antonis A, Bersohn I: The influence of diet on fecal lipids in South African white and Bantu persons. Am J Clin Nutr 11:142–155, 1962.

137. Hill MJ, Drasar BS, Williams REO, Meade T, Simpson J, Morson BC: Faecal bile acids, clostridia and the etiology of cancer of the large bowel. Lancet i:535–539, 1975.

138. Reddy BS, Wynder EL: Metabolic epidemiology of colon cancer: fecal bile acids and neutral steroids in colon cancer patients with adenomatous polyps. Cancer 39:2533–2539, 1977.

139. Blackwood A, Murray WR, Mackay C, Calman K: Fecal bile acids and clostridia in the etiology of colorectal cancer and breast cancer. Br J Cancer 38:175, 1978.

140. Mudd DG, McKelvey ST, Sloan JM, Elmore DT: Faecal bile acid concentrations in patients at increased risk of large bowel cancer. Acta Gastroenterol Belg 41:241–244, 1978.

141. Moskovitz, M, White C, Floch M: Bile acid and neutral steroid excretion in carcinoma of the colon, other cancers and control subjects. Gastroenterology, 75:1071, 1978.

142. Hill MJ: The effect of some factors on the fecal concentration of acid steroids: neutral steroids and urobilins. J Pathol 104:239–245, 1971.

143. Cummings JH, Wiggins HS, Jenkins DJA, Houston H, Jivraj T, Drasar BS, Hill MJ: Influence of diets high and low in animal fat on bowel habit, gastrointestinal transit time, fecal microflora, bile acid and fat excretion. J Clin Inv 61:953–963, 1978.

144. Hill MJ: Colon cancer: A disease of fibre depletion or dietary excess? Digestion 11:289–306, 1974.

145. Thompson MH, Hill MJ: The effect of dietary fibre on intestinal flora and carcinogenesis. In: Pflanzenfasern-Ballaststoffe in der Menschlichen Ernährung, Rottka H (ed). Stuttgart: Georg Thieme Verlag, 1980, pp 135–142.

146. Irving D, Drasar BS: Dietary fibre and cancer of the colon. Br J Cancer 28:462–463, 1973.

147. Hill MJ: The role of colon anaerobes in the metabolism of bile acids and steroids and its relation to colon cancer. Cancer 36:2387–2400, 1975.

148. Owen RW, Bilton RF, Tenneson ME: The degradation of cholic acid and deoxycholic acid by Bacteroides species under strict anaerobic conditions. Biochem Soc Trans 5:1711–1714, 1977.

149. Tenneson ME, Owen RW, Mason AN: The anaerobic side chain cleavage of bile acids by Escherichia coli isolated from human faeces. Biochem Soc Trans 5:1758–1760, 1977.

150. Goddard P, Fernandez F, West B, Hill MJ, Barnes P: The nuclear dehydrogenation of steroids by intestinal bacteria. J Med Microbiol 8:429–435, 1975.

151. Drasar BS, Goddard P, Heaton S, Peach S, West B: Clostridia isolated from faeces. J Med Microbiol 9:63–71, 1976.

152. Mastromarino A, Reddy BS, Wynder EL: Metabolic epidemiology of colon cancer: enzymic activities of the fecal flora. Am J Clin Nutr 29:1455–1460, 1976.

153. Renwick A. Drasar BS: Environmental carcinogens and large bowel cancer. Nature 263:234–235, 1976.

154. Hill MJ: The etiology of the adenoma–carcinoma sequence. In: The pathogenesis of colorectal cancer, Morson BC (ed). London: Saunders, 1978, pp 153–162.

9. Colonoscopy in the Prevention, Detection and Treatment of Large Bowel Cancer

CHRISTOPHER B. WILLIAMS

Since introduction of the fibreoptic colonoscope, into clinical practice in 1969–70, the investigation and management of colo-rectal disease has been transformed. For the first time since barium contrast radiology became available in the early years of this century, there is an alternative method for inspection of the whole colon and rectum and for the first time biopsies and tissue specimens can be taken from the proximal colon without recourse to operation. Not only will the instrument reach to previously inaccessible areas, but the view obtained in colour, in close-up and from the mucosal aspect is frequently better than that of the radiologist in black and white or that of the surgeon from the serosal aspect of the bowel.

The incidence of large bowel pathology in general and large bowel neoplasia in particular, increases towards the rectum. It was frequently claimed that the rigid proctosigmoidoscope could view most of the 'at risk' area of the colo-rectum. At best this was wishful thinking since there was no way of checking the facts; at worst, it was cruel. In spite of good. intentions the forced insertion of a rigid tube high up the sigmoid colon amounts to torture. With the advent of the fibre-sigmoidoscope and long colonoscope the position is radically changed because the patient should have little or no pain for considerably more bowel examined.

In the past decade a great deal of experience – technical, clinical and pathological – has accumulated about the possibilities and the limitations of colonoscopy [1–9]. This chapter constitutes a personal view of the impact of the technique on the problem of colo-rectal cancer in the Western world.

1. USE AND LIMITATIONS OF COLONOSCOPY AS A DIAGNOSTIC METHOD

Colonoscopic bowel preparation requirements [4, 10] are not different from those for X-ray or surgery, but since the endoscopist sees any residue close-up in colour, and since passage of the colonoscope may be impossible, he has a greater incentive than either radiologist or surgeon to evolve thorough preparation regimes and to be critical about their efficacy. Our experience with different regimes in a large number of patients suggests that there is no 'perfect method'. Regimes based on dietary restrictions and purgatives such as castor oil, senna, magnesium salts and enemas give poor results in 10% of patients and acceptable but less than perfect results in 50%. The saline lavage method [11, 12] by nasal intubation and perfusion of 5–10 litres of normal saline is more effective but very demanding on nursing time and disliked by some patients [13]. The compromise of drinking a smaller volume of saline or mannitol solution [14] gives less good results and is still not tolerated by all patients. Overall the best results are obtained by choosing a 'normal' routine that fits local circumstances and by being prepared to vary it to the needs of the individual. A patient who vomits the preparation or gets a poor result on one occasion will do the same thing again unless the regime is changed.

The endoscopist has the advantage of being able to aspirate and remove any fluid or soft residue. Unlike the radiologist he has no difficulty in telling the difference between faecal residue and tissue masses. If the results of preparation are too bad, he is also likely to abandon the procedure and say so, whereas the radiologist still obtains pictures of a kind and the surgeon can continue his procedure, at a risk. These points are unglamorous but important for the certain diagnosis or exclusion of neoplastic lesions. The bowel preparation regimes evolved for colonoscopy should give better results for the other disciplines as well.

Detailed technical aspects of colonoscopy are not [1–5, 9, 15, 16] relevant to this chapter. Some general points must be recognised. A colonoscopic examination is relatively acceptable to the patient if he knows it is the means of early diagnosis of cancer or avoiding abdominal surgery; nonetheless it is an invasive procedure, usually feared, unwelcome and often made tolerable only by heavy sedation. It is occasionally impossible. Colonoscopy is also a manual technique that depends on the dexterity of the performer; its propagandists are usually virtuosos or enthusiasts who make light of the difficulties sometimes encountered and make it seem that total colonoscopy is effortless and routine. Even an expert will find about 25% of colonoscopies technically difficult or at least transiently painful for the patient. The non-expert may have to cut short or compromise on the procedure, or may increase the sedation and convert his difficulty into potential danger for the patient. These problems are of little importance in patients at high risk for cancer, compared to the gains in accuracy made by colonoscopy, but they should be borne in mind in thinking of the fibre-scope as a 'routine' or 'screening' procedure of the whole colon of any patient by any doctor.

Colonoscope design has evolved very rapidly; improvements in glass technology have lead to smaller glass fibres and therefore smaller fibre-bundles, which makes possible a high resolution and wide-angle view. The small bundle also allows more space in the instrument shaft for stronger angling-wires and a larger instrument channel for biopsy-taking, suction, etc. By a process of trial and error, more flexible colonoscopes have proved easier for the non-expert to handle than the original stiffer models and this 'softness' of the shaft is the main characteristic of the colonoscope compared to the gastroscope. The flexibility and pronounced tip-angulation of the modern colonoscopes make it possible to pass with relative ease flexures that were difficult or required difficult manoeuvres (such as the so-called alpha manoeuvre [3, 9]) only a few years ago. With more agile instruments it is thus possible to divorce colonoscopy from dependence on fluoroscopy and to make it an 'office procedure' [7].

Further advances in design and technology will presumably occur and there is even research into the possiblity of self-propelled colonoscopes, although the great variability in the physical characteristics and attachment in each individual colon make the 'ideal colonoscope' as unlikely as the 'perfect' bowel preparation. For the moment, insertion of a colonoscope is an unpredictable business, sometimes easy, sometimes difficult and also difficult to teach except by experience. Many, but not all, doctors find that they can manage the technique satisfactorily; many but not all patients prove to be suitable for re-examination if necessary. Some who are very difficult to colonoscope are better managed radiologically.

The use of sedative-analgesic combinations, usually diazepam 5–15 mg i.v. and meperidine 25–75 mg i.v., mean that the patient will have little or no recollection of even a difficult procedure. Over-sedated patients can be rapidly revived with naloxone (Narcan) i.v. or i.m. In our experience about one in three patients can be satisfactorily examined without sedation, which is useful for repeated follow-up examinations. Some endoscopists always use sedation, some never do. There should be no after-effects except for the occasional individual with air-distension, which can be easily avoided by using carbon dioxide insufflation for the procedure.

Patient questionnaires usually show preference for colonoscopy compared to the rigid procto-sigmoidoscopy or barium enema previously experienced. This preference should not induce any sense of false security, for there is a small but definite complication rate for colonoscopy [17–24], amounting to about one perforation in about 500 examinations in previous large cumulated series, and the rate is higher in the learning phase and with older intruments. Hopefully, the increased flexibility and agility of the newer instruments will be reflected in lower complication figures, providing that they are not counter-balanced by the problems encountered by the large numbers of doctors now taking up colonoscopy with little guidance or chance to learn from the mistakes of their predecessors.

2. THE RELATIONSHIP OF COLONOSCOPY TO THE AIR-CONTRAST BARIUM
   ENEMA

One of the contributions of colonoscopy has been to highlight the inadequacy of the poorly-prepared single-contrast barium enema offered as the
'standard' procedure in many hospitals, compared to the impressive accuracy
of a well-performed double- or air-contrast enema [25–30]. As more radiologists accept this possibility of improving their technique, and as a new generation of radiologists is trained to it, there should be a change from the present
feeling of competition between 'rival' techniques of endoscopy and radiology
to an atmosphere in which co-operation is possible to ensure that the patient
benefits from what both techniques have to offer [31] (Figure 1). Clearly, local
circumstances will always dictate the 'best-buy' and for a few more years not
enough centres will have both enthusiastic G-I radiologists and competent
endoscopists to allow a free choice.

Essentially, an air-contrast enema is easier to perform than a colonoscopy
but more difficult to interpret: it offers a permanent image, a better view of
topography and the patients are not given sedation. The colonoscope is more
difficult to insert, but the colour close-up view of each area is extremely easy
to interpret and biopsies can be taken for proof. Each technique has its
problems. Barium enema is safer technically but less accurate than colonoscopy in the danger area of the left colon, missing some polyps and cancers in

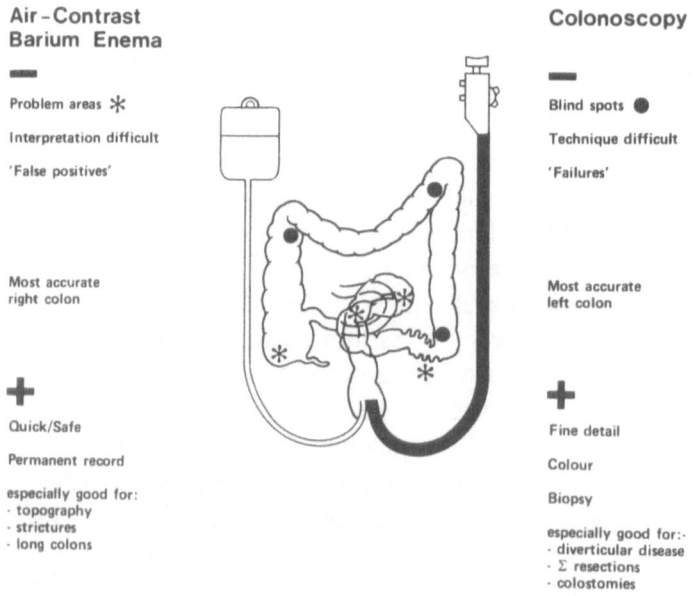

Figure 1. The plus and minus points of air-contrast barium enema and colonoscopy in colonic
diagnosis.

the overlapping loops or diverticular deformations of the sigmoid colon and wrongly committing some patients to colonic surgery, usually due to the confusing appearances of diverticular disease simulating possible cancer.

Colonscopy has 'blind-spots' [32–39] as well as technical difficulties, the capacious and haustrated right colon may be poorly seen and lesions missed [27, 29, 40]. Every honest endoscopist will remember a few 'misses' of his own as well as a large number of the radiologists'! An obvious future combination of the virtues of both techniques (endoscopy easy and accurate in the left colon, barium enema easy and relatively accurate in the right colon) might be for each new patient to have fibre-sigmoidoscopy at his initial visit for gastrointestinal investigation, a decision then being taken on technical and clinical grounds as to whether the rest of the colon is to be screened by barium enema, colonscopy or a combination of the two. Obviously a barium-filled colon cannot be endoscoped without further preparation and an air-filled colon is difficult to coat with barium. However by insufflating carbon dioxide during colonoscopy all the gas is absorbed within 15–20 minutes and barium enema can be performed almost immediately after the endoscopy. The increased accuracy of this double procedure might be justified, for instance, in the follow-up of high-risk patients or to check the right colon if total colonoscopy has proved difficult.

Purely from a mechanical point of view, certain patients select themselves for barium enema or colonoscopy respectively. Colonoscopy to the caecum will be difficult in a patient with a very redundant colon, but total colonoscopy is extremely easy after sigmoid resection. Air-contrast barium enema is usually unsatisfactory in patients with a colostomy or poor anal sphincters, resulting in inability to hold contrast and air so as to obtain satisfactory coating of the mucosa. The barium enema is easy to perform but often impossible to interpret in the presence of diverticular disease, colonoscopy being indicated if there is any reason (bleeding, etc.) to suspect polyps or cancer.

3. THE ROLE OF FIBRE-SIGMOIDOSCOPY

The popularity of fibre-sigmoidoscopy as a screening procedure [41–47] to some extent reflects the difficulty of total colonoscopy but also the limitations of rigid procto-sigmoidoscopy. It does, however, have important virtues of its own compared to total colonoscopy. Fibre-sigmoidoscopy requires no bowel preparation other than a disposable phosphate enema, which evacuates all stool from the distal colon with 90% efficiency, but is not effective in diverticular disease. No sedation is needed for fibre-sigmoidoscopy since the procedure is quick, and terminated if there is undue difficulty or pain. The proximal sigmoid colon is reached in 90% of cases and the descending colon or even the splenic flexure in some. Finally the yield over rigid proctosigmoidoscopy of pathology such as polyps is increased two-to-four fold.

Fibre-sigmoidoscopy does, however, require some patience and skill since the sigmoid colon is the most tortuous part of the bowel and there is likely to remain a major role for the rigid instrument for limited examination in non-specialist centres. Ideally, however, all at-risk patients should have fibre-sigmoidoscopy as part of their work-up unless colonoscopy is planned at a later date. Present fibre-sigmoidoscopes are only 60–70 cm long and relatively stiff; there are certain to be many changes and improvements in instrument design to achieve a comfortable, easy-to-pass short instrument for 'screening' use. Preliminary experience with longer, small-diameter and floppy instruments suggest that such instruments are more acceptable to the patient and will usually reach to the splenic flexure in a maximum of 7 or 8 minutes without sedation. With such instruments the physician will be performing 'limited colonoscopy' rather than fibre-sigmoidoscopy, with a corresponding increase in the usefullness of the examination. The general use of such instruments in symptomatic or follow-up patients should make a major contribution to cancer prevention and detection. Whether limited colonoscopy can be acceptable as a true 'screening procedure' in normal patients remains to be seen.

4. SELECTION OF PATIENTS FOR COLONOSCOPY

4.1. A First-Line Procedure?

Colonoscopy may sometimes be the first-line procedure, performed before, or more likely instead of, barium enema. The least satisfactory reason for this would be the non-availability of high-quality air-contrast barium enema. Other patients may be selected because barium enema has previously been a failure for mechanical reasons, incontinence, diverticular disease, etc. or because colonoscopy is likely to be technically easier, as after sigmoid resection, colostomy. It is also logical to select endoscopy as the investigation of choice for any patient where biopsies are important (chronic ulcerative colitis, ureterosigmoidostomy surveillance) or if colonoscopy is likely to be requested whatever the result of the barium enema (persistent or severe rectal bleeding). The accuracy of endoscopy in seeing minute lesions may be valuable in screening relatives in an adenomatosis (familial polyposis) or colon cancer family, where identification and biopsy of 1–2 mm adenomas may diagnose the condition or place the patient in a 'high-risk' group at a stage when the barium enema would appear normal.

4.2. Abnormality on Barium Enema

When an existing barium enema shows an uncertain abnormality, colonoscopy is important to obtain biopsies or, in the case of a polyp, to perform an excision biopsy of the whole lesion. Even when a 'definite' cancer can be seen on X-ray there may be an indication for colonoscopy, both to make the diagnosis absolute with histological confirmation and to ensure that no synchronous (co-existing) neoplastic lesion has been missed [48]. It is disturbing to find unexpected multiple adenomas on a resection specimen and worse to find them in the remaining bowel post-operatively pointing out, too late, the need for a more extensive resection. In such patients colonoscopy can be attempted in the pre-operative period after surgical bowel preparation and thus fits conveniently into the routine management of the patient.

Strictures demonstrated radiologically merit endoscopic examination [50, 51] with biopsies and/or cytological specimens obtained by brushing or washing [52]. If a standard colonoscope will not pass a stricture, a paediatric colonoscope or paediatric gastroscope, will usually do so or allow passage of a guide-wire for dilatation with subsequent inspection. The most important role of colonoscopy in the examination of strictures usually turns out to be the constructively-negative one of proving that no malignancy is present, therefore avoiding surgery. In chronic ulcerative colitis, for instance, the orthodox view is that any stricture should be assumed to be malignant, whereas colonoscopy and biopsy shows that this is actually rarely the case [49]. An uncommon but important catch for the endoscopist is his inability to exclude *extra*-colonic pathology unless invading neoplasm has penetrated the colonic mucosa; the colonoscopist can only report on the colonic mucosa and in a few circumstances the clinician must make his own judgement based on the combination of the radiological appearances, colonoscopic findings and the overall clinical picture.

Diverticular disease presents a problem for the endoscopist [49, 53–55] as well as the radiologist; characteristically the endoscopic difficulties are technical whereas the radiologist's are interpretative. Patients with diverticular disease are difficult to prepare and to examine endoscopically because of the combination of circular muscle spasm, tortuous lumen with confusing diverticular orifices, and peri-colic adhesions which make the bowel difficult to straighten. Although the colonoscope can be successfully passed in over 90% of patients and a very good view obtained, the examination is likely to be slow and traumatic to both patient and instrument.

Some thought should therefore be given to the indications for examination before colonoscoping a patient with diverticular disease. If the symptoms are those of pain or altered bowel habit compatible with diverticular disease, not accompanied by bleeding, with no previously demonstrated polyps and no radiological suspicion of neoplasm, colonoscopy should be avoided. On the other hand, if there is suspicion and the alternative possibility is surgery, there is a clear indication for colonoscopy, which will usually prove the diverticular disease to be uncomplicated. As with strictures it may be sometimes be necessary to use a paediatric instrument in order to traverse severe diverticular disease, not because of narrowing, which is virtually never a problem, but because of the fixed angulations encountered.

4.3. After Normal Barium Enema

Persistent rectal bleeding with a normal barium enema or apparently uncomplicated diverticular disease has been shown in a number of studies to constitute a major indication for colonoscopy [36–39, 56]. Around 10% of such patients referred for colonoscopy are found to have carcinoma missed on X-ray and a further 15–18% have missed polyps, most of these missed lesions being in the sigmoid colon. These figures reflect a combination of poor X-ray technique and careful clinical selection. The majority of the barium enemas in these series are single-contrast or poorly performed 'air-contrast' examinations. Personal experience suggests that very often the lesion is visible on the films but not reported.

Furthermore, analysis of patients attending a colo-rectal clinic suggests that although the majority mentioned bleeding amongst their presenting symptoms the clinician is usually satisfied that the source of bleeding is local (haemorrhoids, fissure, etc.) and rarely proceeds to further investigation [57]. Only 10% of patients, including those with persistent, darker or mixed-in blood, often seen on sigmoidoscopy, are referred for barium enema and a lesser percentage for colonoscopy. With fibre-sigmoidoscopy available in the clinic the pick-up rate for colonoscopy will fall again, but even with iron deficiency anaemia alone, and after high-quality air contrast enema, there is still a small pick-up of missed right colon or caecal carcinoma.

If prior procto-sigmoidoscopy and barium enema have been normal, patients with abdominal pain or altered bowel habit without bleeding do not merit colonoscopy. To cause obstructive symptoms such as these, a carcinoma must be relatively advanced and will be seen on the X-ray.

4.4. Chronic Ulcerative Colitis Surveillance

In 1967 Morson introduced the concept of rectal-biopsy dysplasia, or pre-cancer, as a marker of potential malignancy in patients with chronic ulcerative colitis [58–60], comparable to the precancerous changes seen in the uterine cervix or the bronchial epithelium. The advent of the colonoscope extended the range of the biopsy forceps throughout the colon, which gives a unique opportunity for repeated examinations to observe the natural history of dysplasia as well as to provide more accurate surveillance for the patient [61–70].

A history of 8–10 years or more of extensive or total colitis is accepted as conferring increased risk for development of colon cancer. There are several problems: at-risk patients may be entirely symptomless and require some persuasion to come for checks at all; a high proportion of cancers are intra-mucosal or flat and likely to be missed on conventional examinations including air-contrast barium enema or colonoscopy without biopsy. Some are only visible on microscopy of the resected colon. Notwithstanding this, at any one time the majority of at-risk patients have neither cancer nor pre-cancerous change and, contrary to previous opinion, most probably never will have. There is therefore no indication for routine colonic excision on the grounds of cancer-risk alone and it is equally unjustified to frighten patients unduly or to submit them to over-rigorous follow-up.

A number of different centres have now reported success in the use of screening for dysplasia in identification of high-risk patients [62, 64, 68–71], up to one half of those with severe dysplasia on biopsy being found to have cancer, usually at a resectable stage. Extremely few patients are described with cancer following ulcerative colitis without associated dysplasia. Conceptually it seems better to risk late diagnosis in a few patients than to commit larger numbers of unselected patients to the significant mortality rate of colo-rectal surgery. It is well recognised that dysplasia may be a patchy abnormality, necessitating multiple biopsies to find or to exclude it [60]. The proportion of patients without rectal involvement when dysplasia is found proximally varies from 10 to 70% in different series but these figures justify the routine use of colonoscopy.

Understandably centres with a high yield from rectal biopsy recommend prime reliance on proctosigmoidoscopy at 6–12 monthly intervals with colonoscopy every 18 months or 2 years, whereas others with a poor yield from rectal biopsy favour annual colonoscopy, taking rectal biopsies during the procedure. Barium enema is not routinely used for, although with high-resolution air-contrast technique it might help to localise areas of interest for endoscopic biopsy [72], which means two procedures for the patient.

The colon is deliberately examined in a quiescent phase if possible because of the difficulty of histological interpretation when the mucosa is actively regenerating during or after a relapse. Perhaps because examination occurs in remission there are very few problems resulting from the formal colonoscopic bowel preparation (using castor oil, senna, etc.) that is necessary for accurate examination. In an experience of several hundred such patients, including a small prospective series where careful observations were made after colonoscopy [73], no severe relapse occurred although several patients required extra medication. Technically colonoscopy may be extremely quick and easy if the colitis has resulted in a tubular shortened colon, examination then being possible in a few minutes and without any sedation. Some examinations are, however, difficult and traumatic and the patient must be protected with heavy sedation if he is to agree to future procedures.

There is a wide range of mucosal appearances in chronic colitis patients, a few returning to normal (transparent, shiny epithelium with visible underlying vascular pattern), many showing thickened 'atrophic' mucosa (pale and feature less and sometimes matt-surfaced) and some having numerous post-inflammatory polyps or mucosal excrescences. The endoscopist needs to take at least 10–15 biopsies at intervals around the colon, with extra biopsies or cytology of any suspicious area [74]; each biopsy can take a minute or more and any ability to localise areas of possible abnormality would be most desirable.

Japanese endoscopists have described the use of 'dye-spray technique' with methylene blue or indigo-carmine, which respectively opacifies the surface and fills up any irregularities or interstices [75]. The dye can be used only in a perfectly clean colon, is time consuming and usually only adds to the problem by highlighting mucosal irregularity, which then shows no dysplasia on biopsy. Severe dysplasia can occur in apparently flat and featureless mucosa but never when there is a visible vascular pattern. Dysplasia is sometimes described histologically as having a villous surface but this is usually not apparent to the endoscopist, who may see only varying degrees of nodular or micro-nodular surface irregularity not strikingly different from the rest of the surface.

There is a problem in differentiating between possibly dysplastic areas and the various shapes of post-inflammatory polyps, sometimes characteristically shiny and wormlike but occasionally irregular and covered in exudate. The most suggestive endoscopically visible lesion is a raised and sometimes plaque-like area 1–3 cm in diameter, the edges of which are indistinct and merge into smaller 'satellite nodules'. Any other polypoid lesion, neoplastic or non-neoplastic, has a discrete edge where it reaches normal mucosa.

In addition to the mucosal biopsies, representative forceps biopsies must be taken of raised lesions other than the most characteristic post-inflammatory polyps. Snare polypectomy or snare loop biopsies will give more material for the pathologist. True adenomas appear to be relatively rare in ulcerative colitis [76] and any pathological report of 'adenomatous tissue' should be assumed to be colitis-associated dysplasia until proved to the contrary. To any but the most experienced pathologist, the microscopic appearances of dysplasia and adenomatous epithelium are identical, the difference between the two lesions being one of macroscopic structure, which is not apparent on a biopsy specimen. The tiny colonoscopic biopsies are thus perfectly adequate for dysplasia screening providing that enough are taken. A map is made at the time of the examination to show the approximate site of biopsies. If the colonoscope has reached the caecum and has been straightened out (usually

70–80 cm) the withdrawal distance will reasonably accurately reflect the position of the tip, 60 cm being transverse colon, 50 cm splenic flexure and 40 cm descending colon. Only the most excessively long or shortened colon deviates from these mapping rules. A report of dysplasia of any grade on any biopsy, particularly if taken from a raised lesion, means that the patient should be considered as high-risk and re-endoscoped within a period of a few months so that extra biopsies can be taken in the relevant area.

The finding of severe, or possibly even moderately severe, dysplasia on repeated biopsies should probably be taken as an indication for surgery. There is circumstantial evidence to suggest that severe dysplasia is indeed an early warning and there is no need for undue haste. Some patients may need 4–6 months of gentle education to the prospect of surgery and modified anatomy, a period which in any case may be necessary for repeat checks before the decision is finalised. With the perfection of various ileal-pouch procedures, particularly the pelvic pouch [77] allowing ileo-anal anastomosis with continence, surgery is in any case much more acceptable.

The combination of an endoscopic-pathological surveillance routine with the possibility of curative surgery in selected patients gives hope that the future management of cancer risk in colitis can be on a rational basis which is also reasonable for the patient. Although from the endoscopist's point of view repetitive surveillance is tedious and unrewarding in about 90% of examinations, the gains to the patient easily jutify the work involved.

4.5. Uretero-colic Anastomoses

The possibility of ureteric implantation into the distal colon (ureterosigmoidostomy) was described over 100 years ago [78] but was most frequently performed from the 1930s to the 1950s, both for older patients with carcinoma of the bladder and for children with congenital bladder anomalies. The operation gave problems with severe chronic renal infection and metabolic acidosis due to colonic absorption of chloride and was therefore superseded by the introduction of the ileal conduit procedure in 1950 [79]. The unexpected long-term complication of ureterosigmoidostomy (and possibly of the ileal-conduit as well) is that colonic cancer may arise at the site of implantation. This was first reported in 1928 [80] and since then there have been numerous case reports of adenomas or adenocarcinomas mostly occurring with a latent interval of between 10 and 30 years after operation [81–85], and the soonest being two years. Since most of the cases reported are between 16 and 35 years of age, it is scarcely surprising that the risk of development of colon carcinoma has been estimated as being from 100 to 2000 times the expected incidence in a normal population of the same age [83, 85]. The reason for this tendency to develop neoplasia is uncertain. Various factors have been suggested, from local trauma, the effect of urinary carcinogens, urinary modification of colonic immune mechanisms to a direct irritant effect of urine.

The importance of follow-up of these patients is obvious and it has been suggested that all patients should be examined every two years until 15 years after operation and annually after that [82, 86]. The potential for malignant change in the non-functioning residual stoma appears to continue even if the urinary stream has been diverted to an ileal conduit many years previously, such patients requiring surveillance of both bowel and conduit.

Previously the suggested mode of screening was by sigmoidoscopy and barium enema. Clearly such patients are now ideal for fibre-sigmoidoscopy and this has proved practicable and acceptable to the patient [84]. Only a single phosphate enema is needed and since sedation is usually unnecessary the procedure is normally completed in a few minutes. Technically the examination is sometimes more difficult than anticipated due to post-operative fixation of the colon; a very flexible endoscope is preferable to one of the large and stiff models of fibre-sigmoidoscope.

It may sometimes be difficult to identify a small stoma but this can be overcome by an intravenous injection of methylene blue before the examination.

The appearance of the normal ureteric stoma may vary enormously from a slit to an ampulla-like blob. Non-neoplastic enlargement may also occur due to cystic dilatation of entrapped mucus; this entirely benign condition may produce a 2–3 cm friable and irregular tumour, endoscopically indistinguishable from a malignant lesion [87].

If adenomatous change occurs it seems to arise in the immediate vicinity of the stoma, which is usually involved in the large tumour which results and surgery is therefore necessary rather than snare polypectomy if the stoma is functional [87, 88].

Having located the stoma, whether normal or enlarged, the endoscopist takes one or more biopsies from both stoma and adjacent mucosa for histological assessment. One or more confirmed dysplastic biopsies presumably warrants surgery as it does in chronic colitis; negative results in an enlarged stoma should lead to a repeat examination and multiple check biopsies after a short interval.

Searching out ureteric-implant patients for check examintion promises to be a highly rewarding field for the endoscopist, with a more accurate and comfortable single procedure for the patient than rigid sigmoidoscopy and barium enema which it replaces. These patients are often young, fit and reluctant to submit to further checks that may at first seem to them to be irrelevant; the risk of not performing regular checks is however, so great that no effort should be spared to achieve compliance.

5. COLONOSCOPY AND THE POLYP PROBLEM

The somewhat sterile argument that raged about whether carcinomas of the colon arise 'de novo' or from pre-existing adenomas seems to have been resolved in favour of general acceptance of the adenoma–carcinoma sequence [89–93]. With the exception of ulcerative or schistosomal colitis and ureteric implants there are no other obvious precursor conditions. Environmental considerations suggest that genetic, nutritional and possibly bacterial factors contribute [94] to determine adenomas. Thereafter the adenoma bulk (size and number) [89] type (tubular, tubulo-villous or villous) and degree of dysplasia (average, moderate, severe) influence the likelihood of cancer being present or being likely to develop in the future. The practical importance of some of these factors to the endoscopist will be mentioned later in this section, but his role is primarily to remove all possible polyps, because most (in Western countries) will be adenomas and some will contain carcinoma.

The problem is mainly that polyps are common, become more frequent with age and are usually an incidental finding during investigation for other reasons. The exact incidence is unknown, depending on the accuracy of the means of study (barium enema, post mortem, etc.) and the age of the population studied [95–98]. Probably over 10% of the population develop one or more adenomas during their life-time and one study calculated that 4% will have an adenoma over 1 cm diameter [99]. A small proportion of these adenomas — 5% in most endoscopic series — contain invasive carcinoma; others, but the minority, might have become malignant at a later date. The time taken for malignant change has been estimated as 3–5 years for a 2 cm adenoma [93] but the evidence for this is, at best, circumstantial. The estimate represents a plausible average rate, some adenomas taking longer and a few a shorter time. Once removed, follow-up studies suggest a 30–40% incidence of further adenomas at an average of 8–10 years follow-up [100–104], but again the results are averaged out without relation to different factors (number of adenomas, degree of dysplasia, family history, etc.) that may put some patients at higher risk [103–105].

The colonoscope has resulted in new-found accuracy in detecting polyps of any size but as colonoscopic snare polypectomy anywhere in the colon is so easy, any chance of new data on the natural history of adenomas is destroyed; a control group would be unethical. Procto-sigmoidoscopic observation of unremoved polyps shows that some grow, some remain stationary, and some disappear. Barium enema demonstrates great variation in the growth rates of adenomas [106–108], a study made possible before colonoscopy became available by the policy of performing repeated radiological follow-up until the polyp was seen to change in size or configuration [109]. Colonoscopy proves the danger of this policy since a significant number of innocuous-looking adenomas on thin stalks are found already to contain invasive malignancy.

6. COLONOSCOPIC POLYPECTOMY

Probably the biggest single advance in the management of colo-rectal disease in recent years has been the ability to remove polyps out of reach of the
sigmoidoscope without recourse to surgery. Not only is it possible [110–113]
but it is also usually easy to do so, thanks to the extreme manoeuvrability
and wide-angle view of current instruments. A polypectomy adds only a few
minutes to the examination, which in most cases is performed on an outpatient basis. Large series are reported [114–121].

Selection of patients presents no great problem since any polyp proximal to
the rectum is suitable for attempted colonoscopic removal and only 3%
(usually large sessile villous adenomas) prove impossible to snare [122]. Fortunately the largest villous adenomas occur in the rectum, where they are
accessible to local surgical removal. Even rectal polyps can be more easily
snared with the fibre-endoscope than with the rigid instrument except for
those within 5–7 cm of the anus where anaesthesia may be needed because
the anal canal is pain-sensitive. The only major exception to the rule of
colonoscopic removal is in a patient with biopsy-proven adenomatosis coli
(familial polyposis coli) where, unless there is some unique reason against it,
colectomy is absolutely indicated.

Bowel preparation for colonoscopic polypectomy can be by one of the methods
previously described except that the danger of employing mannitol, sorbitol or
lactulose must be recognised. These non-absorbed sugars form a perfect
substrate for bacterial fermentation, producing hydrogen [123]. Several studies
have confirmed this risk [124, 125], the highest hydrogen concentration
recorded being 12%, three times the explosive concentration in air. There is
one report of a fatal explosion during polypectomy after mannitol preparation [126]. Although there are several contrary papers in the literature [127–129] suggesting that there is no explosion hazard after colonoscopic
bowel preparation with castor oil, only small numbers of patients were studied
and with the rapid insertion possible with modern instruments there may
occasionally be a small risk of encountering a pocket of hydrogen or methane
not diluted by normal instrumental insufflation and aspiration. Care must be
taken, especially if any faecal residue is present, either to aspirate and re-
insufflate several times before polypectomy or to use carbon dioxide for
insufflation throughout the procedure. If polypectomy is to be performed after
limited bowel preparation for fibre-sigmoidoscopy the use of carbon dioxide is
particularly important because there is a very serious risk of explosive gas
concentrations from the undisturbed faecal content in the proximal bowel.

The technique of colonoscopic polypectomy [9, 113] requires a fair degree of
competence in handling the endoscope, because polyps around acute bends or
in regions fixed by adhesions may be exceedingly difficult to visualise. An

inexperienced endoscopist may get an incomplete view of a polyp and not realise that he has left part of it behind; he may also miss seeing it altogether. The snare wires used are usually commercially available models with a convenient handle, making it possible to estimate how far open the loop is. It is also possible to fabricate home-made snares using a teflon tube and a double length of braided stainless steel wire[112]. Both types of wire give a very good 'feel' to indicate how tightly the polyp is being strangulated. The loop is made relatively thick to avoid any danger of premature cutting as it is closed. Manoeuvring the snare loop into the best position, usually near the top of the polyp stalk, requires some practice; the higher position is safer when snaring because it leaves room for a safe length of electrocoagulation in the centre of the stalk, whereas the base is often wider and more difficult to coagulate.

Electrocoagulation of the stalk vessels (using a high-frequency 'coagulation' or 'blended' current) is the critical part of the procedure[130], since the major complication of polypectomy is haemorrhage[17–22, 24]. If bleeding does occur it is much harder for the endoscopist to stop it than for the surgeon, who has haemostats and sutures at his disposal. The stalk vessels are a leash of arteries and veins derived from the submucosal plexus of the bowel wall and may be at the centre or the periphery of the stalk, so that it is important to see thorough evidence of 'cooking' of the whole polyp stalk (whitening, swelling, boiling or smoke) as or before the wire cuts through. This is more difficult to achieve in stalks over 1 cm diamter, both because large polyps have large muscular feeding vessels, which are difficult to electrocoagulate, and because the volume of tissue to be heated is so much greater.

Patients with large polyps are therefore usually admitted to the hospital for polypectomy, with haematological checks and blood available, whereas most other polypectomies can be arranged on an ambulatory basis. Large polyp stalks may rarely result in a secondary or delayed haemorrhage occurring at 5–14 days due to separation of the slough at the polypectomy site. At-risk patients must be warned of the possibility in case transfusion is required. Haemorrhage at the time of polypectomy is normally self-limiting but can be rapidly controlled by re-closing the snare loop onto the remaining stalk for 15–30 minutes, by which time the feeding vessels will have coagulated. Overall haemorrhage rates after polypectomy are reported of around 1 in 50 patients, very few requiring surgery or arteriographic management[131]. Although immediate or delayed perforations have been reported they are rare, presumably due to the relatively low power (25–35 W) required for most polypectomies.

6.1. Large Polyps

While the majority of colonic polyps are either stalked or semi-pedunculated and snareable, there are occasional large broad-based or sessile lesions that present problems to the endoscopist. Some, such as an extremely flat villous adenoma found in the thin right colon, are clearly unsnareable and probably too hazardous even for more sophisticated techniques such as laser photo-coagulation.

A sessile lesion may be situated on an angle or haustral fold in such a way that it is technically impossible to remove or destroy all parts of it in spite of acute angling or retroversion. A few large polyps in the sigmoid colon can be caught with the snare-loop and removed after snare-intussusception to the anus [132]; others, whilst large, can relatively easily be removed piecemeal by repeated snaring (on different occasions if necessary) [133–136].

The endoscopist may be faced with a dilemma between what is possible and what is wise. Piecemeal removal may cause difficulty if the pathologist cannot be sure whether a focus of invasive carcinoma is from the apex or base of the tumour, and therefore whether it is adequately removed (see below). There is also the theoretical danger that a malignant focus could be left behind unrecognised in the disorganised base of a polyp removed piecemeal. It is also necessary to balance the endoscopic problems against the risks of operation; the rate of growth and malignant change of colonic polyps can be so slow that some older patients with an apparently benign lesion may be best served by doing nothing, and thus avoiding any risk of precipitating a complication. In younger patients it may simply be quicker and surer to opt for surgery at an early stage rather than to attempt heroic endoscopy.

6.2. Small Polyps

Polyps of 2–5 mm in diameter in the rectum are most frequently found to be hyperplastic (metaplastic), but the same is not true of the colon where 35–70% of small polyps are found to be adenomas [122, 137, 138]. Many endoscopists thus adopt the policy of routine biopsy and electrocoagulation of even small lesions using the electrically-insulated 'hot-biopsy forceps' [139]. The chance of such small lesions having any focus of invasive cancer is insignificantly small and there is not even any certainty that they will develop into larger lesions. It may however, be useful in deciding on further follow-up regimes to know the total number of adenomas a patient has, regardless of size, a patient with one or two adenomas being at lower future risk than one who has a total of 5 or 10 [103, 104, 140]. Uncontrolled personal observation suggests that the presence of multiple small adenomas in one segment of colon is not infrequently followed by the development of carcinoma in that segment; multiple adenomas may perhaps reflect an 'unstable' epithelium, or there may have been undetected intramucosal 'microadenomas', as are known to exist in familial adenomatosis (polyposis) coli [141, 142].

6.3. *Multiple Polyps*

The importance of colonoscopy in the diagnosis or exclusion of familial adenomatosis coli at an early stage has already been mentioned, including the enhancement of endoscopic detection of tiny polyps by using the dye-spray technique. This technique may be equally relevant in the few patients seen to have 15–20 obvious polyps during a colonoscopy, because in this situation it may be more important to rule out the presence of future generations of minuscule adenomas than to undertake multiple polypectomies when surgical resection might be more logical. Seeing small polyps is of course no proof without biopsies to confirm that they are adenomas, since multiple hyperplastic (metaplastic), hamartomatous (retention) polyposis also occur [143].

Technically speaking, there is no quick and satisfactory way of snaring multiple polyps and retrieving them whilst keeping them separately identified in case one is malignant. Fortunately only 2% of patients have over 5 adenomas [122] so that this does not present much of a problem, especially if the 'hot-biopsy' technique is used on those of 5–6 mm diameter. The usual practice for retrieving polyps is to suck them onto the instrument tip or pick them up again with the snare-loop, and then to withdraw the whole instrument. Since most polyps are left-sided, re-insertion is usually quick but if not, for instance in a patient with severe diverticular disease, it may be necessary to retrieve the biggest or most suspicious-looking polyp and to attempt to wash out the remainder with a saline enema. The chance of successful evacuation can be increased by infusing the saline down the instrument proximal to the polypectomy sites before it is withdrawn. Although from personal and reported experience [144] there is no technical difficulty in performing 60–70 polypectomies in a patient with non-neoplastic Juvenile or Peutz-Jeghers polyps, there is clearly no indication for attempting such a feat on adenomatous polyps.

7. MALIGNANT ADENOMAS AND POLYPOID CANCERS

Although the endoscopist may have his suspicions that a particular polyp will prove to be an adenoma containing invasive carcinoma, the proof-positive lies with the histopathologist. Contrary to radiological dogma, many malignant adenomas (a colloquially accepted term although pathologically inexact) and even a few polypoid carcinomas are on narrow stalks. Large head size, irregular surface and firmness are features suggesting malignancy, but infarction and entrapment of the regenerating epithelium (misplaced epithelium, pseudo-invasion) can mimic the histological features as well as the endoscopic features of malignancy. If malignancy is suspected, the endoscopist must try to snare the stalk lower down than usual in order to increase the chance of resecting below the level of invasion and to give the pathologist the best possible specimen for interpretation. If malignancy is endoscopically obvious (broad-base and shaggy, ulcerated, friable outline) it is necessary only to obtain a large forceps biopsy or a small snare-biopsy and not to do anything to put the patient at risk before inevitable surgery, other than to check the rest of the colon if this is technically possible. There is no firm evidence to suggest that passage of a colonoscope is more risky than passage of stool in releasing metastatic cells, whereas the gain from checking for synchronous cancer or coexisting polyps is obvious, especially if the rest of the colon has not been well shown on air-contrast barium enema.

The histological definition of malignancy in an adenoma has become more precise since most pathologists have agreed that carcinoma must be seen to be invading across the level of the muscularis mucosae (Figure 2). The previous inclusion of 'focal cancer' or 'carcinoma in situ' was pathologically inexact, since the surface epithelium of any benign adenoma is neoplastic and may show varying degrees of dysplasia, sometimes in patchy distribution. It was also clinically incorrect since, almost without exception, unless there is invasion across the muscularis mucosae, metastases do not occur and the lesion is therefore not clinically malignant. This is ascribed to the fact that the lymphatics within a polyp head are limited by the muscularis mucosae and thus, whatever their malignant potential, severely dysplastic epithelial cells remain benign until they cross the muscularis mucosae.

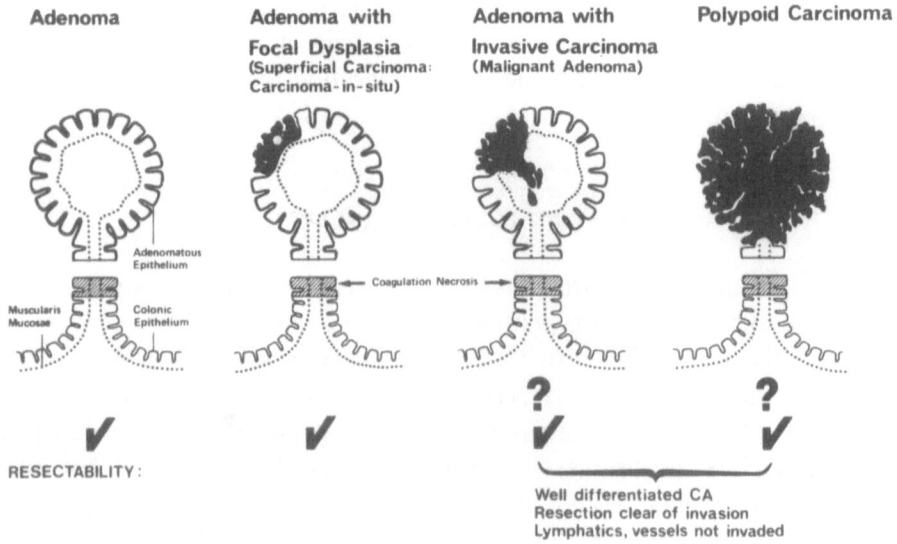

Figure 2. A schematic representation of benign and malignant polypoid neoplasms of the colon and their endoscopic resectability.

Even correcting for this source of error the frequency of malignant adenomas in different colonoscopic series, around 4–5% overall[119, 122, 145], is only half that of the generally accepted figure of 10% malignancy for a large 'surgical' series[93], even if corrected for size or type of adenoma. The colonoscopic figure is more likely to be correct, since the surgical series may be more liable to sources of bias such as the inclusion of adenomas from cancer-resection specimens or a longer period of observation before surgical polypectomy. Even the endoscopic figure may in future tend to fall as series are 'diluted' by a higher proportion of small polyps found at follow-up or as a result of increasing use of the more accurate air-contrast barium enema.

Polypoid carcinomas, composed completely of cancer tissue without evidence of adenoma, add a further 1–2% of malignancies to the endoscopic series. Some of these polypoid carcinomas are pedunculated, and many are 'semi-pedunculated; meaning that after closure of the snare loop at their base they can be lifted up onto a 'pseudo-pedicle' though which the snare can cut safely, leaving a coagulated basal ulcer.

8. CAN MALIGNANCY BE ENDOSCOPICALLY EXCISED?

Formerly, the surgical approach with broad-based or possibly malignant lesions would have been to perform local resection. The endoscopist's ability to resect most lesions encountered, including those subsequently shown by the pathologist to contain invasive carcinoma, brings into new prominence the controversy of local removal versus resection of rectal carcinoma[146–148]. The histopathological rules evolved for rectal lesions apply also to malignant colonic lesions, local removal being judged adequate (Figure 2) if:
1. The carcinoma is of low or average grade malignancy.
2. Invasion is clear of the resection line.
3. Lymphatics and blood vessels are not invaded.

In the rectum there are few exceptions where these rules are satisfied but metastatic carcinoma subsequently develops. Many surgeons therefore accept the principle of attempted local removal on the basis that in the elderly population involved the immediate mortality of colo-rectal surgery is probably at least equal to the longer-term mortality of those that have metastasised[149]. Since so many colonic lesions are pedunculated, conservatism is probably even more justified[122, 145, 158] and though again there are rare exceptions[149, 150], there are also surgical series where local excision of malignant colon polyps resulted in 100% 5-year survival[148]. In our own colonoscopic series of 36 patients with either malignant adenoma or polypoid carinoma satisfying the above rules only one patient is known to have developed metastases with an average of over 4 years follow-up; since this patient died after 9 months, distant metastases may already have been present at the time of excision. The results of those few endoscopists [151–153] who argue for the more aggressive policy of subsequent resection in the hope of removing undetected local spread and nodes will only be justified if their 5–10 year survival rates of matched patients are significantly better than those of the majority taking a more conservative view. In the meantime, it seems commonsensical that any risk of death should be borne by those with spread of cancer rather than as a result of surgery, which will often prove to have been unnecessary.

The colonoscope may also have an occasional role in the palliation of advanced cancer, either in reducing tumour bulk in a patient unfit for any form of surgery, or even in endoscopic dilation of a semi-obstructed patient with insertion of a tube, as is so successful in the oesophagus.

9. POLYP FOLLOW-UP

Whatever the reason for the discovery of a polyp (usually chance) the first colonoscopy presents no logistical problem; the problem lies thereafter. To do annual or even two-yearly follow-up on every patient with such a common lesion as an adenoma would result in grotesque numbers of procedures – 'an endless chain of people colonoscoping each other end to end' [154]. Quite apart from the numbers and expense involved in colonoscopy or barium enema, with prior bowel preparation, these are traumatic procedures for the patient. With new-found access to the colon there is a danger of inducing cancer-hysteria in patients or unjustified fervour for cancer-prevention in the doctor. The new-found accuracy of colonoscopic detection must be used to improve on what we already know about risk-factors, rates of recurrence and methods of follow-up so as to produce for the individual patient the most acceptable follow-up regime at the least frequent intervals necessary.

Following polypectomy it may be desirable to perform a check-examination since 2–5% of polyps may be missed at colonoscopy [105], especially after technically difficult procedures, in a long colon or if bowel preparation was poor. On the other hand if the colonoscopy was preceded by a high-quality air-contrast barium enema there should be little risk of having missed anything. If a malignant polyp was excised and resection is not indicated a check examination should possibly be made within 2–3 weeks whilst the tell-tale electrocoagulation ulcer remains; at this time biopsies can be taken of the base and indian ink injected at the site [155] for future location.

Thereafter the method and frequency of follow-up procedures is at present a matter of judgement. The method used is determined to some extent by patient-preference and the technical difficulty and results of previous procedures; an air-contrast barium enema, properly performed, has advantages that have already been mentioned and should not be dismissed for those patients who are difficult to endoscope or in those many centres where a really skilled endoscopist is not available. Fibresigmoidoscopy possibly combined with air-contrast barium enema may provide a useful compromise procedure but neither occult blood nor CEA estimations appear to have sufficient specificity to form a reliable screening method for detecting polyps [156].

Although the purpose of follow-up is to prevent cancer or to detect it at its earliest and preferably endoscopically resectable stage for practical purposes this means finding adenomas. It has already been pointed out that present follow-up data [100–104] make no allowance for risk factors which might help to separate out for more frequent surveillance those patients at higher risk, and presently recommended 1–3 yearly routines are not based on hard evidence. One useful principle that emerges from previous literature [100, 103] is the concept that finding a polyp-free or 'clean' colon on repeated follow-up justifies a longer interval between examinations, and that a patient with 1–2 polyps removed may in fact be at lower risk than other 'normal' subjects. Follow-up may therefore sometimes be abandoned.

On the other hand, finding numerous recurrent adenomas implies high risk and the need for continued frequent checks. Whether the finding on the initial colonoscopy of numerous (more than 3–5) adenomas, severe dysplasia, malignancy, or villosity always justifies extra surveillance remains to be proved. For the moment most centres would concur with 2–3 yearly checks on patients with 1–2 tubular adenomas [118, 122] with an initially more frequent but gradually reducing rate of check examinations in those at probable higher risk (large, numerous or dysplastic polyps) [103–105]. Even with such regimes, whether because of human error or quirks of nature, unexpected and symptomatic cancers may develop between follow-up examinations and patients must be told to report as usual bleeding or unexplained alterations of bowel habit.

10. CAN COLONOSCOPY PREVENT COLON CANCER?

From the foregoing remarks it will be apparent that there are many reasons why colonoscopy is likely to make only a small dent in the massive colon cancer problem confronting Western physicians. If prevention is the goal (earlier detection is a more likely one), the polyp hunt must be of massive proportions. It has been postulated that about 7 000 000 patients a year in the USA must have new polyps so that, not allowing for negative examinations or those for other reasons, each of perhaps 3000 endoscopists in the country would have to perform 2500 colonoscopies annually with escalating numbers of follow-ups. The morbidity and even the mortality of such an absurd programme would become significant as more and more undertrained endoscopists were enrolled. The financial implications would also be ridiculous.

Some encouragement is brought by the demonstration that regular proctosig-moidoscopy will greatly reduce the expected incidence of rectal cancer in a normal population [157, 158] and the relatively modest expenses of these examinations could be justified against the saving on cancer operations avoided.

If, as seems likely, the key to making good use of the accuracy and thera-peutic efficacy of colonoscopy lies in selecting the highest-risk groups for surveillance it is most unlikely that it will be possible to prove cancer prevention (as opposed to detection) unless a matched control group can be provided. Even if a large number of cancers *are* prevented in a high risk group the observed cancer incidence is unlikely to fall to that expected for the normal population. In certain small and defined groups, such as those with chronic extensive ulcerative colitis or ureterosigmoidoscomies control popula-tions will be possible and good results likely. In the rest of the population it is more likely that the major yield of colonoscopy will be in the avoidance of unnecessary surgery (and thus the occasional death) and in the detection of colon cancer at the Dukes A or B stage when the long-term prognosis is favourable [159]. Without doubt, the problem deserves tackling, colorectal cancer results having not improved over the past 25 years in spite of better surgical technique, and mortality being similar to that of automobile acci-dents [160]. With the advent of colonoscopy, intelligently used, and making a contribution to prevention, early diagnosis [161] and cure it is difficult to imagine that the position cannot be improved [162].

REFERENCES

1. Deyhle P, Demling L: Colonoscopy: technique, results and indications. Endoscopy 3:143–151, 1971.
2. Overholt BF: Flexible fiberoptic sigmoidoscopy — technique and preliminary results. Can-cer 28:123–126, 1971.
3. Sakai Y: The technique of colonofiberscopy. Dis Col Rectum 15:403–412, 1972.
4. Williams CB, Teague RH: Progress report: colonoscopy. Gut 14:990–1003, 1973.
5. Overholt BF: Colonoscopy: a review. Gastroenterology 69:1308–1320, 1975.
6. Shinya H, Wolff WI: Colonoscopy. Surg Ann 8:257–295, 1976.
7. Gaisford WD: Fibreoptic colonoscopy — total colonoscopy — an office procedure. Dis Col Rectum 19:388–394, 1976.
8. Waye JD: Colitis, cancer and colonoscopy. Med Clin N Am 62:211–224, 1978.
9. Cotton PB, Williams CB: Practical gastrointestinal endoscopy. Oxford: Blackwell Scientific, 1980.
10. Teague RH, Manning AP: Preparation of the large bowel for endoscopy. J Int Med Res 5:374–377, 1977.
11. Hewitt J., Reeve J, Rigby J: Whole-gut irrigation in preparation for large bowel surgery. Lancet 2:337–340, 1973.
12. Levy AG, Benson JW, Hewlett EL, Herdt JR, Dopmann JL, Gordon RS: Saline lavage: a

rapid effective and acceptable method for cleansing the gastrointestinal tract. Gastroenterology 70:157–166, 1976.

13. Downing R, Dorricott NJ, Keighley MR, Oates GD, Alexander-Williams J: Whole gut irrigation: a survey of patient opinion Br J Surg 66:201–220, 1979.

14. Rhodes JB, Zvargulis JE, Williams CH, Gonzales G, Moffat RE: Oral electrolyte overload to cleanse the colon for colonoscopy. Gastroint Endosc 24:24–26.

15. Deyhle P: A plastic tube for the maintenance of the straightening of the sigmoid colon during coloscopy. Endoscopy 4:224–226, 1972.

16. Gaisford WD: Fibrendoscopy of the cecum and terminal ileum. Gastrointest Endosc 21:13–18, 1975.

17. Berci G, Parish JF, Shapiro M, Corlin R: Complications of colonoscopy and polypectomy: report of the Southern California Society for Gastrointestinal Endoscopy. Gastroenterology 67:584, 1974.

18. Gathright JB: Evaluation of the colonoscopic examination — complications. Dis Col and Rectum 18:374–375, 1975.

19. Meyers MA, Ghahreman GG: Complications of fiberoptic endoscopy: colonoscopy. Radiology 115:301–307, 1975.

20. Rogers BHG, Silvis SE, Nebel OT, Sugawa C, Mandelstam P: Complications of fiberoptic colonoscopy and polypectomy. Gastrointest Endosc 22:73b–77, 1975.

21. Smith LE: Complications of colonoscopy and polypectomy. Dis Col Rectum 19:407–412, 1976.

22. Chabanon R: Accidents in course of colonoscopy and colonoscopic polypectomy. Ann Gastr Hepat 13:65–73, 1977.

23. Ecker MD, Goldstein M, Hoexter B: Benign pneumoperitoneum after fiberoptic colonoscopy: a prospective study of 100 Patients. Gastroenterology 73:226, 1977.

24. Frühmorgen P, Demling L: Complications of diagnostic and therapeutic colonoscopy in the Federal Republic of Germany. Results of an enquiry Endoscopy 11:146, 1979.

25. Loose HW, Williams CB: Barium enema versus colonoscopy. Proc R Soc Med 67:1033–1036, 1974.

26. Williams CB: Evaluation of the colonoscopic examination: results of 3 studies. Dis Col rectum 18:366–368, 1975.

27. Laufer I, Smith NCW, Mullens JE: The radiological demonstration of colorectal polyps undetected endoscopy. Gastroenterology 70:167–170, 1976.

28. Miller RE, Lehman G: The barium enema — is it obsolete? J.A.M.A. 235:2842–2844, 1976.

29. Miller RE, Lehman G: Polypoid colonic lesions undetected by endoscopy. Radiology 129:295–297, 1978.

30. Wolff WI, Shinya H, Geffen A, Ozoktay S, deBeer R: A comparison of colonoscopy and the contrast enema in 500 patients with colorectal disease. Am J Surg 129:181–186, 1975.

31. Tedesco FJ, Waye JD: Colonoscopy and barium enemas — reply. Ann Int Med 90:857, 1979.

32. Kronborg O, Ostergaard A: Evaluation of the barium enema examination and colonoscopy in diagnosis of colonic cancer. Dis Col Rectum 18, 8:674–677, 1975.

33. Kobayashi S, Yoshii, Y, Kasugai T: Fibercolonoscopy — effective use in symptomatic patients with negative barium enema. Endoscopy 7:63–67, 1975.

34. deBeer RA, Geffin A, Ozoktay S, Shinya H, Wolff WI: Comparison of colonoscopy and contrast X-ray study in diagnosis of 500 cases of colorectal disease. J.A.O.A. 7:569–574, 1976.

35. Thoeni RF, Menuck L: Comparison of barium enema and colonoscopy in the detection of small colonic polyps. Radiology 124:631–635, 1977.

36. Tedesco FJ, Waye JD, Raskin JB, Morris SJ, Greenwald RA: Colonoscopic evaluation of rectal bleeding: a study of 304 patients. Ann Intern Med 89:907–909, 1978.
37. Knoepp LF, McCulloch JH: Colonoscopy in the diagnosis of unexplained rectal bleeding. Dis Col Rectum 21:590–593, 1978.
38. Teague RH, Thornton JR, Manning AP, Salmon PR, Read AE: Colonoscopy for investigation of unexplained rectal bleeding. Lancet 1, 8078:1350–1351, 1978.
39. Swarbrick ET, Fevre DI, Hunt RH, Thomas BM, Williams CB: Colonoscopy for unexplained rectal bleeding. Br Med J 2:1685–1686, 1979.
40. Gelfand DW, Wu WC, Ott DJ: Extent of successful colonoscopy — implication for the radiologist. Gast Radiol 4:75, 1979.
41. Bohlman TW, Katon RM, Lipshutz GR, McCool Mf, Smith FW, Melnyk CS: Fiberoptic pansigmoidoscopy. An evaluation and comparison with rigid sigmoidoscopy. Gastroenterology 72:644–649, 1977.
42. Marino AW: Types of flexible sigmoidoscopes and preparation of the patient. Dis Col Rectum 20:91–93, 1977.
43. Talbott TM: Evaluation of the new flexible sigmoidoscopes Dis Col Rectum 20:88–90, 1977.
44. Lambert R, Olive C, Lange ME, Chabanon R: Fibrorectosigmoidoscopy: results of 476 cases. Nouve Presse Med 7:4213–4215, 1978.
45. Crespi, M, Casale V, Grassi A: Flexible sigmoidoscopy: a potential advance in cancer control. Gastrointest Endosc 24:291–292, 1978.
46. Carter HG: Routine office use of the 60 cm flexible fiberoptic sigmoidoscope Dis Col Rectum 21:101–103, 1978.
47. Manier JW: Fiberoptic pansigmoidoscopy: an evaluation of its use in an office practice. Gastrointest. Endosc 24:119–120, 1978.
48. Marks G., Boggs HW, Castro AF, Gathright JB, Ray JE, Salvati E: sigmoidoscopic examinations with rigid and flexible fiberoptic sigmoidoscopes in the surgeons office. Dis Col rectum 22:162–168, 1979.
49. Heald RJ, Lockhart-Mummery HE: The lesion of the second cancer of the large bowel. Br J Surg 59:16–19, 1972.
50. Hunt RH, Teague RH, Swarbrick ET, Williams CB: Colonoscopy in the management of colonic strictures. Br Med J 2:360–361, 1975.
51. Rozen P, Ratan J, Gilat, T: Colonoscopy in the differential diagnosis of colonic strictures. Dis Col Rectum 18:425–429, 1975.
52. Kline TS, Yum KK: Fiberoptic colonoscopy and cytology. Cancer 37:2553–2556, 1976.
53. Dean ACB, Newell JP: Colonoscopy in the differential diagnosis of carcinoma from diverticulitis of the sigmoid colon. Br J Surg 60:633–635, 1973.
54. Glerum J, Agenant D, Tytgat GN: value of colonoscopy in the detection of sigmoid malignancy in patients with diverticular disease. Endoscopy 9:228–230, 1977.
55. Max MH, Knutson CO: Colonoscopy in patients with inflammatory colonic strictures. Surgery 84:551–556, 1978.
56. Hunt RH: Rectal bleeding. Clin Gastroenterol 7:719–740, 1978.
57. Williams JT, Thomson JPS: Anorectal bleeding — a study of causes and investigative yield. The Practitioner 219:327–331, 1977.
58. Morson BC, Pang LSC: Rectal biopsy as an aid to cancer control in ulcerative colitis. Gut 8:423, 1967.
59. Riddell RH: Endoscopic recognition of early carcinoma in ulcerative colitis. J.A.M.A. 237:2811, 1977.
60. Riddell RH, Morson BC: Value of sigmoidoscopy and biopsy in detecting carcinoma and pre-malignant change in ulcerative colitis. Gut 20:575–580, 1979.

61. Shearman D.J.C.: Colonoscopy in ulcerative colitis. Scand J Gastroenterol 8:289–291, 1973.
62. Cook MG, Goligher JC: Carcinoma and epithelial dysplasia complicating ulcerative colitis. Gastroenterology 68:1127–1136, 1975.
63. Crowson TD, Ferrante WF, Gathright JP: Colonoscopy: inefficacy for early carcinoma detection in patients with ulcerative colitis. J.A.M.A. 236:2651–2652, 1976.
64. Lennard-Jones JE, Morson BC, Ritchie JK, Shove DC, Williams CB: Cancer in colitis — assessment of the individual risk by clinical and histological criteria. Gastroenterology 73:1280–1289, 1977.
65. Rossini FP, Ferrari A: Colonoscopic evaluation in high risk lesions of the large bowel. Giorn Gastroent End 1:69–79, 1978.
66. Waye JD: Colitis, cancer and colonoscopy. Med Clin. North Am 62:211–224, 1978.
67. Yardley JH, Bayless TM, Diamond MP: Editorial: Cancer in ulcerative colitis. Gastroenterology 76:221–225, 1979.
68. Nugent FW, Haggitt RC, Colcher H, Kutterruf GC: Malignant potential of chronic ulcerative colitis. Preliminary report. Gastroenterology 76:1–5, 1979.
69. Blackstone MO, Rogers BHG, Levin B, Riddell RH: Dysplasia associated masses detected by colonoscopy in long-standing ulcerative colitis. Gastroenterology 74:1009, 1978.
70. Grandqvist S, Gabrielsson N, Sundelin P, Thorgeirsson T: Precancerous lesions in the mucosa in ulcerative colitis. A radiographic, endoscopic and histopathological study. Scand J Gastroenterol 15:289–296, 1980.
71. Myrvold HE, Kock NG, Ahren C: Rectal biopsy and precancer in ulcerative colitis. Gut 15:301–430, 1974.
72. Frank PH, Riddell RH, Feczko PJ et al.: Radiological detection of colonic dysplasia (precarcinoma) in chronic ulcerative colitis. Gastrointest Radiol 3:209–219, 1978.
73. Gould SR, Williams CB: Gastrointest Endosc (in press).
74. Grandqvist S, Granberg-Ohlman I, Sundelin P: Colonoscopic biopsies and cytological examinations in chronic ulcerative colitis. Scand J Gastroenterol 15:23–28, 1980.
75. Miyaoka T, Nakajima M, Misaki F, Mirakami K, Kohli Y, Tada M, Koboyashi A, Kawai K: Comparative study of clinical and endoscopical observation of ulcerative colitis. Endoscopy 6:169–175, 1974.
76. Teague RH, Read AE: Polyposis in ulcerative colitis. Gut 16:792–795, 1975.
77. Nicholls RJ, Parks AG: Proctocolectomy without ileostomy for ulcerative colitis. Br Med J 2:85–88, 1978.
78. Simon J: First ureterosigmoidostomy. Lancet 2:568, 1852.
79. Bricker AM: Bladder substitutions after pelvic evisceration. Surg. Clin N Am 30:1511–1521, 1950.
80. Hammer E: Cancer du colon dix ans après implantation des uretères d'une vaissie extrophiée. J Urol Nephrol 28:260–263, 1929.
81. MacGregor AMC: Mucus-secreting adenomatous polyp at the site of ureterosigmoidostomy. Br J Surg 55:591–594, 1968.
82. Haney MJ, McGarity WC: Ureterosigmoidostomy and neoplasms of the colon. Arch. Surg 103:69–72, 1971.
83. Eraklis AJ, Folkman MJ: Adenocarcinoma at the site of ureterosigmoidostomies for exstrophy of the bladder. J Pediatr. Surg 13:730–734, 1978.
84. Rossini FP, Ferrari A, Rizello N: Fiberendoscopic evaluation of ureterosigmoidostomies. Endoscopy 11:249–252, 1979.
85. Thompson PM, Hill JT, Packham DA: Colonic carcinoma at the site of ureterosigmoidostomy: What is the risk? Br J Surg 66:809, 1979.
86. Urdaneta JA, Duffel D, Aust JB: Late development of carcinoma of the colon following ureterosigmoidostomy. Ann Surg 164:503–513, 1966.

87. Markowitz AM, Koontz P: The development of colonic polyps at the site of ureteral implantation. Surgery 60:761–767, 1966.
88. Williams CB, Gillespie PE: Accidental removal of ureteral stoma at colonoscopy. Gastrointest. Endosc 25:109–110, 1979.
89. Enterline HT, Evans GW, Mercado-Lugo R, Miller L, Fitts WT: Malignant potential of adenomas of the colon and rectum. J.A.M.A. 179:322–330, 1962.
90. Morson BC, Bussey H.J.R.: Predisposing causes of intestinal cancer. Current problems in surgery (February), Year Book Medical Publishers, 1970.
91. Potet F, Soullard J: Polyps of the rectum and colon. Gut 12:468–482, 1971.
92. Morson BC: The polyp–cancer sequence in the large bowel. Proc Roy Soc Med 67:451–457, 1974.
93. Muto T, Bussey HJR, Morson BC: The evolution of cancer of the colon and rectum. Cancer 36:2251–2270, 1975.
94. Hill MJ: The etiology of colon cancer. Crit Rev Toxicol 31:82, 1975.
95. Atwater JS, Bargen JA: Pathogenesis of intestinal polyps. Gastroenterology 4:395–408, 1945.
96. Blatt LJ: Polyps of the colon and rectum: incidence and distribution. Dis Col Rectum 4:277–282, 1961.
97. Chapman I, Adenomatous polypi of large intestine: incidence and distribution. Ann Surg 157:223–226, 1963.
98. Hughes LE: The incidence of benign and malignant neoplasms of the colon and rectum: a post mortem study. Austral N Z J Surg 38:30–35, 1968.
99. Arminski TC, McLean DW: Incidence and distribution of adenomatous polyps of the colon and rectum based on 1000 autopsy examinations. Dis col Rectum 7:249–261, 1964.
100. Kirsner JB, Rider JA, Moeller HC, Palmer WL. Gold SS: Polyps of the colon and rectum; statistical analysis of a long-term follow-up study. Gastroenterology 39:178–182, 1960.
101. Weakley FL, Swinton NW: Follow-up study of patients with benign mucosal polyps of the rectum. Dis Col Rectum 5:345–355, 1962.
102. Brahme F, Ekelund GR, Norden JG, Wenckert A: Metachronous colorectal polyps. Dis Col Rectum 17:166–171, 1974.
103. Henry LG, Condon RE, Schulte WJ, Aprahamian C, De Cosse JJ: Risk of recurrence of colon polyps. Ann Surg 182:511–515, 1975.
104. Deyhle P: Results of endoscopic polypectomy in the gastrointestinal tract. Endoscopy (suppl) 35–46, 1980.
105. Panish JF: State of the art: management of patients with polypoid lesions of the colon — current concepts and controversies. Am J Gastroent 71:315–324, 1979.
106. Knoernschild HE: Growth rate and malignant potential of colonic polyps: early results. Surg Forum 14:137, 1963.
107. Welin S. Youker J, Spratt J.S.: The rates and patterns of growth of 375 tumours of the large intestine and rectum observed by double contrast enema study (Malmö technique). Am J Roentgenol Rad Ther Nucl Med 90:673–687, 1963.
108. Figiel LS, Figiel SJ, Wietersen FK: Roentologic observations of growth rates of colonic polyps and carcinoma. Acta Radiol 3:417–429, 1965.
109. Martel W, Robins JM: The barium enema: technique, value and limitations. Cancer 28:137–143, 1971.
110. Deyhle P, Seuberth K, Jenny S, Demling L: Endoscopic polypectomy in the proximal colon. Endoscopy 3:103–105, 1971.
111. Williams CB, Hunt RH, Loose H, Riddell RH, Sakai Y, Swarbrick ET: Colonoscopy in the management of colon polyps. Br J Surg 61:673–682, 1974.
112. Sugarbaker PH, Vineyard GC: Snare polypectomy with the fiberoptic colonoscope. Surg Gynecol Obstet 138:581–583, 1974.

113. Williams CB, Riddell RH: Colonoscopic polypectomy: Topics in gastrointestinal endoscopy, Salmon PR, Schiller KFR (eds). London: Heinemann Medical, 1976.

114. Wolff WI, Shinya H: Endoscopic polypectomy — therapeutic and clinicopathologic aspects. Cancer 36:683–690, 1975.

115. Vanheuverzwyn R *et al.*: Colonoscopy in the diagnosis and treatment of colonic polyps. Acta Gastroenterol Belg 39:104–114, 1976.

116. Theuerkauf FJ: Rectal and colonic polyp relationships via colonoscopy and fibersigmoidoscopy. Dis Col Rectum 21:2–7, 1978.

117. Frimberger E, Kuhner W, Seib HJ, Ottenjann R: Colorectal adenoma: relationships among histological structure dimensions of the polyps and age distribution. Minerva Med 69:3979–3985, 1978.

118. Gabriellson N, Grandqvist S, Ohlsen H, Sundelin P. Malignancy of colonic polyps. Diagnosis and management. Acta Radiol (Diag) Stockh 19:479–495, 1978.

119. Wolff WI, Shinya H: The impact of colonoscopy on the problem of colorectal cancer. Prog Clin Cancer 7:51–69, 1978.

120. Brule J, Emerit J: Colonoscopic polypectomy — histopathologic features and course. Presse Med 8:1575–1578, 1979.

121. Coutsoftides T, Sivak MV, Benjamin, SP. Jagelman D: Colonoscopy and management of polyps containing invasive carcinoma. Annls Surg 188:638–641, 1979.

122. Gillespie PE, Chambers TJ, Chan KW, Doronzo F, Morson BC, Williams CB: Colonic adenomas — a colonoscopic survey. Gut 20:240–245, 1979.

123. Bond JH, Levitt MD: Use of pulmonary hydrogen measurements to quantitate carbohydrate absorption. J Clin Invest 51:1219–1225, 1972.

124. Williams CB, Bartram CI, Bat L, Milito G: Bowel preparation with mannitol is hazardous Gut 20:A933, 1979.

125. Le Brooy SJ, Avgerinos A, Fendick CL, Williams CB, Misiewicz JJ: Potentially explosive colonic concentrations of hydrogen after bowel preparation with mannitol. Lancet i: 634–636, 1981.

126. Bigard MA, Gaucher P, Lasalle, C: Fatal colonic explosion during colonoscopic polypectomy. Gastroenterology 77:1307, 1979.

127. Ragins H, Shinya H, Wolff WI: The explosive potential of colonic gas during colonoscopic electrosurgical polypectomy. Surg Gynecol Obstet 138:554–556, 1974.

128. Bond JH. Levitt MD: Factors influencing the concentration of combustible gases in the colon during colonoscopy. Gastroenterology 68:1445–1448, 1975.

129. Fruhmorgen P, Joachim G: Gas chromatographic analyses of intestinal gas to clarify the question of inert gas insufflation in electrosurgical endoscopy. Endoscopy 8:133, 1976.

130. Curtiss LE: High frequency currents in endoscopy: a review of principles and precautions. Gastrointest Endosc 20:9–12, 1973.

131. Carlyle DR, Goldstein HM: Angiographic management of bleeding following transcolonoscopic polypectomy. Am J Dig Dis 20:1196–1201, 1975.

132. Gillespie PE, Nicholls RJ, Thomson JPS, Williams CB: Snare polypectomy by sigmoid-rectal intussusception. Br Med J 1:1395, 1978.

133. Christie JP: Colonoscopic excision of sessile polyps. Am J Gastroenterol 66:23–28, 1976.

134. Dagradi AE: Colonoscopic polypectomy excision of a huge villous adenoma. Am J Gastroenterol 66:464–466, 1976.

135. Christie JP: Colonoscopic removal of sessile colonic lesions. Dis Col Rectum 21:11–14, 1978.

136. Buhler H, Nuesch HJ, Kobler E, Deyhle P: Large colonic polyps: endoscopic or surgical removal? Schweiz Med Wochenschr 109:619–620, 1979.

137. Grandqvist S, Gabrielsson N, Sundelin P: Diminutive colonic polyps — clinical significance and management. Endoscopy 11:36–42, 1979.
138. Waye JD, Frankel A, Braunfeld SF: Abstract: The histopathology of small colon polyps. Gastrointest Endosc 26:80, 1980.
139. Williams CB: Diathermy-biopsy — a technique for the endoscopic management of small polyps. Endoscopy 5:215–218, 1973.
140. Spencer RJ, Coates HL, Anderson MJ: Colonoscopic polypectomies. Mayo Clin Proc 49:40, 1974.
141. Bussey HJR: Familial polyposis coli. Baltimore: Johns Hopkins university Press, 1975.
142. Maskens AP: Histogenesis of adenomatous polyps in the human large intestine. Gastoenterology 77:1245–1251, 1979.
143. Morson BC, Dawson IMP: Gastrointestinal pathology. Oxford: Blackwell Scientific, 1972.
144. Kropp G: Massenpolypectomien und Bergungsmodus in Kolon. Dtsche Med Wochenschr 101:19–20, 1976.
145. Nivatvongs S, Goldberg SM: Management of patients who have had polyps containing invasive carcinoma removed via colonoscope. Dis Col Rectum 21:8–11, 1978.
146. Carden ABG, Morson BC: Recurrence after local excision of malignant polyps of rectum. Proc Roy soc Med 57:559–561, 1964.
147. Morson BC: Factors influencing the prognosis of early cancer of the rectum. Proc Roy Soc Med 59:607, 1966.
148. Shatney CH, Lober PH, Gilbertsen VA, Sosin H: The treatment of pedunculated adenomatous colorectal polyps with focal cancer. Surg Gynaecol Obstet 139:845, 1974.
149. Hermanek P: In: Operative endoscopy: past and future, Demling L, Koch H (eds). Stuttgart: Schatteneur Verlag, 1979.
150. Wolff WI, Shinya H: Definitive treatment of malignant polyps of the colon. Annls Surg 182:516–525, 1975.
151. Hedberg SE: In discussion of Coller, Corman and Veidenheimer paper, Am J Surg 131:494, 1975.
152. Montori A et al.: Endoscopic and surgical treatment of the colonic polyps. Acta Hepatogastroenterol (Stuttgart) 23:459–465, 1976.
153. Coutsoftides, T, Lavery I, Benjamin SP, Sivak MV: Malignant polyps of the colon and rectum — a clinicopathologic study. Dis Col Rectum 22:82–86, 1979.
154. Kern F: Good news and bad news, Presidential address. Gastroenterology 71:537–542, 1976.
155. Ponsky JL, King JF: Endoscopic marking of colonic lesions. Gastrointest. Endosc 22:42–43, 1975.
156. Winawer SJ, Sherlock P, Schottenfeld D, Miller DG: Screening for colon cancer. Gastroenterology 70:783–789, 1976.
157. Gilbertsen V: Proctosigmoidoscopy and polypectomy in reducing the incidence of rectal cancer. Cancer 34:936–939, 1974.
158. Sherlock P, Winawer SJ: The role of early diagnosis in controlling large bowel cancer. Cancer 40 (suppl) 2616–2619, 1977.
159. Penfold JC: Early detection of colonic cancer by colonoscopy. Dis Col Rectum 20:85–88, 1977.
160. Bassett ML, Goulston KJ: Colorectal cancer: the challenge of early detection. Med J Aust 1:489–493, 1978.
161. Buchanan ID, Lightfoot A, Thornton JR, Teague RH, Williams CB, Milton-Thompson GJ, Hunt RH: Abstract: Prognosis of colonic carcinomas diagnosed by colonoscopy. Gut 21:A454.
162. Kronborg O: Review: Polyps of the colon and rectum: approach to prophylaxis in colorectal cancer. Scand J Gastroenterol 15:1–5, 1980.

10. Cancer in Inflammatory Bowel Disease

THEODORE M. BAYLESS and JOHN H. YARDLEY

The term idiopathic inflammatory bowel disease is used to denote several illness including ulcerative proctitis, chronic ulcerative colitis and Crohn's disease of the small intestine or colon.

A markedly increased risk of developing cancer of the colon is now a well accepted fact of life for patients with ulcerative colitis[1]. Although the magnitude of the problem is less ominous, the cancer incidence is also increased in patients with Crohn's disease in the small bowel and colon [2, 3].

1. INFLAMMATORY BOWEL DISEASE

1.1. Definitions and Descriptions

1.1.1 Ulcerative proctitis is a chronic relapsing disorder with rectal bleeding as the main problem, which is more of an annoyance than a major illness. It comprises about 20% of patients diagnosed as ulcerative colitis. In over 80% of the patients the severe inflammation remains localized to the rectum or rectosigmoid and does not become more generalized. Patients with proctitis are not thought to be at increased risk of colon cancer development.

1.1.2. Ulcerative colitis affects individuals at all ages with a peak incidence in teenage and early adult life with another somewhat lower peak incidence in the 50s and 60s. There are variations in the extent of bowel that is inflamed as well as the severity of the disease manifestations [4]. The colitis may involve just the recto-sigmoid or may extend proximally to involve the left half of the colon or even the entire colon, in which case it is usually referred to as pancolitis. In some series, 40% of patients have pancolitis. When ulcerative colitis begins in childhood or adolescence, most patients have universal colonic involvement. Active colitis causes rectal bleeding and diar-

rhea and usually follows an acute intermittent course with relapses and remissions. Five percent have no further attacks over the next 10 or 15 years.
Most of the others can be kept in prolonged remission on long term sulfasalazine therapy. Some patients with pancolitis or with left sided colitis have
either mild disease or go into prolonged spontaneous remissions. Other
patients, perhaps 15 or 20%, may have a chronic unremitting course, which
does not respond completely to medical therapy. After several years of a
chronic unremitting course, a total proctocolectomy and ileostomy is usually
recommended to provide a cure for the colitis. Obviously this will also
prevent the future occurrence of large bowel cancer. Five to ten percent of
patients manifest severe or fulminant colitis either *de novo* as the first manifestation of the illness or superimposed on either of the other two chronic
courses. Because of the high risk of perforation, emergency total proctocolectomy is often performed for patients with fulminant colitis, with or without
toxic megacolon. Overall, after 10 years of disease, about 20% of patients
with ulcerative colitis will have had a colectomy for colitis-related problems
leaving a large number of patients with both pancolitis and left sided disease
at risk for cancer development.

The etiology of ulcerative colitis is unknown. There is a definite genetic
predisposition and at least 10% of patients give a history of either ulcerative
colitis or Crohn's disease in a close relative. While viral infections, such as
cytomegalovirus, may at times be associated with exacerbations, a primary
viral etiology for ulcerative colitis itself has not been proven. Immunologic
events also occur in the colonic mucosa, but these are often thought to be
secondary to the injury and as yet have not been shown to be primary.
Likewise, psychological factors, although present in some individuals, are not
thought to be the cause or the dominant pathogenic mechanism in ulcerative
colitis.

The damaged colonic mucosa is a site of both acute and chronic inflammation, often with mucosal erosions and superficial ulceration. Plasma cells and
lymphocytes are prominent features of the inflammatory reaction. It is not
surprising that such a mucosa is permeable to various antigenic materials as
well as being a source of intestinal protein loss. Presumably carcinogens
would have enhanced access to these damaged tissues.

1.1.3 Crohn's disease is primarily a disorder of young people with the
average age at onset of 27 years [5]. Fifteen percent of the patients note the
onset of their illness before age 15 and a great majority have the illness
appear before the age of 40. Although there are exceptions, it is unusual to
see Crohn's disease appearing *de novo* in the elderly. This chronic inflammatory condition of unknown etiology may affect any portion of the gastrointestinal tract. The most common areas of involvement are the terminal ileum,

cecum and right colon. The term regional enteritis is often applied to such patients with predominantly terminal ileal disease. In other patients, with so-called 'Crohn's colitis', the inflammation may involve part or all of the colon without obvious small bowel disease. Sarcoid-like granulomas can be found in the colon or small bowel of 1/4 of the patients with Crohn's disease, while additional patients will show non-specific inflammation with granulomatous features. Most investigators currently believe that Crohn's disease begins as a focal mucosal inflammation in many parts of the small and large bowel and later becomes transmural with ulcerations and deep fissuring. A specific causative agent has not been identified.

Although the etiology of Crohn's disease is unknown, there does appear to be a genetic predisposition to this disorder: 10 percent of patients have a family history of inflammatory bowel disease. In addition, all of the idiopathic inflammatory bowel diseases seem to be more common among the Jewish population than would be expected.

Medical therapy of Crohn's disease usually involves adrenocorticosteroids, sulfasalazine, antibiotics and at times moderate but long-term courses of azathioprine, 6-mercaptopurine or metronidazole. None of these therapies are curative; they are at best suppressive of active inflammation and are most effective in the early phases of the illness or for recurrences after a surgical resection.

Surgical therapy for Crohn's disease was used in the past as the initial and presumably curative treatment for the disease but because of the very high recurrence rates, reaching 50% at 5 years and almost 100% after 20 years, the role of surgical therapy has been revised to one of palliation and correction of mechanical problems such as obstruction and fistula formation.

In the 1940s and early 1950s, terminal ileal bypass with the creation of an ileo-transverse colostomy was used for patients with obstruction. However, this did not provide long-term control of the disease and in addition it has recently become clear that this type of bypass and anastomosis resulted in an increase of risk of small bowel cancer development in the bypassed segment [3]. Bowel resection has now become the standard surgical approach, usually removing only the obviously diseased or obstructed portions. Mildy diseased or grossly normal bowel is retained in order to conserve as much bowel function as possible. At times portions of defunctionalized colon or rectum are left in place after a diverting ileostomy or colostomy.

The natural history of Crohn's disease in the colon may include development of short strictures as well as large masses of inflammatory polyps. Both lesions can be very difficult to distinguish radiographically from neoplasms.

Up to the present, the moderately increased cancer risk for patients with Crohn's disease has not usually dictated surgical therapy; that is, prophylactic large or small bowel resections have not been advised, the key exception being the bypassed ileal segments, which are now either avoided or usually are taken down and removed if there is another indication for operation. There are probably a number of patients who have had rectal or colonic bypasses in whom these segments become inactive and have not been removed.

Approximately 20% of patients with inflammation of the colon without obvious small bowel disease present a seemingly unsolvable problem in differential diagnosis. In some it is not possible for the radiologist, endoscopist or pathologist to make a firm distinction between ulcerative colitis and Crohn's disease of the colon so that the term 'indeterminant colitis' is applied.

2. ULCERATIVE COLITIS AND COLORECTAL MALIGNANCIES

2.1. Even in the face of the high frequency of colorectal cancer development in the United States, Scandinavia and the United Kingdom, there is general agreement that patients with chronic ulcerative colitis have an 8 to 30 fold increased likelihood of developing large bowel cancer. Risk factors for cancer include extent of colonic involvement with colitis, the duration of disease and perhaps a childhood onset of ulcerative colitis. Chronic injury of the mucosa in ulcerative colitis might predispose to neoplastic change or alterations in the repair process. It is also possible that a common factor may predispose individuals to both ulcerative colitis and colorectal cancer. Such processes might occur independently or synergistically. The pathogenetic mechanisms presumably are complex since ulcerative colitis accounts for only a small fraction of all cancers of the colon and rectum, and conversely, only a minority of the patients who had ulcerative colitis go on to develop large bowel cancer. Despite these limitations there are certain features in the epidemiologic pattern of each disease which are parallel. Both are generally regarded as a disease of industrialized countries. The mortality for both may be more frequent in the northeast and north central regions of the United States[6].

Cancer of the colon and rectum in patients with ulcerative colitis generally tends to occur at an earlier age than cancer in the general population. The average age of the usual patient with ulcerative colitis who develops cancer is 40 in contrast to the average age of 62 in the non-colitic population with colon cancer. However, a second peak incidence of colorectal cancer in ulcerative colitis patients occurs at about 70 years of age, with most of the tumors in the recto-sigmoid[7]. In most series the prognosis for cancer in ulcerative colitis tends to be quite poor with an average 18% survival rate after surgery in contrast to a 50% five year survival rate with ordinary colorectal cancer. The dismal prognosis is due in part to delay in diagnosis. Factors contributing to this delay before cancer recognition will be a major focus of this chapter.

2.2. Pathology of Cancer and 'Precancer' in Ulcerative Colitis

2.2.1. Site. Cancer in ulcerative colitis differs from conventional (non-colitic) colorectal cancer in that the recto-sigmoid is less often involved (50% vs 70% of non-colitic tumors) while right-sided and transverse colonic locations are more common. Cancer in ulcerative colitis may also be multi-centric, the reported frequency of multiple carcinomas ranging from 5 to 42%.

There have been some reports of carcinoma in the terminal ileum in patients with ulcerative colitis, colon cancer and 'backwash' ileitis and other types of ileal inflammation [8–10]. Primary carcinoma involving ileostomies many years after colectomy for ulcerative colitis has been observed at least twice [11, 12].

2.2.2. Gross or macroscopic features. While macroscopic features of some carcinomas associated with ulcerative colitis are comparable to those in non-colitis cancer, many times the tumor in colitis is a scirrhous, flat lesion that can either be small or occupy long segments of colon (Figure 1). The mucosal surface in such lesions often looks irregular, heaped-up, thickened and is nodular or rough-looking. When the carcinoma involves a long segment of colon, it is usually impossible to identify a precise point of origin, suggesting

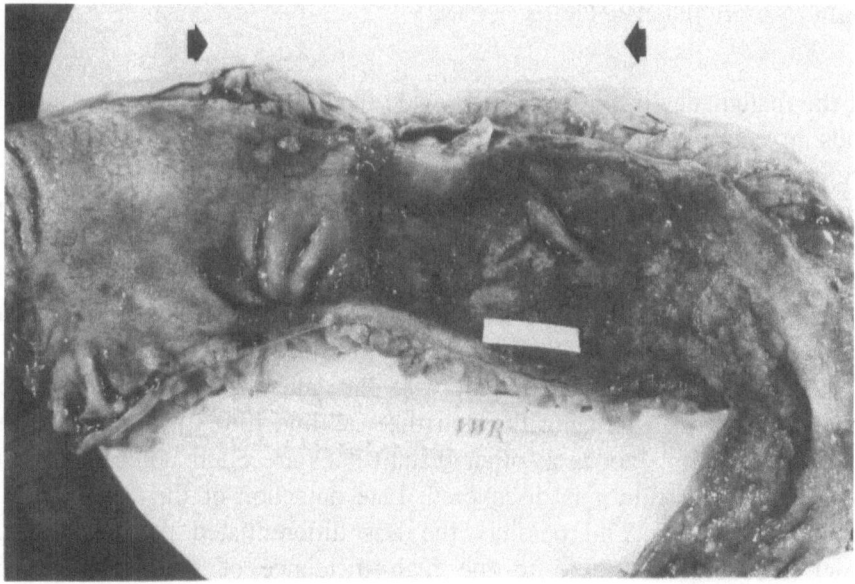

Figure 1. Carcinoma of ascending colon in ulcerative colitis. Lesion was detected as persistently narrowed segment during a bout of fulminant colitis. The cancerous region (between arrows) measured about 15 cm. Note thickened wall, puckering, narrowing, and absence of intraluminal mass but with mucosal thickening.

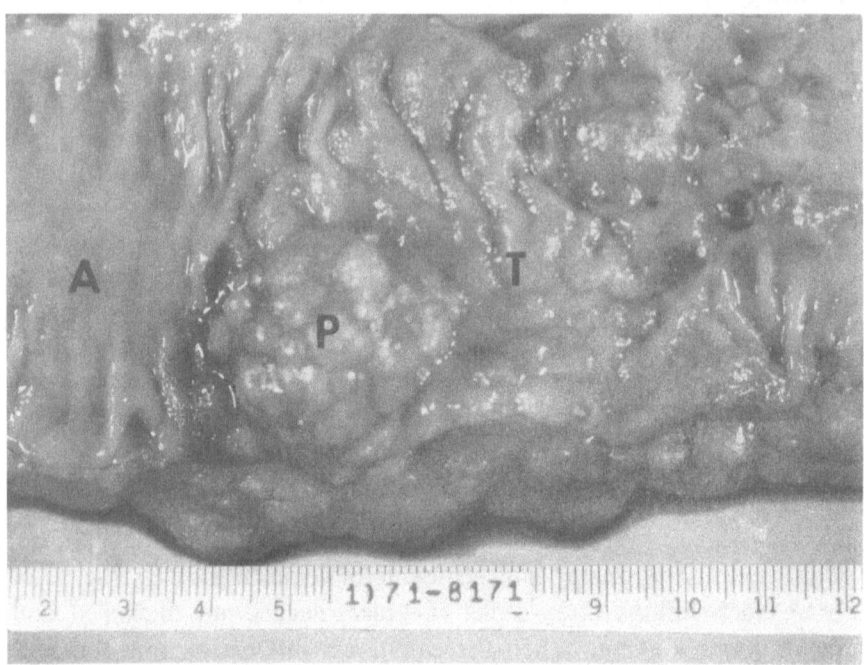

Figure 2. Cancer in ulcerative colitis. Atrophic colitic mucosa (A) is clearly contrasted with thickened, tumor-bearing area (T) and associated polyp (P). Reprinted with permission from the journal *Cancer*, ref. [19]. Also Figures 3, 4 and 5.

that the malignancy has arisen over a wide field of altered mucosa. All of this stands in contrast to conventional (non-colitic) carcinoma, which tends to have much sharper limits and more often grows into the lumen as an exophytic lesion or as a short stricture. These contrasting features are especially evident in non-colitic cancers that have demonstrably originated in an adenomatous polyp. While cancer in ulcerative colitis can present as a polyp or other mass projecting into the lumen, even these lesions are typically associated with malignant transformation of the surrounding mucosa (Figure 2).

Cancer occasionally arises in otherwise flat and atrophic-looking mucosa. Whatever its form, extension through the wall and into surrounding fat and metastasis to lymph nodes at other distant sites are often noted at the time when the primary tumor is discovered. Late detection of the often unobtrusive primary tumor, and possibly the less differentiated colloid form (see below), probably contribute to the high incidence of metastases on first detection.

2.2.3. Microscopic Features. Carcinoma in ulcerative colitis, in keeping with its gross appearance, often is seen as a heaped-up, adenocarcinoma replacing a

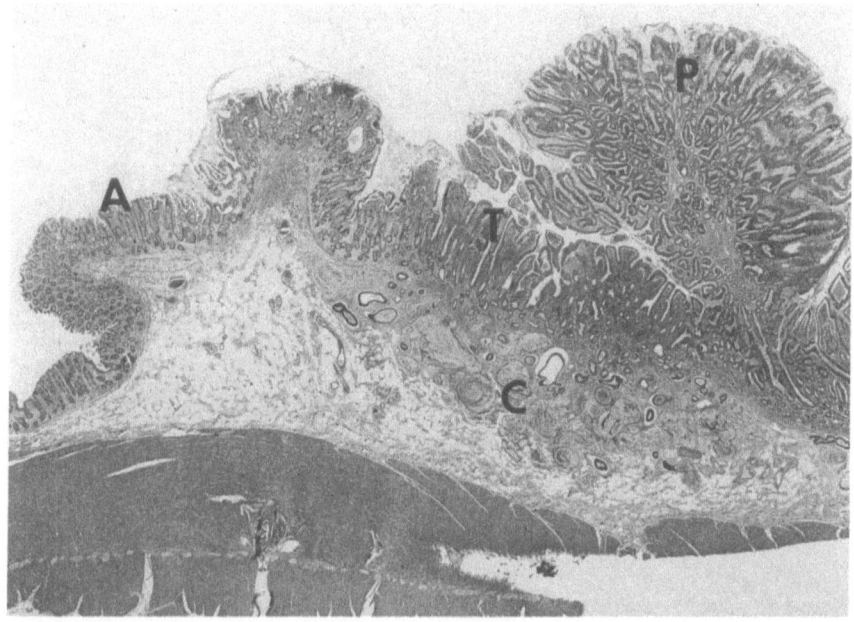

Figure 3. Cross-section through specimen shown in Figure 2 [19].Invasive colloid carcinoma (C) is present beneath a villiform and polypoid adenocarcinoma in mucosa. Other symbols as in Figure 2 (10×).

large area of mucosa (Figure 3). In other respects there are no significant microscopic differences from non-colitic carcinomas. The growth pattern is often villous but may be predominantly glandular. The invasive component may seem to 'drop away' into the underlying structures over a wide field and poorly differentiated and colloid (mucinous) forms are common (Figure 3). Cytologically, the usual features of nuclear irregularities, reduced mucin and dedifferentiation are present.

2.2.4. Mucosal Dysplasia ('Precancer'). The terms 'precancer,' 'precancerous change,' 'dysplasia' (usually further characterized as moderate, severe, high grade, etc.) and 'adenomatous epithelium' have been employed by various authors to characterize the neoplastic transformation in the mucosa that almost always accompanies large bowel cancer in ulcerative colitis [13, 14].

'Precancer' consists primarily of dysplastic cytologic changes in the epithelium (Figure 4 and 5) comparable to those found in pre-invasive neoplastic transformation in the epithelium of other organs such as the cervix or bronchus. Dysplasia is usually, but not always, seen in the context of a glandular or villiform growth pattern like that of non-colitic adenomas (Figure 4 and 8).

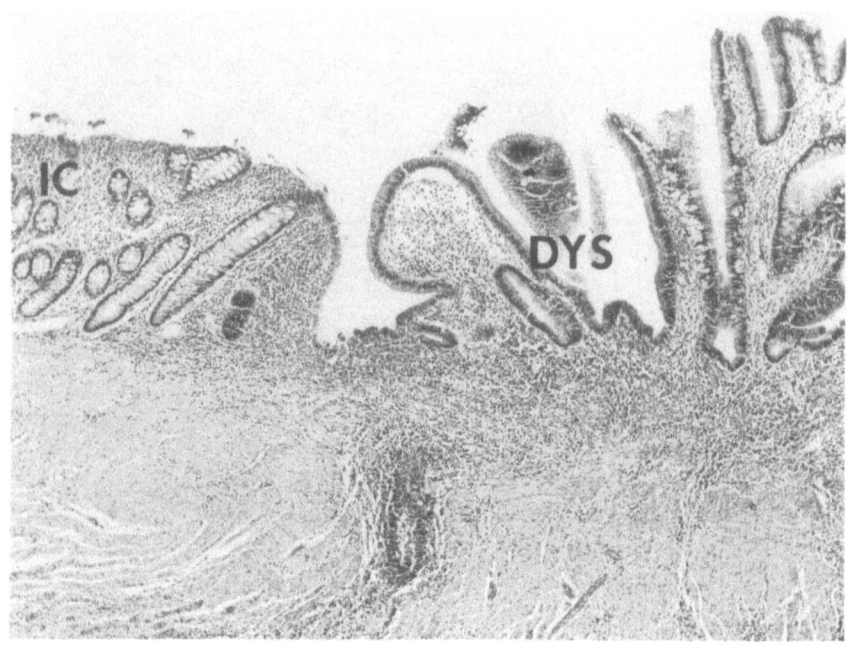

Figure 4. Distinctions between inactive colitis (IC) and dysplastic mucosa (DYS) are well seen at the juncture [19]. Note villiform character, decreased mucus and loss of nuclear polarity in dysplastic area (45 ×).

Morson and Pang[15], who first brought wide notice to the concept of 'precancer,' found dysplastic changes in about 20% of colectomy specimens from patients without carcinoma who had had colitis for more than ten years, as well as in 100% of patients who had carcinoma with their colitis. Observations of this type have been repeatedly verified by others, and Dobbins[16], has summarized the literature in this regard. Since ulcerative colitis itself has not been shown to lead inevitably to colon cancer, it would also be wrong to infer that 'precancer' always culminates in cancer. However, in early studies at various medical centers, at least half of the patients undergoing colectomy for biopsy-diagnosed 'precancer' had one or more foci of invasive cancer somewhere in their colon [14, 17, 18].

Although precancerous lesions may on the average have less severe dysplasia than invasive carcinoma in colitis, there is no clear line between the two histologically except for the invasion itself. Similarly, their gross appearances overlap. Dysplasia can occur in mucosa which shows no distinguishing gross features from those commonly encountered in longstanding ulcerative colitis. While thickening of the wall and lumenal narrowing will usually be absent in precancer, raised and roughened areas in the mucosa may stand out in

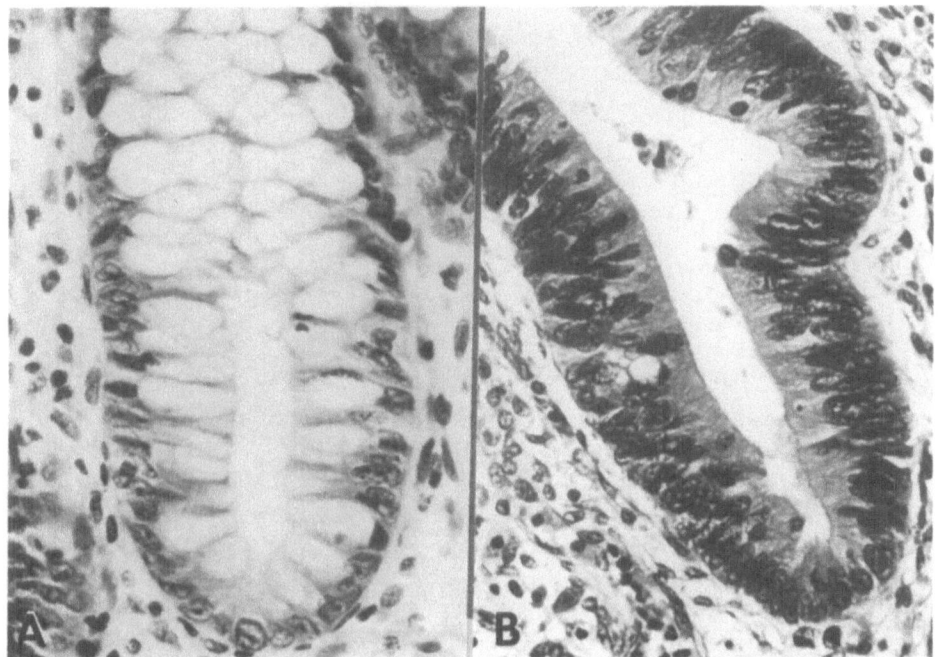

Figure 5. A Crypt from mucosa in inactive colitis. B. Severe dysplasia showing nuclear changes and loss of mucin (both 100×) [19].

contrast to atrophic looking non-precancerous mucosa when a colectomy specimen is opened (Figure 6). Some precancerous lesions are described as verrucose while others have a velvety appearance (Figure 7). Polypoid precancerous masses may be seen, but it may not be possible to distinguish inflammatory polyps from precancerous or cancerous areas grossly. Histologically, however, inflammatory pseudopolyps are usually distinguishable from precancerous changes, and pseudopolyps are not themselves considered premalignant.

The problem most regularly faced by the pathologist is in interpreting epithelial atypia in the context of the inflammation and injury associated with active colitis. The loss of mucin, enlarged nuclei and increased mitoses, sometimes accompanied by glandular irregularities or villiform changes that occur in active colitis, may be very difficult to distinguish from true dysplasia [19].

Carcinoma complicating ulcerative colitis must be distinguished from the rare occurrence of non-specific inflammation behind a benign or malignant colonic obstruction such as a tumor, stricture, diverticulitis or even Hirschsprung's disease. At times, acute colonic inflammation has been seen as a complication of obstructing carcinoma as well.

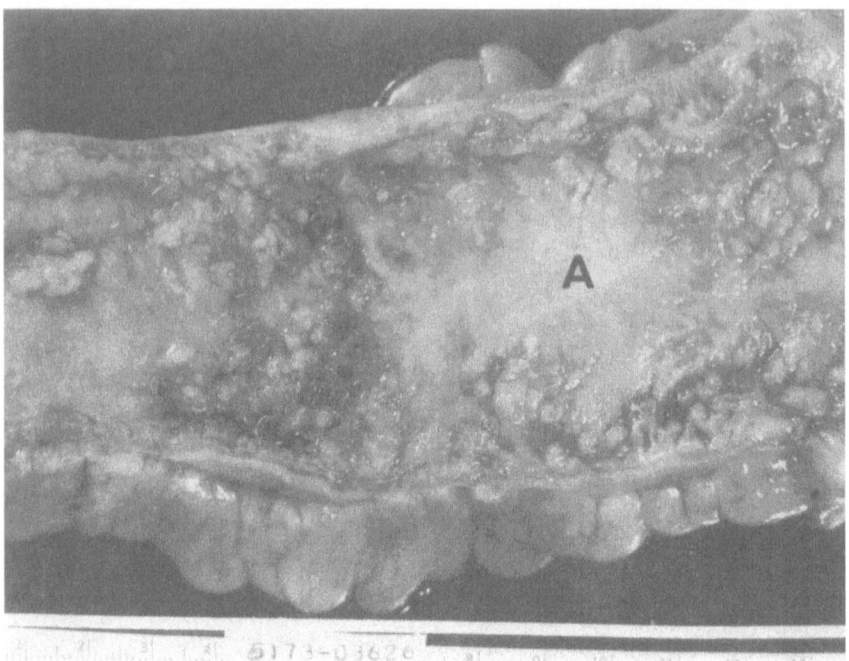

Figure 6. Transverse colon from a patient with colitis and carcinoma in the ascending colon. Multiple irregular, polypoid nodules in dysplastic areas contrast sharply with atrophic mucosa (A).

Precancerous change occurs in many histologic and cytologic patterns and degrees. In addition, however, there is also variation in interpretation and terminology among pathologists. A lesion described as moderate dysplasia by one pathologist might be described by another as severe. Inconsistency in grading comes about in part because grading is subjective and inherently inexact, but it also results from differences in the grading scales. Some pathologists have used a mild to severe scale in which only 'severe dysplasia' is viewed as the point at which colectomy was advised. Others define 'moderate dysplasia' as ominous. To develop terms and definitions for describing high risk histologic changes and for distinguishing them from non-neoplastic findings in a standardized way, organized exchanges of material and ideas among pathologists are needed. Such exchanges are currently taking place among a group of pathologists with the ultimate goal of publishing the results.

2.2.5. Miscellaneous Malignancies and Ulcerative Colitis. Squamous cell tumors of the rectum have rarely been found in some patients with ulcerative colitis. The tumors are not brought to arise from the squamous epithelium of

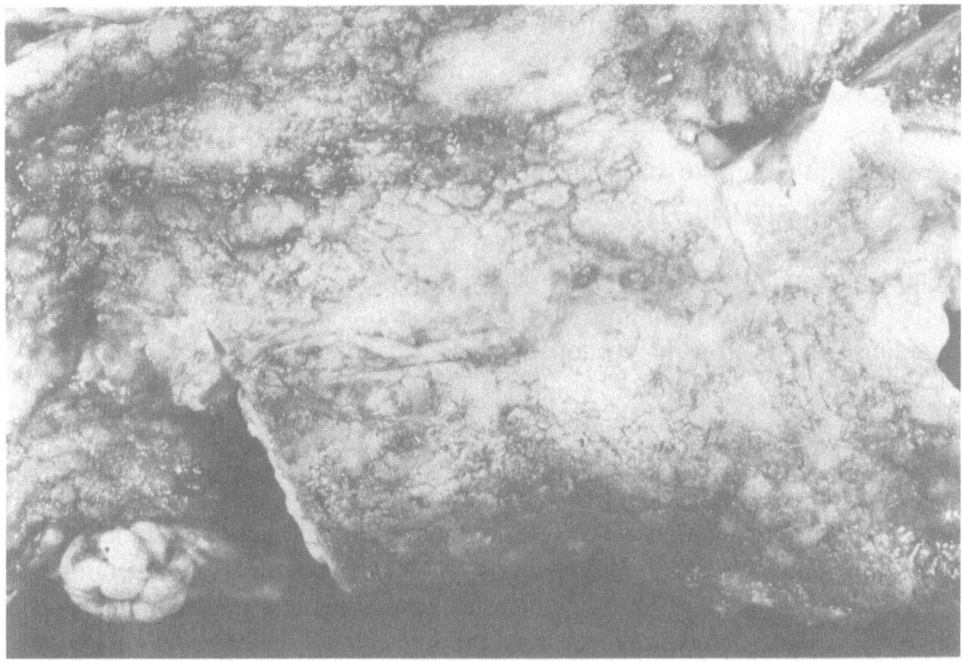

Figure 7. Close up of fixed, washed area of dysplastic mucosa to emphasize irregular, roughened appearance. The endoscopist finds it difficult to see these changes because of overlying mucus, lighting and limitations of resolution by the fiberscope.

the anus but rather from the cellular epithelium proximal to the dentate line and they are probably a result of epithelial metaplasia [20].

Other malignancies that have been seen in association with colitis include lymphoma of the colon [21] (see Chapter 12); premalignant changes and adenocarcinomas in backwash ileitis [10]; Kaposi's sarcoma [22]; biliary tract carcinoma and other intrabdominal malignancies. There is some concern that some of these other malignancies as well as the adenocarcinoma of the colon might be in some way related to radiation exposure as a result of the numerous diagnostic procedures performed in these patients with chronic ulcerative colitis.

2.2. Risk Factors for Developing Colon Cancer

2.2.1. Extent of Colitis. A generally accepted figure for the incidence of carcinoma in all patients with ulcerative colitis using an inception cohort is between 3 and 4.5%. The incidence of carcinoma appears to be directly proportional to the extent of colonic involvement with ulcerative colitis. With pancolitis, the incidence range is from 13 to 24% at 20 years, while in patients with distal colitis affecting only the rectosigmoid there is a less than

1% chance that cancer will develop[23]. The incidence of carcinoma in patients with ulcerative proctitis is so low as to be undetectably greater than in the general population.

Those with radiologic evidence of involvement of only the left portion of the colon are also at increased risk of colon cancer but the onset of cancer development seems to be delayed approximately 10 years as compared to patients with pancolitis[1, 24]. After 20 years of colitis, the frequency of colon cancer increases at a rate comparable to that for patients with extensive colitis. The relative contribution of the extent of colitis to cancer risk is difficult to separate from the age of onset and the duration of colitis. As mentioned above, the proportion of ulcerative colitis patients with total or very extensive involvement would be greater in a series of patients with childhood-onset colitis compared to an adult-onset series.

The methods of ascertainment of extent of colonic involvement have changed over the last several decades. Most of the data in the literature was based upon radiographic studies utilizing single contrast barium enemas. Use of the currently popular double contrast enemas utilizing air and barium, as well as colonoscopy with multiple biopsies have illustrated that many patients thought to have involvement of only the left colon usually have inflammation in the right colon as well. In addition, some patients with presumed proctitis with normal barium enemas may also have mild to moderate degrees of histologic involvement of the recto-sigmoid and descending colon as well. It is not clear what significance in terms of risk of colon cancer development should be attached to these histologic changes in radiographically normal portions of bowel since the data showing that patients with only left sides disease developed their cancer approximately 10 years later than those with pancolitis was developed using only single contrast barium enema findings[1, 24]. It will have to be left to future research to decide whether a person who has histologic involvement of pancolitis as developed through colonoscopy and multiple biopsy examination should be considered to be at increased risk of early cancer development or whether this patient can safely be placed in a category of left-sided colitis based on the X-ray findings and therefore the theoretic possibility of a delayed onset of risk.

2.2.2. Duration of Ulcerative Colitis. The risk of colon cancer development seems to be related directly to the duration of the colitis, increasing exponentially after 10 years of disease. When the two factors of duration and extent of disease are combined, as, for example, in patients with pancolitis for over 20 years, a greater than 24% probability of developing colon cancer has been estimated[23]. A long-term study from the Mayo Clinic of 296 children who developed ulcerative colitis before age 14, indicated that 20% of the remaining patients developed cancer at each decade beyond the first 10 years of disease with a probability of 43% that any individual would develop cancer by 35 years from the onset of colitis[1]. A recent Scandinavian study of 234 patients presented almost identical figures on the risk of colon cancer development in patients with adult onset of pancolitis, with a cumulative incidence of 24.2% at 20 years[25].

The average age at the time of death from cancer of the colon was 46 years in a series of 118 patients reported between 1949 and 1962. Twenty-two percent had ulcerative colitis for less than 10 years before the diagnosis of cancer was made. Forty-seven percent had colitis for 10–19 years and 31% had had inflammatory bowel disease for more than 20 years[26].

2.2.3. Age at Onset of Ulcerative Colitis. There are conflicting answers to the question as to whether patients whose ulcerative colitis which began in childhood are at greater cancer risk than those with an adult-age onset. Though there are apparently insufficient cases to provide statistical significance, one has the impression that individuals in their late teens or earlier 20s seem to have a shorter duration between the onset of ulcerative colitis and the occurrence of carcinoma[25, 27, 28]. Current statistical evidence would suggest that the risk per year of colitis is the same for both children and adults with equal extent of disease. Those with onset in childhood differ only in that the majority have universal involvement so that their risk of cancer is therefore higher than in all adult patients with ulcerative colitis.

2.2.4. Colitis Activity. There are some authors who believe that carcinoma arises more frequently in chronic continuously active forms of ulcerative colitis than in patients with intermittent disease activity. This is thought to be due, in part, to the slightly higher incidence of colon cancer in those patients who have a severe initial attack. Goligher, DeDombal and their associates felt that the degree of activity of colitis had an important influence on the cancer risk. They related cancer risk to 'patient years' of activity. They urge prophylactic colectomy for patients with severe pancolitis after the initial episode[29]. This view is not, however, universally accepted and some workers, including our own group, feel that a likelihood of carcinoma is as great in the patient with no recent symptoms as in the patient with continuous active disease. Patients with chronic ulcerative colitis who developed colon cancer had less active and milder disease than the patients who underwent colectomy for ulcerative colitis uncomplicated by cancer. The latter patients were more likely to be operated for severe disease at earlier stages in their illness and thus were removed from the at risk group before they had had the illness for 10 years. It should be empathically stated that quiescence of colitis is no guarantee that carcinoma will not develop. Carcinoma occurs in patients with ulcerative colitis who have been asymptomatic for as long as 16 years.

Inactive colitis creates the problem of a false sense of security in both the patient and his physician, so that the carcinoma risk may either be overlooked or ignored. Eight of 16 patients with ulcerative colitis and colon cancer diagnosed at our institution had not been seen in the past eight years and had gone for prolonged periods, often over 5 years, without proctoscopy, colonoscopy or barium enema examination. Thus this inactivity and false sense of security lead to a delay in the diagnosis of colon cancer.

2.2.4. Genetics. Although it seems clear that there are polygenetic factors affecting the incidence of ulcerative colitis itself, there is very little information on the role, if any, of genetics in determining the incidence of colon cancer development in ulcerative colitis. Since the relatives of patients with adenomatous polyps and with ordinary colon cancer unassociated with colitis are at increased risk of polyp and colon cancer development, respectively, one would assume this would apply equally if not to a greater degree to patients with ulcerative colitis whose relatives had polyps or colon cancer. Data on this question may be very difficult to obtain because there may be a natural tendency for the physician and his patient to feel that the presence of a strong family history of colon cancer would place the individual patient with ulcerative colitis of long duration at an increased risk. Thus prophylactic colectomy might be more easily considered and this patient is then removed from the pool of patients at risk for colon cancer development.

2.2.5. Geographic Differences. It has not been settled whether there are differences in the risk of colon cancer occurring in ulcerative colitis in varying areas of the world. Some workers report that the risk of colon cancer is less in Central Europe, Turkey, Israel and Japan as compared to Scandinavia, the United States and the United Kingdom where non-colitis associated colorectal cancer is also high.

Since epidemiologic observations indicate that variations in the incidence of non-colitic colorectal cancer correlate significantly with prevailing dietary habits of those areas, it has been suggested that diet may play some role in these geographic ulcerative colitis-cancer differences. Differences in diet might be associated with alterations in colonic bacterial flora and resultant variations in the processes of metabolism of various lumenal materials and these metabolic variations might be associated with differing concentrations of carcinogenic metabolites. If these dietary and bacterial metabolic factors are shown to be significant in the etiology of usual colon cancer, they would certainly deserve consideration in the etiology of cancer in patients with inflammatory bowel disease since the injured mucosa might be more permeable or sensitive to carcinogens and might help explain the earlier age of cancer appearance in ulcerative colitis. In fact, study of those factors in patients with ulcerative colitis who are at enhanced risk of colon cancer, might provide clues for the general colon cancer problem. In addition in the past decades, diets highly restrictive in fiber and roughage have been used for patients with ulcerative colitis, perhaps providing another etiologic factor for colon cancer in a patient with ulcerative colitis.

2.2.6. Mucosal Dysplasia. Since ulcerative colitis itself is not known at this time to inevitably lead to colon cancer, it would obviously be wrong to infer that severe dysplasia or 'precancer' would always lead to cancer. Information on how often colon cancer will be found when the presence of severe dysplasia or 'precancer' is the indication for total colectomy, is still being determined. At least one half of the reported patients who underwent colectomy because of biopsy evidence of 'precancer' had foci of colon cancer at some point in their colon.

Thus, based on all available data, it seems reasonable to assume that the patient with ulcerative colitis who has well-documented areas of severe or high grade dysplasia scattered throughout the colon, its at high risk of colon cancer development. The risk of co-existent carcinoma seems to be even greater if the dysplasia is associated with mass lesions in contrast to dysplastic flattened areas of mucosa. Since as many as 50% of the patients with high grade dysplasia have been found to have small and often unsuspected carcinomas, it is unlikely that a control trial will be performed to determine the natural history of this lesion.

Information is now being gathered to determine if the risk factors for 'precancer' are the same as those for cancer and how often patients with various degrees and extent of ulcerative colitis develop this premalignant change. Our 'average' patient with ulcerative colitis who has an area of 'precancer' found in his colectomy specimen without evidence of cancer in the colon, has had the colitis for 13 years. Some patients have had pancolitis for as short as seven years.

The question of how long it takes for an area of severe dysplasia to become malignant is going to be difficult to answer because of the spectrum of degrees of dysplasia that has been found in ulcerative colitis as well as the lack of evidence for an evitable progression from mild or low grade up to severe or high grade dysplasia to cancer. Also, the dysplastic areas may be distributed in a patchy fashion and may go undetected even on very careful colonoscopic examination and biopsy. In addition, the natural history of the process is often interrupted by colectomy since the presence of multiple areas of severe dysplasia or dysplasia on a mass or stricture is now being used by several centers as an indication for recommending colectomy. Thus accurate information on the lag time between the appearance of dysplasia and cancer development may never be ascertained with accuracy. There are, however, some general figures which one can consider. Patients who have had a colectomy that contains only 'precancer' have, on the average, had colitis for six or seven years less than those with colon cancer. Anecdotally, one patient had 'precancer' in a random rectal biopsy nine years before colon cancer was found in the left colon. As an analogy, the limited data available on the time for progression of adenomatous colonic polyps to colon cancer suggests at least a seven or eight year lag for an identifiable polyp to become malignant.

2.2.7. Radiation Exposure. Cumulative radiation effects of numerous barium enema examinations, upper gastrointestinal series and other abdominal X-rays that are performed on patients with chronic inflammatory bowel disease should probably be listed as the first paragraph in any discussion of the possible etiology of neoplastic degeneration in these disorders. The combination of continued radiation exposure with the chronic injury and reparative processes in inflammatory bowel disease would theoretically provide a fertile ground for oncogenesis. Rogers and Kirkpatrick have specifically raised the issue of radiation exposure from the diagnostic procedures in inflammatory bowel disease as a factor in the later heightened risk of cancer formation and have suggested one keep a log of the X-ray examinations performed on patients with inflammatory bowel disease throughout their lifetime, so that the amount of radiation delivered to the abdomen could be estimated [30]. The risk is not restricted to the colon but includes the interabdominal organs, including bone marrow, which are within the field of radiation.

Radiation exposure is an important area for further education of physicians who deal with patients with inflammatory bowel disease. Many of these patients became ill during adolescence or early adult life and thus have at least another 30 or 40 years of risk time for further radiation exposure. Since inflammatory bowel disease is often very difficult to treat and therapeutic decisions are often not clear cut, the physician might find himself ordering extra radiographic studies as a way to decrease his own insecurity and without gaining information necessary for a decision. Although there has been a report of identification of the 'precancer' lesions by high magnification air contrast barium enemas [31], it should be strongly emphasized however that annual X-rays in a patient in whom there is no specific reason to suspect carcinoma are not to be recommended as a method of following the high risk ulcerative colitis patient. It would be very important to try to resolve the issue of how often barium enemas, with their low sensitivity for neoplasia in inflammatory bowel disease but with their attendent radiation exposure, should be performed before the risk of cancer induction outweighs the diagnostic value. It would seem somewhat analogous to the issue of mammograms in terms of detection versus induction of breast cancer.

2.2.8. Exposure to Medications for Inflammatory Bowel Disease. The medications used to suppress the active disease of ulcerative colitis have the potential for altering immunocompetence as well as the possibility of inducing changes in the fecal flora. Because some alteration in immune surveillance has been suggested as a problem in the pathogenesis of colon cancer in ulcerative colitis, prednisone, azathioprine, 6-mercaptopurine and metronidazole are worthy of some consideration in this regard. In addition local hydrocortisone enemas and suppositories are used in the therapy of ulcerative colitis, thus exposing the injured rectal area directly to this medication. Salicylazosulfapyridine or sulfasalazine (Azulfadine®) is also concentrated in the tissues of the colon as well as having a potential effect on the colonic flora. Also, three of the agents used in the management of inflammatory bowel disease of the colon, metronidazole, azathioprine, and 6-mercaptopurine have been considered mutagenic and potentially oncogenic. These medications are currently being used for long-term therapy by some physicians for colonic inflammatory disease and especially for patients with rectal and perianal disease.

2.3. Clinical Features of Colorectal Cancer in Patients with Ulcerative Colitis

The symptoms of the neoplasms are similar to those of the underlying inflammatory bowel disease. The clinical manifestation of a cancer may so closely imitate those of ulcerative colitis as to be interpreted as only a mild exacerbation. The patient may believe the cancer related symptoms to be only a recurrence of colitis and not seek medical attention for a number of months or years. Unfortunately his physician may also fall into this same trap of blaming the tumor symptoms on the underlying bowel disease. Before the onset of surveillance programs for precancer and early cancer, most patients who were found to have colon cancer were quite symptomatic at the time of diagnosis. All 14 patients who presented to our institution with symptoms referable to colon cancer were dead with two years of cancer diagnosis.

One reason for late diagnosis of colon cancer complicating ulcerative colitis is that some patients who go on to develop cancer have relatively inactive colitis. Both they and their physicians tend to develop a false sense of security, which may result in a reluctance to undergo colectomy or even diagnostic procedures that could serve as some form of surveillance. In our experience, half of the patients who have been encountered with colon cancer complicating ulcerative colitis had inactive disease for over 5 years, some for more than 10 years, and most had not undergone proctoscopy or barium enema prior to the appearance of colon cancer related symptoms.

2.4. Diagnosis of Colorectal Cancer in Chronic Ulcerative Colitis

The diagnosis of colorectal cancer in a patient with ulcerative colitis is usually quite difficult, especially at early stages when the tumors are small and flat. Even when polypoid, they could be mistaken for inflammatory or pseudopolyps and vice versa [32].

2.4.1. Radiography. Barium enema examinations, even double contrast techniques, may miss both well developed carcinoma of the colon as well as potentially curable lesions in patients with ulcerative colitis. There are some suggestions that arteriography may be a useful technique in neoplasm detection in this setting but this is unproven. Finding a new stricture in ulcerative colitis definitely is a point of concern, since this is not a usual complication of ulcerative colitis and would require colonoscopy and multiple biopsies of that area, both for carcinoma and for premalignant or 'precancer' changes.

2.4.2. Endoscopy. Proctosigmoidoscopy is of limited value because the cancers do not have the tendency to localize in the rectum. Only 5 of 19 cancers in our patients were within reach of the proctoscope. Flexible sigmoidoscopy permits examination of up to 50 cm of left colon and this should prove helpful in the surveillance of patients with ulcerative colitis. Colonoscopy has proven quite helpful as a method of gross examination as well as a source of multiple biopsy specimens and is discussed in detail in the chapter by Dr. Williams in this book.

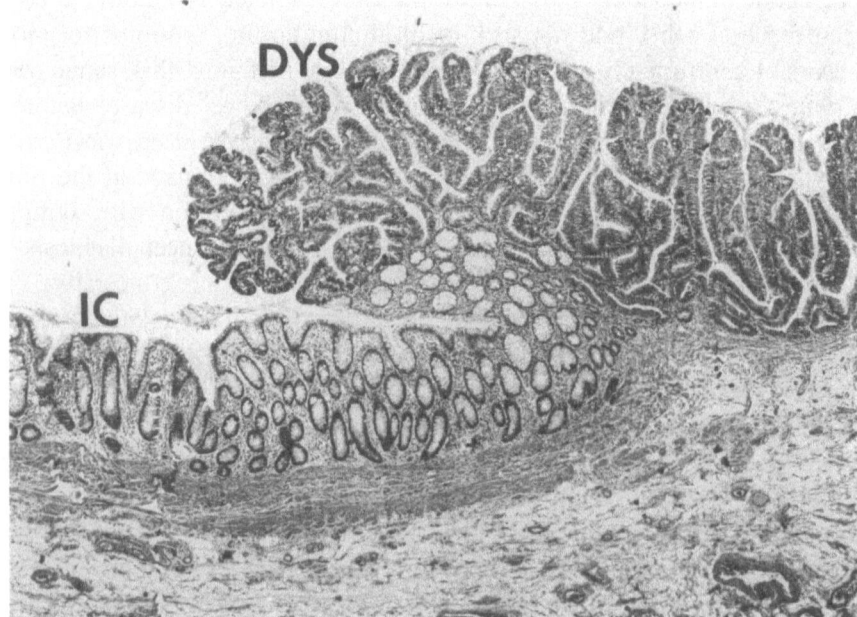

Figure 8. An example of dysplastic adenomatous mucosa with villiform growth pattern (DYS). Note heaping up and contrasting histologic appearance of adjacent inactive colitis (IC) (26×).

2.4.3. Biopsy. Biopsy of suspicious lesions through the proctosigmoidoscope, flexible sigmoidoscope, or colonoscope, is still one of the most useful
techniques for the diagnosis of adenocarcinoma of the colon. Inadequate
sampling of a lesion can be an important problem when using the small
biopsy forceps that will fit through most colonoscopes and flexible sigmoidoscopes since frank carcinoma may be below the surface of the mucosa and
may not be reached by superficial biopsies (Figures 3 and 9). Physicians using
these techniques must be aware of the fact that negative biopsies of a polyp
or a mass do not rule out carcinoma in the patient with ulcerative colitis. As
discussed in detail earlier in the chapter by Williams, the finding of severe
dysplastic or 'precancer' changes on biopsy may be helpful in recognizing the
fact that the mucosa of this particular patient with ulcerative colitis has the
propensity for neoplastic change.

2.4.4 Cytology. Cytology is a vastly underused technique that may be
helpful at times in detecting early carcinoma of the colon in patients with
ulcerative colitis. Techniques of continued irrigation and lavage via the sigmoidoscope or colonoscope, using a pulsatile dental irrigating unit, have made

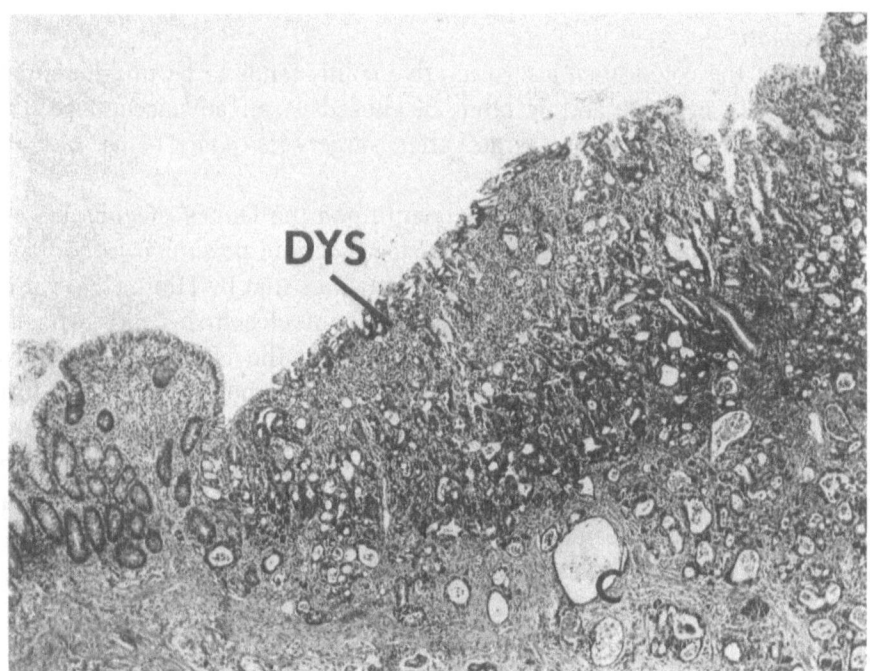

Figure 9. Area in mucosa showing invasive carcinoma (C) and overlying severe dysplasia. A
shallow biopsy would have revealed the dysplasia but may not have shown the invasion, leading
to the incorrect conclusion that only 'precancer' was present (35×).

it possible to obtain samples for cytologic analysis and there are some reports of successful diagnosis of colon cancer in ulcerative colitis via this method [33].

It should seem possible however that there might be a difficulty in separating cancer cells from the atypical hyperplastic cells of ulcerative colitis which would originate and actively multiply in cells at the base of the crypts. Active inflammation might limit the use of cytologic techniques just as occurs in the search for severe dysplasia by biopsy.

2.4.5. Biomarkers. Carcinoembryonic antigen (CEA) levels are elevated with advanced colon cancer but are unfortunately not a reliable detector of early carcinoma of the large bowel. In addition the majority of patients with active inflammatory bowel disease have elevated plasma levels of CEA without evidence of carcinoma. The lack of sensitivity for early cancer and the association of elevated levels with active colitis limits the use of this plasma biomarker as a screening test for detecting early cancer in ulcerative colitis. If an individual had normal levels of CEA and a gradual or sudden rise occurred in the absence of any evidence of disease activity, it certainly would bear further investigation in terms of cancer development (see Chapter 11).

2.5. Prognosis

Cancer of the colon arising in ulcerative colitis tends to be undifferentiated and extremely invasive and is often diagnosed at an advanced stage. Generally, the five year survival rate after surgery is poor, being less than 20%.

The survival rate seems to be dependent upon the Dukes' staging just as in the general population and the rates for stage seem to be similar to non-colitic patients. There are a few favorable reports such as that by Hinton [34] with an overall survival rate of 40–75% in patients with ulcerative colitis who were treated at St. Mark's Hospital. A recent study at the University of Chicago also reported approximately a 50% survival [35]. It is hoped that in the future as better surveillance techniques are employed, the colon cancers that do develop will be found at an early and surgically curable stage. This has been the experience in programs that have instituted multiple colonoscopic and rectal biopsies for 'precancer' as a form of surveillance. Cancers found in these centers generally have been Dukes' A or B tumors [17, 18, 36].

2.6. Strategies to Prevent Colorectal Cancer in Ulcerative Colitis

2.6.1. Prophylactic Proctocolectomy. Since a total proctocolectomy will not only cure ulcerative colitis but also obviously prevent colon cancer, physicians caring for patients with severe, extensive, unresponsive, longstanding ulcerative colitis are always looking for an excuse to urge a proctocolectomy. There are some who would urge prophylactic colectomy for cancer prevention, i.e. the removal of the entire colon and rectum in all patients with extensive colitis either early in the course of the disease for acute symptoms, or after 10 years in patients with mild disease [29, 37].

Because of the alternative of surveillance for precancer, there is some opinion that in the context of a premalignant disease, ulcerative colitis does not carry a high enough risk of cancer, perhaps 5% in total population after 20 years, to justify a routine proctocolectomy and ileostomy with its associated morbidity and mortality and inconvenience. Even when one is speaking of the population with pancolitis and a 25% cancer risk at 20 years, it is difficult to justify carrying out proctocolectomy routinely at 10 years when there is a reasonable chance that some patients may not develop carcinoma for many years, if at all [23].

Although there is actuarial data on the risk of colon cancer in patients with pancolitis, the physician has very little information with which to base individual decisions in the patient with X-ray evidence of only left-sided disease. It is these patients with limited disease and those in whom colitis has gone into complete remission that one finds it hard to recommend prophylactic colectomy.

It should be pointed out that it has become much easier recently to consider colectomy for the patient with other indications for colon removal. Ileostomy techniques have improved as has the ostomy equipment. Ostomy management has been aided by the knowledge and experience of stomal therapists and, quite importantly, by the presence of large groups of patients in Ostomy associations who serve as sources of information and counseling for other patients. In addition, the advent of the continent ileostomy has made it easier to recommend colectomy for patients with ulcerative colitis. Recently, there has been increased surgical experimental interest in ileo-anal anastomoses with complete removal of the rectal mucosa.

2.6.2. Early Cancer Diagnosis. The fact that it is very difficult to recognize colon cancer early in its course in the patient with ulcerative colitis makes this option undependable. The physician cannot rely on early cancer detection as one does in breast cancer. Routine use of early air contrast barium enemas would be insufficient for early cancer diagnosis and would also be exposing the patient to the risks of repeated radiation exposure. Cytologic studies have not been applied extensively, but even segmental lavage studies are inadequate to regularly detect early carcinomas in patients with ulcerative colitis. Rectal and colonoscopic biopsies may also fail to reveal the presence of carcinoma and cannot be used to exclude the presence of malignant change in the person with a suspicious lesion or stricture. Plasma carcinoembryonic antigen levels and stool examinations for occult blood are also not helpful in the detection of early carcinoma development in the patient with ulcerative colitis.

2.6.3. Surveillance for 'Precancer'. Regularly scheduled programs seeking evidence of dysplasia are being evaluated in patients with extensive colitis of over eight years duration to try to decide which patients are at greatest risk of cancer development and should be urged to undergo total proctocolectomy [13, 14, 17, 18]. The success of this type of surveillance program in place of colectomy requires careful followup of every patient and the availability of experienced and devoted clinicians, endoscopists, pathologists and surgeons as well as cooperative and understanding patients. Theoretically, it is hoped that one will be able to advise surgery at a time when dysplasia is present but before frank cancer has developed, or if it has, when the tumor is still at a curable stage. Dr. Williams outlines the role of colonoscopy and multiple colonic biopsies in chapter 9. Surveillance in place of colectomy is not reasonable in patients with severe or unremitting ulcerative colitis or for patients whose colon shows evidence of neoplastic potential as judged by histological criteria or for patients who are uncooperative. Colectomy would also be urged for patients who have suspicious lesions or multiple polyps and in whom the presence of carcinoma cannot be excluded. While the procedures may be somewhat unpleasant and inconvenient, the risks of colonoscopy and the other procedures are actually quite low in patients with chronic inactive ulcerative colitis. There have been reports of a few patients having some increase in disease activity after preparation for colonoscopy but no reports of perforation of the colon. Analogy with the use of routine Papanicoleau cervical smears is sometimes helpful in explaining the surveillance program to the patient. It should also be absolutely clear that one cannot guarantee that colon cancer will not develop during the years of surveillance, especially if the examinations are not performed at regular relatively frequent intervals.

A surveillance program to detect 'precancer' and/or early colon cancer should be considered in all patients with ulcerative colitis with the possible exception of those with proctitis or proctosigmoiditis. The risk of cancer development in patients with proctitis or with disease limited to the rectosigmoid, does not seem to be great enough to require as extensive a followup program as other patients with ulcerative colitis. Patients who have had a partial colectomy for ulcerative colitis but in whom the rectum is retained after surgery, should also be included in a regular followup program. At least 60 patients are known to have developed rectal cancer in the stump left after partial colectomy [38].

Once the total duration of ulcerative colitis exceeds eight years, a regular followup with sigmoidoscopy or flexible sigmoidoscopy should be supplemented by colonoscopy with multiple biopsies every one or two years, depending on the presence or absence of any suspicion of dysplasia. Biopsies should be taken from suspicious areas and in addition, 2 to 3 random biopsies should be taken from 5 to 7 different levels of the bowel.

Biopsies obtained via proctosigmoidoscopic examination have been positive for dysplasia in some patients who already have colon cancer[15, 18] but seem to be inadequate at earlier stages in precancer development[17, 19].

Colonoscopy allows the endoscopist the potential for seeing and biopsying scattered patches of precancerous changes in the early stages of transformation when the rectum is less likely to be involved. Colonoscopy can also reach the more proximal carcinomas which would also go undetected by conventional barium enema. Also the precancerous dysplasia in the proximal colon may be more readily distinguished histologically from active colitis because the inflammatory changes are often less marked than in the left colon. The endoscopist must learn to perform biopsies in the areas that are most likely to result in precancer detection, such as thickened, plaquelike or nodular areas of mucosa. Dysplasia containing biopsies that are from a mass are more likely to be associated with an underlying carcinoma than dysplasia from a flat mucosa (Figure 2)[39].

Obvious polyps of 1 cm in size are usually excised through the colonoscope. It is important, however, to take additional biopsies from the base of polypoid lesions as well as on the elevation itself, since the changes of severe dysplasia or 'precancer' may be most easily identified at the edge of a polypoid lesion. A number of biopsies in the surrounding thickened areas may also be quite helpful. Williams (in Chapter 9) discusses the technique of 'hot biopsy', which provides large amounts of material for examination. It is quite important that the exact site of the biopsy specimen be ascertained if at all possible and this be noted on a pathology department form for correlation with the microscopic changes as well as radiographic landmarks. Use of a number of biopsy bottles may be helpful in trying to establish this clinical-pathologic correlation. Endoscopic photographs also aid in the communication process.

2.6.4. Difficulties in Identifying Precancer: The technical problems involved in trying to identify various degrees of dysplasia in rectal and colonoscopic biopsies are compounded by the very small size of the biopsies obtained through the colonoscope, as well as difficulties in orienting these specimens for embedding.

Technical problems for the endoscopist include the presence of mucus and debris which obscure the mucosa, and the lack of topographic relief in the end-on view through the colonoscope and the further hindering of having only direct lighting without access to angled lighting. Most physicians involved in the colonoscopic examination of patients with ulcerative colitis who have gone to the surgical pathology department to view the subsequent colectomy specimen were chagrined to find very obvious areas of elevation and plaque-like lesions when they are shown a pinned-out and fixed colon specimen. These lesions were often not appreciated through the colonoscope. Dye scattering techniques such as those used for carcinoma of the stomach by the Japanese have been suggested but no formal report of their usefulness was known to us.

Interpretive problems that confront the pathologist were discussed earlier in terms of the spectrum of changes that can be found as well as the different definitions and nomenclature systems that have been applied. Some of the more difficult interpretive problems occur with biopsies from areas of active disease with its resultant atypia. The patchy nature of the dysplastic changes also cause sampling problems. Thus the small superficial biopsies miss an area of dysplasia and in addition may also not reveal underlying carcinoma. It is essential that the endoscopist, the pathologist and the radiologist communicate very clearly so that the histologic findings can be correlated with the gross appearance.

In terms of anticipated results of surveillance programs, it is not yet clear how frequently 'precancer' will be found in the rectums or colons of patients with chronic ulcerative colitis. Prospective study with strict definitions of the extent of involvement of the colon with ulcerative colitis as well as the duration of disease are necessary before this type of information will be available. In a 1977 review of the literature, precancer was found in the rectal biopsies of 53 of 937 patients with chronic ulcerative colitis, or 5.7% [16]. Seventeen of these 53 patients were found to have colon cancer at the time of colectomy. Twenty-six of the patients with 'precancer' had no obvious evidence of carcinoma and were still under followup at the time of that report. Thus, 5.7% of patients with ulcerative colitis undefined as to duration or extent, were found to have 'precancer' on rectal biopsy. One third of those patients already had colon cancer. Forty-two percent of the patients who had precancer in both the rectum and in the colon had evidence of cancer.

Nugent and his colleagues from the Lahey Clinic reported that 17 of 86 patients (21%) with chronic ulcerative colitis of over five years duration had evidence of colonic dysplasia on rectal and colonoscopic biopsies [18, 40]. Four of the ten who underwent colectomy because of the finding of dysplasia already had unsuspected colon cancer which was metastatic in 2. In a prospective study of a larger number of patients by Lennard-Jones et al., 13 of 229 patients (5.7%) with chronic ulcerative colitis were found to have evidence of severe dysplasia. Four of the seven who underwent colectomy because of the finding of severe dysplasia were found to have carcinoma. Fortunately five of the six cancers were Dukes' A stage, one was a Dukes' B. At the University of Chicago Clinics, Levin and his colleagues have performed 196 colonoscopies in 91 patients [41]. The mean duration of symptoms in the 54 still actively involved in the study is 19.7 years with a range of 7 to 38 years. Ten patients (11%) have had significant dysplasia on colonoscopic biopsies. Rectal biopsies were 'positive' in only four. Six underwent colectomy and three had cancer, one suspected preoperatively, the other two unsuspected.

2.6.5. Frequency of Surveillance Examination. There is no firm basis currently available for determining the optimal frequency of cancer surveillance in pancolitis [41]. Two or three years may be too long a waiting period because one colonoscopic examination may not provide a complete view of the colon and carcinoma arising or progressing between surveys and could easily reach an untreatable stage in two or three years. If colon biopsies from a patient with pancolitis are negative for any degree of dysplasia, a followup study the next year will help to insure a representative sampling of most of the colon. If this second study was also negative for dysplasia, then intervals of two or perhaps even three years between studies would seem reasonable. Flexible sigmoidoscopy with biopsies up to 50 cm could be used in the intervening years.

If low grade dysplasia (mild or moderate by some criteria) were identified in flat areas of mucosa without an obvious polypoid lesion, a repeat colonoscopy in 6 to 12 months would be in order and then continued surveillance at at least yearly intervals. Proctosigmoidoscopy or flexible sigmoidoscopy with multiple biopsies at regular interspersed times would also be part of the surveillance program. Followup visits would also include history review, physical examination, examination of stool for occult blood, blood counts, liver function tests and carcino-embryonic antigen levels.

At the present there are no data on which to decide on a cost effective surveillance program in patients whose radiologic changes of ulcerative colitis are limited to the left half of the colon. This group is at increased risk of colon cancer development but the onset of the risk seems to be delayed for approximately 10 years when compared to the patients with pancolitis [1, 24]. Morson and Pang did not find any evidence of 'precancer' in the colectomy specimens from 17 people with subtotal colitis of over 10 years duration [15]. In our own recent experience with patients with 'left-sided' colitis as determined by X-ray, 3 of 17 (not randomly selected) had evidence of precancer. Two of the three had both colon cancer and 'precancer.' Histologically there was evidence of total colonic involvement with colitis in two of the three patients. To put these findings in patients with left-sided colitis in perspective, one-third of the patients with pancolitis for more than five years, but without evidence of invasive cancer, who underwent colectomy at our institution had evidence of 'precancer' in the resection specimen. As a working approach to surveillance for patients with 'left-sided' colitis, one might consider an air contrast barium enema as a baseline and colonoscopy with multiple biopsies to obtain histologic information on the extent of involvement, which is usually beyond that seen on X-ray. Whether the onset of this program could be delayed until the person has had colitis for 15 years is not yet known. Patients with easily controlled proctitis or even proctosigmoiditis are reportedly not at increased risk of cancer development and presumably an occasional proctosigmoidoscopy or flexible sigmoidoscopy with mucosal biopsies would seem to be a reasonable course of action.

It has been assumed in this discussion that all of the patients have remained asymptomatic. Obviously any changes in symptomatology would be investigated as would the appearance of occult blood in stool, anemia or a rise in serum carcino-embryonic antigen levels. Any recurrence of active colitis would interfere with the interpretation of both studies as well as search for histologic evidence of dysplasia. Determination of the significance of dysplasia can be quite difficult in the presence of any degree of active inflammation or reactive hyperplasia [19].

2.6.6. Indications for Proctocolectomy in Patients with Definite Evidence of Precancer. Guidelines for advising proctocolectomy are still somewhat flexible and will probably continue to change as more experience accumulates with colonoscopy, multiple biopsies and pathologic detection of 'precancer.' The finding of definite dysplasia on a grossly polypoid lesion or in a strictured area would usually be considered an indication for colectomy. Investigators at St. Mark's Hospital in London advocate proctocolectomy if severe dysplasia is found at multiple sites in the colon or on repeated examination [17]. Nugent and Haggitt from the Lahey Clinic recommend proctocolectomy for all patients with evidence of moderate or severe dysplasia [40]. Finding dysplasia in the presence of marked inflammation is considered insignificant by most observers.

If definite severe dysplasia is found on only one biopsy from a flat area or on one biopsy from an unknown area, an air contrast barium enema might be used to look for a lesion which might have been unappreciated on colonoscopy. Followup studies in six months would be indicated.

The finding of a single adenomatous polyp also raises questions as to management. If there was severe dysplasia in the polyp, this would then be considered an indication for colectomy. It is not clear what the proper management should be if a single adenomatous polyp is found with only very mild dysplasia and with no evidence of dysplasia elsewhere in the colon.

Other indications for colectomy include: obvious carcinoma; undefined polypoid masses; an individual at high risk of cancer development who is unable or unwilling to participate in a regularly scheduled surveillance program and a patient who is at high risk because of extent and duration of disease who has developed a stricture that prevents adequate colonoscopy and biopsy surveillance. We have also had difficulty following patients with a large number of pseudopolyps because of the concern that areas of dysplasia might not be appreciated on endoscopic examination and thus not biopsied. A strong family history of colon cancer has also been considered in decision making.

2.7. Surgical Treatment of Ulcerative Colitis

Complete proctocolectomy is indicated as the treatment of choice because any rectal tissue that is left behind is still at increased risk of cancer development. A number of patients who have had an ileoproctostomy to preserve their rectum have had carcinoma occur in the rectal stump [38]. If an ileorectal anastamosis is to be performed with retention of rectal mucosa, intensive surveillance with repeated biopsies would obviously be in order. If a patient with carcinoma of the colon superimposed on ulcerative colitis had obvious metastases, a more limited resection would presumably be justified. Based on very limited experience, it would seem best to avoid formation of a continent ileostomy in a patient with known carcinoma who may need chemotherapy. Pouch disruption was a problem in one of our patients who received repeated courses of chemotherapy.

There is increasing recent interest in ileoanal anastamosis with removal of the entire rectal mucosa with a pull through type procedure attaching the ileum to the rectal musculature. This operation has been performed mainly in children but there are some reports of its use in adults as well. This may provide another option for gut restoration after total proctocolectomy.

2.8. Other Malignancies and Ulcerative Colitis

2.8.1. Backwash Ileitis. There are at least three cases of carcinoma in backwash ileitis, all in patients who also had colon cancer [8–10]. One 27-year-old patient with an 8-year history of pancolitis with a dilated terminal ileum thought to be due to 'backwash ileitis' was found to have multiple plaques of adenocarcinoma and precancer in the small bowel as well as in the sigmoid colon [10]. Although it is difficult to absolutely rule out Crohn's disease in such patients [9], the possibility of premalignant changes in the small bowel of a patient with ulcerative colitis may have to be considered in terms of future followup. This might include biopsies of the small intestine, searching for premalignant change. In addition this might cause further concern in a patient with colonic cancer or precancer if one was constructing a continent ileostomy with its attendant stasis and perhaps carcinogen formation in the static loop.

2.8.2. Lymphoma. Primary malignant lymphoma appearing in patients with longstanding ulcerative colitis occurs but is unusual (see Chapter 12). The lymphomas have occurred anywhere in the large intestine including the cecum and rectum; in both sexes; in an age range of 26–64 years; and with a duration of ulcerative colitis of from 5 to 16 years. Malignant lymphomas seem to have a propensity for invading the muscularis and being quite destructive. The muscle necrosis is said to be more extensive than that seen with the invasion of adenocarcinoma. Fifteen patients with malignant lymphoma complicating ulcerative colitis were cited as of 1977 [21]. Two patients with sarcoma in ulcerative colitis were not included because of the lack of a histologic classification. At least 6 of the 15 patients had two or more separate lesions or diffuse involvement of a portion of colon. Both lymphoma and adenocarcinoma were found in three other patients. Only five had a single focus of lymphoma. Histologic classification of the reported cases of malignant lymphoma complicating ulcerative colitis is difficult because of the lack of uniform nomenclature. The age of onset of lymphoma and the survival data that are similar to that of primary colonic lymphoma suggest to some authors a coincidental occurrence of lymphoma in ulcerative colitis [21]. The lymphoma might be modified in the direction of multiplicity by pre-existing inflammatory disease. However, Lightdale and his colleagues have hypothesized that there is a relationship between ulcerative colitis and lymphoma and that there may be a premalignant state related to abnormal lymphoid tissue in the lamina propria [42].

2.8.3. Squamous Carcinoma of the Rectum. There are several reports of squamous carcinoma of the rectum complicating ulcerative colitis. The squamous cell epithelium is seen to arise not from the anal or perianal tissues but from the mucosa proximal to the dentate line. It is postulated that the regenerating mucosa has produced squamous cells instead of columnar cells. Radical surgical extirpation was the treatment for these patients [20].

2.8.4. Kaposi's Sarcoma. A patient with Kaposi's sarcoma superimposed on ulcerative colitis and diverticulitis presented with hemorrhagic diarrhea. There was no other evidence of Kaposi's sarcoma on the skin or in the abdominal cavity. The association with ulcerative colitis was thought to be fortuitous [22].

2.8.5. Biliary Tract Carcinoma. Biliary tract carcinoma in patients with ulcerative colitis has been reported as being 8 to 21 times more frequent than in the general population. In general these tumors have been associated with longstanding (mean 15 years), relatively inactive pancolitis. Several have been discovered 10 to 20 years after colectomy so that removal of the colon did not prevent their progression [43]. Differential diagnosis between sclerosing cholangitis and bile duct carcinoma is always difficult because the tumors may be very slow growing and may incite an intense fibrotic reaction. Since both of these conditions seem to appear more frequently in ulcerative colitis than might be expected, there presumably are some common etiologic factors. Also diagnostic difficulties may arise and may be very difficult to resolve even at surgery.

2.8.6. Other Intrabdominal Malignancies. Carcinoma of the esophagus, stomach, pancreas and kidney and leukemia have been reported in patients with ulcerative colitis. The relationship of these tumors to radiation exposure as part of the diagnosis and followup management of patients with inflammatory bowel disease bears further investigation by careful epidemiologic studies.

3. CROHN'S DISEASE AND GASTROINTESTINAL MALIGNANCIES

3.1. Colorectal Cancer

There is apparently an increased frequency of colorectal cancer as well as small intestinal cancer in patients with Crohn's disease involving the colon or small bowel respectively [44]. With Crohn's disease of the colon the incidence ranges from 1.8 to 3.7 and the risk is thought to be at least 20 times that of the general population [2, 45]. Extent and duration of disease are risk factors, with many of the cancers being located in the transverse and ascending colon. Some are in association with fistulae [42]. There are also a number of reports of precancer and premalignant changes being found in various areas of the bowel in patients with Crohn's disease who have developed cancer [39, 46, 47]. Some findings in the rectum have led to colectomy, which revealed unsuspected carcinoma [45].

If surveillance for 'precancer' via endoscopy and multiple biopsies were to be considered for patients with Crohn's disease, it would be much more difficult than with ulcerative colitis. Many of the patients with Crohn's disease have perianal disease and strictures of the rectal area as well as strictures in other areas of the colon that would make examination quite difficult. In addition there seems to be an increased risk of perforation of the colon by colonoscopy in patients with Crohn's disease as compared to ulcerative colitis and to the general population, especially if the colon has previously been defunctionalized as a form of management.

In general, most physicians have not been recommending prophylactic colectomy for Crohn's disease in terms of cancer prevention. This might be kept in mind as one factor when trying to decide whether to perform a bowel resection or a colonic defunctioning procedure. Although the role of the defunctionalized colon and rectum in the pathogenesis of cancer is not as clear as in the small intestine, there are some hints in the literature that it might be best to avoid leaving defunctionalized loops of bowel in place for a long period. Whether one should reoperate on patients with Crohn's disease with an ileostomy who have a defunctionalized and inactive rectal stump is not known.

3.2. Crohn's Disease and Small Bowel Cancer

There is an approximately 300 fold increased frequency of distal small bowel cancers in patients with longstanding Crohn's disease as compared with the general population in which primary carcinoma of the small intestine is rare and is usually found in the duodenum [48]. The adenocarcinoma of the small bowel in association with Crohn's disease were often found incidentally in the ileum when surgery was performed for bowel obstruction associated with the inflammatory bowel disease itself. The other common setting for cancer in Crohn's disease of the ileum has been in the surgically bypassed loops of diseased small bowel [3]. This type of surgery was quite popular thirty and forty years ago. It is presumed that stasis in the bypassed loop plus the diseased state of the mucosa combine to lead to increased tumorogenesis. This creates a clinical problem because the bypassed loops of bowel cannot be examined and the tumors do not become symptomatic until very late in their course. Fortunately this type of bypass surgery is no longer recommended as a surgical option for Crohn's disease and is probably performed only rarely. If a patient is encountered who has had this type of bypass many years ago, it would probably be best to advise reoperation and resection of the bypassed loop at some convenient time.

Patients with Crohn's disease have been reported with Non-Hodgkin's lymphoma as well as with carcinoid tumors of the ileum and appendix. However a major diagnostic dilemma is sometimes presented by the patient with primary or secondary lymphoma involving the small or large intestine in whom the radiographic and endoscopic appearance mimic Crohn's disease. A number of such patients have been mistakenly treated as Crohn's disease for weeks or months before the correct diagnosis was appreciated. In the United States, lymphoma of the small bowel or colon is probably one of the most important differential diagnostic considerations when confronted with a patient with Crohn's disease and a laparotomy may be required to resolve the dilemma.

REFERENCES

1. Devroede GJ, Taylor WF, Sauer WC, Jackman RJ, Stickler GB: Cancer risk and life expectancy of children with ulcerative colitis. New Engl J Med 285:17–21, 1971.
2. Weedon DD, Shorter RG, Idstrup DM, Huizenga KA, Taylor WF: Crohn's disease and cancer. New Engl J Med 289:1099–1103, 1973.
3. Greenstein AJ, Sachar D, Pucillo A, Kreel I, Geller S, Janowitz HO, Aufses A Jr: Cancer in Crohn's disease after diversionary surgery. Am J Surg 135:86–90, 1978.
4. Edwards FC, Truelove SC: The course and prognosis in ulcerative colitis: carcinoma of the colon. Gut 5:1–22, 1964.
5. Bayless TM, Yardley JH, Huang SS, Greene CC: Crohn's disease. So Med J 71:825–830, 1978.
6. Schottenfeld D, Haas JF: Epidemiology of colorectal cancer. In: Gastrointestinal tract cancer, Lipkin M, Good RA (eds). New York: Plenum Medical, 1978, 228–230.
7. Welch CE, Hedberg SE: Colonic cancer in ulcerative colitis and idiopathic colonic cancer. J Am Med Assoc 191:815–818, 1965.
8. Brown Ch, Diaz RJ, Michener WM: Carcinoma of the colon and ileum in chronic ulcerative colitis with reflux ileitis. Report of a case of a sixteen-year old boy. Gastroenterology 47:306–312, 1964.
9. Jalan KM, MacLean N, Ross JM, Sircus W, Butterworth STG: Carcinoma of the terminal ileum and sarcoidosis in a case of ulcerative colitis. Gastroenterology 56:583–588, 1969.
10. Schlippert W, Mitros F, Schulze K: Multiple adenocarcinomas and premalignant changes in 'backwash' ileitis. Am J Med 66:879–882, 1979.
11. Sigler L, Jedd FL: Adenocarcinoma of the ileostomy occurring after colectomy for ulcerative colitis. Dis Colon Rectum 12:45–48, 1969.
12. Cuesta MA, Donner R: Adenocarcinoma arising at an ileostomy site: report of a case. Cancer 37:949–952, 1976.
13. Riddell RH: The precarcinomatous lesion of ulcerative colitis. In: The gastrointestinal tract, Yardley JH, Morson BC, Abell MR (eds). Baltimore: Williams & Wilkins, 1977, pp 109–123.
14. Yardley JH, Bayless TM, Diamond MP: Cancer in ulcerative colitis. Gastroenterology 76:221–225, 1979.
15. Morson BC, Pang LSC: Rectal biopsy as an aid to cancer control in ulcerative colitis. Gut 8:423–434, 1967.
16. Dobbins WO III: Current status of precancer lesion in ulcerative colitis. Gastroenterology 73:1431–1433, 1977.
17. Lennard-Jones JE, Morson BC, Ritchie JK, Shove DC, Williams BM: Cancer in colitis: assessment of the individual risk by clinical and histological criteria. Gastroenterology 73:1280–1289, 1977.
18. Nugent FW, Haggitt RC, Colcher H, Kutteruf GC: Malignant potential of chronic ulcerative colitis: preliminary report. Gastroenterology 76:1–5, 1979.
19. Yardley JH, Keren DF: 'Precancer' lesions in ulcerative colitis: A retrospective study of rectal biopsy and colectomy specimens. Cancer 34:835–844, 1974.
20. Hohm WH, Jackman RJ: Squamous cell carcinoma of the rectum complicating ulcerative colitis: report of two cases. Mayo Clinic Proc 39:249–251, 1964.
21. Wagonfeld JB, Platz CE, Fishmen FL, Sibley RK, Kirsner JB: Multicentric colonic lymphoma complicating ulcerative colitis. Am J Dig Dis 22:502–508, 1977.
22. Gordon HW, Rywlin AM: Kaposi's sarcoma of the large intestine associated with ulcerative colitis: a hitherto unreported occurrence. Gastroenterology 50:248–253, 1966.
23. Whelan G: Cancer risk in ulcerative colitis: why are the results in the literature so varied?

Clinics in gastroenterology 9:469–476, 1980.
24. Greenstein AJ, Sachar DB, Smith H, Pucillo A, Papateśtas AT, Kreel I, Geller SA, Janowitz HD, Aufses A Jr: Cancer in ulcerative colitis: factors determining risk. Gastroenterology 77:290–294, 1979.
25. Kewenter J, Ahlman H, Hulten L: Cancer risk in extensive ulcerative colitis. Ann Surg 188:824–828, 1978.
26. de Dombal FT, Watts JM, Watkinson G, Goligher JC: Local complications of ulcerative colitis: stricture, pseudopolyposis and carcinoma of colon and rectum. Br Med J 1:1442–1447, 1966.
27. Diamond MP, Yardley JH, Bayless TM: Colon carcinoma and severe epithelial dysplasia in patients with ulcerative colitis. Gastroenterology 74:1120, 1978.
28. MacDougall IPM: The cancer risk in ulcerative colitis. Lancet 2:655–658, 1964.
29. Goligher JC, Hoffman DC, deDombal FT: Surgical treatment of severe attacks of ulcerative colitis with special reference to the advantages of early operation. Br Med J 2:703–706, 1970.
30. Rogers AG, Kirkpatrick JR: The need for a radiation history in patients with gastrointestinal disease: case reports. Gastroenterology 76:1228, 1979.
31. Frank PH, Riddell RH, Feczko PJ, Levin B: Radiological detection of colonic dysplasia (precarcinoma) in chronic ulcerative colitis. Gastrointest Radiol 3:209–219, 1978.
32. Martinez CR, Siegelman SS, Saba GP, Diaconis JN, Yardley JH: Localized tumor-like lesions in ulcerative colitis and Crohn's disease of the colon. Johns Hopkins Med J 140:249–259, 1977.
33. Katz S, Katzka I, Platt N, Hajdu EO, Bassett E: Cancer in chronic ulcerative colitis. Diagnostic role of segmental colonic lavage. Am J Dig Dis 22:355–363, 1977.
34. Hinton JM: Risk of malignant change in ulcerative colitis. Gut 7:427–432, 1966.
35. Hughes RG, Hall TJ, Block GE, Levin B, Moossa AR: The prognosis of carcinoma of the colon and rectum complicating ulcerative colitis. Surg Gyn Obst 146:46–48, 1978.
36. Bayless TM, Yardley JH, Diamond MP, Paulson M: Colon cancer and precancer in ulcerative colitis. In: Colorectal cancer: prevention, epidemiology and screening, Winawer S, Schottenfeld D, Sherlock P (eds). New York: Raven Press, 1980, pp 397–401.
37. Bonnevie O, Binder RV, Anthonisen P, Riis P: The Prognosis of ulcerative colitis. Scand J Gastroenterol 9:81–91, 1974.
38. Kurtz LM, Flint GW, Platt N, Wise L: Carcinoma in the retained rectum after colectomy for ulcerative colitis. Dis Colon Rectum 23:346–350, 1980.
39. Riddell RH: Dysplasia in inflammatory bowel disease. Clin Gastroenterol 9:439–458, 1980.
40. Nugent FW, Haggitt RC: Long term follow-up, including cancer surveillance, for patients with ulcerative colitis. Clin Gastroenterol 9:459–468, 1980.
41. Levin B, Riddell RH, Frank P, Gilpin JE: Evaluation of cancer risk in chronic ulcerative colitis: University of Chicago experience. In: Colorectal cancer: prevention, epidemiology and screening, Winawer S, Schottenfeld D, Sherlock P (eds). New York: Raven Press, 1980, pp 381–385.
42. Lightdale CJ, Sternberg SS, Posner G, Sherlock P: Carcinoma complicating Crohn's disease. Am J Med 59:263–268, 1975.
43. Ritchie JK, Allan RN, Macarthey J, Thompson H, Hawley PR, Cooke WT: Biliary tract carcinoma associated with ulcerative colitis. Quart J Med 170:263–279, 1974.
44. Devroede G: Risk of cancer in inflammatory bowel disease. In: Colorectal cancer: prevention, epidemiology and screening, Winawer S, Schottenfeld D, Sherlock P (eds). New York: Raven Press 1980, pp 325–334.
45. Perett AD, Truelove SC, Massarella GR: Crohn's disease and carcinoma of the colon. Br

Med J 2:466–468, 1968.

46. Thompson H: Malignancy in Crohn's disease. In: The management of Crohn's disease, Weterman IT, Pena AS, Booth CC (eds). Amsterdam: Excerpta Medica, 1976, pp 146–152.

47. Burbidge EJ, Bedine MS, Handelsman JC: Adenocarcinoma of the small intestine in Crohn's disease involving the small bowel. Western J Med 127:43–45, 1977.

48. Fielding JF, Prior P, Waterhouse JA, Cooke WT: Malignancy in Crohn's disease. Scan J Gastroenterol 7:3–7, 1972.

11. Role of CEA in Large Bowel Cancer

THOMAS A. COLACCHIO and PAUL LOGERFO

1. INTRODUCTION

Adenocarcinoma of the colon and rectum is a disease of considerable proportions that affects more than 100,000 adults in the United States each year [1]. This incidence is second only to cancer of the skin, and its resultant mortality is second only to cancer of the lung [2]. Unfortunately, with the possible exception of Turnbull's no-touch technique, there has been no real improvement in survival during the past three decades [3]. Surgical treatment has been suboptimal with about 80% of patients being resectable, but less than one half of this group are cured. Survival is related closely to stage of disease at time of therapy, and the only improvement has come from earlier detection and improved peri-operative care. The five year survival rates of patients based upon the Dukes' classification of their disease generally range from 75 to 90% for Dukes' A; from 45 to 65% for Dukes' B and from 25 to 35% for Dukes' C lesions; with those patients having distant metastases (Dukes' D) rarely surviving 5 years [3]. Even these figures are optimistic since the gross survival of large mixed populations is somewhat less. Of 1687 patients with colon cancer at Charity Hospital in Louisiana, the determinate 5 year survival was only 23% and the gross survival only 17% [4].

The majority of these patients die from residual, recurrent or metastatic disease. In addition, the incidence of multiple or second colon primaries ranges from 0.2 to 12% [4, 5] and the incidence of multiple organ primaries ranges from 11 to 56% [4]. The postulated mechanisms for development of recurrence include: 1) development of a metachronous primary lesion; 2) presence of an overlooked synchronous lesion; 3) inadequate resection with continued growth and; 4) implantation at the site of the anastomosis [5]. Unfortunately, in patients with advanced disease, there exists no single or multidrug regimen which is capable of significant tumor regression with improvement in survival or quality of life [8].

J. J. DeCosse and P. Sherlock (eds.), Gastrointestinal cancer 1, 289–309. All rights reserved.
Copyright © 1981 Martinus Nijhoff Publishers, The Hague/Boston/London.

Thus, when Gold and Freedman [9] identified an antigen (called carcinoembryonic antigen – CEA) in 1965 that appeared to be 'tumor-specific' for colon cancer, there was great enthusiasm that this would herald a new era of earlier diagnosis both of primary lesions and recurrent tumors. This was further heightened by the development of a radioimmunoassay [10] that could detect serum levels of circulating CEA. The criteria for clinical usefulness of such an antigen were described by Lawrence [1] and included: 1) the antigen or tumor product must pass from the tumor into body fluids; 2) the more tumor- or tissue-specific the antigen is, the more useful it will be; 3) serum levels of the antigen should bear some relationship to the amount of tumor present; and 4) the assay should be reproducible by routine techniques. Although the CEA has met these criteria at least in part, Goldenberg stated at the First International Conference on the Clinical Uses of CEA, that since its discovery, we have come to realize that no tumor antigens are truly tumor-specific but rather are tumor-associated. Further, despite all the activities and publications from research on CEA, many of the basic issues facing the practitioner regarding the interpretation of CEA results are still not resolved [1]. It is our goal to address these various issues regarding CEA, review the data in order to provide answers where they exist and, more importantly, to focus and direct further investigation in those areas where answers are unknown.

2. CEA-SUBSTANCE

Carcinoembryonic antigen (CEA) was first described by Gold and Freedman in 1965 [9] as a tumor-specific antigen contained in pooled tumor extracts but not present in normal colonic tissue. Its name was derived when it was also noted to be present in the gut and digestive organs of embryos and first and second trimester fetuses. Since that time, further studies have defined, categorized and quantified it in various organs, tumors and disease states [6, 9, 10, 12–17]. To summarize, CEA is a typical acid glycoprotein of molecular weight approximating 200,000 and is about 50% carbohydrate. It exhibits beta-globulin electrophoretic activity and has a sedimentation coefficient of 7.0–8.0 S. Using electron microscopy, it is of uniform size with a complex secondary structure, and even highly purified preparations of CEA manifest a degree of both intermolecular and intramolecular heterogeneity.

CEA is a peripheral membrane glycoprotein within the fluid mosaic of the cell membranes in which it is found. It is indigenous to the cancer cell and not simply absorbed or interiorized by these cells. From this site on the cell surface, it is easily released into surrounding body fluids. Once in circulation, it is rapidly catabolized and serum values fall to undetectable levels within 2–14 days postoperatively. All Animal studies suggest that the liver is the major site for this activity, and some human investigations have shown CEA to be produced by normal intestinal mucosa, extracted from the circulation by the liver and partially excreted into the bile.

Various methods of radioimmunoassay have been described and CEA as defined by the circulating material that binds to these antibodies in available radioimmunoassay is probably a mixture of related glycoproteins. In addition, a number of subfractions and materials have been described in these assays that are distinct from but cross react with CEA. All these factors have been reviewed and analyzed in relation to Hansen's commercially available method of radioimmunoassay [15]. It was found to have a sensitivity of 0.5 ng/ml and a coefficient of variation of 4.96–7.39% within the range of 2.5–12 ng/ml; and it has been accepted as sensitive and reproducible in intralaboratory studies, but less so in interlaboratory comparisons.

3. CEA IN NON-MALIGNANT TISSUES

Since its original description, the use of more sensitive techniques of detection have identified CEA to be present in normal colon, lung, pancreas, liver, breast and serum. As a result, benign conditions of these organs (primarily of an inflammatory nature) can lead to elevated serum levels [6]. There are some data to suggest that the CEA from these different organ sources may have different antigen specificity [12]. CEA or CEA-like activity has also been detected in saliva, GI secretions, feces, urine, bronchial washings and fluids and secretions of other organ systems. In addition, intestinal perfusion techniques have quantified the secretion of CEA-like activity in the GI tract of healthy humans [17]. This CEA-like material has chromatographic and immunologic properties similar to purified CEA and is highest in the colon, and next highest in pancreaticobiliary secretions. Winawer et al. [17] showed the concentration of CEA in colonic lavage specimens to range from 0 to 4450 ng/ml. Patients who had colon carcinoma or adenomatous polyps were in the highest range, followed by patients with ulcerative colitis, and finally, normals were in the lowest range. In addition, Martin et al. [13] showed that patients having colonic polyps and an elevated serum CEA had their serum levels fall to normal after their polyps were removed. Thus CEA is produced by malignant and non-malignant colonic neoplasms, and also normal colonic mucosa.

Abnormal urine concentrations of CEA have been measured in patients with bladder cancer and also in those with urinary tract infections. In addition, although CEA in pancreatic secretions cannot distinguish between normals and those with pancreatic disease, cholecystokinin stimulation led to an increase in CEA concentration of pancreatic secretions in one third of patients with pancreatic carcinoma and 20% of those with chronic pancreatitis [17].

Thus CEA is present in and released by a variety of organs other than the colon in both normal and non-malignant diseased states.

4. SERUM LEVELS OF CEA IN PATIENTS WITHOUT MALIGNANCY

In an attempt to define the sensitivity and specificity of CEA in relation to colon cancer, many groups of patients with varying disorders have been screened with serum assays for CEA. Unfortunately, this has led to the discovery that there are a variety of conditions which cause an elevation of serum CEA. Part of the difficulty arises in deciding what concentration of CEA will be considered abnormal. As always, sensitivity and specificity vary inversely with higher and lower limits of normal serum CEA levels. Using 2.5 ng/ml (Hansen method) as the upper limit of normal, LoGerfo et al. [6] found 11.6% of normal subjects without a history of smoking to have a serum CEA greater than this level. If the normal range was increased to 5 ng/ml, the false positive rate decreased to 1.3%. Cooper et al. [18] describes a collected series of more than 10,000 normal subjects who has a 3% incidence of a CEA over 2.5 ng/ml. Martin et al. [13] reported similar results and also noted a 3% incidence among pregnant women and, like LoGerfo, showed a significant increase in subjects more than 50 years old (3–5% in 10–20 ng/ml range [6]. All groups [6, 13, 17–19] have noted a marked rise in serum CEA in heavy smokers. LoGerfo et al. [6] reported that 20% of smokers had CEA levels higher than 2.2. ng/ml and, interestingly, a group of former smokers had only 6.6% of levels higher than 2.5 ng/ml, as opposed to only 3% of non-smokers in this selected population.

Aside from these non-pathologic causes for increased CEA, elevated levels have been seen in a variety of benign disorders of the GI and respiratory tracts – particularly the liver. Since CEA is rapidly excreted by the liver in animals and humans, it is not surprising that liver disease can lead to decreased excretion and increasing serum CEA levels. This has been shown by several authors [6, 12, 13, 17, 19–21] with elevated CEA in the presence of cirrhosis ranging from 20 to 70%. Other hepatic disorders, including biliary obstruction, cholangitis and hepatitis, have shown similarly high incidences of abnormal CEA levels. An interesting report by Molnar et al. [16] showed that 28% of recipients of CEA-positive, HB_sAg-negative blood developed acute hepatitis and increased CEA levels versus only one of 39 with CEA-negative, HB_sAg-negative blood. Other GI disorders, including pancreatitis, Crohn's disease, ulcerative colitis, peptic ulcer disease, and adenomatous polyps, have shown varying incidence of increased serum CEA. Interestingly, Gardner et al. showed increased CEA levels in 37 of 57 patients with ulcerative colitis and demonstrated a significant correlation ($p < 0.005$) with extent and severity of disease. Similarly, Martin *et al.* [13] showed that patients with adenomatous polyps and increasing CEA had return of CEA to normal after polypectomy.

Patients with bronchitis and emphysema had a 30–60% incidence of elevated serum CEA [6, 17, 19]. Similarly, alcohol addiction was associated with a 50–60% incidence of increased CEA [6, 23]. The loss of specificity for malignant disease could be improved by increasing the normal range to 5.0 or even 10.0 ng/ml, but there would then be a significant and concomitant fall in the assay's sensitivity for malignancy.

5. CEA IN MALIGNANT DISORDERS

CEA has been found to be elevated in the sera and also to be present in the tissues of many patients with malignant neoplasms of both enteric and non-enteric origin. Once again, the determined upper limit of normal will affect the incidence of positivity (i.e. sensitivity) of serum CEA levels. Table 1 shows the major published series of serum CEA levels in various enteric neoplasms. All these groups used 2.5. ng/ml as their upper limit of normal except for Lawrence *et al.* [19] whose value of 12.5 [11] is equivalent to 2.5 ng/ml and Beatty *et al.* [20] who used 5.0 ng/ml as their upper limit of normal. Patients with colorectal cancers ranged from 65% to 81% in positivity; somewhat higher than gastric cancer (46–75%); and somewhat lower than pancreatic cancer (64–91%). As expected, both hepatomas and biliary carcinomas had a high incidence of elevated CEA levels.

Table 2 depicts the findings by several authors of elevated CEA levels in patients with non-enteric neoplasms. There are a considerable number of tumors with elevated serum CEA levels, although lung and breast have the

Table 1. Percentage of positive preoperative CEA assays in patients with enteric neoplasms.

	Cooper [18] (%)	Martin [13] (%)	Lawrence [19] (%)	Beatty [20] (%)	LoGerfo [6] (%)
Colorectal	79	81	69	65	72
Gastric	59	75	46	67	61
Pancreatic	81	90	90	64	91
Hepatoma	75	40	100	—	—
Biliary	73	80	—	—	—
Small bowel	83	30	—	—	—
Esophageal	61	27	—	—	—

Positive values: >2.5 ng/ml.

Table 2. Percentage of positive preoperative CEA assays in patients with non-enteric neoplasms.

	Cooper [18] (%)	Martin [13] (%)	Lawrence [19] (%)	LoGerfo [6] (%)
Lung	67	25	66	76
Breast	69	60	46	47
Kidney	68	—	27	—
Bladder	60	37	49	—
Prostate	67	22	44	—
Testes	50	25	75	—
Ovary	—	20	40	—
Uterus/cervix	67	13	37	—
Thyroid	50	0	0	—
Head and neck	—	6	—	—
Lymphoma	18	9	37	35
Sarcoma	0	—	—	31
Skin	30	9	20	—
Brain	—	—	—	28
Leukemia	—	—	57	37

Positive values: >2.5 ng/ml.

most significant incidence of positivity (25–76% and 47–68% respectively). In those series with analysis of multiple variables there was no relationship between age, sex or size of the lesion and the incidence of CEA positivity. Conversely, those authors who compared the stage of disease with the incidence of CEA positivity frequently found a significant correlation between positivity and advancing stage of disease, not only in colorectal lesions, but also in breast, lung, pancreas, stomach and bladder tumors. Similarly, Joyce *et al.* [23], by using direct measurement of CEA levels and comparing mean pretreatment values, found much higher levels (in descending order) with colorectal, bronchogenic and pancreatic as compared to esophageal or breast neoplasms.

It is this relative lack of specificity that made Beatty *et al.* [20] state that in the general population, CEA$\geq$5 ng/ml is a nonspecific indicator of disease, either benign or malignant, and a CEA level >10 ng/ml is a non-specific indicator of malignancy. In the case of breast cancer, however, he concluded that a preoperative CEA>10 ng/ml is suggestive of and a level >25 ng/ml is highly suspicious for metastatic disease.

A caution was offered by Gold [14] to explain in part this lack of specificity. He stated that the CEA-like material found in tissues and serum from patients with non-enteric neoplasms has not been shown to be identical to CEA. In fact, the difficulty in specificity may not be with the antigen but rather with the radioimmunoassay, which is merely identifying CEA-like activity in other substances. It should be noted however, that no assay for CEA has ever been shown to be specific; and a specific 'CEA' antigen may not really exist.

6. CEA IN LARGE BOWEL CANCER

6.1. Screening

Although virtually all authors agree that CEA lacks the specificity and sensitivity to allow for screening of large asymptomatic populations, the question of its use in that capacity still occasionally arises [12]. For an assay to be effective in screening, the predictive value of a positive result must be greater than the prevalence of the disease sought, and must be high enough to be cost-effective and minimize the number of patients without malignant disease undergoing further and sometimes extensive investigation. The difficulties with using CEA in this capacity include: 1) the difficulty of interlaboratory reproducibility [6, 15] since a 95% confidence level of $+/-2.0$ ng/ml would change the result of 20% of the tests from one lab to the next; 2) a false positive rate of 15% [6]; and 3) a false negative rate of 40–60% in non-metastatic disease [1, 6, 20, 23, 24]. In a highly selected group of patients reviewed by Costanza et al. [6] who underwent barium enema for various clinical criteria, 116 of 576 patients had CEA levels greater than 2.5 ng/ml. Of this group 15 of 16 had documented cancer, nine had CEA levels greater than 5.0 ng/ml, and only two of these 15 were Dukes' B lesions. Five additional cancers had normal CEA levels including only two Dukes' B lesions. Thus even in this highly selected population 25% of cancers including half of the early lesions would have been missed with CEA screening. Chu et al. [1] screened a population of 1800 business executives and detected two previously unsuspected cancers – one colon and one pancreas, for a cost of $36,000 per tumor found. Finally, Cooper et al. [18] projected the predictive value for CEA testing on a proposed population with a 2% prevalence of malignant disease. He found that the predictive value for a positive test was 3.1% if the normal value was <2.5 and 10.6% if the normal was <10 ng/ml. The predictive value of a negative test was 99% and 98.6% respectively for the different normal values. Thus even if you used a normal value for CEA of <10.0 ng/ml, only one of ten patients identified in this proposed population would have malignant disease and you would still miss the majority of early lesions.

These projected data, based on the measured sensitivity and specificity of CEA, would strongly mitigate against its use in screening large populations for cancer. Similarly, there is no evidence to support the use of serum CEA levels in screening high risk populations (i.e. patients with ulcerative colitis or adenomatous polyps) for the likelihood of developing malignancy [1, 16] Studies need to be performed to test the efficacy of using CEA levels in colonic lavage samples for screening of these high-risk populations.

6.2. Prognosis

The prognostic value of careful histologic staging of disease (Duke's Classification, TNM Classification, Astler-Coller modification) has long been established, and any potential prognostic indicator must be compared with these techniques. The more complex issue of the usefulness of prognostic indicators as criteria for additional or adjunctive therapy will be discussed later. Some authors have claimed that preoperative CEA levels increase one's ability to estimate recurrence, and others state that CEA merely mirrors the pathologic staging and does not improve upon it. Table 3 compares the incidence of positive preoperative levels of CEA as determined by various authors with the standard Dukes' Classification Staging system. There is clearly a higher incidence of elevated preoperative CEA in the Dukes' B and C lesions as compared with Dukes' A. There is, however, a much less clear distinction between Dukes' B and C lesions, despite the acknowledged marked difference in survival between these two groups. The possible causes for this discrepancy are: 1) a much greater, or lesser, sensitivity of CEA in these groups; or, 2) a lack of sensitivity of Dukes' Classification versus TNM or the Astler-Coller modification system for these two groups. This question could be answered in part if the investigators had compared survival within each classification, as some have done; and if they compared CEA with TNM or Astler-Coller systems of staging, as none have done. Regarding the former comparison, some data do exist, but they unfortunately conflict.

LoGerfo et al. [6] studied the incidence of recurrence at three years and found that for each stage of Dukes' Classifications, the incidence of recurrence was 1.8 times greater in those patients with preoperative CEA higher

Table 3. Percentage of positive preoperative CEA assays versus Dukes' classification.

	Dhar [26] (%)	(%)	LoGerfo [6] (%)	Wanebo [7] (%)	Slater [49] (%)	(%)	Lawrence [19] (%)
Dukes' A	19[a]	6[b]	19[a]	4[c]	23[a]	4[c]	44[a]
Dukes' B	53	24	59	25	46	33	75
Dukes' C			75	44	54	30	60
Dukes' D	100	61	90	65	87	87	—

[a] Positive values >2.5 ng/ml.

[b] Positive values >10 ng/ml.

[c] Positive values >5 ng/ml.

than 4.0 ng/ml, and they concluded that preoperative CEA correlated with prognosis. In a somewhat different type of analysis, Wanebo et al. [7] found that disease-free survival at 30 months in Dukes' B and C patients was correlated with preoperative CEA values with a statistical significance of $p < 0.02$ for B lesions and $p < 0.001$ for C lesions. He found that 78% of Dukes' B patients with CEA levels less than 5.0 ng/ml but only 44% with CEA levels greater than 5.0 ng/ml were disease free at 30 months; and 41% of Dukes' C patients with CEA levels less than 5 ng/ml but only 15% with CEA greater than 5.0 ng/ml were disease-free at 30 months. In this latter group, results became even more striking if they used 10 ng/ml as the cut-off: 21% with a CEA greater than 10 ng/ml and 88% with a CEA less than 10 ng/ml were disease-free at 30 months. Esposito et al. [25] had similar findings among Dukes' C patients: 60% with a preoperative CEA less than 10 ng/ml and 20% with a CEA greater than 10 ng/ml were alive at 24 months ($p < 0.05$).

Conversely, Slater et al. [24] found little difference in preoperative CEA in Dukes' B and C patients and concluded that the CEA did not compare stage for stage with recurrence rates. Similarly, Beatty et al. [20] found a 2.1 fold increase in incidence of recurrence in patients with preoperative CEA greater than 5 ng/ml; however, he found Dukes' staging to be more discriminating and not enhanced by preresection CEA levels in assessing prognosis. These findings were substantiated by Evans et al. [27], who found preoperative CEA was not additive to Dukes' classification and not more predictive than TNM staging.

Chu et al. [47] had a somewhat different assessment and felt that CEA and Dukes' staging were additive in value with the former being a more sensitive marker within the first two years and the latter more useful after that time. He also stated that postoperative CEA values were prognostic with a higher recurrence rate among patients with persistent elevations postoperatively. Alsabti [28], in a short follow-up period of 15 months, noted a marked difference in recurrence in patients with persistent elevation of CEA. In those with increased CEA preoperatively but normal postoperatively, there was a 30% recurrence at 15 months; however, in those with persistently elevated CEA post-operatively, the recurrence at 15 months was 90%. Wanebo et al. [29] compared Dukes' B and C patients in relation to persistently elevated postoperative CEA and found that 67% of patients with B lesions and 100% of patients with C lesions had recurrence if CEA levels remained greater than 5 ng/ml postoperatively. Koch et al. [30] noted similar findings with 89% of patients with persistently elevated CEA greater than 5 ng/ml postoperatively developing recurrence versus 29% of those with CEA less than 5 ng/ml within the first six months after resection.

Clearly the available data do not resolve the question of the prognostic value of preoperative CEA levels, although most authors agree that a persistent elevation of CEA after resection (i.e. failure to fall to normal) is associated with a high incidence of recurrence.

Gunderson et al. [2] reported on the predictive value of the Astler-Coller modification of the Dukes' classification in a large series of patients. He showed a very high correlation between the extent of original disease with regard to penetration of the bowel wall and number and pattern of lymph node involvement not only for incidence but also for pattern of recurrence of colorectal cancer. He used this system to indentify high-risk groups who might benefit by some form of adjuvant therapy.

Unfortunately, the real value of preoperative and postoperative CEA levels for prognosis will not be known until they are compared to this modified system of tumor staging, since it is individuals at higher risk within large groups who need to be identified.

6.3. Marker for Recurrence

The concept of using serial CEA in surveillance for recurrent colorectal carcinoma was first mentioned in the literature by Thompson et al. [10] in 1969 when he described his radioimmunoassay for CEA. At that time, he stated that if CEA fell to zero postoperatively, then return of elevated CEA levels should indicate recurrent disease. Since that time there have been many studies to test that premise, and many articles published both supporting and refuting it. The difficulty with undertaking a comparative analysis of these series is that they are frequently incomplete, retrospective, overlapping and occasionally arrive at conflicting conclusions from a single institution. There are several major series that address this issue and attempt to arrive at some conclusions. The questions that exist are: 1) Is CEA a sensitive marker for recurrence; 2) Is CEA specific for recurrence in the population post-resection of colorectal cancers; 3) Will it detect recurrence before other means of evaluation (physical examination, serum chemistries, scintigraphy, radiography); 4) Will it recognize recurrence in a more frequently localized (i.e. treatable) state than other techniques; and, 5) Will it have any effect on survival in this population? Unfortunately, many data in this area are anecdotal with only two or three prospective studies, relatively short follow-up and no randomized, prospective series. Nevertheless, some implications can be drawn from the data available.

The largest prospective study is by Attiyeh et al. [31], who reported on 32 patients post-resection of Dukes' B and C lesions who developed elevated CEA levels postoperatively without any other signs of recurrence. Twenty-eight had documented metastases of which 17 were hepatic and 11 were regional. Of this group, 14 were resected and 10 are still alive 2–55 months post-reexploration. One patient had metastatic disease not found at operation and three had presumed false positive CEA elevations. From the same institution, Wanebo et al. [29] reported on 98 cases of recurrent tumor of whom 52 had liver metastases and 48 of this group (92%) had a CEA greater than 5.0 ng/ml. The other 46 had local recurrence and only 23 (50%) had a CEA greater than 5.0 ng/ml. He also described the rate of CEA rise to be more rapid in those with hepatic metastases.

Another study, partly prospective, was reported by Martin et al. [13, 21, 23, 32, 33] in which he began by stating that careful physical examination was the most reliable way of detecting recurrence in those patients without elevated CEA. He stated that two-thirds of recurrences will occur within 18 months, and that in those patients who have increasing CEA greater than 2.5 ng/ml preoperatively which then falls to below 2.5 ng/ml postoperatively, the most sensitive and reliable indicator of recurrence was a rising level of CEA. His group has derived a normogram for CEA that applies the patient's previously normal serum for control and is able to distinguish significant CEA rise from laboratory error. Using this method he retrospectively reviewed 22 patients who underwent re-operation for presumed recurrence. Nineteen were found to have recurrence at operation and another two developed metastatic disease later despite negative laparotomy. Of this group, six had resectable tumor, and there was one false positive CEA elevation. He then described a second group of 18 patients who prospectively underwent reoperation for a significantly elevated CEA. Of this second group there was one false positive value and 13 had localized resectable disease. He emphasized that the delay between increasing CEA and operation averaged 4.5 months in the unresectable group and only 1.4 months in the resectable patients. He concluded that this short interval of delay was responsible for his high percentage of resectable recurrences. From the same center, Joyce et al. [23] reported on eight cases of liver recurrence who had preoperative CEA levels greater than 20 ng/ml, none of whom fell below 5 ng/ml postoperatively. In this group, seven had normal liver scans an four had normal alkaline phosphate levels at the time recurrence was documented. Thus, CEA seems to be as efficacious as these other modalities in detecting liver metastases.

Rau et al. [34] and Steele et al. [35] reported on 75 patients who were followed post-resection of Dukes' B and C lesions. Of this group 18 developed recurrence, and 15 of these were first diagnosed by an elevated CEA. Two patients had discovery of recurrence simultaneously with an increasing CEA, one patient had recurrence with a normal CEA, and one patient with an increasing CEA had no recurrence detected at exploration. They emphasize that those patients with regional metastases generally had a slower rate of rise in CEA than those with extensive or distant metastases. Four of seven of the former group were resectable as compared to only one of eight in the latter group.

Three other patient groups were reported from that same center. The first was a group of 25 patients [36] who had significant CEA elevations according to the criteria of Martin's nomogram [21] and were therefore eligible for re-operation for presumed recurrence. However, in nine of these patients the rise was transient for only two consecutive determinations and eight more demonstrated no clinical evidence of recurrence. Sugarbaker *et al.* [37] reported on the other two groups: in one, 11 of 33 patients with persistently increasing CEA postoperatively have shown no evidence of recurrence after two to four years; and in the other, six of 12 patients with recurrence had an increase in CEA as their first manifestation, but another four had normal CEA levels when their recurrence was diagnosed.

Evans *et al.* [27] described a fourth prospective study in which 14 patients underwent re-operation for elevated CEA levels. Of these, 11 had recurrent disease, but only one was resectable. He also stated that 15% of their patients had spurious transient CEA elevations on two consecutive occasions and that all patients with a single elevation greater than 25 ng/ml had recurrence, as did all patients with a 5 ng/ml rise on two consecutive determinations. In a retrospective review, Moertel *et al.* [38] reported on 36 patients with recurrent tumor, of whom 20 (56%) had a CEA less than 25 ng/ml and 27 (75%) had a CEA less than 5 ng/ml, despite the fact that all had symptomatic recurrence at the time of CEA determination.

Finally, in a retrospective analysis of 15 patients with recurrence by Beatty *et al.* [20], 13 had a CEA greater than 5.0 ng/ml at the time of diagnosis and in eight the CEA rise preceded diagnosis of recurrence by a mean of 7.9 months. From these several reports and the other data summarized in Table 4, there is considerable variation among investigators as to the value of CEA determinations in surveillance for recurrent cancer, not only among different groups, but also within the same institution. Until such time when randomized, prospective studies are completed to answer these questions regarding CEA's usefulness in this area, some general impressions can be made. First. CEA is more effective in identifying extensive and hepatic metastases than in local recurrence. Secondly, a rapidly rising postoperative CEA level or a level greater than 25 ng/ml is highly suggestive of extensive recurrence, frequently hepatic. Thirdly, a post-operative CEA level that remains above 5 ng/ml and does not return to normal is associated with a higher incidence of recurrence. Fourthly, normal postoperative CEA levels do not preclude the presence of recurrent disease and do not replace careful clinical and laboratory follow-up in search for recurrence. Finally, CEA elevations postoperatively do not diagnose recurrent tumor, but may be spurious or due to other factors.

In summary, CEA may be helpful in surveying for recurrence but to date has not been clearly shown to improve or replace careful clinical follow-up of patients at risk for developing recurrence.

Table 4. CEA in patients with recurrent colorectal cancer.

	No. pts. followed	No. pts. with recurrence	% pos. CEA	% false pos. CEA	% false neg. CEA	% local recurrence
Attiyeh [31]	32	29	100	9	3	38
Minton [32]	22	21	100	5	0	43
Martin [21]	18	17	100	5	0	76
Sugerbaker [37]	33	22	100	33	0	—
Rittgers [36]	25	8	100	68	0	—
Evans [27]	14	11	100	21	0	—
McKay [38]	220	53	100	32	32	11
Ratcliffe [39]	148	37	97	10	3	46
Steele [34, 35]	75	18	94	5	5	—
Mach [40]	66	19	89	41	11	5
Beatty [20]	15	15	87	0	13	—
Staab [41]	31	31	90	0	10	—
Herrera [1]	23	23	87	—	13	—
Neville [1]	82	82	77	0	23	—
Wanebo [29]	98	98	72	0	28 [a]	47
Sugarbaker [37]	12	12	67	0	33	—
Moertel [38]	36	36	25	0	75 [b]	25

[a] Includes half of the patients with local recurrence.
[b] Includes all of the patients with local recurrence.

6.4. CEA and Second-Look Operations

The efficacy of 'second-look' operations in the management of patients post-resection of colorectal carcinomas was first investigated in a prospective manner by Wangensteen *et al.* [42] in 1948. He reported on 153 patients with Dukes' C lesions of the colon and rectum who underwent 'blind' second-look operations six to 12 months after initial resection. Ninety-seven patients who had carcinoma of the colon developed 50 recurrences, of which 43 were discovered at reoperation. Four in this group were resectable for cure and there were nine operative deaths. Thirty-five of 56 patients who had rectal lesions developed recurrence and 27 of these were noted at reexploration. There were two operative deaths and only two were amenable to reresection. With an operative mortality of 7% and a conversion to cure rate of only 7%, this concept was not popularized. Despite the low cure rates, the survival of both groups was prolonged after second operation with increased survival at one and two years for rectal lesions and at one year for colonic lesions. Gunderson *et al.* [2] at the University of Minnesota reported on a second group of 74 patients, of whom 52 developed recurrence. Forty-six of these were diagnosed at reoperation with four operative deaths (5% and only four patients converted to a disease-free state (15%). Once again, these figures were not very encouraging. Similarly poor results were reported by Machman et al. [3] in a group of patients who received adjuvant chemotherapy before blind reoperation. Despite a 76% reported two year survival, only five patients (5%) were considered cured at five years.

Polk et al. [43] reported a series of patients with recurrence who received either no therapy, radiotherapy or reresection. None of the first two groups were alive at three years, and 25% (three of 12) of the resected group survived more than five but less than ten years. In a review of other series, he noted an 8–41% rate of reresection. One of these groups, described by Bacon, was a selected group of patients with recurrence: 79 had local pelvic recurrences and 14 occurred outside the pelvis. thirty-two of the local recurrences were resected: 11 patients were alive at five years and of the six with distant metastases who were resected, four were alive at five years. The operative mortality was zero with a conversion rate of 16%. Although this was a selected group, the results of 50% resectability, with associated increased survival and 16% cure are more acceptable. Pemberton [44] and Wanebo et al. [29] published series of selected patients with hepatic metastases who underwent resection. The survival was 29% (two to five years) in the former and 40% (more than five years) in the latter. From these series, we can see that although blind reexplorations may not be efficacious, directed reoperation in selected patients with recurrence should result in a 15–30% incidence of improved survival with minimal operative mortality.

Since the limiting factor for success at reoperation is the extent of recurrence and/or presence of distant metastases, there has been considerable enthusiasm generated over the possibility of using CEA to identify 'earlier' recurrence and thereby improve results of reoperation. As noted in the previous section, there is no clear data to show that monitoring of CEA levels in post-resection patients enables recognition of recurrence either more often or sooner than careful clinical follow-up. Nevertheless, several authors have studied prospective groups of patients who have undergone reoperation for suspected recurrence on the basis of rising CEA levels post-resection; and their results are summarized in Table 5. As shown, the results vary and the percentage of resectability ranged from 9 to 76% with the percentage of 'cure' ranging from 9 to 35%. Unfortunately, the follow-up of all these groups is less than five years and often less than three years. which makes their presumption of cure on the basis of resectability somewhat optimistic. The authors of these series emphasize several points that may or may not be validated by long-term follow-up.

Martin et al. reviewed two groups, one prospective [21] and one retrospective [45], and found striking differences in resectability and cure rates between them: 76% and 35% respectively in the former versus 27% and 0% respec-

Table 5. Results of reoperation for recurrent colorectal cancer.

		No. of reops.	% recurrence at op.	% false neg. op.	% operative mortality	% resect-ability	% cure/ conver.	Follow-up
A	Gunderson [2]	74	70	11	5	—	5	—
	Wangensteen [42]	153	46	10	7	—	7	1–10 yr
	Machman [3]	96	33	3	—	5	5	5 yr
B	Pemberton [44]	31	100	0	16	100	29	2–5 yr
	Wanebo [18]	24	100	0	—	100	40	5 yr
	Bacon [43]	93	100	0	0	41	16	2–5 yr
C	Attiyeh [31]	32	88	3	—	55	34	2–55 mo
	Savrin [21]	18	95	—	—	76	35	1–5 yr
	Martin [45]	22	86	14	—	27	0	5 yr
	Evans [27]	14	79	—	—	9	9	—
	Rau [34]	16	94	—	—	24	13	13–24 mo
	Staab [41]	28	100	0	—	14	14	—

A : Blind second look operations.
B : Clinically directed second look operations.
C : Rising postoperative CEA directed second look operations.

tively in the latter. He emphasizes that the mean delay between increasing CEA, as determined by normogram, and operation in the retrospective group was 7 months as compared to 1.4 months in the prospective group. He claims that this factor is responsible for the difference in resectability and 'cure' rates.

Attiyeh *et al.* [31] reported on a group of 32 patients with a resectability rate of 55% and a presumed cure in 34%. They stress that although 53% of these recurrences were hepatic metastases, all 32 patients were asymptomatic without clinical evidence for disease at the time of operation. Unfortunately, for the five hepatic resections considered to be free of disease, the follow-up has only been 3–14 months. Of the 31 patients reported by Staab *et al.* [41] to have developed recurrence, 28 had rising CEA levels an average of four months before diagnosis of recurrence and there was no false positive. However, of the nine patients reoperated upon solely for rising CEA levels, none was resectable; and of the four patients resectable for cure, one had a normal CEA level and the remaining three had other evidence for recurrence in addition to a rising CEA.

· Rau *et al.* [34] emphasized that although the mean interval before operation was two months after an increased CEA level, it was the rate of CEA rise that correlated with resectability and survival. Only one of seven 'fast rising' patients was resectable versus three of the eight 'slow rising' patients; and of the remaining five patients in this latter group, four were alive at 10 months compared to none of the unresectable patients in the former group. Despite a 25% incidence of resectability only two patients (13%) were still disease free at 13 and 24 months. Finally, only one of the patients in the group explored by Evans *et al.* [27] for a rising CEA had resectable disease.

The short follow-up and lack of randomization in these later series of directed second look operations in patients with rising CEA levels makes comparison with the previous series of blind reexploration impossible. Nevertheless, there is no clearly demonstrated advantage over careful clinical follow-up to monitoring of CEA levels in order to identify patients for second look operations. Similarly, there is no evidence that this method of follow-up and reexploration will result in improved survival in patients at risk for developing recurrent cancer. This impression is supported by Kjaer[46], who reviewed seven prospective studies using CEA levels in the follow-up of patients who were postresection of colorectal cancers. Despite a 67–100% incidence of elevated CEA levels at the time of recurrence (100% in five of the series), these increased CEA levels were of therapeutic consequence in only 2.2% of the patients. Larger randomized studies with longer follow-up are needed to answer these questions.

6.5. *Identification of High Risk Groups*

The identification of those patients who are at higher risk for developing recurrent disease is a justifiable endeavor only if it is being done for more than mere assessment of prognosis. With this assumption, identification of high risk groups might allow for more cost effective follow-up, potentially provide a population for adjuvant therapy (chemotherapy, radiotherapy, immunotherapy, reoperation), and might possibly discriminate between those patients who are more likely to develop local versus distant metastases. Various authors have described pathologic characteristics of the primary tumor that correlate with a higher incidence of recurrence. Certainly the stage of disease, regardless of the system used, is correlated with recurrence and survival. Polk *et al.* [43], after affirming that the only reason for any system of follow-up is if one intends to treat recurrent disease, noted that 65% of recurrences occur within 24 months and 85% within 48 months. Within these categories, however, they found that 89% of patients with either infiltrating tumor margins or absence of surrounding inflammatory response manifested recurrence within eighteen months of operation, and thereby comprised a high risk population. We have already reviewed Gunderson's series[2] in which he used the Astler-Coller modification of Dukes' Classification for staging. Using this system he found that in patients with invasion through the bowel wall (B2, B3, C2, C3) and in patients with more than three positive nodes, there was a greatly increased incidence of recurrence (85% and 55%

respectively). If both factors were present, the incidence of recurrence rose to 80–100%. In addition, he was able to correlate this system with the likelihood of developing local versus distant metastases.

We have also already reviewed the data concerning the usefulness of preoperative CEA versus pathologic staging of the primary lesion in establishing prognosis. Although there is some disagreement regarding its efficacy, some statements can be made concerning the role of postoperative CEA and the risk of developing recurrence. Go [17], Wanebo et al. [7], Joyce et al. [23], Evans et al. [27], and Chu [47] concur that a CEA elevation >25 ng/ml is almost certainly associated with metastatic disease which is usually extensive and/or hepatic in nature. Several authors have also noted that a postoperative CEA that does not fall below 5 ng/ml is also associated with a significantly higher incidence of recurrence. Alsabti showed that a group of patients whose CEA was <2.5 ng/ml preoperatively and <2.5 ng/ml postoperatively had a 30% incidence of recurrence at 15 months; whereas those patients with CEA levels <5 ng/ml pre- and postoperatively had a 90% incidence of recurrence at 15 months. Wanebo et al. [7] found that in a group of Dukes' B patients, 78% of those patients with normal CEA levels and only 44% of those with elevated CEA levels were free of disease at 30 months ($p < 0.02$). Similarly, 88% of Dukes' C patients with CEA levels >10 ng/ml and only 21% with CEA <10 ng/ml were disease free at 30 months ($p < 0.001$). Furthermore, 12 of 14 (85%) patients whose postoperative CEA never fell below 5 ng/ml developed recurrence.

Koch et al. [30] noted that during the first six months postoperatively 89% of patients with CEA levels greater than 5 ng/ml developed recurrence versus only 29% of those with CEA levels less than 5 ng/ml. After six months, the incidence of recurrence was: 6.4% with CEA <5 ng/ml, 67% with CEA >5 ng/ml and 87% for patients with CEA levels >10 ng/ml. Steele et al. [35] has reported that the rate of rise of postoperative CEA levels is correlated with the extent of disease found at reoperation. Seven of nine patients in his group with resectable recurrences had an increasing CEA rate of less than 2.1 ng/ml/30 days, whereas all six of those with unresectable recurrences had a rising CEA rate greater than 2.1 ng/ml/30 days. He proposed that this latter group might best forego reoperation entirely and be given alternative therapy.

Thus, we see that although the evidence is not conclusive, there certainly exist identifiable groups which are at high risk for developing recurrent cancer. Wanebo et al. [29] summarizes them as: Astler-Coller Class B1, B2, C1, C2, and some D patients in whom all gross tumor has been resected. In addition to these, they add all patients who have both pre- and postoperative CEA levels >5 ng/ml. It remains to be shown whether identification of these high risk patients and their subsequent incorporation into adjuvant protocols will lead to improved survival.

6.6. *Monitoring Response to Therapy*

As with the other potential applications of monitoring serial CEA levels, there is conflicting evidence that the CEA is efficacious in following the response of patients to nonsurgical therapy. Go[17] cautions that there other factors in addition to tumor response to chemotherapy which may cause CEA levels to rise or fall. He states that various chemotherapeutic agents may alter the synthesis or secretion of CEA without affecting progression of the tumor; conversely, CEA levels may rise due to liver toxicity without actual progression of disease. Al-Sarraf *et al.* [48] reported that 16 of 18 patients achieving partial remission of their metastatic colon cancer with chemotherapy had a fall in CEA. Further, they noted that survival correlated in an inverse fashion with the change in CEA regardless of the clinical evaluation of response. These results were corraborated by Ravry [48] who noted that the response to chemotherapy correlated with the change in level of CEA (i.e. those with increasing CEA had progression and those with decreasing CEA had improvement). Herrera [1] noted a correlation between survival and CEA response: 16 of 29 CEA responders were alive at the time of follow versus only six of 46 CEA nonresponders. However, 20% of the patients in his series with clinical progression of their disease had a false decrease in CEA levels.

Shani *et al.* [49] found in their series that although there was generally a good correlation between serial CEA levels and objective responses ($p < 0.05$), there were a number (11 of 53) of discordant values of CEA when compared to response. He also found that although there was a very good correlation between survival and objective response ($p < 0.001$), this was not as significant when comparing survival to CEA levels ($p < 0.07$). Mayer *et al.* [50] concurred that although CEA frequently correlated with response, the prognostic value of this information was minimal.

Unlike the response in patients receiving chemotherapy, Sugarbaker *et al.* [51] and others [48] found a direct and sensitive correlation between serial CEA levels and the dosage of and response to radiotherapy. They used this parameter to determine if the bulk of the tumor was within the radiotherapy port. They also noted this decrease in CEA to be shortlived, and felt that this indicated that in the case of preoperative radiotherapy, surgery should be performed within eight weeks to obtain maximal benefit.

In sum, it appears that although CEA levels correlate with response in most cases, serial levels have not been shown to have any advantage over objective measurement of response in predicting prognosis and survival.

7. OTHER APPLICATIONS OF CEA

Finally, there are potential uses of CEA in the management of colorectal cancer patients that have yet to be explored. One such area was recently studied by Kom *et al.* [53]. They labelled anti-CEA IgG and tested its accuracy as a radioimmunodetector in patients with primary and metastatic colon cancer. They found the sensitivity (true positive result) to be 90% in patients with both primary and metastatic disease. The specificity of the test was 94% and the overall accuracy was 93%. They also noted that high serum levels of CEA did not hinder the localization of disease and suggested use of this technique for determining the source of antigen in patients with rising CEA titres.

In closing, it is the responsibility of surgeons and oncologists caring for patients with colorectal cancer not only to initiate randomized, prospective studies to test the efficacy of monitoring CEA in the areas we have discussed but also to develop and test other modalities of adjuvant/curative therapy in order to improve the prognosis and survival for this highly lethal disease.

REFERENCES

1. Holyoke E, Cooper EH: CEA and tumor markers. Semin Oncol 3:377–397, 1976.
2. Gunderson LL, Sosin H: Areas of failure found at reoperation (second or symptomatic look) following 'curative surgery' for adenocarcinoma of the rectum. Cancer 34:1278–1292, 1974.
3. Mackman S, Ansfield FJ, Ramirez G, Curreri AR: A second look at the second look operation in colonic cancer after the administration of fluorouracil. Am J Surg 128:763–766, 1974.
4. Travieso CR, Jr, Knoepp LF Jr, Hanley PH: Multiple adenocarcinomas of the colon and rectum. Dis Colon Rectum 15:1–6, 1972.
5. Zer M, Mukamel E, Dintsman M: Long-term survival following repeated resections of the colon for multiple or current carcinoma. Am J Procto Gastroenterol Colon Rectal Surg :23–27, 1979.
6. LoGerfo P, Pennington G: Current status of carcinoembryonic antigen. In: Progress in clinical cancer, Ariel IM (ed). New York: Grune & Stratton, vol VI, pp 65–72, 1975.
7. Wanebo HJ, Rao B, Pinsky CM, Hoffman RG, Stearns M, Schwartz MK, Oettgen HF: Preoperative carcinoembryonic antigen level as a prognostic indicator in colorectal cancer. New Eng J Med 299:488–451, 1978.
8. Valdivieso M, Mavligit GM: Chemotherapy and chemoimmunotherapy of colorectal cancer. Role of the carcinoembryonic antigen. Surg Clin North Am 58:619–631, 1978.
9. Gold P, Freedman SO: Demonstration of tumor-specific antigens in human colonic carcinomata by immunological tolerance and absorption techniques. J Exp Med 121:439–462, 1965.
10. Thomson DMP, Krupey J, Freedman SO, Gold P: The radioimmunoassay of circulating carcinoembryonic antigen of the human digestive system. Med SCi 64:161–167, 1969.
11. Goldenberg D: Introduction to the international conference on the clinical uses of carcinoembryonic antigen. Cancer 42:1397–1398, 1978.

12. Green JB, Trowbridge AA: The use of carcinoembryonic antigen in the clinical management of colorectal cancer. Surg Clin North Am 59:831–839, 1979.

13. Martin EW Jr, Kibbey WF, DiVecchia L, Angerson G, Catalano P, Minton JP: Carcinoembryonic antigen. Clinical and historical aspects. Cancer 37:62–81, 1976.

14. Gold P, Shuster J Freedman SO: Carcinoembryonic antigen (CEA) in clinical medicine. Historical perspectives, pitfalls and projections. Cancer 42:1399–1405, 1978.

15. Reynoso G: The analytical reliability of the zirconyl phosphate method of plasma carcinoembryonic antigen. Cancer 42:1406–1411, 1978.

16. Loewenstein MS, Zamcheck N: Carcinoembryonic antigen (CEA) levels in benign gastrointestinal disease states. Cancer 42:1412–1418, 1978.

17. Go VLM: Carcinoembryonic antigen. Clinical application. Cancer 37!37:562–566, 1976.

18. Cooper MJ, Mackie CR, Skinner DB, Moossa AR: A reappraisal of the value of carcinoembryonic antigen in the management of patients with various neoplasms. Br J Surg 66:120–123, 1979.

19. Laurence DJR, Stevens U, Bettelheim R, Darcy D, Leese C, Turberville C, Alexander P, Johns Ew, Nevill AM: Rose of plasma carcinoembryonic antigen in diagnosis of gastrointestinal, mammary, and bronchial carcinoma. Br Med J 3:605–609, 1972.

20. Beatty JD, Romero C, Brown PW, Lawrence W Jr: Clinical value of carcinoembryonic antigen. Diagnosis, prognosis, and follow-up of patients with cancer. Arch Surg 114:563–567, 1979.

21. Savrin RA, Cooperman M, Martin EW Jr: Clinical application of carcinoembryonic antigen in patients with colorectal carcinoma. Dis Colon Rectum 22:211–215, 1979.

22. Meeker WR Jr: The use and abuse of CEA test in clinical practice. Cancer 41:854–862, 1978.

23. Joyce S, Lobe T, Cooperman M, Martin EW Jr: Direct carcinoembryonic antigen assay in diagnosis and prognosis. Surgery 86: 627–631, 1979.

24. Slater G, Papatestas AE, Aufses AH Jr: Preoperative carcinoembryonic antigen levels in colorectal carcinoma. Arch Surg 114:52–53, 1979.

25. Esposito M, Rubagotti A, Aste H, Porcile GF: Carcinoembryonic antigen level as a prognostic factor in colorectal cancer. Cancer 7:437, 1979.

26. Dhar P, Moore T, Zamcheck N. Kupchik HZ: Carcinoembryonic antigen (CEA) in colonic cancer. Use in preoperative and postoperative diagnosis. JAMA 221:31–35, 1972.

27. Evans JT, Mittelman A, Chu M, Holyoke ED: Pre- and postoperative uses of CEA. Cancer 42:1419–1421, 1978.

28. Alsabti E: Carcinoembryonic antigen (CEA) as prognostic marker in colonic cancer. J Surg Oncol 12:127–129, 1979.

29. Wanebo HJ, Stearns M, Schwartz MK: Use of CEA as an indicator of early recurrence and as a guide to a selected second-look procedure in patients with colorectal cancer. Ann Surg 188:481–493, 1978.

30. Koch M, McPherson TA: Predictive value of plasma CEA in patients with colorectal carcinoma. J Surg Oncol 12:319–25, 1979.

31. Attiyeh FF, Stearns MW Jr: Second look laparotomy based on CEA elevations in colo-rectal cancer. Abstract presented at Annual Meeting for Society of Surgical Oncology, San Francisco, Calif., May 1980.

32. Minton JP, Martin EW Jr: The use of serial CEA determinations to predict recurrence of colon cancer and when to do a second-look operation. Cancer 42:1422–1427, 1978.

33. Minton JP, James KK, Hurtubise PE, Rinker L, Joyce S, Martin EW JR: The use of serial carcinoembryonic antigen determinations to predict recurrence of carcinoma of the colon and the time for a second-look operation. Surg Gyn Obs 147:208–210, 1978.

34. Rau UP, Steele G, Mayer RJ, Wilson RE, Zamcheck N: The rate of post operative CEA

rise in selecting treatment for recurrent colorectal cancer. Gastroenterology 76:1223, 1979.

35. Steele G Jr, Zamcheck N, Wilson R, Mayer R, Lohich J, Rau P, Maltz J: Results of CEA-initiated second-look surgery for recurrent colorectal cancer. Am J Surg 139:544–548, 1980.

36. Rittgers RA, Steele G Jr, Zamcheck N, Loewenstein MS, Sugarbaker PH, Mayer RJ, Lokich JJ, Maltz J, Wilson RE: Transient carcinoembryonic antigen (CEA) elevations following resection of colorectal cancer: a limitation in the use of serial CEA levels as an indicator for secondlook surgery. JNCI 61:315, 1978.

37. Sugarbaker PH, Zamcheck N, Moore FD: Assessment of serial carcinoembryonic antigen (CEA) assays in postoperative detection of recurrent colorectal cancer. Cancer 38:2310–2315, 1976.

38. Moertel CG, Schutt AJ, Go VLM: Carcinoembryonic antigen test for recurrent colorectal carcinoma. Inadequacy for early detection. JAMA 239:1065–1066, 1978.

39. Ratcliffe JG, Wood CB, Burt RW, Malcolm AJ, Blumgart LH: Patterns of change in carcinoembryonic antigen (CEA) levels in patients after 'curative' surgery for colorectal cancer. In: Carcino-embryonic proteins: chemistry, biology, clinical applications, Lehmann FG (ed). New York: Elsevier/North Holland Biomedical, vol II, 1979.

40. Mach JP, Vienny H, Jaeger P, Haldemann B, Egely R, Pettavel J: Long-term follow-up of colorectal carcinoma patients by repeated CEA radioimmunoassay. Cancer 42:1439–1447, 1978.

41. Staab HJ, Angerer FA, Stumpf E, Fischer R: Carcinoembryonic antigen follow-up and selection of patients for second-look operation in management of gastrointestinal carcinoma. J Surg Oncol 10:273–282, 1978.

42. Cohen AM, Wood WC: Carcinoembryonic antigen levels as an indicator for reoperation in patients with carcinoma of the colon and rectum. Surg Gyn Obs 149:22–26, 1979.

43. Polk HC Jr, Spratt JS Jr: Recurrent colorectal carcinoma: detection, treatment, and other considerations. Surgery 69:9–23, 1971.

44. Pemberton M: Assessment and management of recurrences of carcinoma of the large intestine. Proc Roy Soc Med 65:663–670, 1972.

45. Martin EW Jr, Cooperman M, King G, Rinker L, Carey LC, Minton JP: A retrospective and prospective study of serial CEA determinations in the early detection of recurrent colon cancer. Am J Surg 137:167–169, 1979.

46. Kjaer M: Carcinoembryonic antigen (CEA) test. A review of its possible applications in cancer of the colon and rectum. Ugeskr Laeger 141:2297–2302, 1979.

47. Chu Tm, Lavin P, Day J, Eans JT, Mittleman A, Holyoke ED, Vincent R: Carcinoembryonic antigen: prognosis and monitoring of cancer. Medicine 141:55–64, 1979.

48. Al-Sarraf M, Baker L, Talley RW, Kithier K, Vaitkevicius VK: The value of serial carcinoembryonic antigen (CEA) in predicting response rate and survival of patients with gastrointestinal cancer treated with chemotherapy. Cancer 44:1222–1225, 1979.

49. Shani A, O'Connell J, Moertel CG, Schutt AJ, Silvers A, Go VLM: Serial plasma carcinoembryonic antigen measurements in the management of metastatic colorectal carcinoma. Ann Intern Med 88:627–630, 1978.

50. Mayer RJ, Garnick MB, Steele GD Jr, Zamcheck N: Carcinoembryonic antigen (CEA) as a monitor of chemotherapy in disseminated colorectal cancer. Cancer 42:1428–1433, 1978.

51. Sugarbaker PH, Bloomer WD, Corbett ED, Chaffey JT: Carcinoembryonic antigen (CEA): Its role as a monitor of radiation therapy for colorectal cancer. Cancer 42:1434–1436, 1978.

52. Kim EE, Deland FH, Casper S, Corgan RL, Primus FJ, Goldenberg DM: Radioimmunodetection of colorectal cancer. Cancer 45:1243–1247, 1980.

12. Lymphomas of the Gut

DANIEL N. WEINGRAD, JEROME J. DE COSSE, PAUL SHERLOCK,
DAVID J. STRAUS and PHILIP H. LIEBERMAN

1. INTRODUCTION: CURRENT PROBLEMS

Lymphomas involving the gastrointestinal tract comprise a heterogeneous group of uncommon neoplasms that are often a challenge to the skills of both clinician and pathologist. Among 23 000 new cases of lymphoma projected for 1980 in the United States, fewer than 1200 new cases of primary gastrointestinal lymphomas can be expected [1, 2]. However, there is a much larger group of cases with secondary gastrointestinal involvement from both Hodgkin's and non-Hodgkin's lymphomas.

Primary lymphoma is relatively uncommon in the stomach and large bowel compared to other primary neoplasms but is relatively frequent in the small bowel, where other malignant neoplasms are uncommon. When contiguous structures or nodal groups are involved, the distinction between primary and secondary lymphoma is difficult.

Differentiation of primary gut lymphoma from other histologically similar lesions can occasionally be difficult for even the experienced pathologist. Lymphoma must be distinguished from other lesions, including lymphoid hyperplasia, leukemic infiltrate, plasmacytoma, non-epithelial tumors, undifferentiated adenocarcinoma and histiocytic tumors [3–6]. Precise histological subclassification may present additional difficulties.

The application of sophisticated histochemical, cytological, genetic and immunologic techniques to pathological diagnosis has led to the recognition of distinct subtypes of lymphomas and several proposed classification systems. Earlier reports from Memorial Sloan-Kettering Cancer Center employed the subclassification then in vogue, which was little more than a nominal division of cases. Ideally, a system of classification should be sufficiently precise scientifically and effective prognostically to provide a basis for rational therapy. Presently only compromises exist. The need to evaluate and compare the potentially toxic and complex modern treatment regimens for lymphomas

J. J. DeCosse and P. Sherlock (eds.), Gastrointestinal cancer 1, 311-341. All rights reserved.
Copyright © 1981 Martinus Nijhoff Publishers, The Hague/Boston/London.

has underscored the importance of careful staging of the disease. Although staging of nodal lymphomas seems appropriate by the current schemes, staging of extranodal lesions is less well adapted. This is especially true for gut lesions where precise staging is often difficult because of local extension of disease and involvement of multiple intraabdominal nodal groups.

During the past three decades, treatment of lymphomas has evolved rapidly to the current strategies of sophisticated radiation therapy and combination chemotherapy. Except for lymphomas of the gut, the role of surgery has been limited to diagnosis and staging with occasional adjunctive resection as part of primary therapy. At Memorial Hospital, emphasis has shifted from exclusively regional therapy towards intensive local treatment followed by vigorous systemic therapy for all except the most confined gut primary lymphomas.

In this review previous reports about primary gut lymphomas are considered in the perspective of the Memorial Hospital experience with these lesions from 1949 to 1978. The charts of all adults with clinical primary gastrointestinal lymphoma of stomach, small bowel or large bowel were reviewed. The diagnosis of lymphoma was then histologically confirmed. Cases where extraabdominal dissemination existed were included if the predominant lesion was confined to the gut. Patients with late secondary involvement of the gastrointestinal tract by lymphoma were excluded. Information was not complete for all determinants on all patients: the number for whom information is available is therefore indicated. Current treatment regimens that have evolved from previous experience at Memorial Hospital are presented.

Although Dawson's [7] criteria are followed in many reports of gut lymphoma [8–12], they may exclude more advanced lesions with primary origin in the gastrointestinal tract. For this reason we employed the criteria of Lewin [13] and Herrmann [14], which included lesions confined to or arising primarily from the gastrointestinal tract. Mesenteric and nodal primary lesions were excluded. Cases were staged retrospectively according to the Ann Arbor classification with modification according to Musshoff [15] as outlined below.

2. INCIDENCE

Primary gastrointestinal lymphomas comprise about 1% of all gastrointestinal cancers [16] and 3.9–8.7% of large series of non-Hodgkin's lymphomas [8, 14, 17–19].

An earlier review of lymphoma from Memorial Hospital [20] has reported that 11.1% of patients had secondary gastrointestinal tract involvement at the time of presentation. Jones [21] reported that 45 of 405 patients, or 11.1%, had secondary gastrointestinal involvement. In an earlier report from Memorial Hospital [20], 30% of patients who died with lymphoma and gastrointestinal involvement at autopsy. Other postmortem studies[14, 17] have suggested that secondary involvement of the gut may ultimately occur in over 40% of cases. No instance of Hodgkin's disease primary in the stomach, small bowel or large bowel could be confirmed. Other exhaustively staged and carefully reviewed series corroborate this experience[22]. Sherlock[23] has emphasized the rarity of primary Hodgkin's disease of the gastrointestinal tract.

3. GUT LYMPHOMA: GENERAL CLINICAL FEATURES AND DIAGNOSIS

Of 104 Memorial Hospital patients, 60% presented in the fifth and sixth decade. The average age of the total series was 59 years with a range from 21 to 83 years (Table 1). Most primary gut lymphomas occur in middle-aged or elderly patients usually in their fifth or sixth decade[9, 10, 12–14, 19, 24].

Of the Memorial Hospital cases, 64% were male. Other studies[9, 10, 12–14, 18] have confirmed a male predominance that persisted when cases were divided by site of occurrence. In contrast to the earlier Memorial Hospital experience which showed 54% of lesions to be gastric, in the present review of 104 patients, we found 73% of the lesions in the stomach, 14% in the small bowel and 13% in the large bowel. In all series, except those reporting on so-called Mediterranean lymphoma, the stomach has been the most frequent site of occurence[1, 8–10, 12, 13, 18, 19, 24]. In the review of 360 cases by Berg, 51% occurred in the stomach, 33% in the small bowel and 16% in the colon. In Freemann's series[18] there was an even greater proportion of gastric cases.

The clinical presentation of gastrointestinal lymphoma was generally indistinguishable from a variety of other infiltrative and neoplastic conditions of

Table 1. Gut lymphoma. Age, sex, site and size in patients for whom information was available out of total of 104 patients.

	All patients	Stomach	Small bowel	Large bowel
Number	104	76	15	13
Age				
Mean	59	58	57	61
Range	21–83	21–83	40–73	31–79
Sex (M : F)	1.7 : 1	1.7 : 1	1.1 : 1	2.3 : 1
Size				
Number	71	54	9	8
Mean (cm)	9.0	9.2	7.7	8.9
Range (cm)	1–20	1–20	4–14	3–16

the primary organ site. In 83% of our cases, a definitive diagnosis was not made until laparotomy. However, most of the cases were collected before the extensive use of fiberoptic gastroscopy. In all except small bowel primaries, adenocarcinoma was the most frequent preoperative diagnosis.

3.1. Gastric Lymphoma

3.1.1. Clinical Features. Previous studies from Memorial Hospital [25] showed that primary gastric lymphoma represented less than 3% of all gastric cancers. In a recent review of patients from 1958 to 1969, less than 3% of all non-Hodgkin's lymphomas occurred primarily in the stomach. In the same series, the incidence of secondary involvement of the stomach at initial presentation was 10%.

The most common symptoms were non-specific pain, weight loss, nausea and vomiting and anorexia (Table 2). Gross bleeding occurred in less than 25% of the patients. Occult or gross melena was detected in 35% on physical examination. An abdominal mass was found in only 18%. Ulcer-type pain characterized by relief on ingestion of food or antacids occurred in only 30%. More commonly, food exacerbated or had little effect on the pattern of pain.

Table 2. Gut lymphoma. Symptoms and findings in all 87 stage I and II patients.

Symptom or finding	Stomach		Small bowel		Large bowel	
	No.	(%)	No.	(%)	No.	(%)
	66		10		11	
Pain	53	(80)	7	(70)	8	(73)
Dysphagia	3	(5)	—		—	
Ulcer pain	20	(30)	—		—	
Colic	0		4	(40)	1	(9)
Nausea/vomiting	26	(39)	4	(40)	2	(18)
Weight loss	41	(62)	5	(50)	3	(27)
Diarrhea	3	(5)	2	(20)	3	(27)
Bleeding	15	(23)	2	(20)	3	(27)
Fatigue	17	(26)	5	(50)	3	(27)
Altered bowel habits	8	(12)	5	(50)	5	(45)
Anorexia	30	(45)	2	(20)	1	(9)
Asymptomatic	1	(2)	1	(10)	0	
Blood in stool	23	(35)	2	(20)	3	(27)
Mass	12	(18)	5	(50)	9	(82)
Hepatomegaly	12	(18)	1	(10)	1	(9)
Splenomegaly	1	(2)	2	(20)	0	
TOTAL	66		10		11	

It has been suggested that the chronic inflammation and lymphoid hyperplasia associated with long-standing peptic ulcer disease are related to the
pathogenesis of gastric neoplasms [26]. Of our 66 patients, seven had an
antecedent history of ulcer disease. In one patient, lymphoma occurred in the
gastric remnant after subtotal gastrectomy for peptic ulcer disease.

Of five tumors located in the cardia and distal esophagus, three were
associated with dysphagia and often a startling degree of weight loss. Of all
patients, 62% reported weight loss, of whom nearly 50% lost more than 9 kg
and 17% more than 14 kg.

3.1.2. Diagnosis. The definitive diagnosis of primary lymphoma of the
stomach was most often made at laparatomy undertaken for diagnosis and
treatment of presumptive primary gastric adenocarcinoma (Table 3). With the
advent of flexible fiberoptic gastroduodenoscopy the diagnosis has been made
more frequently before exploration. Foreknowledge of the diagnosis has
proven to be extremely important by permitting accurate staging, offering
alternative operative approaches and enlisting early participation of a multi-
disciplinary team in treatment decisions [10, 13, 26–30].

Endoscopic features helpful in the diagnosis of gastric lymphoma have been
defined at Memorial Hospital [27] and elsewhere [26, 30, 31]. In a prospective

Table 3. Gut lymphoma. Diagnostic features and initial diagnosis in 87 stage I and II patients.
For all categories: number positive/number for whom information available.

	All patients No. (%)	Stomach No. (%)	Small bowel No. (%)	Large bowel No. (%)
Initial diagnosis				
Adenocarcinoma	63/83 (77)	57/66 (86)	1/7 (14)	5/10 (50)
Lymphoma	9/83 (11)	4/66 (6)	2/7 (29)	3/10 (30)
Leiomyosarcoma	2/83 (2)	1/66 (2)		1/10 (10)
Appendicitis	1/83 (1)			1/10 (10)
Peptic ulcer	4/83 (5)	4/66 (6)		
Carcinoma of pancreas	1/83 (1)		1/7 (14)	
Leiomyoma uteri	1/83 (1)		1/7 (14)	
Mechanical obstruction	2/83 (2)		2/7 (29)	
Diagnostic studies				
UGI series		59/61 (97)	2/4 (50)	
Barium enema			1/3 (33)	5/6 (83)
Acid study		3/13 (23)		
Cytology		5/15 (33)		
Means of Diagnosis				
Endoscopic biopsy	15/87 (17)	9/66 (14)	1/10 (10)	5/11 (45)
pre 1970		3/55		
1970-1978		6/11		
Laparotomy	72/87 (83)	57/66 (86)	9/10 (90)	6/11 (55)

study of 40 patients with gastric leymphoma at M.D. Anderson Hospital, Nelson and Lanza [31] reported the correct diagnosis by endoscopy alone in 13 of 21 patients; by endoscopic biopsy in 35 of 40 patients; by conventional radiology in seven of 21 patients; and by brush cytology in four of 20 patients. The gastroscopic findings were divided into three groups: 1) large folds or masses; 2) large folds or masses with ulcers including a peculiar volcano-like crater observed in nine of 30 patients with reticulum cell sarcoma; and, 3) atypical findings including mucosal alterations of gastritis and multiple benign-appearing ulcerations.

In five of our 15 patients who had gastric cytology by a nasogastric tube, the diagnosis of malignant neoplasm was suggested. Other recent reports using gastric washings [32, 33], brushings alone [34], and combined washings with brushing [35] have yielded substantially better results. In one report [33], four of five cases of gastric lymphoma were diagnosed as lymphoma solely from cytology. Improvements in the methodology and interpretation of cytology have made recognition of even histological subtypes of lymphoma possible. Present experience suggests that endoscopic recognition coupled with aggressive biopsy, brushing and cytology will yield a correct diagnosis in the majority of cases. If the lesion is exophytic, the diagnosis is more likely to be made by biopsy or cytology than if the lesion is infiltrative [36].

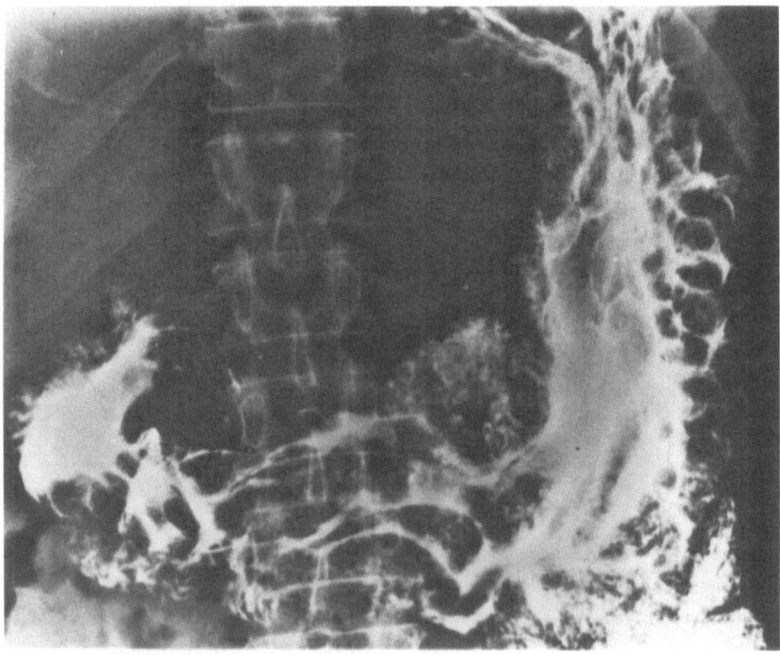

Figure 1. Barium upper gastrointestinal series showing thickened mucosal folds and intraluminal filling defects in a stomach involved by lymphoma.

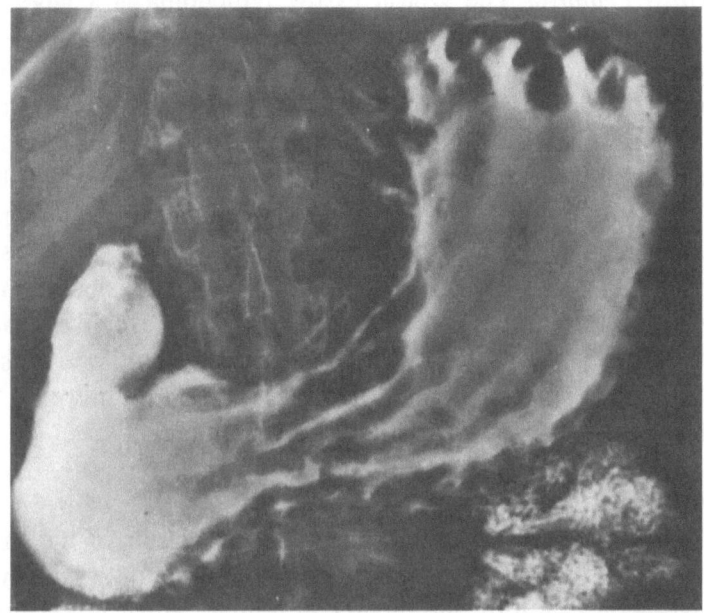

Figure 2. Barium upper gastrointestinal series showing thickened mucosal folds in a stomach diffusely involved by lymphoma.

In the 13 of our patients for whom acid studies were available, only three were achlorhydric. Although the majority of patients with gastric adenocarcinoma may be expected to have little or no gastric acid, this was not necessarily the case in gastric lymphoma [10, 12, 25, 26, 37, 38].

The single most frequency positive study in patients with gastric lymphoma was the barium upper gastrointestinal X-ray series (Figures 1 and 2). In 97% of our patients, some diagnostic abnormality was recognized: only two patients had normal findings. Although abnormal findings were regularly found on radiographic examination, the specific diagnosis of lymphoma was made in only 10–15% of cases [39]. Recent retrospective reviews [39–41] have better defined the specific radiological attributes of gastric lymphoma. Menuck [39] concluded that gastric lymphomas often presented as lesions larger than carcinomas. Lymphoma frequently involved the adjacent duodenum or esophagus and presented commonly with multiple radiographic patterns. Privett [40] concluded that there was no single accurate pattern for recognition of gastric lymphoma, but found several distinguishing radiographic characteristics: a distensible stomach in the presence of the mass; mucosal hypertrophy in the presence of the mass; mucosal hypertrophy associated with large or multiple gastric ulcers; contiguous spread of the abnormality into the duodenal bulb; and, duodenal ulceration associated with a gastric mass.

3.1.3. Gross Features. The typical gastric lymphoma is a large, ulcerated lesion completely infiltrating through gastric wall and serosa, and involving the stomach in more than one area. Infiltration into surrounding structures and organs occurred in 41% of cases. These findings are similar to the earlier report by McNeer and Berg [25]. Ulcers were usually superficial, ranging from small to large, and were single or multiple. The earliest lesions usually had an intact mucosa. Infiltration of the gastric wall was extremely common, ranging from small plaque-like lesions to diffuse lesions similar to linitis plastica. Most tumors had some element of infiltration with a cobblestone pattern disrupting the gastric mucosa. A polypoid or nodular exophytic pattern was prominent in only 14%. In 16%, the lesion was multifocal arising from separately identified sites. Joseph and Lattes [37] found multicentric lesions in 20% of their series of primary gastric lymphoma.

3.2. Small Bowel Lymphoma

3.2.1. Clinical Features. Although malignant neoplasms of the small intestine comprise only 3–5% of all gastrointestinal tumors [42], nearly 20% of these are lymphomas [43]. In one report [18] primary small bowel lymphomas comprised 1.3% of all non-Hodgkin's lymphomas. In an earlier Memorial Hospital report [17], primary small bowel lymphoma accounted for 1.4% of all lymphomas. A more recent review of cases revealed four instances of primary small bowel lymphoma among 494 patients with lymphoma.

Pain, weight loss, nausea, vomiting, altered bowel habits, fatigue and abdominal mass were the most common clinical expressions in our ten patients. Most often pain was colicky with vomiting, suggesting obstruction. Weight loss occurred in one half of the patients and ranged from 9 to 34 kg. Diarrhea was not a prominent symptom, being present in only two of ten patients, of whom one also had celiac sprue.

In older reports [44–48], intussusception has been found in 5–25% of adult cases; one of our stage IV patients presented in this way. In the pediatric population with primary or secondary lymphoma, intussusception has occurred frequently in patients with small bowel or ileocecal involvement.

3.2.2. Diagnosis. The definitive diagnosis was made at laparotomy in nine of ten patients who had primary small bowel lymphoma (Table 3). The single instance of duodenal lymphoma was diagnosed by endoscopic biopsy. Of seven patients for whom information was available, two were explored for obstruction and two were diagnosed as lymphoma preoperatively.

The role of endoscopic biopsy of small bowel lesions is undefined. Biopsy of duodenal lesions with fiberoptic gastroduodenoscopy is readily possible. Even lymphoma in the terminal ileum has been visualized and biopsied [49]. Peroral capsule biopsy has established the diagnosis of so-called Mediterra-

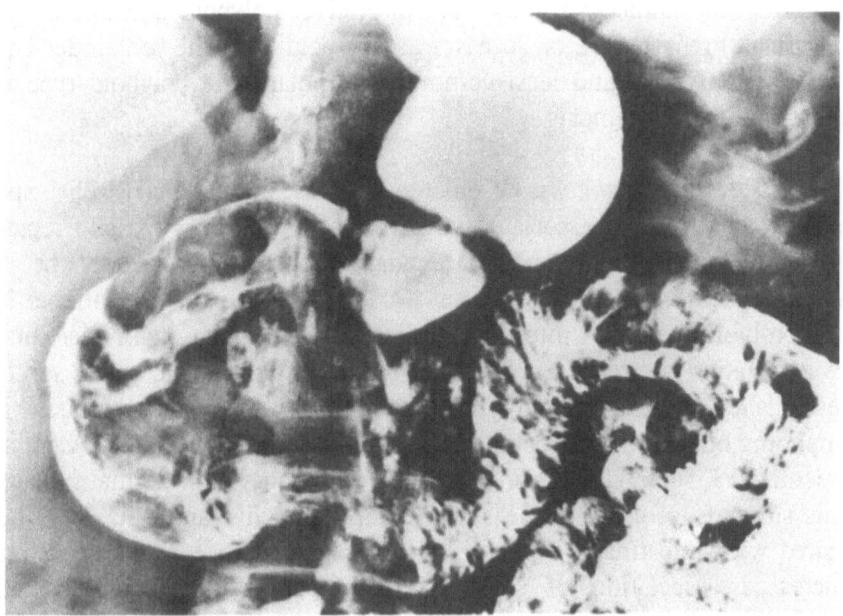

Figure 3. Barium upper gastrointestinal series showing multiple nodular filling defects in duodenum involved with lymphoma.

nean-type lymphoma in the upper small bowel [13].

The correct preoperative diagnosis of primary small bowel lymphoma was made infrequently [13, 24, 48, 50, 51]. Recently Marshak [41] reviewed the radiologic features of small bowel lymphoma and classified abnormalities as: multiple nodular defects (Figure 3); infiltrating form; endo-exoenteric form with excavation and fissure formation; and prominence of mesenteric invasion with large extraluminal masses or a sprue pattern. In Balikian's review [50] of small intestinal lymphoma, the infiltrating form was most common.

3.2.3. Gross Features. The predominant lesion seen in primary small intestinal lymphoma was a large, ulcerated, infiltrating tumor arising from more than one focus. Size ranged from 4 to 14 cm. Of the ten small bowel tumors, four occurred in the jejunum, four in the ileum, one in the duodenum and one involved multiple sites in the small bowel. The site of lymphoma in the small intestine has been thought to vary directly with the amount of lymphoid tissue present [1, 5, 9, 13, 48]. However, the incidence of jejunal tumors was higher both in our series as well as in the reports of Loehr [12] and Naqvi [10].

Of the many gross classifications of small bowel lymphomas [7, 44, 52], the one proposed by Wood [52] has been cited most often. There were four characteristic appearances; aneurysmal, ulcerative, polypoid and annular. Fu and Perzin [48] reported 12 of 26 cases as polypoid with the remainder being ulcerative, aneurysmal and least commonly annular. The polypoid type had the most favorable prognosis.

3.2.4. Associated Conditions. Of our ten patients, only one had celiac sprue (gluten-enteropathy) and associated small bowel lymphoma. Despite regional lymph node involvement and extranodal extension of disease, he has remained without recurrence for over two years. None of our patients had immunoproliferative small intestinal disease or were alpha chain secretors.

The association between primary abdominal lymphoma and celiac sprue is well established (Table 4) [53–56]. The small bowel was the most frequent site of lymphoma but gastric, retroperitoneal and mesenteric lymphomas were also documented [53, 56, 57]. At least two-thirds of patients with dermatitis herpetiformis suffer from celiac sprue [54, 65]. Familial celiac sprue has also been associated with intestinal lymphoma [62]. Recent evidence has demonstrated an increased association of similar histocompatibility antigens in celiac sprue [97, 98] and some lymphomas [99].

Ulcerative jejunitis with malabsorption is a well-documented presentation of intestinal lymphoma [53, 61, 100, 101]. The association of celiac sprue and abdominal lymphoma may be higher than previously recognized because of the difficulty of distinguishing benign ulcerative jejunoileitis complicating celiac sprue from malignant ulcerative lymphoma [54]. Celiac sprue presenting later in life should be investigated for lymphoma as the primary cause.

The majority of lymphomas occurring in association with celiac sprue have been classified as diffuse histiocytic lymphoma. Recently Isaacson and Wright [100, 101] proposed that the majority of lesions associated with ulcerative jejunitis are in fact malignant histiocytosis of the small intestine. Malabsorption can result from intestinal lymphoma [102], but Thompson [53] has cautioned against the suggestion that celiac disease is a complication of

Table 4. Conditions with reported etiologic association with small bowel lymphoma.

Celiac sprue [53–64]
Dermatitis Herpetiformis [54, 65, 66]
Immunoproliferative small intestinal disease [67–86]
  (so-called 'Mediterranean abdominal lymphoma' and alpha-chain disease)
Primary immunodeficiency diseases [87–89]
Lymphoid hypertrophy [90–92]
Familial occurrence [62, 71, 93]
Crohn's disease [94, 95]
Thymoma [96]

malignant neoplasm. Typically, many years elapse between the diagnosis of celiac sprue and the appearance of lymphoma with an age of onset of lymphoma similar to that found in other gut lymphomas [53, 54, 56, 58]. It was originally suggested that adherence to a gluten-free diet may diminish the risk of subsequent malignant neoplasm [56, 103], but a later series with long-term follow-up has failed to corroborate this observation [104].

Immune defects have been found in patients with celiac disease. Mac-Laurin [105] demonstrated both diminished levels of lymphocyte proliferation upon stimulation with phytohemagglutinin as well as decreased lymphocyte cytotoxicity *in vitro*. A serum inhibitor of both phytohemagglutinin stimulation and cytotoxicity was also demonstrated. Ferguson [59] investigated the plasmacytes and lymphocytes in the lamina propria and epithelium of jejunal biopsies from celiac sprue patients, including 16 patients who subsequently developed primary intestinal lymphoma. Specimens were obtained at variable intervals before the diagnosis of lymphoma. When compared with untreated celiac sprue patients without lymphoma, lymphoma patients had lower plasma cell counts in the lamina propria and lower lymphocyte counts in the epithelium. Both MacLaurin as well as Ferguson speculated that a deficiency in immune surveillance may have permitted development of neoplasms in the gut.

Since recognition by Azar [67] in 1962 of the high frequency of small bowel lymphomas in the Middle East, immunoproliferative small intestinal disease has been widely reported. Although frequently referred to as Mediterranean abdominal lymphoma, the presently-accepted designation of the World Health Organization is immunoproliferative small intestinal disease [106]. This condition occurs in association with malabsorption and has a high incidence of alpha-heavy chain paraproteinemia [74, 85]. Occurrence is not limited to Mediterranean countries but appears to be ubiquitous with the greatest number of reports emanating from Middle Eastern countries and South Africa [82].

Typically, men under 30 years of age of lower socioeconomic status are affected. In addition to abdominal pain and diarrhea, there is a high frequency of clubbing and osteoarthropathy [74, 82]. A combination of chronic abdominal pain, diarrhea and clubbing in a young patient is nearly pathognomonic for immunoproliferative small intestinal disease.

Cases documented from Israel occur almost exclusively in Arabs and Jews of North African or Sephardic origin while sparing Jews of European or Ashkenazi origin [75, 84]. Cases from South Africa are confined largely to the black and mulatto population [68, 74]. Novis [68] has suggested that local geographic factors may be important. Immunoproliferative small intestinal disease is frequently associated with bowel infestation by pathogenic microorganisms and parasites which may contribute to malabsorption [107].

Ramos [108] has reviewed the radiographic findings in immunoproliferative small intestinal disease and concluded that none is diagnostic for the condition. Peroral biopsy has resulted in a diagnosis in more than 60% of cases [80, 82, 84]. Lesions occur proximally in the jejunum and are characterized grossly by diffuse thickening of the mucosa often involving considerable lengths of bowel [109]. Single or multiple nodules may be present. There may be loss of the plicae circulares. The disease is usually confined to the intestine and mesenteric lymph nodes but extraabdominal lymph node involvement and rarely distant organ involvement occur. Salem [74] has stressed the importance of staging by laparotomy and offered a new system of staging.

Rappaport [109] characterized the histologic picture as a diffuse plasma cell infiltrate of the mucosa and submucosa along with malignant lymphoma of the bowel wall. Four of his 20 patients had a plasma cell infiltrate without lymphoma. Rappaport suggested the plasma cell lesions was responsible for the malabsorption. It has also been suggested that the plasma cell infiltrate may represent a reversible premalignant phase. Lewin [80] proposed that lymphoma in immunoproliferative small intestinal disease, which he designates as pleomorphic lymphoma, is in fact immunoblastic sarcoma in accord with the designation of Lukes and Collins [110].

This condition has been treated by various combinations of surgical resection, radiotherapy and multiple drug chemotherapy. Few have survived more than three years [74, 80].

Paraproteinemia with IgA heavy-chain pattern (alpha-chain disease) is a frequent but not invariable concomitant of immunoproliferative small intestinal disease [85]. Salem [74] found nine patients with alpha-chain disease among 16 with immunoproliferative small intestinal disease. Two with alpha-chain disease did not have lymphoma. Whether the alpha-chain disease in these two patients was a premalignant phase of lymphoma or an isolated condition was uncertain.

Alpha-chain disease can occur both in a pulmonary as well as in an intestinal form [85]. It has been reported from North America in a patient with polypoid lymphoma without malabsorption [92]. In contrast to other small bowel lymphomas, alpha-chain lymphoma appears most often in the duodenum and proximal jejunum [28, 85]. Seligman and Rambaud [85] have suggested that the majority of cases of lymphoma and immunoproliferative small intestinal disease are a late malignant stage of alpha-chain disease.

3.3. Large Bowel Lymphoma

3.3.1. Clinical Features. Primary lymphoma of the large bowel is a rare tumor representing 0.3% of all colon and rectal neoplasms [16, 111]. In our study, as in most other series, the large bowel was the least frequent site of primary extranodal lymphoma [1, 9, 10, 12–14, 17–19, 24]. Pain, altered bowel habits, and abdominal or rectal mass were the most significant features in our cases (Table 2). Bleeding and weight loss were observed less commonly than in other series [13, 14, 112]. Pain was typical of that caused by other tumors located at similar sites in the colon. In one case of a cecal primary lymphoma, the patient presented with findings typical of appendicitis.

3.3.2. Diagnosis. Proctoscopic rectal or sigmoid biopsy established the diagnosis of lymphoma in all five rectal cases (Table 3). For more proximal lesions, laparotomy was required for a diagnosis. Six patients were studied with barium enema examinations: five showed abnormalities but none was diagnostic. As with other sites in the gastrointestinal tract, flexible fiberoptic endoscopy should make earlier diagnosis possible. A case report by Green [113] has illustrated the important role of endoscopy.

Review of the radiographic appearances of colonic lymphoma have appeared with the aim of achieving a more diagnosis on barium enema examination [41, 112, 114]. Marshak [41] described two major forms of colonic lymphoma: discrete or localized tumor presenting as a single mass and, extensive diffuse infiltrating tumor involving long segments of bowel. O'Connell [114] used a modification of Marshak's scheme for small intestinal lymphoma to retrospectively characterize the radiographic features of 34 patients with colonic lymphoma: mucosal nodularity; endoexoenteric; intraluminal mass; mural infiltration; and, mesenteric invasion. The endoexoenteric pattern was the most common, consisting of a large extended mass with mural infiltration and mucosal destruction.

3.3.3. Gross Features. The usual appearance of primary colonic lymphoma in our patients was a large unifocal, circumferential, infiltrating and ulcerated mass. Unlike other reports [5, 112, 115, 116], annular lesions were common in our series; diffuse or multifocal lesions were not found. Multiple lesions have been reported in up to 20% of cases [116].

In six of our patients the cecum was the primary site. Cecal primaries were common in other series reporting colonic lymphomas [9, 12, 13, 112].

3.3.4. Associated Conditions. Primary lymphoma of the large bowel has been reported in association with ulcerative colitis [6, 112, 115, 117–122] and as a complication of immunosuppressive therapy for both transplantation [123] as well as treatment of macroglobulinemia [124]. No example was found among our patients.

Morgan [6] reviewed the evidence for malignant neoplasms associated with inflammatory bowel disease. Although adenocarcinoma was reported commonly, lymphoma was less frequent. Wagonfeld [117] found fewer than 20 adequately documented cases. Although Friedman [121] was uncertain if ulcerative colitis gave rise to lymphoma or if lymphoma occurred simultaneously with ulcerative colitis, Wagonfeld found that the age of onset, distribution, cell types and survival were similar to other large bowel lyphomas. In addition, large bowel lymphoma can mimic ulcerative colitis or both conditions may occur simultaneously [119].

The duration of antecedent ulcerative colitis before development of lymphoma was usually very long, ranging from 12 to 30 years [117, 118, 120]. As with lymphoma in celiac sprue, the repeated episodes of lymphoid hyperplasia commonly seen in ulcerative colitis may predispose to development of lymphona [122]. Sherlock [125] has proposed that abnormal lymphoid tissue in the lamina propria may represent a premalignant phase of colonic lymphoma.

4. HISTOLOGICAL CLASSIFICATION

The histopathological classification on non-Hodgkin's lymphoma is a subject of considerable controversy [126–128]. Ideally a classification should be scientifically correct, clinically useful with respect to treatment and prognosis, and readily reproducible among pathologists. In the United States the currently popular scheme is the Rappaport classification [129]. Other systems have been proposed by Lukes and Collins [110, 130], Lennert (Kiel classification) [131], Dorfman [132], Bennett [133] and the World Health Organization [134].

The Rappaport classification has been demonstrated clinically useful with a prognostically significant division of cases (Table 5) [21]. The older literature on primary gut lymphomas used terms such as giant follicular lymphoma, lymphosarcoma, and reticulum cell sarcoma. There is some overlap of the older terms with those used in the Rappaport scheme, but the former are too imprecise to correlate exactly with the latter.

The Rappaport classification is derived from presumed morphogenesis from normal cell types [129]. Immunological marker data have shown this concept to be inaccurate [135, 136]; nonetheless, clinical correlations with respect to survival between those histologies identified as favorable or unfavorable have been well documented [137]. Favorable histologies are nodular, well-differentiated lymphocytic; nodular, poorly differentiated lymphocytic; nodular, mixed; and, diffuse, well-differentiated lymphocytic lymphomas. Unfavorable histologies include: diffuse, poorly differentiated lymphocytic (rare); diffuse histiocytic; nodular histiocytic; diffuse mixed; and, diffuse undifferentiated lymphomas.

Only a few recent series of primary gut lymphomas employ the Rappaport classification [13, 14, 24, 138–140]. Of 327 patients reported, 55% had diffuse histiocytic lymphoma with the proportion of this histology ranging from 20 to

Table 5. Classification of Non-Hodgkin's lymphomas.

Rappaport	Lukes and Collins (1977)	Kiel (1974)
Malignant lymphoma*	U-cell (undefined)	Low-grade malignancy
Well-differentiated lymphocytic		Malignant lymphoma,
Poorly differentiated lymphocytic	T-cell	Lymphocytic (chronic lymphocytic
Mixed cell	Small lymphocyte	leukemia, others)
Histiocytic	Convoluted lymphocyte	Lymphoplasmacytoid (immunocytic)
Undifferentiated	Sezary cell-mycosis fungoides	Centrocytic
Lymphoblastic	Immunoblastic sarcoma	Centroblastic- centrocytic,
	Lennert's lymphoma	Follicular,
* Nodular or diffuse		Follicular and diffuse,
	B-cell	and diffuse; with or
	Small lymphocyte	without sclerosis
	Plasmacytoid lymphocyte	
	Follicular center cell	High-grade malignancy
	(Follicular or diffuse,	Malignant lymphoma,
	with or without sclerosis)	Centroblastic
	Small cleaved	Lymphoblastic
	Large cleaved	Burkitt's type
	Small transformed (non-cleaved)	Convoluted cell type
	Large transformed (non-cleaved)	Others
	Immunoblastic sarcoma	Immunoblastic
	Hairy cell leukemia	
	Histiocytic	

67%. Diffuse poorly differentiated lymphocytic lymphoma was the next most frequent type. It is difficult to conclude from the available reports if histology affects survival in primary gut lymphoma. Novak [24] and Lewin [13], found that the histological subtype had little influence on survival. Lim [139] reported that nodular lymphoma in the stomach and a better outcome. Herrmann [14] concluded that diffuse histiocytic lymphoma has a more favorable prognosis when compared to other types.

Lukes and Collins [110, 130] have proposed a functional classification of malignant lymphoma presupposing that various immunologic cell types may be recognized by morphology. The major premise behind this classification has yet to be proven. There are scant data available on primary gut lymphoma classified according to Lukes and Collins.

The Kiel classification by Lennert [131] is also a functional classification with separate terminology based on a morphological definition of cells. Malignant lymphomas are divided into high grade or low grade neoplasms (see Table 5). In a recent review of primary lymphomas of the gastrointestinal tract, Buget [11] observed a poorer survival of patients with high grade malignant lymphoma as classified by Lennert.

The terminology of the Bennett [133], Dorfman [132], and World Health Organization [134] classifications are for the most part descriptive and can be found in the works cited.

Recent reports have appeared questioning the reported morphogenesis of many primary gastrointestinal lymphomas. Henry and Farrer-Brown [3] reported that 49 of 125 cases of gastrointestinal lymphomas were in fact plasma cell lesions, which they considered to be extramedullary plasmocytomas. Most of these lesions appeared in the ileocecal region. Other authors [109], however, conclude that the plasma cell infiltrate might be reactive rather than part of the neoplastic process.

Isaacson [4] applied light microscopic and immunohistochemical techniques to classify 66 cases of primary gastrointestinal lymphoma. He found 50% to be malignant histiocytic neoplasms as opposed to lymphocyte-derived neoplasms. Lightdale [141] reviewed Isaacson's paper and expressed doubt about his contentions. It is important to ascertain that the cells being studied are in fact neoplastic and not part of an inflammatory infiltrate: studies on fresh material and cell suspensions will be required to settle this issue [142].

5. STAGING

The currently recommended scheme for non-Hodgkin's lymphoma is the Ann Arbor classification adopted in 1971 [143, 144] (Table 6). In relation to both the time of evaluation as well as the methods used, the staging of

Table 6. Current staging of non-Hodgkin's lymphomas.

I   Involvement of a single lymph node region or of a single extralymphatic organ or site (I_E).

II Involvement of two or more lymph node regions on the same side of the diaphragm (II) or localized involvement of an extralymphatic organ or site of one or more lymph node regions on the same side of the diaphragm (II_E). *Suggested modification by Musshoff*[15]: Stage II divided into cases with involvement of regional lymph nodes (II_{1E}) and involvement of regional but non-confluent lymph nodes (II_{2E}).

III Involvement of lymph node regions on both sides of the diaphragm (III) which may also be accompanied by localized involvement of extralymphatic organ or site (III_E) or by involvement of the spleen (III_S) or both III_{E+S}.

IV Diffuse or disseminated involvement of one or more extralymphatic organ or tissue with or without associate lymph node enlargement. The stage IV patient is identified further by specifying sites.

lymphoma is specified as: 1) clinical-diagnostic; 2) surgical-evaluative; 3) postsurgical treatment-pathological; and, 4) treatment. In this report and other publications, survival is generally expressed in terms of the post-surgical-pathological staging. Rosenberg[145] points out that satisfactory support for the application of the Ann Arbor staging classification in Hodgkin's disease exists, but there is no proof of the prognostic value of this classification when applied to the non-Hodgkin's lymphomas.

Gut lymphoma presents special problems in staging. Primary gut lymphoma often infiltrates adjacent organs. Our own experience (Table 7) showed that extranodal involvement is prognostically important. Relapse-free survival in patients with involvement of adjacent structures was 28.3% at five years and without involvement was 58%. This may reflect differences in adequacy of treatment and stage of disease. The frequency of adjacent organ involve-

Table 7. Postsurgical treatment — pathologic stage of 104 patients with gut lymphoma I+ and II+ designate patients with adjacent organ involvement. II_{1E} and II_{2E} are the substages of stage II according to Musshoff's modification of Ann Arbor staging[15]. Substage and status of adjacent organ involvement unknown in one patient.

	Total	Stomach	Small intestine	Colon
I_E	37	29	3	5
I+	7	6	0	1
II_E	50	37	7	6
II+	26	21	2	3
II_{1E}	38	29	4	5
II_{2E}	11	7	3	1
III_E	1		1	
IV	16	10	4	2
All stages	104	76	15	13

ment increases with advancing stage. Furthermore, in gastric lymphoma, the primary tumor size was larger in those cases with adjacent organ involvement and higher stage.

Hermann[14] found local infiltration of adjacent structures to be prognostically unimportant, whereas Lim[139] suggested that adjacent organ involvement by gastric lymphoma represented an advanced stage of disease with a poorer prognosis. The number of their patients involved was too small for firm conclusions.

Nodal involvement occurred in 57% of our 87 stage I and stage II patients. Musshoff[15] concluded that the location of nodal involvement by primary gut lymphoma is prognostically significant. The Ann Arbor classification does not distinguish cases of gut lymphoma by involvement of primary draining nodal groups (II_{2E}). This distinction is important to predict the prognosis and determine effective therapy; compare cases; and analyze results. Our experience is similar to that of Musshoff[15] and Herrmann[14]. Five year relapse-free survival was 49.2% for stage II_{1E} compared with 0% for stage II_{2E} cases.

With the recognition of the weaknesses inherent in the Ann Arbor classification as applied to gut lymphomas, other staging schemes have been proposed [9, 14, 139]. These do not seem an improvement over the modified Ann Arbor staging.

Reasons for the importance of any staging system are provided by Rosenberg[145]: 1) to furnish prognostic data for site and extent of disease; 2) to assist in choosing treatment regimens; 3) to provide a standardized means of comparison of results; and, 4) to establish an accepted descriptive form that communicates the extent of disease. In terms of the first and third reasons stated above, these proposals would make both comparison with lymphoma at other sites difficult as well as comparison with other institutions using the Ann Arbor classification.

TNM staging has not been widely used for staging lymphoma because of the ambiguities between primary tumor, nodes and metastases in these lesions. Lim[139] has applied the TNM system to a carefully studied group of patients with primary gastric lymphoma when compared to gastric adenocarcinoma and found that both serosal penetration and perigastric nodal involvement were important in prognosis. Patients with nodular histology had longer survivals. Analysis of the survival curve, however, showed that there is little benefit to this system when compared with the Ann Arbor classification. The TNM classification does not account for other important prognostic variables such as histological sub-type, cytogenetic studies and immunological markers.

The appropriate place for staging laparotomy in the diagnostic evaluation of patients with non-Hodgkin's lymphoma is controversial [146–151]. Using laparoscopy, Lightdale [152] was able to demonstrate hepatic involvement by lymphoma. Chabner [146] reported that Stage III or IV disease was often established by non-surgical procedures. Without requiring staging laparotomy, these patients then received systemic as opposed to regional therapy. Chabner also defined a group of patients with diffuse histiocytic lymphoma who have localized, Stage I and II, disease. Diffuse histiocytic lymphoma has been found in up to 56% of patients in some series of gastrointestinal lymphoma [14].

Unlike Hodgkin's disease, laparotomy for primary non-Hodgkin's gut lymphomas is often more than a diagnostic procedure. Some recent series [153, 154] have reported high complication rates from bleeding and bowel perforation at tumor sites in the gut of patients undergoing treatment for diffuse histiocytic lymphoma. Hande [153] reported massive intestinal hemorrhage or perforation from tumor necrosis in 38% of treatment failures. Rosenfelt [154] found that 25% of his patients had bleeding or perforation as a result of therapy. Earlier surgical resection or debulking might be therapeutically important in these cases.

Formal staging in instances of primary gastrointestinal lymphoma seems useful for clinical-diagnostic stage I and II cases. Identification of noncontiguous involvement of spleen, liver or non-draining nodal groups should offer important information in planning modern treatment. Staging laparotomy should be carried out after lymphangiography: unfortunately, as in our series,

Table 8. Staging procedures at Memorial Sloan-Kettering Cancer Center for non-Hodgkin's lymphoma (NHL-4, NHL-5, NHL-6). Baseline studies.

1. Histologic verification with cell markers, terminal deoxynucleotidyl transferase and, whenever possible, kinetic studies and electron microscopy.
2. Detailed history and physical examination.
3. Laboratory studies: Complete blood count; differential; platelet count; chemical profile (SMA 12) including LDH, 5'nucleotidase, quantitative immunoglobulins (NHL-4), serum immunoglobulin electrophoresis, sedimentation rate (NHL-4).
4. Radiograph and radionuclide studies: Chest X-ray; lymphangiogram, gallium scan (NHL-5).
5. Bilateral bone marrow aspiration and biopsy.
6. Spinal tap (NHL-5).

Additional studies when indicated by protocol or clinical situation:
1. Intravenous pyelogram.
2. Liver/spleen scan.
3. Liver biopsy.
4. Formal staging laparotomy with splenectomy and sampling paraaortic, iliac and porta hepatis lymph nodes. If laparotomy not feasible, liver biopsy with laparoscopic visualization, if possible.
5. Baseline ECG (NHL-6).
6. Abdominal CT scan and upper GI series for head and neck primaries (NHL-6) and others when indicated.

diagnosis is often made only at laparotomy. With advances in cytologic technique, endoscopic recognition and biopsy, and intraoperative frozen section diagnosis, the surgeon should be prepared to carry out a formal staging laparotomy including multiple node sampling, liver biopsies, bone marrow biopsy, and possibly splenectomy in all patients with lymphoma primary at gastrointestinal sites. Only in this way can the efficacy of various treatment regimens be assessed meaningfully.

Table 8 presents the current diagnostic work-up required by treatment protocols (NHL-4, NHL-5, NHL-6) for non-Hodgkin's lymphoma at Memorial Hospital.

6. TREATMENT AND RESULTS

Life table survival results for 97 patients with primary gastrointestinal lymphomas (excluding seven postoperative deaths) are presented in Table 9.

Table 9. Life table survival of patients with gut lymphoma at Memorial Hospital: 1949–1978. Seven postoperative deaths excluded. Substage and status of contiguous involvement unknown in one patient.

	Number	Absolute (%)		Relapse-free (%)	
		5 yr	10 yr	5 yr	10 yr
Cohorts (Stage I, II)					
1949–1958	32	47.3	43.7	42.5	38.6
1959–1968	31	52.6	47.3	44.5	44.5
1969–1978	18	74.4	—	58.4	—
All cases	97	44.0	40.3	36.9	35.1
Stages I, II	81	53.0	48.6	44.2	42.0
Stage I	33	72.5	58.8	63.6	57.8
Stage II	48	40.8	40.8	31.4	31.4
Stage II$_{1E}$	37	60.7	60.7	49.2	49.2
Stage II$_{2E}$	10	0	—	0	—
Stage IV	16	0	—	0	—
Contiguous involvement					
I$_E$+, II$_E$+	35	35.0	18.1	28.3	22.0
I$_E$−, II$_E$−	45	71.4	71.4	58.0	58.0
Site (Stage I+II)					
Stomach	60	47.2	41.1	37.1	32.5
Small intestine	10	68.4	68.3	68.4	68.4
Colon	11	58.3	58.3	35.0	35.0
Treatment (Stage I+II)					
Surgery-only	29			57.3	57.3
Surgery and RT	32			41.7	35.7
Primary RT	10			40.0	40.0
Other	10			—	—

Over the three decades reviewed, there was a trend toward improved survival with five year absolute and relapse-free survival for the 1949-1958 group as 47.3% and 42.5% respectively; for the 1959–1968 group as 52.6% and 44.5%; and, for the 1969–1978 group as 74.4% and 58.4%. In the last group, virtually all patients received some form of adjunctive treatment in addition to surgery.

Stage, involvement of adjacent structures and location of nodal involvement in stage II patients all affected prognosis and survival. Although it would appear that large bowel and small intestinal primaries have a better prognosis when compared to gastric primaries, there is no agreement on this point when compared to other reports [10, 12, 14, 19, 24].

The respective places for surgery, radiation and chemotherapy have yet to be defined for localized lymphoma. Analysis of our survival results showed an advantage to the surgery alone group; however, this was due in part to the greater proportion of advanced cases who received postoperative radiotherapy, namely patients with stage IIE disease and those with continuous organ involvement (IE+, IIE+). Traditionally, aggressive surgical resection with extensive lymphadenectomy and en-bloc excision of clinically involved adjacent structures has been practiced at Memorial Hospital. In our series, the postoperative death rate was less than 6%, with the majority of deaths occurring before 1960. Since 1960, the postoperative death rate has been less than 1%.

Overall local control was 72% (Table 10). Surgery alone achieved local control in 83% of patients. Primary radiotherapy given at greater than 3000 rads achieved similar results in 86% of a smaller number of patients. It appeared from our data that in selected cases with localized disease, both surgery and radiotherapy were equally effective in achieving local control. Two patients had massive bleeding episodes: one during primary radiation therapy and another during treatment with chemotherapy for recurrent disease.

Bitran [155] reported that radiotherapy can effectively control disease for 5 years in 78% of carefully staged patients with stage IE and IIE diffuse histiocytic lymphoma.

Lipton and Lee [156] from Memorial Hospital reported local control in all patients with stage I disease who received adequate radiotherapy of at least 3500 rads. Fuks and Kaplan [157] reported approximately 80% local control in patients receiving more than 4400 rads. Fuller [158] stressed the importance of over 3000 rads of large volume radiation to achieve local control.

Specific information on the use of radiotherapy in the treatment of primary gastrointestinal lymphoma suggests that it is effective used alone or in combination with surgery. Bush [19] demonstrated marked improvement in five year survival in 'early' cases of patients receiving postoperative radiotherapy.

Table 10. Recurrence, failure of local control and dose of radiation in stage I and II patients excluding seven postoperative deaths out of total of 87 patients. In some cases tumor recurred at multiple sites. Results of nine patients treated with chemotherapy in addition to radiotherapy excluded from analysis of treatment and recurrence. They are included in the analysis of adjunctive radiotherapy when information is available.

		Treatment and recurrence				
Primary treatment	Number treated	Recurrent and resistant disease No. (%)	Local No. (%)	Other abdominal No. (%)	Distant No. (%)	Unknown site No. (%)
Surgery	29	10 (34)	5 (17)	2 (7)	3 (10)	5 (17)
Surgery + radio- therapy	32	20 (63)	12 (38)	6 (19)	13 (41)	1 (3)
Radiotherapy	10	5 (50)	3 (30)	0	2 (20)	0
Total	71	35 (49)	20 (28)	8 (11)	18 (25)	6 (8)

Dose of radiotherapy and failure of local control

Dose	Adjunctive radiotherapy			Primary radiotherapy	
	Number treated	Recurrence No. (%)	Local failure No. (%)	Number treated	Local failure No. (%)
<3000 rads	15	10 (67)	5 (33)	3	2 (67)
≥3000 rads	23	15 (65)	8 (35)	7	1 (14)
Total	38	25 (66)	13 (34)	10	3 (30)

More recently, Herrmann[14] cited radiotherapy as a prognostically important feature, with better survival in those patients who received radiotherapy with or without operation.

In our experience (Table 10), of 35 patients with recurrence disease, 26 had involvement outside the primary site. As in other series[14, 137, 154, 155, 159, 160], most recurrences occurred in the first two years following diagnosis. This was especially true in patients with diffuse histiocytic lymphoma.

There is evidence that in non-Hodgkin's lymphoma, perhaps unlike Hodgkin's disease, relapse often occurs at sites other than those contiguous with the primary site, namely missed foci[159, 161, 162]. In a recent report from Sweden, Landberg[159] achieved an 86% relapse free survival at 30 months in a group of non-laparotomized patients by adding adjuvant chemotherapy (cyclophosphamide, vincristine, and prednisone) for nine cycles following extended field radiotherapy (4000 rads in 20 fractions). The group receiving

Table 11. Current treatment regimens for non-Hodgkin's lymphoma at Memorial Hospital.

NHL-4

Stages II, III, IV patients with 'favorable' histology (excluding diffuse well-differentiated lymphocytic)

1. *Chemotherapy*

   Regimen I: Thiotepa

              Vincristine (Oncovin)

              Prednisone

              Chlorambucil (Leukeran)

   Regimen II: (given if no complete response on Regimen I)

              Cyclophosphamide (Cytoxan)

              Doxorubicin (Adriamycin)

              Melphalan (Alkeran)

2. Radiation therapy (started after response assessed for Regimen I) 3000–3500 rads in $3\frac{1}{2}$-4 weeks to sites of initial bulky disease. If total nodal irradiation required, dose limited to 2000 rads.

NHL-5

Comparison of two different chemotherapeutic regimens for stages II, III, IV B-cell type diffuse lymphomas (unfavorable histology)

1. *Chemotherapy*

   Regimen I — CHOP (8 cycles)

              Cyclophosphamide (Cytoxan)

              Doxorubicin (Adriamycin)

              Vincristine (Oncovin)

              Prednisone

              Methotrexate (intrathecal for patients with bone marrow involvement)

   Regimen II — BLEO-CHOP

Bleomycin (Blenoxane) (cycles 1,5)	Cyclophosphamide (cycles
Cyclophosphamide (Cytoxan)	2,3,4,6,7,8)
Vincristine (Oncovin)	Doxorubicin
Doxorubicin (Adriamycin)	Vincristine
Prednisone	Prednisone

2. *Radiation therapy*

   Treatment to areas of bulky disease or in resistant areas after chemotherapy

NHL-6

A randomized trial of adjuvant chemotherapy after regional treatment for patients with stage I non-Hodgkin's lymphomas

1. Standard regional therapy, surgery and/or radiotherapy
2. Randomization to six months of chemotherapy or observation
3. Chemotherapy

Cyclophosphamide (Cytoxan)	Vincristine (Oncovin)
Doxorubicin (Adriamycin)	Prednisone

---

radiotherapy alone had a 41% relapse free survival at 30 months. In 13 of the patients with recurrent disease, 12 recurred outside of the treatment field, with eight recurring on the opposite side of the diaphragm. In the adjuvant chemotherapy group there were no local recurrences.

Present treatment for non-Hodgkin's lymphoma is presented in Table 11. For State I gut lymphomas, protocal NHL-6 has recently been instituted. Adriamycin is given in addition to cytoxan, vincristine, and prednisone in the hope of more effective elimination of subclinical disseminated disease [163]. Patients with more advanced disease are treated under protocols NHL-4 and NHL-5, which involve intensive multimodality therapy employing chemotherapy, radiotherapy and in some cases immunotherapy. Patients are often treated after resection of primary disease with the extent of intraabdominal disease carefully assessed at laparotomy and often marked with clips.

It is hoped that early diagnosis, meticulous staging and multimodality treatment regimens will achieve improved survivals with long-term remission and minimal toxicity. Results over the last decade have suggested some progress in this respect, but many challenges remain for those involved in the diagnosis, treatment and care of patients with primary gut lymphoma.

REFERENCES

1. Berg JW: Primary lymphomas of the human gastrointestinal tract. In: Symposium on comparative morphology of hematopoietic neoplasms, National Cancer Institute Monographs 32, Lingeman CH, Garner FM (eds). United States Government Printing Office, 1969, pp 211–220.
2. Silverberg E: Cancer statistics, 1980. Cancer 30:23–30, 1980.
3. Henry K, Farrer-Brown G: Primary lymphomas of the gastrointestinal tract. I. Plasma cell tumours. Histopathology 1:53–76, 1977.
4. Isaacson P, Wright DH, Judd MA, Mepham BL: Primary gastrointestinal lymphomas. A classification of 66 cases. Cancer 43:1805–1819, 1979.
5. McGovern VJ: Lymphomas of the gastrointestinal tract. In: The gastrointestinal tract, Monographs in Pathology 18, Yardley JH, Morson BC, Abell MR (eds). Baltimore: Williams & Wilkins, 1977, pp 184–205.
6. Morgan CN: Malignancy in inflammatory diseases of the large intestine. Cancer 28:41–44, 1971.
7. Dawson IMP, Cornes JS, Morson BC: Primary malignant lymphoid tumors of the intestinal tract. Report of 37 cases with a study of factors influencing prognosis. Br J Surg 49:80–89, 1961.
8. Lee YN, Spratt JS: Malignant lymphoma: nodal and extranodal diseases. New York: Grune & Stratton, 1974, pp 229–260.
9. Contreary K, Nance FC, Becker WF: Primary lymphoma of the gastrointestinal tract. Ann Surg 191:593–598, 1980.
10. Naqvi MS, Burrows L, Kark AE: Lymphoma of the gastrointestinal tract: prognostic.guides based on 162 cases. Ann Surg 170:221–231, 1969.

11. Bugat R, Voigt JJ, Delsol G, Robert A, Combes PF: Non-Hodgkin's primary lymphomas of the gastrointestinal tract. Clinicopathological correlation. Front Gastrointest Res 4:192–197, 1979.

12. Loehr WJ, Mujahed, Zahn FD, Gray GF, Thorbjarnarson B: Primary lymphoma of the gastrointestinal tract: a review of 100 cases. Ann Surg 170:232–238, 1969.

13. Lewin KJ, Ranchod M, Dorfman RF: Lymphomas of the gastrointestinal tract. A study of 117 cases presenting with gastrointestinal disease. Cancer 42:693–707, 1978.

14. Herrmann R, Panahon AM, Barcos MP, Walsh D, Stutzman L: Gastrointestinal involvement in non-Hodgkin's lymphoma. Cancer 46(1):215–222, 1980.

15. Musshoff K: Klinische Stadieneinteilung der Nicht-Hodgkin-lymphome. Strahlentherapie 153:218–221, 1977.

16. Warren S, Lulenski CR: Primary solitary lymphoid tumors of the gastrointestinal tract. Ann Surg 15:1–12, 1942.

17. Rosenberg SA, Diamond HD, Jaslowitz, Craver LF: Lymphosarcoma: a review of 1269 cases. Medicine 40:31–84, 1961.

18. Freeman C, Berg JW, Cutler SJ: Occurrence and prognosis of extranodal lymphomas. Cancer 29:252–260, 1972.

19. Bush RS, Ash CL: Primary lymphoma of the gastrointestinal tract. Radiology 92:1349–1354, 1969.

20. Ehrlich AN, Stalder G, Geller W, Sherlock P: Gastroenterology 54:1115–1121, 1968.

21. Jones SE, Fuks Z, Bull M, Kadin ME, Dorfman RF, Kaplan HS, Rosenberg SA. Kim H: Non-Hodgkin's lymphomas IV. Clinicopathologic correlation in 405 cases. Cancer 31:806–823, 1973.

22. Kaplan HS: Hodgkin's disease. Cambridge: Harvard University Press, 1972.

23. Sherlock P, Winawer SJ, Lacher MJ, Ehrlich An: Gastrointestinal manifestations of Hodgkin's disease. In: Hodgkin's disease, Lacher MJ (ed). New York: John Wiley, 1976, pp 297–324.

24. Novak S, Caraveo J, Trowbridge AA, Peterson RF, White RR III: Primary lymphomas of the gastrointestinal tract. South Med J 72:1154–1158, 1979.

25. McNeer G, Berg JW: The clinical behavior and management of primary malignant lymphoma of the stomach. Surgery 46:829–840, 1959.

26. Hertzner NR, Hoerr SO: An interpretive review of lymphoma of the stomach. Surg Gynecol Obstet 143:113–124, 1976.

27. Katz S, Klein MS, Winawer SJ, Sherlock P. Disseminated lymphoma involving the stomach. Correlation of endoscopy with directed cytology and biopsy. Am J Dig Dis 18:370–374, 1973.

28. Welborn JK, Ponka JL, Rebuck JW: Lymphoma of the stomach. A diagnostic and therapeutic problem. Arch Surg 90:480–487, 1965.

29. Macon WL: Gastric lymphoma vs. adenocarcinoma. A diagnostic problem. Arch Surg 114:305–306, 1979.

30. Dunn GD, Moeller D, Laing RP: Primary reticulum cell sarcoma of the stomach. Gastrointest Endosc 17:153–158, 1971.

31. Nelson RS, Lanza FL: The endoscopic diagnosis of gastric Lymphoma. Gross characteristics and histology. Gastrointest Endosc 21:66–68, 1974.

32. Prolla JC, Kobayashi S, Kirsner JB: Cytology of malignant lymphomas of the stomach. Acta Cytol 14:291–296, 1970.

33. Kiine TS, Goldstein F: Malignant lymphoma involving the stomach. Cancer 32:961–968, 1973.

34. Rilke F, Pilotti S, Clemente C: Cytology of non-Hodgkin's malignant lymphomas involving the stomach. Acta Cytologica 22:71–79, 1978.

35. Cabre'-Fiol V, Vilardell F: Progress in the cytological diagnosis of gastric lymphoma. A report of 32 cases. Cancer 41:1456–1461, 1978.
36. Posner G, Lightdale CJ, Cooper M, Sherlock P, Winawer SJ: Reappraisal of endoscopic tissue diagnosis in secondary gastric lymphoma. Gastrointest Endosc 21:123–125, 1975.
37. Joseph JI, Lattes R: Gastric lymphosarcoma. Clinicopathologic analysis of 71 cases and its relation to disseminated lymphosarcoma. Am J Clin Pathol 45:653–669, 1966.
38. Salmela H: Lymphosarcoma of the stomach. A clinical study of 39 cases. Acta Chir Scand 134:567–576, 1978.
39. Menuck LS: Gastric lymphoma. A radiologic diagnosis. Gastrointest Radiol 1:157–161, 1976.
40. Privett JTJ, Davies ER, Roylance J: The radiologic features of gastric lymphoma. Clin Radiol 28:457–463, 1977.
41. Marshak RH, Lindner AE, Maklansky D: Lymphoreticular disorders of the gastrointestinal tract: Roentgenographic features. Gastrointest Radiol 4:103–120, 1979.
42. Herbsman H, Wetstein L, Rosen Y, Orces H, Alfonso AE, Swaminath KI, Gardner B: Tumors of the small intestine. Curr Probl Surg 17:121–182, 1980.
43. Mason GR: Tumors of the duodenum and small intestine. In: Davis-Christopher textbook of surgery. The biologic basis of modern surgical practice, Sabiston DC Jr. (ed.). Philadelphia: WB Saunders, 1977, pp 969–976.
44. Faulkner JW, Dockerty MB: Lymphosarcoma of small intestine. Surg Gynec Obstet 95:76–84, 1952.
45. Marcuse PM, Stout AP: Primary lymphosarcoma of small intestine: Analysis of thirteen cases and review of literature. Cancer 3:459–474, 1950.
46. Marshak RH, Wolf BS, Eliasoph J: Roentgen findings in lymphosarcoma of small intestine. Am J Roentgenol Rad Therapy Nucl Med 86:682–692, 1961.
47. Skrimshore JFP: Lymphoma of stomach and intestine. Quart J Med 24L:203–214, 1955.
48. Fu Y, Persin KH: Lymphosarcoma of the small intestine. A clinicopathologic study. Cancer 29:645–659.
49. Katz S, Katzka I, Schneider K, Silverberg M: Ileoscopy in the diagnosis of ileal Lymphosarcoma. Pediatrics 56:127–129, 1975.
50. Balikian JP, Nassar NT, Shamma'a MH, Shahid MH: Primary lymphomas of the small intestine including the duodenum. A roentgen analysis of twenty-nine cases. Am J Roentgenol Rad Therapy Nucl Med 107:131–141, 1969.
51. Welborn JK, Rebuck JW, Ponka JL: Intestinal lymphosarcoma. Arch Surg 94:717–723, 1967.
52. Wood DA: Tumors of the intestine. In: Atlas of tumor pathology, section 6, fascicle 22. Washington, D.C.: US Armed Forces Institute of Pathology, 1967.
53. Thompson H: Necropsy studies on adult coeliac disease. J Clin Pathol 27:710–721, 1974.
54. Freeman JH, Weinstein WM, Shnitka TK, Piercey JRA, Wensel RH: Primary abdominal lymphoma. Presenting manifestation of celiac sprue or complicating dermatitis herpetiformis. Am J Med 63:585–594, 1977.
55. Asquith P: Adult coeliac disease and malignancy. J Ir Med Assoc 67:4–17, 1974.
56. Harris OD, Cooke WT, Thompson H, Waterhouse JAH: Malignancy in adult coeliac disease. Am J Med 42:899–912, 1967.
57. Brunt PW, Sircus W, Maclean N: Neoplasia and the coeliac syndrome in adults. Lancet 1:180–184, 1969.
58. Brandt L, Hagander B, Norden A, Stenstam M: Lymphoma of the small intestine in adult celiac disease. Acta Med Scand 204:467–470, 1978.
59. Ferguson R, Asquith P, Cooke WT: The jejunal cellular infiltrate in coeliac disease com-

plicated by lymphoma. Gut 15:458–461, 1974.

60. Dutz W, Asvadi S, Sadri S, Kohout E: Intestinal lymphoma and sprue: a systemic approach. Gut 12:804–810, 1971.

61. Hourihane DO, Weir DG: Malignant celiac syndrome. Report of two cases with malabsorption and microscopic foci of intestinal lymphoma. Gastroenterology 59:130–139, 1970.

62. Barry·RE, Morris JS, Kenwright S, Read AE: Coeliac disease and Malignancy. The possible importance of familial involvement. Scand J Gastroenterol 6:205–207, 1971.

63. Cooke WT, Thompson H, Williams JA: Malignancy and adult coeliac disease. Gut 10:108–111, 1969.

64. Tönder M, Sörlie D, Kearney MS: Adult coeliac disease. A case with ulceration, dermatitis herpetiformis and reticulosarcoma. Scand J Gastroenterol 11:107–111, 1976.

65. Gould DJ, Howell R: Dermatitis herpetiformis and reticulum cell sarcoma, a rare complication. Br J Dermatol 96:561–562, 1977.

66. Silk DBA, Mowat NAG, Riddell RH, Kirby JD: Intestinal lymphoma complicating dermatitis herpetiformis. Br J Dermatol 96:555–560, 1977.

67. Azar HA: Cancer in Lebanon and the Near East. Cancer 15:66–78, 1962.

68. Novis BH: Primary intestinal lymphoma in South Africa. Israel J Med Sci 15:386–389, 1979.

69. Shahid MJ, Alami SY, Nassar VH, Balikian JB, Salem AA: Primary intestinal lymphoma with paraproteinemia. Cancer 35:848–858, 1975.

70. Alsabati EAK: Paraproteinemia in normal family members of eight cases with primary intestinal lymphomas in Iraq. Oncology 35:68–72, 1972.

71. Haghshenass M, Haghighi P, Abadi P, Kharazmi A, Gerami C, Nasr K: Alpha heavy-chain disease in southern Iran. Am J Dig Dis 22:866–873, 1977.

72. Shaklai M, Mintz U, Pinkhas J, Pick A, Ben-Bassat M, DeVries A: Intestinal lymphoma with unusual sequence of serum IgA changes. AM J Dig Dis 19:279–286, 1974.

73. Nasr K, Haghighi P, Bakhshandeh K, Abadi P, Lahimgarzadeh A: Primary upper small intestinal lymphoma. A report of 40 cases from Iran. Am J Dig Dis 21:313–323, 1976.

74. Salem PA, Nassar VH, Shahid MJ, Hajj AA, Alami SY, Balikian JB, Salem AA: Mediterranean abdominal lymphoma, or immuncproliferative small intestinal disease. Part I: Clinical aspects. Cancer 40:2941–2947, 1977.

75. Ramot B, Many A: Primary intestinal lymphoma: clinical manifestations and possible effect of environmental factors. Rec Results cancer Res 39:193–199, 1972.

76. Al-Khateeb AK: Primary malignant lymphoma of the small intestine. Int Surg 54:295–300, 1970.

77. Al-Saleem T, Zardawi IM: Primary lymphomas of the small intestine in Iraq: a pathological study. Histopathology 3:89–106, 1979.

78. Doe WF: Alpha chain disease clinicopathological features and relationship to so-called Mediterranean lymphoma. Br J Cancer 31 (suppl II): 350–355, 1975.

79. Kharazmi A, Haghighi P, Haghshenas M, Nasr K, Abadi P, Rezai HR: Alpha-chain disease and its association with intestinal lymphoma. Clin Exp Immunol 26:124–128, 1976.

80. Lewin KJ, Kahn LB, Novis BH: Primary intestinal lymphoma of 'Western' and 'Mediterranean' type, alpha chain disease and massive plasma cell infiltration. A comparative study of 37 cases. Cancer 38:2511–2528, 1976.

81. Ramot B, Hulu N: Primary intestinal lymphoma and its relation to alpha heavy chain disease. Br J Cancer 31 (suppl II):343–349, 1975.

82. Haghighi P, Nasr K: Primary upper small intestinal lymphoma (so-called mediterranean lymphoma). Pathol Annu 8:231–255, 1973.

83. Rambaud JC, Matuchancky C: Alpha-chain disease. Pathogenesis and relation to Mediter-

ranean lymphoma. Lancet I 817:1430–1432, 1973.

84. Selzer G, Sherman G, Callihan TR, Schwartz Y: Primary small intestinal lymphomas and α-heavy-chain disease. A study of 43 cases from a pathology department in Israel. Isr J Med Sci 15:111–123, 1979.

85. Seligmann M, Rambaud J: α-chain disease: a possible model for the pathogenesis of human lymphomas. In: The immunopathology of lymphoreticular neoplasms, Twomey JJ, Good RA (eds). New York: Plenum Medical, 1977, pp 425–447.

86. Rambaud JC, Bognel C, Prost A, Bernier JJ, LeQuintrec Y, Lambling A, Danon F, Hurez D, Seligmann M: Clinico-pathological study of a patient with 'Mediterranean' type of abdominal lymphoma and a new type of IgA abnormality ('alpha chain disease'). Digestion 1:321–336, 1968.

87. Spector BD, Perry GS III, Good RA, Kersey JH: Immunodeficiency diseases and malignancy. In: The immunopathology of lymphoreticular neoplasms, Twomey JJ, Good RA (eds). New York: Plenum Medical , 1978, pp 203–222.

88. Shackelford GD, McAlister WH: Primary immunodeficiency diseases and malignancy. Am J Roentgenol Rad Therapy Nucl Med 123:144–153, 1975.

89. Faraci RP, Hoffstrand HJ, Witebsky FG, Blaese RM, Beazley RM: Malignant lymphoma of the jejunum in a patient with Wiskott-Aldrich syndrome. Surgical treatment. Arch Surg 110:218–220, 1975.

90. Whitehead R: Primary lymphadenopathy complicating idiopathic steatorrhea. Gut 9:569–575, 1968.

91. Kahn LB, Novis BH: Nodular lymphoid hyperplasia of the small bowel associated with primary small bowel reticulum cell lymphoma. Cancer 33:837–844, 1974.

92. Cohen HJ, Gonzalvo A, Krook J, Thompson TT, Kremer WB: New presentation of alpha heavy chain disease: North American polypoid gastrointestinal lymphoma. Clinical and cellular studies. Cancer 41:1161–1169, 1978.

93. Maurer HS, Gotoff SP, Allen L, Bolan J: Malignant lymphoma of the small intestine in multiple family members. Association with an immunologic deficiency. Cancer 37:2224–2231, 1976.

94. Lee GB, Smith PM, Seal EME: Lymphosarcoma in Crohn's disease: report of a case. Dis Col Rect 20:351–354, 1977.

95. Collins WJ: Malignant lymphoma complicating regional enteritis. Case report and review of the literature. Am J Gastroenterol 68:177–181, 1977.

96. Gould TS, Tanguay PR, Delellis RA: Thymoma and primary lymphoma of the small intestine. Cancer 40:1755–1758, 1977.

97. Stokes PL, Asquith P, Holmes GKT: Histocompatability antigens associated with adult celiac disease. Lancet 2:162–164, 1972.

98. Falchuk ZM, Rogentine GN, Strober W: Predominance of histocompatability antigen HL-A8 in patients with gluten-sensitive enteropathy. J Clin Invest 51:1602–1607, 1972.

99. Morris PJ, Forbes JF: HL-A in follicular lymphoma, reticulum cell sarcoma, lymphosarcoma and infectious mononucleosis. Transplant Proc 3:1315–1316, 1971.

100. Isaacson P, Wright DH: Malignant histiocytosis of the intestine. Its relationship to malabsorption and ulcerative jejunitis. Hum Pathol 9:661–667, 1978.

101. Isaacson P, Wright DH: Intestinal lymphoma associated with malabsorption. Lancet 1 8055:67–70, 1978.

102. Ramot B: Malabsorption due to lymphomatous disease. Annu Rev Med 22:19–24, 1971.

103. McCrae WM, Eastwood MA, Martin MR, Sircus W: Neglected coeliac disease. Lancet 1 7900:187–190, 1975.

104. Holmes GKI, Stokes Pl, Sorahan TM, Prior P, Waterhouse JAH, Cooke WT: Coeliac disease, gluten-free diet, and malignancy. Gut 17:612–619, 1976.

105. MacLaurin BP, Cooke WT, Ling NR: Impaired lymphocyte reactivity against tumour cells in patients with coeliac disease. Gut 12:794–800, 1971.

106. World Health Organization report on α-heavy chain disease meeting, Geneva, 1975, pp 10–13.

107. Russell RM, Abadi P, Ismail-Beigi F: Role of bacterial overgrowth in the malabsorption syndrome of primary small intestinal lymphoma in Iran. Cancer 39:2579–2583, 1977.

108. Ramos L, Marcos J, Illanas M, Hernández-Mora M, Pérez-Payá F, Picouto JH, Santana P, Chantar C: Radiological characteristics of primary intestinal lymphoma of the 'Mediterranean' type: observations on twelve cases. Radiology 126:379–385, 1978.

109. Rappaport H, Ramot B, Hulu N, Park JK: The pathology of so-called Mediterranean abdominal lymphoma with malabsorption. Cancer 29:1502–1511, 1972.

110. Lukes RJ, Collins RD: immunological characterization of malignant lymphomas. Cancer 34:1488–1503, 1974.

111. Perry PM, Cross RM, Morson BC: Primary malignant lymphoma of the rectum (22 Cases). Proc R Soc Med 65:72, 1972.

112. Wychulis AR, Beahrs OH, Wollner LB: Malignant lymphoma of the colon: a study of 69 cases. Arch Surg 93:215–225, 1966.

113. Greene FL, Livstone EM, McAllister WB Jr, Passarelli NM, Troncale FJ: Reticulum cell sarcoma of the large intestine. The role of fiberoptic colonoscopy. Am J Dig Dis 19:379b–384, 1974.

114. O'Connell DJ, Thompson AJ: Lymphoma of the colon: the spectrum of radiologic changes. Gastrointest Radiol 2:377–385, 1978.

115. Messinger NH, Bobroff LM, Beneventano TC: Lymphosarcoma of the colon. Am J Roentgenol Rad Therapy Nucl Med 117:281–286, 1973.

116. Allen AW, Donaldson G, Sniffen RC, Goodale F: Primary malignant lymphoma of the gastrointestinal tract. Ann Surg 140:428–438, 1954.

117. Wagonfeld JB, Platz CE, Fishman FL, Sibley RK, Kirsner JB: Multicentric colonic lymphoma complicating ulcerative colitis. Am J Dig Dis 22:502–508, 1977.

118. Vieta JO, Delgado GE: Chronic ulcerative colitis complicated by colonic lymphoma: report of a case. Dis Colon Rectum 19:56–62, 1976.

119. Myerson P, Myerson D, Miller D, DeLuca VA, Lawson JP: Lymphosarcoma of the bowel masquerading as ulcerative colitis: report of a case. Dis Colon Rectum 17:710–715, 1974.

120. Renton P, Blackshaw AJ: Colonic lymphoma complicating ulcerative colitis. BR J Surg 63:542–545, 1976.

121. Friedman HB, Silver GM, Brown CH: Lymphoma of the colon simulating ulcerative colitis: report of four cases. Am J Dig Dis 13:910–917, 1968.

122. Cornes JS, Smith JC, Southwood WFW: Lymphosarcoma in chronic ulcerative colitis with report of two cases. Br J Surg 49:50–53, 1961.

123. Pinkus GS, Wilson RE, Corson JM: Reticulum cell sarcoma of the colon following renal transplantation. Cancer 24:2103–2108, 1974.

124. Levy M, Stone AM, Platt N: Reticulum cell sarcoma of the cecum and macroglobulinemia: a case report. J Surg Oncol 8:149–153, 1976.

125. Sherlock P, Winawer SJ, Goldstein MJ, Bragg DG: Malignant lymphoma of the gastrointestinal tract. Prog Gastroenterol 2:367–391, 1970.

126. Berard CW: Discussion II: Round table discussion of histopathologic classification. Cancer Treat Rep 61:1037–1048, 1977.

127. Sweet DL, Golomb HM: The non-Hodgkin lymphomas. Curr Probl Cancer 4:1–35, 1980.

128. Nathwani BN: A critical analysis of the classification of non-Hodgkin's lymphomas. Cancer

44:347–384, 1979.

129. Rappaport H: Tumors of the hematopoietic system. In: Atlas of tumor pathology, section 3, fascicle 8. Washington, D.C.: US Armed Forces Institute of Pathology, 1966.
130. Lukes RJ, Collins RD: New approaches to the classification of the lymphomata. Br J Cancer 21 (suppl II):1–28, 1975.
131. Lennert K, Mohri N, Stein H, Kaiserling E: The histopathology of malignant lymphoma. Br J Haematol 31 (suppl):193–203, 1975.
132. Dorfman RF: Classification of non-Hodgkin's lymphomas. Lancet 1:1295–1296, 1974.
133. Bennett MH, Farrer-Brown G, Henry K, Jelliffe Am: Classification of non-Hodgkin's lymphomas. Lancet 2:405–406, 1974.
134. Mathe G, Rappaport H, O'Conor GT, Torloni H: Histological and cytological typing of neoplastic diseases of haematopoietic and lymphoid tissues. International histological classification of tumours 14. Geneva: World Health Organization, 1976, pp 37–42.
135. Musshoff K, Schmidt-Vollmer H: Prognostic significance of primary site after radiotherapy in non-Hodgkin's lymphomata. Br J Cancer 31 (suppl II):425–433, 1975.
136. Filippa DA, Lieberman PH, Erlandson RA, Koziner B, Siegal FP, Turnbull A, Zimring A, Good RA: A study of malignant lymphomas using light and ultramicroscopic, cytochemical and immunologic technics. Correlation with clinical features. Am J Med 64:259–268, 1978.
137. Jones SE: Non-Hodgkin lymphomas. J Am Med Assoc 234:633–638, 1975.
138. Ho F, Gibson JB: Gastrointestinal lymphomas in Hong Kong Chinese Israeli J of Med Sci 15:382–385, 1979.
139. Lim FE, Hartman AS, Tan EGC, Cady Bm Meissner WA: Factors in the prognosis of gastric lymphoma. Cancer 39:1715–1720, 1977.
140. Cox JD: Prognostic factors in malignant lymphoreticular tumors of the small bowel and ileocecal region: a review of 50 case histories. Int J Radiat Oncol Biol Phys 5:185–190, 1979.
141. Lightdale CJ: Classifying gastrointestinal lymphomas. Gastroenterology 78:1641–1642, 1980.
142. Siegal FP, Filippa DA, Koziner B: Surface markers in leukemias and lymphomas. Am J Pathol 90:451–460, 1978.
143. Carbone PP, Kaplan HS, Musshoff K, Smithers DW, Tubiana M: Report of the committee on Hodgkin's disease staging classification. Cancer Res 31:1860–1861, 1971.
144. American Joint Committee for Cancer Staging and End Results Reporting: Manual for staging of cancer 1978. Whiting Press, 1978.
145. Rosenberg SA: Validity of Ann Arbor staging classification for the non-Hodgkin's lymphomas. Cancer Treat Rep 61:1023–1027, 1977.
146. Chabner BA, Johnson RE, Young RC, Canellos GP, Hubbard SP Johnson SK, DeVita VT: Sequential nonsurgical and surgical staging of non-Hodgkin's lymphoma. Ann Intern Med 85:149–154, 1976.
147. Goffinet DR, Warnke R, Dunnick NR, Castellino R, Glatstein E, Nelson TS, Dorfman RS, Rosenberg SA, Kaplan HS: Clinical and surgical (laparotomy) evaluation of patients with non-Hodgkin's lymphomas. Cancer Treat Rep 61:981–992, 1977.
148. Veronesi U, Musumeci R, Pizzetti F, Gennari L, Bonnadonna G: The value of staging laparotomy in non-Hodgkin's lymphomas (with emphasis on the histiocytic type). Cancer 33:446–459, 1974.
149. Goffinet DR, Castellino RA, Kim H, Dorfman RF, Fuks Z, Rosenberg SA, Nelson T, Kaplan HS: Staging laparotomies in unselected previously untreated patient with non-Hodgkin's lymphomas. Cancer 32:672–681, 1973.
150. Hanks GE, Terry LN, Bryan JA, Newsome JF: Contribution of diagnostic laparotomy to

staging non-Hodgkin's lymphoma. Cancer 29:41–43, 1972.

151. Heifetz LJ, Fuller LM, Rodgers RW, Martin RG, Butler JL, North LB, Gamble JF, Shullenberger CC: Laparotomy findings in lymphangiogram-staged I and II non-Hodgkin's lymphomas. Cancer 45:2778–2786, 1980.

152. Lightdale CJ, Winawer SJ, Kurtz RC, Knapper WH: Laparoscopic diagnosis of suspected liver neoplasms. Value of prior liver scans. Dig Dis Sci 24:588–593, 1979.

153. Hande KR, Fisher RI, DeVita VT, Chabner BA, Young RC: Diffuse histiocytic lymphoma involving the gastrointestinal treact. Cancer 41:1984–1989, 1978.

154. Rosenfelt F, Rosenberg SA: Diffuse histiocytic lymphoma presenting with gastrointestinal tract lesions. The Stanford experience. Cancer 45:2188–2193, 1980.

155. Bitran JD, Kinzie J, Sweet DL, Variakojis D, Griem ML, Golomb HM, Miller JB, Oetzel N, Ultmann JE: Survival of patients with localized histocytic lymphomas. Cancer 39:342–346, 1977.

156. Lipton A, Lee BJ: Prognosis of stage I lymphosarcoma and reticulum cell sarcoma. N Engl J Med 284:230–233, 1971.

157. Fuks Z, Kaplan HS: Recurrence rates following radiation therapy of nodular and diffuse malignant lymphomas. Radiology 108:675–684, 1973.

158. Fuller LM: Results of large volume irradiation in the management of Hodgkin's disease and malignant lymphomas originating in the abdomen. Radiology 87:1058–1064, 1966.

159. Landberg TG, Hakansson Ig, Möller TR, Mattsson WKI, Landys KE, Johansson BG, Killander DCF, Molin BF, Westling PF, Lenner PH, Dahl OG: CVP-remission-maintenence in stage I or II non-Hodgkin's lymphoma. Preliminary results of a randomized study. Cancer 44:831–838, 1979.

160. Peckham MJ, Guay JP, Hamlin IME, Lukes RJ: Survival in localized nodal and extranodal non-Hodgkin's lymphomata. Br J Cancer 31 (suppl II):413–424, 1975.

161. Han T, Stutzman L: Mode of spead in patients with localized malignant lymphoma. Arch Intern Med 120:1–7, 1967.

162. Rudders RA, Ross ME, DeLellis RA: Primary extranodal lymphoma. Response to treatment and factors influencing prognosis. Cancer 42:406–416, 1978.

163. Coltman CA, Luce JK, McKelvey EM, Jones SE, Moon TE: Chemotherapy of non-Hodgkin's lymphoma: 10 Years' experience in the southwest oncology group. Cancer Treat Rep 62:1067–1078, 1977.

13. Functioning Tumors of the Gut

STANLEY R. FRIESEN and JOSEPH B. PETELIN

1. INTRODUCTION

It has been a traditional clinical observation that tumors, in general, and specifically of the gastrointestinal tract, produce symptoms because of their mass encroachment upon surrounding structures (pressure symptoms), upon a lumen (obstructive symptoms), and upon the mucosa (erosive bleeding symptoms). In the instance of functioning tumors these physical and pathologic features are often entirely overshadowed and masked by the systemic manifestations due to their excessive elaboration of humoral products. Neuroendocrine tumors are thus characterized, not so much by their histologic appearance, as by their functional capabilities[1].

The neuroendocrine system, central and peripheral, is composed of several functional groups such as the central hypothalamic–pituitary axis, the pituitary–thyroid–adrenocortical–gonadal endocrine axis, and the entero-insular paracrine axis of the peripheral diffuse gastro-enteropancreatic (GEP) system. The discussion in this chapter is limited to the humoral tumors of the GEP system.

1.1. Characteristics of the Neuroendocrine System

1.1.1. The Endocrine Cell and its Humoral Products. The tumor cell, as well as its normal cell of origin, has ultrastructural evidence of secretory granules that store the synthesized amines or peptides for the process of secretion directly into the contiguous blood stream of capillaries (a process of emiocytosis). Normal neuroendocrine cells, having this capacity to synthesize, store and secrete hormonal substances, are sensitive to stimulation and/or suppression for regulatory homeostatis; tumor cells, on the other hand, secrete their products excessively and autonomously, usually independent of stimulatory or suppressive influences. If the pathologic process is one of hyperplasia, the normal influences of stimulation and suppression are maintained, at least

J. J. DeCosse and P. Sherlock (eds.), Gastrointestinal cancer 1, 343-385. All rights reserved.

until neoplastic autonomy supersedes that responsiveness.

There are three general types of humoral substances: steroids from the adrenal cortex and gonadal organs; amines from the adrenal medulla, thyroid and the gut, including the neurotransmitters; and, the largest group, the polypeptides from the brain and the gut. The latter two types are present almost universally in the autonomic and central nervous systems, the brain and 'the gastro-entero-pancreatic (GEP) system. Together the three types of humoral substances are responsible for normal maintenance of functional homeostasis by the regulation and control of responses to the internal and external human environment. Another characteristic of the neuroendocrine system is the functional necessity of an end-organ (target cell) response to the neuro-humoral substance which is mediated through appropriate specific receptors. Thus a tumor's elaboration of a peptide hormone produces its effect only if the receptor on the target cell is receptive, unblocked or unoccupied, which allows the end-organ to produce its systemic biologic clinical syndrome. Autoantibodies or pharmacologic receptor-blockers or even other peptides may block the receptor so that there is no exocrine response to the endocrine product, a circumstance probably accountable for silent, 'non-functional' endocrine tumors. For some polypeptides a function or end-organ cell has not yet been identified and they are thus termed 'candidate' hormones.

1.1.2. The APUD Concept, Entopia and Ectopia. Most of the neuroendocrine cells that secrete amines and peptides have common cytochemical characteristics, as described by Pearse [2]. The cells contain amines, take up precursor amines and are capable of decarboxylation (amine precursor uptake, decarboxylation). The resulting acronym has been applied to the APUD system, the APUD concept, APUD cells and their tumors, Apudomas. The common cytochemical properties are probably owing to their common embryologic origin from the various components of the neuroectoderm, including the neural crest. The precursor cells of the APUD system, having 'arrived' in the mucosa of the gut and the islets of the pancreas, mature to function normally and thus entopically secrete a single amine or peptide. Normally there has been a repression of other precursor cell functions. This intracellular process requires enzyme(s), a peptidase, to act on the large molecular 'prohormones' to form smaller molecular peptides that circulate normally.

When dysplastic changes occur in these cells for whatever reason, genetic or acquired, an excessive elaboration of amines and/or polypeptides occurs to produce clinical syndromes through the hormonal action on receptive end-organ target cells. When the morphologic change is hyperplastic or adenomatous, the endogenous hypersecretion is usually the peptide hormone which

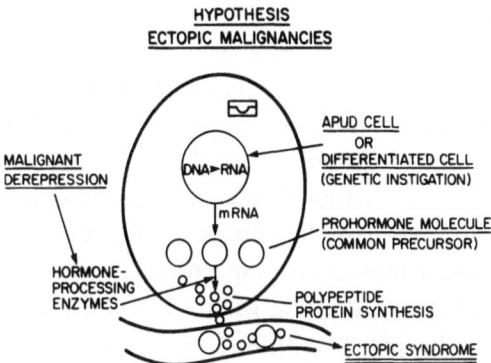

Figure 1. Diagrammatic representation of the hypothesis of ectopic phenomena in which malignant derepression of peptidase activity results in the secretion of large molecular polypeptides into the circulation. The malignant APUD cells thus function in a toti-potential primitive manner to produce a kaleidoscopic array of ectopic clinical syndromes.

normally is synthesized by those cells, an entopic phenomenon that occasionally occurs also in endocrine carcinomas. On the other hand, when there has been a malignant change is these cells, it has been postulated that there is a derepression back to the primitive totipotential capability of the precursor APUD cells; this results in either hypersecretion of the normal (entopic) small molecular polypeptide and/or one or more of the large molecular precursor prohormones that are elaborated *ectopically* from that site. The derepression may be due to a peptidase failure to convert the large molecule (prohormone) to the smaller molecule (hormone) (see Figure 1).

Because of these conceptual considerations, a generality can be expressed concerning pathologic abnormalities of neuroendocrine system: Hyperplasias and adenomas usually hypersecrete one entopic hormone, while malignancies usually hypersecrete one or more prohormones entopically or ectopically, resulting in kaleidoscopic clinical syndromes [3]. Furthermore, endocrinopathies may occur in either a sporadic or genetic fashion. Most sporadic endocrinopathies are adenomatous (single benign adenomas) while most genetic, familial endocrinopathies cover the whole pathologic spectrum from hyperplasia to malignancy and are multiple in highly predictable associations. For instance, the multiplicity of involved cells leads to diffuse hyperplasias and multifocal, bilateral, multiple micro- or macro-adenomas or even carcinomas. The multiple systems include the pituitary, parathyroid and pancreatic islets in Multiple Endocrine Adenopathy (MEA), type I [4], or in the instance of MEA type II complexes [5, 6], the adrenal medullary and thyroid medullary tumors. Multiplicity is also evident in families affected with the abnormal gene as a dominant trait in multiple members of the families [7].

1.2. Historical Considerations

The humoral expression of endocrine tumors became apparent only after years of sporadic observations. For instance, the clinical picture associated with insulin-secreting tumors was not recognized as such until after insulin was synthesized, administered and observed in patients as an 'insulin reaction'. Moreover, to this day, although secretin was described as a biologically functional humoral substance in the duodenal mucosa years ago (1902) by Bayliss and Starling[8], a proven secretin-producing duodenal tumor has yet to be described. Furthermore, the first gastrin-secreting tumors to be reported (1955) were found in the pancreas[9] and not in the gastric antrum, where 'gastric secretin' (gastrin) was postulated to be biologically present 50 years earlier in 1905[10]. The ulcerogenic tumor of the Zollinger-Ellison syndrome was thus an ectopic humoral manifestation – a spectacular clinical phenomenon that stimulated a surge of scientific investigations, both basic and clinical.

1.3. Diagnostic Features

The observable clinical picture of an endocrinopathy depends upon the stimulated exocrine function of the end-organ system involved; the major diagnostic parameters relate thus to the abnormal exocrine effect of the endocrine stimulation. For instance, the clinical appearance associated with tumor hypergastrinemia will actually consist of severe acid-peptic duodenal/jejunal ulcer disease due to the hypersecretion of hydrogen ion as gastric hyperacidity from the gastric parietal cells. Most diagnostic events are thus directed to demonstration of the ulcer(s), the acid hypersecretion and then confirmed by the elucidation of the excessive circulating peptide, gastrin, and finally, localization of the tumor. Whereas bioassays, originally devised to identify the hormone by its effect of the exocrine end-organ, are useful and circumstantially corroborative, absolute diagnostic identification is now more confirmatory by means of radioimmunoassay of the polypeptide. Final substantiation is attained by cytochemical identification of the peptides and/or amines in the tumor cells and granules by immunofluorescence, immunoperoxidase and radioimmunochemical assays.

1.4. Therapeutic Considerations

The most beneficial therapeutic modality, that of surgical excision of the hyperfunctioning tumor, depends upon the localization and presence of a removable single benign hypersecreting tumor (adenoma). Such fortunate circumstances may be present in most entopic and sporadic occurrences, of which insulinoma is a classic example. Such direct approaches are not always possible when the hyperfunctioning tissue is diffusely multiple (hyperplasia or multifocal microadenomata) as in the genetic multiple endocrinopathy syndromes, or when the tumor is metastatic as in many of the ectopic malignancies such as the Zollinger-Ellison syndrome. Therefore, in the instance of hyperplasia, subtotal excision may suffice to numerically reduce the number of hypersecreting cells, but when metastatic disease is non-resectable, surgical excision of the end-organ, such as total gastrectomy in metastatic pancreatic gastrinoma, may be the most practical palliative and beneficial therapeutic procedure. Non-surgical treatment of any of the endocrinopathies are also directed to the tumor, usually by specific chemotherapeutic agents (streptozotocin, chlorozotocin, or mithramycin), inhibition of humoral release (diazoxide, somatostatin), blockade of the end-organ receptors (cimetidine), or by palliative symptomatic treatment of the exocrine effects of the endocrinopathy.

In the following descriptions of the endocrinopathies of the GEP system, it will be noted that functional, rather than morphologic characteristics take precedence in their recognition, diagnosis and treatment. The clinical syndromes are presented according to their functional origin as either entopic or ectopic phenomena. The entopic syndromes include: the carcinoid syndromes due to the release of amines and polypeptides from enterochromaffin tumors (EC cells of the midgut and foregut, including the pancreas); glucagonoma syndrome due to elaboration of glucagon from tumors of the alpha cells of the pancreas and gut; insulinoma syndrome from tumors of the beta cells of the pancreas; somatostatinoma syndrome due to secretion of somatotrophin release-inhibiting factor (SRIF) or somatostatin (SST) from the delta cells of the pancreas; and, the multiple endocrine adenopathy syndrome (MEA, I) in which the entopic pancreatic polypeptide (hPP) is elaborated from pure PP apudomas and appears to be a marker for the pancreatic component of the syndrome. The ectopic syndromes are those due to excessive elaboration of ectopic polypeptides from pancreatic tumors, which include the Zollinger-Ellison syndrome (gastrin), the Verner-Morrison or watery diarrhea syndrome (vasoactive intestinal polypeptide (VIP)), the ectopic Cushing's syndrome (ACTH), and the ectopic hyperparathyroidism syndrome (parathyrin).

2. CLINICAL SYNDROMES

2.1. Entopic

2.1.1. The Carcinoid Syndromes. The carcinoid syndromes encompass a group of clinical manifestations including vasomotor, gastrointestinal, and cardiopulmonary phenomena that occur when the humoral products of a carcinoid tumor enter the systemic circulation. Although serotonin was initially thought to be responsible for these effects, extensive research has revealed that a number of amines, polypeptides and other substances, including kallekrein, bradykinin, histamine, motilin, and prostaglandins, play an integral role in production of the symptom complex known as the carcinoid syndrome. In fact, it is becoming more clear that a number of atypical variants of this syndrome exist and that the key to the understanding of them is intimately linked to the APUD concept.

History. In 1888, Otto Lubarsch published what is generally credited as being the first description of a carcinoid tumor [11]. This report described the autopsy findings on two patients, one of whom had two small tumors of the ileum, and the other who had six. He showed that these 'little carcinomata' arose from the crypts of Lieberkuhn. Shortly thereafter, a patient with massive liver metastases from an ileal carcinoid was reported but it received little attention [12]. Oberndorfer, in 1909, emphasized the benign nature of this slow-growing, usually small tumor, even though it had the appearance of a carcinoma, by coining the term, 'Karzenoide' [13]. In 1914, Masson demonstrated that the granules of the Kultschitsky cells, or 'enterochromaffin' cells of Ciaccio, present in the crypts, had an affinity for silver stain and proposed that these 'argentaffin' cells were the cells of origin of the carcinoid tumor [14]. The functional aspects of these tumors were not recognized until the early 1950s. In 1953–54 serotonin was isolated from a carcinoid tumor and elevated levels of serotonin were found in the blood and urine of two patients with carcinoid [15, 16]. Since then an explosion of information regarding the biochemical (humoral) nature of this tumor has provided a better understanding of the functional aspects of the carcinoid tumor.

Pathology. It is now generally accepted that the enterochromaffin cells are members of the APUD cell population derived from the neuroectoderm, and are ubiquitous throughout the gastrointestinal tract. Understandably then, tumors arising from these cells could be expected to be found in many sites. About three-fourths of all abdominal carcinoid tumors are of midgut origin. Over 40% arise from the appendix, and approximately 30% occur in the small intestine, usually the terminal ileum. These are, in fact, the most common tumors of the small intestine and appendix. The rectum is the third most common site of involvement, accounting for approximately 16% of all abdominal carcinoids. Foregut carcinoids, which are responsible for an atypical presentation of the carcinoid syndrome, occur in the duodenum, stomach, pancreas, biliary tract and lung. Those of bronchial origin are the most common among this group, occurring in 10% of cases. Less frequently, carcinoids have been found in ovarian teratomas, the testis, urethra, larynx, thymus, and sacrococcygeal teratomas [17].

Carcinoid tumors are typically small submucosal growths with discrete borders. They are often multicentric and not infrequently associated with other tumors, many of which are endocrine in nature. Seventy-fiver per cent are less than 1 cm, and only 5% are greater than 2 cm in size [18]. They are usually yellow, owing to their high lipid content, but may be tan or gray. Microscopically, they are composed of small uniform cells arranged in clusters, ribbons, or a scirrhous pattern without a capsule. Since few mitoses are evident, the degree of malignancy is usually determined by the invasiveness of the tumor. Electron microscopy reveals characteristic granules in the cytoplasm.

These tumors generally exhibit slow growth in a stepwise fashion through the muscularis to the serosa and directly into the mesentery. Regional lymph node involvement occurs only after local invasion is present. These metastases often grow to be larger than the primary tumor. The liver is the most common site of distant metastases. The lung is the second most common site and involvement here usually indicates far-advanced disease. Other sites of metastatic spread include bone (osteolytic and osteoblastic), skin, brain, ovary, breast, pancreas, heart, spleen, adrenals, bone marrow, kidney, thyroid, bladder, pleura, nose, testes, epididymis, prostate and cervix.

Although Oberndorfer stressed the relative benignity of these tumors, most extra-appendiceal carcinoids should be considered potentially malignant, as demonstrated by MacDonald in 1956 [19]. The site of origin and the size of the tumor appear to be two important factors useful in predicting the ability of these tumors to metastasize. Those in the appendix metastasize 2–3% of the time, those of the jejuno-ileum 33%, those of the colon 60–70% and those of the rectum 18%. Tumors less than 1 cm in diameter metastasize in less than 2% of cases, while those greater than 2 cm in diameter present with metastatic involvement in more than 80% of cases. Interestingly, it is the presence of distant metastases to the liver, rather than the mass effect of the original tumor, than leads to development of the symptoms characteristic of the carcinoid syndrome.

Classical Carcinoid Syndrome

Pathogenesis. When the secretions of midgut carcinoid tumors (jejunum, ileum and appendix) reach the systemic circulation, the classical carcinoid syndrome appears. Usually this implies significant metastatic spread to the liver or retroperitoneum since the liver and lung are known to metabolize the major product of carcinoids, serotonin, quite effectively. The major manifestations include flushing, cramping abdominal pain, hepatomegaly, and endocardial lesions.

Some of these symptoms are related to the properties and metabolism of serotonin, 5-hydroxytryptamine (5-HT). The chemical synthesis and degradation of serotonin are depicted in Table 1. Serotonin has long been known to be a vasoconstrictor. Another substance felt to be responsible for some of the

Table 1. The synthesis and degradation of serotonin (5HT).

Synthesis	Degradation
Tryptophan ʼ	5HT (serotonin)
↓	↓
5-HTP (5-hydroxytryptophan)	5HA (5-hydroxyindol acetaldehyde)
↓	↓
5HT (5-hydroxytryptamine) (serotonin)	5-HIAA (5-hydroxyindol acetic acid)

Table 2. The formation and metabolic breakdown of bradykinin.

Kininogen
↓
Lysyl-bradykinin
↓
Bradykinin
↓
Inactive peptides and amino acids.

manifestations of the disease is kallikrein, which has been found in some carcinoid tumors. It catalyzes the formation of bradykinin from a serum alpha-2 globulin as shown in Table 2. Bradykinin is known to be an extremely potent vasodilator and also produces bronchoconstriction and increased intestinal motility.

Prostaglandin E (PGE) and a peptide, motilin, have also been isolated from these tumors and do, in fact, produce effects characteristic of the syndrome. PGE may cause flushing and both substances produce increased gastrointestinal motility [20].

Clinical presentation. Diarrhea is the most common and often the most incapacitating feature of the syndrome. Hypermotility of the intestine and abnormal fluid and electrolyte fluxes by the mucosa are considered to be the underlying mechanisms. The result is borborygmus, urgency and the frequent passage of non-bloody, watery diarrhea. These events often accompany or follow attacks of flushing. Hyperserotoninemia seems to correlate best with the diarrhea and anti-serotonin drugs may ameliorate this aspect of the disease. However, other substances, including motilin, bradykinin and prostaglandin, are known to cause hypermotility and may be implicated.

Cutaneous flushing occurs in most carcinoid patients. When produced by the midgut variety of the tumor, the flush may appear deep red or occasionally almost cyanotic. The face and neck are first affected, followed by the trunk and extremities. Episodes are often triggered by emotional stress or ingestion of cheese or alcohol and typically last for only several minutes. Bradykinin appears to be primarily responsible for these flushes and its release is triggered by endogenous or exogenous epinephrine stimulation. Prostaglandin E and serotonin may also be involved in the production of these flushes. At the present time, the exact mediator of the cutaneous flushing of the classic carcinoid syndrome is unknown.

Endocardial lesions occur in 50% of cases and are localized to the right side of the heart. Apparently due to chronic exposure to the products of the carcinoid tumor, the valve cusps, papillary muscles, and chordae tendinae display fibrous thickening, which results in dysfunction and eventual cardiac failure in the form of tricuspid insufficiency and pulmonary stenosis.

Hepatomegaly is common and is secondary to massive replacement by tumor. It is this gross metastatic involvement with systemic release of the humoral products, in fact, that is responsible for the production of the syndrome.

Venous telangiectasias occur in a butterfly pattern on the face in 50% of patients. The pathogenesis is unknown.

Other vasomotor changes are common and may be secondary to bradykinin, serotonin or prostaglandin. Hypotension commonly accompanies attacks of flushing.

Edema occurs in about one half of the patients with carcinoid syndrome and probably relates to hypoproteinemia and right-sided heart failure.

Bronchial constriction presents in 10–20% of cases. Serotonin, prostaglandins and kinins are known to produce this effect.

Pellagra occurs in a small number of patients and although this was initially thought to be secondary to generally poor nutrition, it is likely to be due to niacin deficiency since dietary tryptophan is routed preferentially from niacin biosynthesis to serotonin production.

Retroperitoneal fibrosis is found in some patients. In others, Peyronie's disease, a dense fibrosis of the dorsal shaft of the penis, is present. The agent here is unknown but it is interesting that the anti-serotonin drug, methysergide, is known to produce the same effects.

Atypical Carcinoid Syndrome

Pathogenesis. Carcinoid tumors of the foregut differ biologically, chemically and clinically from their midgut counterparts. The former tumors are generally more aggressive with metastases to bone, skin, brain, lungs, heart, thyroid, kidneys and lymph nodes. They are more often associated with other endocrine tumors. In addition to the production of the usual amines, these foregut tumors produce histamine and other polypeptides including corticotrophin, insulin, gastrin, glucagon and a heterogenous parathyrin. Foregut carcinoid tumors often lack the enzyme 5-HTP decarboxylase so that they may secrete large amounts of 5-HTP and the blood and urine may contain both 5-HT and 5-HTP, while the urinary 5-HIAA levels may be low. Gastric carcinoids have been shown to produce large amounts of histamine and appear to be a special subset of these foregut tumors.

Clinical presentation. Cutaneous flushing is the most common clinical finding. These flushes differ from those secondary to the midgut variety of tumor in that they are more livid, more prolonged and more severe. Marked hypotension, diarrhea, nausea and vomiting and bronchoconstriction accompany these episodes. Periorbital edema and lacrimation are pronounced. The attacks may last up to three or four days. With bronchial tumors the flush is probably related to kinin release, which can be suppressed by corticosteroids, an effect not seen with midgut tumors. Gastric carcinoids, on the other hand, produce a distinctive flush with sharply defined serpentine borders, which is thought to be secondary to histamine release, and which has been shown to be relieved by both histamine-1 and -2 blockers [21]. Additionally, gastric carcinoids are associated with an increased incidence of peptic ulceration with typical attendant symptoms.

Diagnosis of the Carcinoid Syndromes. Carcinoid tumors are occasionally found on routine physical examination long before the functional syndrome is present. This most often occurs when the tumor is in the rectum, testis or ovary. Occasionally a routine chest X-ray will reveal a mass or its secondary atelectatic effects. When the tumor is present in the appendix the diagnosis is usually made during or after appendectomy for appendicitis. Rarely, the jejuno-ileal variety produces symptoms of obstruction by acting as an intussusceptum.

More commonly the patient with an early carcinoid tumor will have non-specific symptoms and may be considered to have a nervous or drinking problem. Once the diagnosis is suspected, however, there are certain specific tests that aid in confirmation and localization of the tumor. The most useful of these is the measurement of 5-HIAA in the urine collected over a 24 hour period. Normal values are 2–9 mg per 24 hour period. During the collection, the patient must abstain from fruits, fruit juices and nuts since these contain serotonin. Falsely elevated values occur in patients taking glyceryl guaiacolate, phenacetin and mephenesin. Falsely low values may be caused by phenothiazines, methenamine mandelate, methyldopa, ethanol and monoamine oxidase inhibitors.

In those patients in whom the tumors lack decarboxylase, 5-HT and 5-HTP levels are useful since urinary 5-HIAA may be high or low in this group. This finding also helps to localize the tumor to the foregut.

Blood serotonin levels may aid in the diagnosis. Histamine, bradykinin and

PGE levels are available in some laboratories. When multiple endocrinopathies or foregut tumors are present, measurement of glucose, calcium, electrolytes, cortisol, gastrin, glucagon, insulin, ACTH, growth hormone, parathyrin and calcitonin may be useful.

Provocative tests include the epinephrine test and calcium infusion test. The epinephrine test may be hazardous, but when it is necessary for diagnosis, increasing doses of epinephrine, beginning at 1 μg, are given at ten minute intervals until a flush occurs. A positive test is thought to be secondary to kallekrein release mediated by epinephrine. The dangers of hypotension, bronchoconstriction and tachycardia make it imperative that the test be done under strict control.

Calcium infusion can produce the same symptoms and is generally considered to be a safer test, although hypotension and bronchoconstriction may still occur. Blood serotonin levels are found to be elevated in patients with carcinoid tumors upon stimulation by calcium.

Localization of the tumor may be accomplished with routine roentgenograms, upper and lower gastrointestinal barium studies, angiography, radionuclide scanning, sonography and computerized tomography. Endoscopy of the upper and lower G.I. tract and tracheobronchial tree is also useful. Caution must be exercised in performing biopsies, however, since carcinoids, especially of bronchial origin, are known to bleed massively when biopsied.

Treatment. The treatment of choice for cure or palliation of carcinoid tumors is surgical. In those patients known to have tumors but without functional symptoms, exploration is associated with little risk to the patient. Operative principles include: 1) Resection of as much of the primary tumor as possible to prevent complications of obstruction and ulceration, and 2) removal of as much of the metastatic tumor as possible. Since these tumors are usually slow growing, the patient is more likely to experience humoral effects of an unresected tumor than from its local mass effect. Lesions greater than 1 cm in diameter should be treated as 'frank carcinomas'. Those less than 1 cm may be adequately treated by local resection. Jejuno-ileal carcinoids should be treated by segmental resection if they are small and by radical resection of all lymph node-bearing tissue if there is any evidence of invasion.

Appendiceal carcinoids that are found incidentally and that appear not to have metastasized are adequately treated with removal of the appendix and mesoappendix. However, if lymph node involvement or local invasion is present, or if the lesion is greater than 1 cm in diameter, a right hemicolectomy with wide node dissection should be performed.

Rectal carcinoids should be excised transanally if they are less than 2 cm in size. Frequent proctoscopic examinations are then suggested. If invasion of the muscularis is present or if the lesion is larger, treatment as for a 'frank carcinoma' is appropriate. Other colon carcinoids behave as malignancies and should be treated as such.

Gastric carcinoids require gastrectomy and node dissection. Associated ulcers should be treated with a standard ulcer operation. Tumors present in the duodenum may be resected if small, but if they are invasive or arise in the head of the pancreas, a radical pancreaticoduodenectomy is indicated.

Bronchial carcinoids may be removed by lobectomy or pneumonectomy. Ovarian tumors can similarly be resected in their entirety.

Palliative resections and/or bypass operations for obstruction may be necessary for the poor risk patient with widespread metastases[22].

In symptomatic patients with a functional carcinoid tumor surgical intervention must be undertaken with caution. Many of these patients exhibit a paradoxic response to endogenous or exogenous epinephrine release, which has become known as 'bradykinin shock'. For this reason all anesthetic agents capable of producing this response should be avoided. Similarly, alpha receptor agonists such as neosynephrine (phenylephrine) and Vasoxyl (methoxiamine) should be available if a vasoconstrictor is needed during induction of anesthesia. An endotracheal tube should be used and curare avoided because of the potential effects of bronchospasm.

The same principles of resection apply in patients with the carcinoid syndrome as in those with only the carcinoid tumor present. Additionally, however, liver metastases will usually be present. Local enucleation of these metastases has been shown to be of some benefit[23]. Formal hepatic lobectomy may be performed if the involvement is confined to one lobe. Hepatic dearterialization or placement of an hepatic artery infusion catheter for chemotherapy are also possible choices for palliation[24–27].

Chemotherapy of carcinoid tumors is of some benefit. Agents that have been used include cyclophosphamide, methotrexate, 5-fluorouracil and streptozotocin. These have been administered peripherally or directly into the hepatic circulation with varying results.

Diarrhea will often respond to narcotics, including paregoric, codeine, tincture of opium or lomotil. Methysergide, a serotonin antagonist, used in doses from 2 mg to 16 mg daily may ameliorate this symptom. Cyproheptadine, an antiserotonin, antihistamine drug, in 1 to 4 mg doses Q.I.D., may be effective in relieving diarrhea. Five-fluorotryptophan, an analog of 5-HTP, has relieved diarrhea and decreased 5-HIAA levels when given in a dose of 200 mg T.I.D. for a year. Tumor size, however, remained unchanged[28]. Parachlorophenylalanine (PCPA) is an inhibitor of tryptophan hydroxylase and available only on an experimental basis.

Flushing may be controlled by the alpha blocker phenoxybenzamine given in doses of 10 to 20 mg per day. Prednisone is effective in treating the flushing associated with bronchial carcinoids. Patients whose tumors secrete 5-HTP may receive symptomatic relief from flushing with the decarboxylase inhibitor, methyldopa. Phenothiazines have also been effective for flushing secondary to foregut carcinoids. The administration of histamine-1 and histamine-2 receptor blockers together has been shown to inhibit the flush associated with gastric carcinoids. Somatostatin may also be effective here. Frolich *et al.* have reported two patients with carcinoid tumors wherein infusion of 100–500 μg of somatostatin per hour completely inhibited pentagastrin-stimulated flushing [29].

Bronchoconstriction may respond favorably to inhalation of beta adrenergic agents such as epinephrine and isoproterenol, but these must be used cautiously because of their known adverse effects of flushing and hypotension in these patients. Pellagra-like symptoms may be relieved by niacin replacement in the form of a simple multivitamin pill daily.

Prognosis. Long term survival is dependent upon the site of the primary tumor, its stage, and the completeness of surgical excision. Appendiceal carcinoids have the best overall prognosis, 99% five-year survival; lung and bronchial and rectal carcinoids average an 85% five-year survival. Colon, small intestine and gastric varieties have the poorest outlook with the five-year survival of approximately 50%.

Tumors demonstrating only local invasiveness are associated with over 90% five-year survival. Those with regional node metastases average 60% five-year survival and where distant spread is present, five-year survival drops to 20% [30].

Many of these patients will live for extended periods with their tumors only to be harassed by the symptoms of this functional syndrome.

2.1.2. The Glucagonoma (Diabetogenic-Dermatitis) Syndrome

History. The presence of mild diabetes mellitus, dermatitis, glossitis, anemia and weight loss associated with a pancreatic tumor was first described in a 45-year-old female by Becker in 1942 [31]. A glucagon-secreting alpha cell tumor of the pancreas was documented by McGavran *et al.* in 1966 as the culprit responsible for similar clinical features found in a 42-year-old housewife [32]. This was made possible, at least in part, by Unger's introduction of a specific radioimmunoassay for glucagon in 1963 [33]. The classic dermatologic description of the rash was defined and named necrotizing migratory erythema by Wilkinson in 1971 [34]. The concept of the glucagonoma syndrome was solidified by Mallinson in 1974 when he reported an additional nine cases and described the clinical manifestations, including dermatitis, diabetes, weight loss and anemia [35]. Since then attention has focused on the relationship between hyperglucagonemia, the tumor and the mechanism for the production of the symptoms. Indeed, many of the details are still unclear.

Pathology. These tumors are found in the sites normally harboring alpha islet cells, notably the tail, body, neck and superior portion of the head of the pancreas. The primary tumor may remain small, but most are greater than 3 cm when found at operation. Metastases to the liver are common and often involve both lobes.

Microscopically, the tumor is composed of variously-sized cells, with some-what enlarged nuclei. Mitoses are infrequent. Cells may be arranged in trabe-cular, glandular, follicular or haphazard patterns, interwoven with variable amounts of connective tissue, depending on the level of differentiation. A rich vascular network is generally present in the more malignant tumors. Histochemically, tumor cells react as do normal alpha cells.

Electron microscopy reveals numerous secretory granules, averaging 200 nm in diameter, which are somewhat smaller than beta cell granules and are limited by an agranular membrane. The granules differ from those of normal alpha cells only in that they vary more in size.

Indirect immunofluorescent studies generally reveal only glucagon reac-tivity.

Although it is uncertain whether all glucagonomas produce glucagon at an excessive rate, it is clear that they release it in an abnormal way. The tumors themselves may contain variable amounts of the hormone and this may reflect differences in storage and secretory rates.

Glucagon is a polypeptide that has been found to exist in human plasma in a number of molecular sizes. All of these have identical immunoreactivity, suggesting a common terminal peptide. Biologic activity, on the other hand, may be different and may be responsible, in part, for the variety of clinical presentations. Glucagon is catabolic, lowers plasma amino acids, and enhances hepatic uptake and deamination of amino acids, resulting in gly-cogen and glucose formation. Its lypolytic effects result in increased gluco-neogenesis. It appears to be intimately involved in the regulation of the entero-insular axis and glucose metabolism. Glucagon suppresses gastric secretory activity and inhibits gastric, jejunal and colonic motility. It lowers serum calcium by inducing hypercalcuria and stimulating release of calcitonin. It also exerts direct chronotropic and inotropic influences on the heart.

Most patients with glucagonomas present with various manifestations of the cutaneous syndrome, which consist of necrotizing migratory erythema, glossitis, anemia, weight loss, diabetes mellitus, depression and venous thrombosis. However, there are patients who present only with diabetes and hyperglucagonemia who have malignant glucagonoma. Others with pluriglan-dular syndromes show alpha cell hyperplasia, adenomatosis, adenomas or carcinomas without elevated glucagon levels and with a clinical picture characteristic of one of the other endocrine tumors. Of the 47 patients reported in the literature, 28 have been females. Patients have ranged in age from 20 to 73 with a mean age of 56 at the time of diagnosis [36].

The rash commonly involves the perineum, lower abdomen and lower extremities and has a tendency to migrate. Glossitis and angular cheilitis are usually present. It begins as a slightly raised erythematous patch, which is extremely friable and easily rubbed off, with resultant secondary infection. As the lesion migrates, the old central areas heal, displaying brown pigmentation while the erythematous boundaries lend a geographic appearance. The lesions are easily confused with atypical forms of psoriasis, pemphigus or eczema and resemble acrodermatitis enteropathica. Histologically the superficial epidermis shows necrosis with underlying vesicles or bullae.

The diabetes associated with the syndrome is usually mild and most often responds to oral hypoglycemic agents. No known reports of the usual complications of diabetes, such as ketoacidosis, retinopathy, neuropathy or nephropathy have been recorded. In most patients there is an associated hyperinsulinism, which is probably partially responsible for the mildness of the diabetic state.

A normochromic, normocytic anemia almost always accompanies the rash in these patients. The pathogenesis of this finding is not clear but more than one half of the patients have had normal erythropoiesis and iron stores on marrow examinations. Hemoglobin concentration returns to normal with control of the rash.

Weight loss is universal in this population and is thought to be related to the catabolic effects of glucagon which result in hypoaminoacidemia. In the later stages of the disease, malnutrition and massive liver replacement by tumor exacerbate the situation.

Deep vein thrombosis has been reported in 30% of cases and pulmonary embolism has also occurred. One-third of all patients have been described as severely depressed. This is considered secondary to the humoral products of the tumor but the exact mechanism is unknown. Some patients may exhibit episodic diarrhea or constipation, but these are by no means constant findings.

Diagnosis. The diagnosis of this syndrome begins with a high index of suspicion on the part of the clinician when confronted with a patient displaying the characteristic rash, diabetes mellitus and anemia. This should lead to a determination of the plasma glucagon level. Traditionally, fasting samples have been used but this requirement is not necessary. Dilantin and cytotoxic drugs lower glucagon levels and can be diagnostically confusing in interpretation of results. All patients reported thus far, however, have had consistently

358   S.R. FRIESEN and J.B. PETELIN.

high values.

Stimulation tests include the glucose tolerance test, tolbutamide infusion test, arginine infusion test and the glucagon provacative test. The glucose tolerance test yeilds blood glucose levels in the diabetic range. Oral administration of glucose in these patients leads to a marked increase in plasma glucagon, whereas normal subjects show a modest depression of plasma glucagon. Intravenous glucose, however, produces a decline in the glucagon levels in the glucagonoma patient. Tolbutamide given intravenously normally depresses glucagon thereby lowering blood glucose; however, patients with glucagonoma display a sharp rise in glucagon, a slow rise in insulin and a modest fall in glucose. Arginine infusion normally stimulates insulin and glucagon release but in these patients the increase is dramatic in absolute and relative terms. The intravenous administration of glucagon in a patient with a glucagonoma does not significantly raise the blood sugar or insulin concentration (i.e. flat glucose tolerance curve) as it does in normal patients.

Localization of the tumor and possible metastases may be effectively achieved by radionuclide scans, sonography, computerized tomography, angiography or endoscopic retrograde cholangiopancreatography (ERCP). Alternatively, pancreatic venous and arterial assays may define the location of the tumor.

Treatment. The treatment of choice for all glucagonomas is surgical excision. When the tumor is in the head of the pancreas this will entail pancreaticoduodenectomy. Focal metastases to the liver should be excised, if possible, and if localized to one lobe, may be amenable to hepatic lobectomy. When the primary tumor, but not the metastases can be removed, it is prudent to do so, along with consideration of placement of an hepatic artery catheter for subsequent chemotherapy.

Chemotherapy has most commonly involved streptozotocin. A number of reports have shown its effectiveness in reducing plasma glucagon levels, decreasing the rash and improving the patient's well-being. The most successful regimen consists of intravenous administration of 1.5 g/M^2 of streptozotocin daily for six weeks [37]. 5-Fluorouracil and diaminotrizaineimidazole carboxamide (DTIC) have been used empirically. DTIC effectively lowered the glucagon levels and improved the necrolytic migratory erythema in one patient [38].

Diphenylhydantoin given as 1 g daily for 5 days has been shown to have antisecretory effects thereby lowering glucagon levels. This may be used as an adjunct to other chemotherapy.

Somatostatin has been shown to suppress glucagon production by the tumor [39].

The necrolytic migratory erythema (NME) has been treated successfully with methotrexate, corticosteroids, tetracycline, zinc and somatostatin. Topical antiseptic and antifungal agents are useful for proven superinfection.

Prognosis. Little is known about the prognosis for patients with glucagonoma. The tumor itself is considered slow-growing and in Mallinson's review, 1974, histories spanning ten years were documented prior to diagnosis [35]. Higgins reported survivors eight and 12 years after the diagnosis was made. In one case a subtotal pancreatectomy had been done five years before documentation of liver metastases and 12 years before death and in the other case only biopsies of a huge pancreatic mass were performed [36].

2.1.3. The Insulinoma (Hypoglycemic) Syndrome

History. In 1902 the anatomic features of an islet cell adenoma were described by Nicholls [40]. Twenty years later Banting and Best discovered insulin [41]. In 1924 Harris reported three cases of spontaneous hyperinsulinism, the features of which resembled those of overdosage of exogenous insulin, including central nervous system changes in mentation, memory and personality [42]. The demonstration of the presence of insulin in lymph node metastases was made by Wilder in 1927 [43]. The first cure of hyperinsulinism came in 1929 when Graham removed a functioning islet cell tumor [44]. In 1935 Whipple and Frantz added a report of six cases of insulinomas to the existing 11 reported cases and established more firm criteria called, Whipple's Triad, for the diagnosis of insulinoma [45]. Since then considerable knowledge and experience with this syndrome has led to earlier diagnosis and more precise localization of the tumor(s). Advances in the medical management of those cases not amenable to surgery have also been made.

Pathology. Approximately 85% of insulinomas occur as solitary benign adenomas. Multiple tumors are present with an approximate incidence of 10%. There is no usual location of the adenomas having been found to be evenly distributed throughout the pancreas [46]. Occasionally, these tumors are found in the duodenum or periduodenal tissues. Generalized hyperplasia of the islets has also been held responsible for hypoglycemic symptoms.

Grossly, benign adenomas are encapsulated and small, 65% being less than 1.5 cm in diameter. Generally these highly vascular tumors appear reddish brown whereas others appear pale yellow. They are generally firmer than the normal pancreas.

Microscopically, the benign adenomas are composed of small prismatic cells with cytoplasmic secretory granules. The cells are arranged in alveolar patterns with occasional ductal differentiation. Variable amounts of hyalinization and fibrosis are present. Mitotic activity is not a prominent feature and diagnosis of malignancy is usually dependent on the demonstration of invasion.

Immunoreactivity and immunofluorescent studies show that virtually all insulinomas stain with suitably prepared anti-insulin immunochemical stains.

Both insulinomas and normal pancreatic beta cells produce insulin. It is synthesized as its precursor proinsulin in the endoplasmic reticulum, transformed to insulin with connection of the C chain in the Golgi complex, and stored into beta granules. Both insulin and proinsulin are normally secreted into the circulation and although the half-life of proinsulin is much longer than that of insulin, it normally constitutes only 25% of the total plasma immunoreactive insulin. The biological properties of the two peptides are the same but on a molar basis, proinsulin has only 10% to 25% of the activity of insulin.

Insulin is known for its ability to lower blood glucose concentration. This is accomplished through inhibition of gluconeogenesis and glycogenolysis. The net result is restriction of inflow of glucose into the body glucose pool. The free outflow of glucose from the extracellular fluid to dependent tissues appears to be significant only in the case of the red blood cell and the brain, and these demands are usually met by the steady glucose release from the liver, which is only partially inhibited by the small amount of insulin present in the portal blood. The ability of insulin to stimulate glucose uptake by the tissues apparently plays only an insignificant role in the pathogenesis of hypoglycemia secondary to insulinoma.

The amount of insulin released into the blood is under feedback control mechanisms, one of which is the glucose concentration of the blood perfusing the pancreas. As blood glucose falls to the 30–35 mg/dl levels, insulin release normally ceases. This mechanism is uniquely absent in insulinoma cells, such that they function more or less autonomously, allowing the blood glucose to fall to dangerously low levels. Eventually the central nervous system becomes glycopenic and characteristic symptoms follow.

Clinical presentation. The incidence of insulinomas appears to be from one per 10^6 to five per 10^5 persons annually. Women are affected only slightly more often than men – approximately 55% of cases. The average age at the time of diagnosis is 42 [46].

These patients behave normally between attacks of hypoglycemia. However, when exposed to prolonged periods of fasting, such as occurs overnight, or when increased glucose demands are present, such as during exercise, the hypoglycemia syndrome becomes manifest. The clinical presentation during an episode depends largely on the rapidity of the fall in glucose concentration. If it occurs rapidly, epinephrine release will be stimulated and the classical signs of an adrenergic barrage will appear. These include nervousness, tachycardia and sweating. If the fall in glucose concentration is slower, over hours instead of minutes, characteristic central nervous system manifestations will supervene. The symptoms may include bizarre behavior, personality changes, impaired work performance, mental deterioration, amnesia, psychoses (paranoia), seizures and coma. If hypoglycemia occurs repeatedly over a prolonged period of time, permanent idiocy may result.

Many of these patients have been found on psychiatric wards and often their bizarre behavior during attacks has gained for them rather dubious reputations in their community. However, with increased recognition of this entity these sad situations are becoming rare.

Diagnosis. As with other uncommon diseases, the diagnosis of insulinoma begins with a high index of suspicion. This is substantiated by documentation of Whipple's Triad: the presence of central nervous system symptoms associated with a blood glucose level of less than 50 mg/dl, and the relief of those symptoms by glucose administration. But at this point in the diagnostic sequence, even the presence of Whipple's Triad is far from being specific for insulinoma. Indeed, non-pancreatic tumors such as pleural mesothelioma, soft tissue sarcoma, carcinoid, adrenal cortical carcinoma, hepatoma and gastrointestinal carcinoma may produce hypoglycemia.

The test of choice for diagnosis of insulinoma is the measurement of plasma insulin during an episode of spontaneous fasting hypoglycemia. The uncontrolled release of insulin in the face of hypoglycemia is characteristic of insulinoma. The normal range of plasma immunoreactive insulin (IRI) in fasting subjects is reported to be $5-30 \, \mu U/ml$ with an average of $14-19 \, \mu U/ml$. More important than the absolute value of plasma insulin is its relationship to the blood glucose level. This has been characterized as the IRI/glucose ratio, calculated as microunits of insulin/ml and mg glucose/100 ml blood. Under this definition most patients with ratios greater than 0.3 have been proven to have insulinoma [47].

The diazoxide suppression test has been used to demonstrate depression of plasma insulin levels in hypoglycemic patients. The usual dose is 600 mg I.V. over one hour. Failure of response to this infusion suggests either a non-diazoxide suppressible tumor or an error in insulin assay [46].

The ratio of proinsulin to insulin in patients with beta cell tumors is higher than in normals. The highest ratios are generally found in those with malignant tumors.

The tolbutamide stimulation test, which usually produces an exaggerated rise in insulin in patients with insulinoma, is non-specific, dangerous and yields little useful information. It is contraindicated if the blood glucose is 40 mg/dl at the start of the test.

The glucagon stimulation test involves the injection of glucagon 1 mg I.V.

over 2 min with subsequent glucose and insulin measurements. Seventy to 80% of insulinoma patients will have an exaggerated insulinemic response to 150 μU/ml or higher within 5 to 10 min. Because glucagon causes a rise in blood glucose, the test is safer than the tolbutamide test; for that reason the pre-test glucose level need not be known.

Other stimulation tests involve L-leucine, L-arginine and caerulein. The first two tests have little role in establishing the diagnosis today. Caerulein, a pancreozymin-like polypeptide obtained from toad skin, has been shown to stimulate insulin release in insulinoma patients but little is known about its applicability. Glucose tolerance tests are so unpredictable in insulinoma patients that they are of little use; if such a test is performed it should be continued through 6 hours, at which time a low glucose level may be diagnostic.

Localization of the tumor(s) may be attempted in a variety of ways, including celiac angiography, sonography and computerized tomography. Of all the pancreatic apudomas, the insulinoma may be most readily demonstrated by angiography, as is the case in approximately 75 % of instances.

Treatment. Surgical removal of the tumor is the procedure of choice when the diagnosis is insulinoma. With the usual (85%) solitary adenoma simple enucleation is often possible. If such a tumor is deeply embedded within the pancreatic substance a subtotal distal pancreatectomy may be required. When the tumor is present in the head of the pancreas and enucleation is not feasible because of the likelihood of injury and leakage of the duct, a pancreaticoduodenectomy may be necessary. Duodenotomy with local resection may be curative for those tumors located within the wall of the duodenum. In those cases where the tumor cannot be found and a high index of suspicion persists, a distal pancreatectomy may be performed sequentially, removing up to 85–90% of the pancreas. If subsequent microscopic examination of the tissue fails to reveal the tumor(s) and the patient's symptoms do not abate, total pancreatectomy may be necessary. Intraoperative monitoring of glucose levels as an indicator of successful excision or of the presence of a second lesion is a controversial procedure because it is not reliable in all instances [48].

Nonoperative treatment may be indicated for those with nonresectable tumors, those with massive metastases, or for poor surgical risk patients. Dietary adjustments may be of some benefit; multiple small meals, judiciously spaced, with a nighttime snack may avoid hypoglycemia. Some patients do well with a high protein diet. This avoids caloric excess, which commonly leads to obesity in this patient population.

Antihormonal therapy may alleviate some of the symptoms attributed to the tumor. Diazoxide exerts a hyperglycemic effect principally by direct inhibition of insulin release. Although plasma insulin levels return to normal, the hormone accumulates in the beta cell and the tumor continues to grow.

Diphenylhydantoin is also a known hyperglycemic agent which inhibits insulin secretion [49] and has been effective in some insulinoma patients refractory to other therapy. There are many patients, however, who do not respond to this drug.

Somatostatin has been shown to inhibit insulin release. Although it is still available for investigational use only, it promises to be helpful especially in those with inoperable tumors [50]. Corticosteroids have proved useful to reverse hypoglycemia and to potentiate the effects of other modes of therapy. Their long-term use is not without well-known side effects.
Antitumor chemotherapy currently focuses on streptozotocin, a naturally occurring nitrosourea isolated from the fermentation cultures of *Streptomyces achromogenes*. It appears to selectively destroy beta cells. At daily doses of 500 mg/M^2 for five days patients have been effectively treated. Reduction of the tumor mass has been reported in 48% of cases and complete remission in 17% of those with islet cell carcinomas [51]. Adverse effects include renal tubular damage and the production of renal adenomas and hepatomas in rodents. Alloxan is toxic to islet cells, and although it increases blood glucose levels, its overall toxicity is too great to warrant its use in humans. 5-Fluorouracil and alkylating agents met with little success in treating islet cell carcinomas.

Radiotherapy may achieve some measure of palliation but it is not frequently advocated and should probably be used only when all else fails.

Prognosis. The long-term outlook is dependent on the nature of the tumor, whether it is benign or malignant, solitary or multifocal, and whether metastases are present. For those with benign disease, cure rates following surgical treatment approach or exceed 90% [48].

2.1.4. The Somatostatinoma (Inhibitory) Syndrome
History. The association of hypochlorhydria, steatorrhea and diabetes mellitus in a patient with a pancreatic Delta-cell tumor containing large amounts of the polypeptide, somatostatin, was first described by Larrson in 1977 [52]. This report followed only four short years after the isolation and characterization of somatostatin from the hypothalamus by Brazeau, and only two years after its localization to the delta cell population of the pancreas [53]. The syndrome is sometimes called the inhibitory syndrome because of the inhibitory characteristics of somatostatin (SST) or somatotrophin-release-inhibiting factor (SRIF).

Pathophysiology. The delta cells, which store and secrete somatostatin, appear to be located between the alpha and beta cells of the islets, such that much of their function is thought to be of a paracrine nature[54]. However, when neoplastic, elevated levels of somatostatin can be found in the pancreatic and hepatic veins, suggesting true endocrine function. Primary pancreatic tumors are composed of solid nests and cords of cells forming ribbons or follicular patterns surrounded by cuboidal or columnar cells and penetrated by bands of connective tissue. Typically multiple granules are present in the cytoplasm on electron microscopy and stain strongly with somatostatin antiserum. Mitoses are infrequent. Radioimmunoassay shows tumors of this cell type to contain large amounts of immunoreactivity to somatostatin[55].

Having received its name because of its inhibitory effect on the release of growth hormone, the tetradecapeptide somatostatin has since been shown to have many other peripheral effects. These include inhibition of function of alpha and beta pancreatic islet cells, G.I. mucosa, thyroid follicles, and the juxtaglomerular apparatus in the kidney. Somatostatin suppresses the release of gastrin, CCK, secretin, GIP and substances with glucagon-like immunoreactivity. Somatostatin lowers the basal and stimulated levels of insulin, glucagon and pancreatic polypeptide. It decreases splanchnic blood flow, hydrochloric acid secretion, gallbladder contraction, duodenal motility, pancreatic exocrine function and the absorption of glucose and xylose. Physiologically, it is thought to regulate nutrient entry from the gut by a negative feedback mechanism[54].

Clinical presentation. Excessive production of somatostatin may present a variety of gastrointestinal manifestations. Its pharmacologic action on the stomach, including decreased hydrochloric acid response to pentagastrin, histamine and meals, decreased pepsin response to meals, and slowed gastric emptying lead to dyspepsia and postprandial fullness. Intestinal reactions to somatostatin include impaired absorption of amino acids and fat and motility changes. This results in indigestion. Decreased gallbladder contractility leads to bile stasis and cholelithiasis. Somatostatin's effect on the endocrine and exocrine pancreas is responsible for the appearance of diabetes mellitus, maldigestion and steatorrhea[56]. Six patients with somatostatinoma have been reported in the literature[52, 55–59]. The most common clinical findings in this group include diabetes mellitus, steatorrhea, cholelithiasis and weight loss. Hypochlorhydria was found in three of the four patients in whom it was studied. Liver metastases were present in all but one patient at the time of diagnosis.

Diagnosis. Early diagnosis is difficult since initial features, dyspepsia, mild diabetes mellitus and cholelithiasis, are non-specific and common in the older age group (46–70 years) in which the tumor has been found. Stimulation of somatostatin release by tolbutamide administration may reveal early cases. However, a high index of suspicion and localization of the tumor by sonography, CT scanning or angiography may be necessary to identify benign disease. Steatorrhea appears to be a late manifestation of the disease since the only patient reported without metastases had none. An elevated plasma level on assay for somatostatin confirms the diagnosis.

Treatment. Surgical removal of the tumor is currently the treatment of choice. Four of the six reported patients underwent Whipple's procedure of radical pancreaticoduodenectomy. One patient underwent an exploratory laporatomy only, and one patient was treated with streptozotocin. The only known survivor is Ganda's patient who has no metastases, underwent pancreaticoduodenectomy and is asymptomatic four years postoperatively [56].

2.1.5. *The Pancreatic Polypeptide (MEA, I) Syndrome*

History. Pancreatic polypeptide, discovered by Kimmel *et al.* [60] during the process of purification of insulin from chicken pancreas, was shown to be present in mammals by Lin and Chance in 1974 [61]. Floyd *et al.* in 1977 found increased levels of this hormone in the serum of some patients with multiple endocrine adenopathy, type I [62]. Larsson *et al.* have reported on a patient with watery diarrhea and a predominantly hPP-secreting pancreatic tumor [63]; Tomita *et al.* have described a similar clinical picture in a patient with pancreatic islet hyperplasia of hPP cell origin [64]. Polak *et al.* have found elevated hPP levels in the plasma of 18 or 28 patients with pancreatic islet neoplasms, including five of eight with the Zollinger-Ellison syndrome [65]. Recently, plasma hPP elevations have led to the discovery and excision of asymptomatic pure polypeptide and mixed pancreatic apudomas in three MEA, I patients; moreover, exaggerated plasma hPP response to a protein meal is indicative of familial islet cell hyperplasia [66]. Thus, plasma hPP determinations appear to be important in the detection of the pancreatic component of MEA, type I.

Pathology. Human polypeptide-containing cells have been identified only in the pancreas. These F (or D_1) cells normally are interspersed in the islets and parenchyma of the posterior portion of the pancreatic head. Pancreatic apudomas, however, occur in all portions of the pancreas and the cells containing hPP have been isolated not only in tumors, but also in extratumoral islets, suggesting that hPP may be an additional marker for mixed functioning pancreatic lesions. However, pure primary hPP-cell hyperplasia and hPP-cell tumors have been described. Larsson reported on a patient with a diarrheogenic syndrome indistinguishable from the classical WDHA syndrome of Verner and Morrison. This patient's tumor contained only hPP and plasma levels of hPP were markedly elevated, while vasoactive intestinal polypeptide (VIP) levels were normal [63]. Bordi reported on a 45-year-old man with recurrent ulcer and two pancreatic tumors which contained only hPP [67]. Tomita reported on a patient with severe watery diarrhea associated with pancreatic hyperplasia of hPP-containing cells [64]. Admittedly, the role of hPP in sporadic functioning islet cell tumors is less clear than its role in the genetic MEA, I pancreatic endocrinopathy.

While its biological activity is still somewhat elusive, some of the pharmacologic effects of hPP are known. This 36 amino acid polypeptide generally acts in opposition to cholecystokinin-pancreozymin (CCK-PZ). It inhibits pancreatic exocrine function, relaxes the gallbladder, increases choledochal tone and inhibits pentagastrin-stimulated gastric acid secretion [68]. Human pancreatic polypeptide levels normally increase after an ingested meal (enteric response) and in the presence of insulin hypoglycemia (vagal response). Pancreatic popypeptide is also released after bombesin (an amphibian dermal tetradecapeptide) infusion. Bombesin-like peptides have been found scattered throughout the endocrine and nerve cells of the gastrointestinal tract in man. Bombesin's ability to stimulate release of pancreatic polypeptide, gastrin and gastric acid suggest the possibility of a complex neurohormonal regulatory mechanism [68]. Normal levels of hPP increase with the age of the patient, while levels are decreased in patients with cystic fibrosis of the pancreas.

Clinical presentation. Although elevated hPP levels have been found in a variety of settings, no consistent clinical picture has been associated with plasma hPP excess. Commonly, elevated hPP levels are present in association with excess hormone production from mixed pancreatic tumors. In such instances the other hormonal products of the tumor usually give rise to symptoms and thereby mask whatever biologic and clinical effect hPP may have. Larsson, however, in an attempt to unravel the mystery of the WDHA syndrome, suggested that hPP might be responsible for the pancreatic source of the diarrheogenic syndrome, while VIP might be the agent in neurogenous tumors that cause diarrhea [63]. Diarrhea is not a clinical feature of most pure hPP apudomas; therefore Larsson's patient is probably an isolated example. Lamers *et al.* have demonstrated elevated levels of hPP in patients with the Zollinger-Ellison syndrome and also with hyperparathyroidism in MEA, type I, as compared to normal controls; these endocrinopathies are integral components of the MEA, I syndrome and may thus signal an undetected islet abnormality [69].

Diagnosis. In families at risk for the development of endocrinopathies within the MEA, type I syndrome, the use of plasma hPP assays in both basal and stimulated states is diagnostic. Significantly elevated basal and meal-stimulated levels of hPP in these patients suggest the presence of a pancreatic tumor, while a normal basal value with an exaggerated response to a meal indicates islet hyperplasia. Those with normal basal and stimulated values have not been found to have hyperplasia or pancreatic tumors. Thus hPP appears to be a specific marker for the pancreatic component of MEA, type I and may be elevated in approximately 50% of non-familial sporadic pancreatic apudomas. The greatest usefulness of the hPP assay is in the prospective screening of MEA, I patients for the detection of silent pancreatic apudomas, as has been reported in three asymptomatic patients whose basal hPP levels were elevated. By this means early diagnosis has prompted surgical excision before metastases were evident. Confirmation by CT scan and/or angiography is advisable preoperatively. Another indication for the use of plasma hPP assays is in the differentiation between the antral (entopic) and the pancreatic (ectopic) hypergastrinemia of the ulcerogenic syndromes. Basal plasma hPP concentrations are elevated in approximately half of patients with pancreatic gastrinomas of the sporadic Zollinger-Ellison syndrome; a normal basal, but highly elevated stimulated plasma hPP response is indicative of antral G-cell hyperplasia (AGCH) type of the ulcerogenic syndrome, as well as in islet hyperplasia in the familial MEA, I syndrome. Plasma hPP assays are also indicated in the diagnosis of the watery diarrhea syndrome for the differentiation between the pancreatic and a neurogenic source of the secretory diarrhea. Normal levels of basal hPP must be interpreted in light of age-matched controls since the normal levels increase with age. The basal value is not considered abnormal unless it is three and one half or four times the age-matched mean including two standard deviations [66].

Treatment. Surgical excision of the tumor and metastases, if possible, is the treatment of choice in most instances. If the ulcerogenic syndrome is present, then total gastrectomy is probably warranted in addition, depending on patient compliance with cimetidine therapy. Guidelines for specific antitumor or antihormonal therapy in situations where mixed tumors are present should be determined by the nature of the primary product. In patients with hepatic metastases from a resected pure pancreatic polypeptide apudoma of the pancreas, selective (intra-arterial) and systemic (intravenous) administration of streptozotocin has resulted in 'complete' disappearance of the metastases on serial CT scanning, together with a return of elevated plasma hPP values to normal [70].

Prognosis. The prognosis in patients with mixed functioning pancreatic apudomas generally follows that of the specific syndrome present. In those whose hPP levels fall following surgical removal of the tumor or antitumor chemotherapy, the outlook is good, but long-term studies in relation to pure hPP tumors are not complete.

2.2. Ectopic

2.2.1. The Gastrinoma (Ulcerogenic, Z-E) Syndrome

History. In 1905 Edkins speculated that a humoral substance, which be called gastric secretin (gastrin), was released by the antral mucosa upon gastric absorption of certain foodstuffs, and that this hormone, in turn, stimulated gastric parietal cells [10]. Subsequently it was shown that a variety of factors caused elaboration of this hormone, including alkalinization of the antrum, absorption of proteins and distension of the stomach. In 1951, Dragstedt *et al.* demonstrated that experimental hyperfunction of the gastric antrum, sutured to the colon as a diverticulum, caused gastrojejunal ulcers in dogs [71]. Four years later, in 1955, Zollinger and Ellison presented two cases of the ulcerogenic syndrome, pointing out a triad of features, duodenojejunal ulceration, gastric hypersecretion and a non-beta islet cell tumor of the pancreas [9]. This was the first clinical example of an extra-gastric source of the hormone, thus an ectopic phenomenon. In the early 1960s, Gregory purified the substance, 'gastrin' and demonstrated its presence in extracts of the pancreatic tumor and its metastases [72]. Its subsequent characterization has fully accounted for all the manifestations of the tumor and syndrome. Experience and investigation over the last 25 years has led to a better understanding of the pathogenesis, diagnosis and treatment of this and other islet cell tumors of the pancreas.

Pathology. The gastrin-secreting tumor is most often located in the islets of the pancreas. However, tumors have been found in the wall of the duodenum, the stomach, in the hilus of the spleen and rarely in other endocrine organs. Solitary lesions occur in 50% of cases with a head–body–tail ratio of 4–1–4. Multiple sites are present in approximately 30% of cases and diffuse hyperplasia in 15–20%. Duodenal wall tumors were found in 13% of patients with more than half of this group bearing an additional pancreatic tumor site. Benign adenomas account for less than 30% of cases, with the remainder being hyperplasias or metastatic malignant lesions [73].

None of the identified normal entopic islet cells appears to be the parent of the pancreatic gastrinoma except that any of the APUD islet cells may have reverted to its primitive totipotential state for the ectopic secretion of gastrin. The cells contain secretory granules, as seen on electron microscopy, which are 150–250 μm in size. Histochemically the cells contain gastrin and are microscopically similar to the antral G-cells, which also produce gastrin. As with most of the other APUD tumors, mitotic activity is not a prominent histologic feature and these tumors are generally considered to be slow-growing. Metastases occur primarily in adjacent lymph nodes and the liver. Rarely, lung metastases have been observed.

Gastrin in several molecular forms is the primary product of the tumor and its effect upon target cells is responsible for the clinical manifestations of the syndrome. It exists in at least three known forms: G-17 gastrin, G-34 (big) gastrin and big, big gastrin (MW 21,000). The most active form appears to be G-17 gastrin. Physiologically it sprincipal role is stimulation of parietal cell secretion of gastric acids. Pharmacologically it affects almost every gastrointestinal organ. It causes contraction of the lower esophageal sphincter and the smooth muscle of the stomach, small intestine, colon and gallbladder. It inhibits the pyloric sphincter, the ileocecal valve and sphincter of Oddi. Moreover, it may have a trophic effect in that is appears to stimulate growth of gastric and duodenal mucosa. Pathophysiologically it accounts for the hyperplasia of the gastric mucosa, which results in hypersecretion of acid and subsequent severe acid-peptic ulcer disease. The continuous high rate of acid secretion leads to acidification of a much longer length of duodenum and jejunum and is felt to be responsible for ulcers seen in these atypical sites and for the steatorrhea, which is often present [74].

Clinical presentation. Over 1000 cases have been recorded in the Tumor Registry at the Medical College of Wisconsin. The age at onset of the disease is commonly in the third to fifth decade of life. However, approximately 8% of cases occurred in patients less than 20 years of age. Males are affected more often than females with a 6:4 ratio.

The classic triad of findings includes the presence of severe peptic ulceration, gastric hypersecretion and an islet cell tumor of the pancreas. The ulcerrations, usually of the duodenum, also occur in the distal duodenum, jejunum or in 25% of cases as recurrent stomal ulcers [73].

Abdominal pain is the most common symptom due to ulceration in 93% of patients. Vomiting, hemorrhage and perforation may occur in approximately 25% of the patients. Diarrhea (steatorrhea) is present in one-third of the patients and is secondary to the effect of the large volumes of gastric juice on the small bowel mucosa with acid inactivation of the pancreatic fat-splitting enzymes [74].

Although most patients with the Zollinger-Ellison syndrome represent sporadic occurrences, upon prospective endocrine observation and family screening, an increasing number are found to have a genetic, familial basis. The multiplicity of cellular and endocrine organ associations in multiple members of families tends to involve the pancreas, the pituitary and the parathyroid glands in a dominant fashion, called multiple endocrine adenopathy (MEA, type I) syndrome of Wermer [75].

In addition to the usual ectopic Zollinger-Ellison syndrome due to pancreaticoduodenal gastrinoma of both the sporadic and genetic forms, there is an unusual and rare type of the ulcerogenic syndrome that is entopic in origin. In such patients the ulceration, hyperacidity and the hypergastrinemia is the result of the entopic elaboration of excessive gastrin from hyperplastic G-cells of the antrum. This entity, antral G-cell hyperplasia (AGCH), is clinically indistinguishable from the Zollinger-Ellison syndrome, except that a pancreatic gastrinoma is absent. Furthermore, the moderate hypergastrinemia is not further elevated by secretin or calcium stimulation and endoscopic biopsy of the antral mucosa reveals G-cell hyperplasia, all of which differentiate this entopic type from the ectopic pancreatic gastrinoma patients[76].

Diagnosis. The diagnosis of either the ectopic or entopic ulcerogenic syndromes should be suspected in the following individuals: 1) those with onset of severe peptic ulcer disease at a young age; 2) post-bulbar, jejunal or gastrojejunal stomal ulcers; 3) radiographic evidence of gastric hyperrugosity, duodenal nodularity or intestinal hypermotility; 4) unexplained diarrhea; 5) a strong family history of peptic ulcer; and, 6) other endocrine abnormalities or diabetes mellitus.

Documentation of the presence of an ulcer is generally made with upper gastrointestinal barium studies or endoscopy. The X-rays may also reveal prominent gastric rugal folds with a large amount of gastric fluid and hypermotility of the intestine. Gastric secretion in excess of 1000 ml during a 12 hour overnight collection is found in 85% of cases. Similarly, secretion of greater than 100 milliequivalents (mEq) of free acid during the same time period occurs 75% of the time[73]. Basal acid output (BAO) of greater than 15 mEq/hr and a ratio of basal acid output/maximal acid output (BAO/MAO), as determined by histamine stimulation, greater than 0.6 strongly suggests gastrinoma. Patients with Zollinger-Ellison syndrome have fasting serum gastrin concentrations ranging from 300 to 350,000 pg/ml with a median of 2000. Normal fasting serum gastrin levels range from 20 to 160 pg/ml[77].

Provocative tests include the calcium infusion test and the secretin infusion test. Calcium gluconate, given intravenously in a dose of 4–5 mg/kg/hr for three hours produces a twofold or more increase in gastrin levels in the ectopic Zollinger-Ellison patients. Maximum levels are reached in the last hour of the collection. When secretin is given as a bolus injection intravenously (2 units/kg) the serum gastrin rises within 15 minutes. With calcium stimulation, gastrin levels are almost uniformly increased 500 pg/ml or more if a pancreatic gastrinoma is present and secretin stimulation produces increases of 110 pg/ml or more. No rise in serum gastrin concentration is observed in the entopic (antral) type of the ulcerogenic syndrome[78].

The assay of plasma pancreatic polypeptide (hPP) concentration may be helpful in confirming the type and etiology of the ulcerogenic syndrome. It has been shown that 50% of patients with the sporadic pancreatic gastrinoma elaborate excessive hPP in a fasting state; if the pancreatic gastrinoma is due to a genetic, familial etiology the response of hPP to a meal is also usually markedly elevated over the normal response. On the other hand, if a pancreatic gastrinoma is absent (entopic AGCH) the basal hPP level is normal and the response to a meal is exaggerated only if the patient is a member of an MEA family. In other words, an elevated basal level of hPP depends upon the presence of a pancreatic tumor and an elevated response to a protein meal depends upon a genetic familial association [66].

Localization of the pancreatic tumor is often difficult. Both arteriography and computerized tomography may complement each other in improving results since only 40–70% success rates are now achieved with arteriography. Endoscopy is indicated for the detection of duodenal gastrinomas and for antral biopsy for the presence or absence of antral G-cell hyperplasia.

The treatment of choice for the gastrinoma is surgical for its dual role of possible ablation of the tumor and the permanent control of the massive gastric acid hypersecretion by total gastrectomy [76]. The latter objective becomes especially important in patients with multiple or metastatic souces of hypergastrinemia, except in extremely poor risk patients when cimetidine receptor blockade of acid secretion may be preferable. Every attempt should be made to remove all resectable tumor if it can be removed by partial or subtotal pancreatectomy with lymph node excision [79]. Duodenal wall tumors, if detected, are usually resectable but 53% of this group of patients harbor additional gastrinomas [80]. Tumor excision plus total gastrectomy provides the only opportunity for attainment of tumor control and eugastrinemia [76]; occasionally actual regression of metastatic tumor is observed [81]. Before the advent of cimetidine less than total gastrectomy was inevitably followed by recurrent ulceration [80, 82]. Cimetidine, by its antagonistic action on the histamine-2-receptor on the parietal cell effectively suppresses gastric secretion and, combined with antacids, controls ulcer symptoms [83, 84]. Its administration requires careful dose monitoring and complete patient compliance. It has not been shown to have any effect on the tumor itself or on the hypergastrinemia [76, 79]. Patients with proven AGCH are preferably managed by surgical antrectomy, although cimetidine therapy is symptomatically adequate.

Streptozotocin has been infused intra-arterially and intravenously in a number of gastrinoma patients with various results. Encouraging reports from Stadil et al. demonstrated relief of symptoms in two patients and regression of metastases in one patient given 1 to 4 g over 30 to 60 min at 6 and 12 week intervals [85].

Prognosis. Patients with pancreatic gastrinomas may live for extended periods even when metastatic tumor is present if acid hypersecretion is controlled either medically or surgically. Occasionally the course may be fulminant in spite of treatment. Wilson and Ellison reported a 73% survival in patients who had undergone total gastrectomy [86]. One of the two original patients reported by Zollinger and Ellison is alive and well 25 years after total gastrectomy and excision of tumors.

2.2.2. The Vipoma (Watery Diarrhea) Syndrome

History. In 1958 Verner and Morrison reported two patients and cited reports of seven additional patients who presented with profuse watery diarrhea, hypokalemia and non-beta cell tumors of the pancreas [87]. The absence of peptic ulceration in this group led them to the conclusion that this represented a syndrome distinct from the previously reported Zollinger-Ellison syndrome. In 1960 Chears *et al.* resected a non-beta cell adenoma from a patient and thereby cured his diarrhea [88]. The fulminating, relentless diarrhea as a characteristic clinical feature led to the terminology of the syndrome as 'pancreatic cholera' [89]. Murray and Paton in 1961, and Espiner and Beaven in 1962 demonstrated achlorhydria as an accompanying feature of the syndrome [90, 91].

Subsequently, the term WDHA (Watery Diarrhea, Hypokalemia, Achlorhydria) was used to describe the syndrome, although Verner and Morrison believe it is more appropriately labeled WDHH since hypochlorhydria is a more constant finding than achlorhydria. More recently, with the advent of a radioimmunoassay for vasoactive intestinal peptide, and the demonstration of elevated levels of this peptide in many patients with the syndrome, the term Vipoma has been used. Admittedly, the pathogenesis, pathophysiology and the ultimate cellular and hormonal culprits are still less than adequately defined, although more than 60 patients have been reported in the literature [92].

Pathology. Lesions responsible for the clinical manifestations have been localized to the pancreas and may exist as a benign adenoma, a carcinoma, or as a diffuse non-beta islet cell hyperplasia. The solitary lesions are most commonly found in the body and tail of the pancreas.

Grossly, the tumors are usually encapsulated and vary in color from yellow-white to fleshy pink. They are generally larger than other islet cell tumors and range in size from 1 cm to 5–6 cm in diameter. When hyperplasia is present the pancreas may appear and feel normal.

Microscopically the tumors are composed of islet cells that are not identified with any of the normal entopic islet cells; thus they are ectopic in location and function. They are arranged in columns or acini, separated by thin-walled blood vessels. Even electron microscopy has failed to reveal the exact identity of these cells, but it has shown the presence of secretory granules ranging in size from 100 to 150 nm [93, 94].

The precise hormonal product has yet to be documented universally. Several hormones have been ruled out as mediators of the syndrome, glucagon, gastrin, serotonin and secretin. Currently the three humoral products receiving most attention are vasoactive intestinal polypeptide, human pancreatic polypeptide and prostaglandin E_2. While the actions of hPP are not known in great detail, those of VIP and PGE_2 include all of those associated with the syndrome. VIP is a peptide neurotransmitter which stimulates intestinal secretion and diarrhea and pharmacologically relaxes gallbladder smooth muscle, augments bile flow, inhibits gastric secretion and motility, enhances glycogenolysis, thereby inducing hyperglycemia, stimulates pancreatic bicarbonate secretion, produces peripheral vessel dilatation and hypercalcemia [95]. It has been found elevated in a number of patients with tumors, but not consistently.

Jaffe and Condon reported eight of 21 patients with the WDHA syndrome in whom elevated levels of prostaglandin E (PGE) were found [96]. This compound causes contraction of non-vascular smooth muscle, increases intestinal motility and inhibits intestinal absorption of water and electrolytes. Moreover, they reported successful treatment of a patient with the WDHA syndrome and elevated levels of PGE with indomethacin, an inhibitor of prostaglandin synthesis [97].

Larsson et al. reported four cases in which the WDHA (watery diarrhea) syndrome was associated with a pancreatic tumor. In two of these, equal populations of VIP and hPP cells were found to comprise 5-10% of all tumor cells. In another, hPP cells comprised 90% of the tumor while VIP cells were scarce. Moreover, the serum levels of VIP were within normal range while hPP levels were elevated one thousandfold [63].

It appears at this point that the WDHA syndrome is a somewhat collective description of more than one diarrheogenic state which may involve several interrelated hormones.

Clinical presentation. The major clinical manifestations include profuse watery diarrhea, massive potassium losses that result in hypokalemia, and hypochlorhydria or achlorhydria. More than one half of the patients exhibit hypercalcemia, steroid-responsive diarrhea and glucose intolerance. Less frequently tetany, in the face of a normal or high calcium, dilated gallbladder, flushing, dermatitis and psychosis are seen. Congestive heart failure and renal failure are late manifestations of the disease. Females are affected three times more frequently than males. The average age at diagnosis is 47 years with a range of 17-72 years.

The diarrhea is the most profound and disabling symptom. Volumes up to six to eight liters daily have been recorded. The output is described often as having the color and consistency of weak tea. Initially it may be an intermittent phenomenon but with time or malignant change it often becomes explosive and relentless. Hypokalemia is routinely associated with the diarrhea, since massive amounts of potassium, up to 300 mEq per 24 hours, may be lost in the stool. Patients commonly present with potassium levels in the 2 to 3 mEq per liter range. This hypokalemic state, if untreated, leads to vacuolar renal tubular degeneration and ventricular fibrillation.

Basal achlorhydria is found in over one half of the patients although gastric biopsies fail to disclose microscopic abnormalities. Temporary rebound hyperchlorhydria has occurred in some patients following successful excision of the pancreatic tumor.

Tetany is not an uncommon finding in these patients, especially during treatment of their hypokalemia. It is possibly due to hypomagnesemia from the diarrhea. It is this magnesium shortage that is also probably responsible for parathyroid stimulation leading to hypercalcemia [92].

Diagnosis. Because of the lack of a specific tumor marker, establishing the diagnosis of the watery diarrhea, hypokalemia, achlorhydria (WDHA) syndrome requires the exclusion of a number of other possibilities in the differential diagnosis in patients with diarrhea. These include villous adenoma, laxative abuse, celiac disease, Zollinger-Ellison syndrome, carcinoid syndrome, medullary carcinoma of the thyroid, parasitic infestation and inflammatory bowel disease. Specific diagnostic maneuvers include the measurement of gastric acidity with response to histamine stimulation. Intestinal perfusion studies appear to be the most specific indicator of increased jejunal secretion and pancreatic cholera. Hormone analyses for VIP, PGE, hPP, secretin, gastrin, serotonin, thyrocalcitonin and urinary 5-HIAA are usually required for accurate diagnosis.

Localization of the tumor can be accomplished with angiography or computerized tomography. Occasionally an upper gastrointestinal series will show displacement secondary to a large tumor.

The ultimate diagnostic procedure is surgical exploration.

Treatment. The specific therapeutic modality for the WDHA syndrome is excision of the tumor. This is a straightforward matter when a solitary mass is present in the body or tail of the pancreas. If the pancreas appears normal on surgical inspection an excision of the tail of the pancreas may reveal islet hyperplasia on frozen section and histological examination and this should then be followed by subtotal distal pancreatectomy. In the rare circumstance that the patient is still symptomatic and no other cause of the diarrhea is forthcoming, a total pancreatectomy may then be considered. If metastases are present an attempt at resection of as much of the gross tumor as possible should be made because significant palliation is possible by such a procedure [92].

For those tumors not amenable to surgical removal, the diarrhea may be controlled, at least temporarily, by corticosteroid administration. In those patients with high PGE levels, indomethacin has been shown to alleviate the diarrhea.

The most encouraging new development in the medical management of this tumor is its response to streptozotocin. When administered intra-arterially to three patients by Gagel *et al.*, two patients showed dramatic clinical response and regression of the tumor mass [94]. Kahn similarly reported two patients with equally impressive results [98].

Although radiotherapy and 5-fluorouracil have been used, these modalities have not been consistently effective to warrant their routine use.

Prognosis. Of the 64 patients reported by Verner and Morrison, 35% had malignant lesions, 41% had adenomata and 24% had diffuse hyperplasia. Those without malignant lesions, treated surgically, responded with an approximately 50% remission rate [92]. There have been reports of those treated with streptozotocin who have experienced tumor regression and absence of symptoms for as long as 12 and 13 months [94, 98].

2.2.3. The Ectopic Corticotrophinoma (Ectopic ACTH) Syndrome

History. The presence of truncal obesity, weakness, osteoporosis, hirsutism, moon facies, buffalo hump, purple striae, acne, arterial hypertension and diabetes associated with a corticotrophin-secreting pituitary tumor with secondary adrenocortical hyperplasia is known as Cushing's *disease.* The same constellation of clinical findings secondary to glucocorticoid excess without a pituitary tumor is described as Cushing's *syndrome.* The syndrome may be due to exogenously administered steroids or to entopic adrenocortical tumors or to ectopic adrenocorticotrophin (ACTH) secreting tumors. Cushing, in the early part of this century, conceived that pituitary hyperfunction, like thyroid hyperfunction, could be due to hyperplastic or adenomatous changes of the entopic organ and that selective surgical excision, even by transsphenoidal approach to the pituitary, could lead to amelioration of the syndrome [99]. However, in his day the pituitary-dependent variety was diagnosed and treated only after the sella had become enlarged; he might reasonably marvel at present-day methods of diagnosing not only early pituitary microadenomas, but the more remarkable non-pituitary, non-adrenal, and therefore ectopic tumors that elaborate a large molecular corticotrophin (ACTH), which stimulates secondary adrenocortical hyperplastic hypercortisolemia. Such ectopic production of ACTH, with the resultant syndrome, is found most commonly in bronchogenic carcinomas [100], but tumors of the pancreas [101, 102], thymus, thyroid, prostate, esophagus and colon that produce Cushing's syndrome have also been reported. Pancreatic islet tumors are the most frequent in this latter group.

Pathology. Islet cell tumors that produce ACTH often secrete other hormones as well, including melanocyte-stimulating hormone (MSH), insulin, gastrin and 5-hydroxytryptamine [103]. These tumors are characteristically highly malignant and will often have metastasized widely by the time clinical expression of the Cushing's syndrome appears. In these cases serum ACTH levels are very high and not suppressible by exogenous corticosteroid administration. Histology of the tumors is typical of apudomas with clusters of cells interspersed among numerous blood vessels. However, these tumors appear more malignant with frequent mitoses, bizarre cells and invasion. Electron microscopy reveals the presence of secretory granules [102].

Clinical presentation. The clinical expression of ectopic ACTH-secreting tumors is often more subtle than that of the classical syndrome. These patients are less likely to exhibit obesity, striae and osteoporosis; however, they frequently are hypokalemic and display easy bruisability and glucose intolerance. Hyperpigmentation is frequent. These patients harbor highly malignant tumors, which are responsible for markedly shortened survival when compared to other islet cell tumors [104].

Diagnosis. The diagnosis of Cushing's syndrome is established by demonstration of elevated urinary free cortisol levels and lack of suppression of cortisol production by the dexamethasone suppression test. The latter involves administration of dexamethasone 1 mg orally at 11 PM and measuring plasma cortisol levels the following morning. While levels in normal subjects will be suppressed to less than $5 \mu g/100$ ml, levels in patients with Cushing's syndrome will not be suppressed below $10 \mu g/100$ ml [105].

Measurement of ACTH levels, combined with the high dose dexamethasone suppression test (2 mg orally every 6 hours times 2 days with concomitant 24 hour urine collection for 17-hydroxycorticosteroid values) will delineate the cause of the syndrome. Low ACTH levels and lack of suppression indicate primary adrenal tumors. Adrenal carcinoma is more likely if urinary 17-ketosteroid levels are elevated. Normal to elevated plasma ACTH levels with partial suppression of 17-hydroxycorticosteroids are found in Cushing's disease. Markedly elevated ACTH levels and lack of suppression with high dose dexamethasone are characteristic of the ectopic ACTH syndrome [106].

Localization of the tumor and its metastases may be accomplished with angiography or computerized tomography.

Treatment. Since most of the tumors causing the ectopic Cushing's syndrome are highly malignant and will probably have metastasized by the time the diagnosis is made, treatment is largely palliative. Those with incurable, but slow-growing tumors may be candidates for bilateral adrenalectomy.

Medical therapy for those patients who are not candidates for surgical extirpation includes metapyrone, aminoglutethimide and cyproheptadine. Metapyrone inhibits adrenal 11-hydroxylase activity where as aminoglutethimide blocks the conversion of cholesterol to pregnenolone. Neither agent affects the growth of the tumor. The efficacy of cyproheptadine in treating hypercortisolism is controversial [107].

Prognosis. The outlook for patients with ectopic ACTH-secreting tumors is dismal because of the highly aggressive nature of the neoplasm itself.

2.2.4. The Ectopic Parathyrinoma (Ectopic Hypercalcemic) Syndrome

History. It is only in the last decade that non-parathyroid tumors were observed to cause hypercalcemia and a hyperparathyroid-like clinical picture [108, 109]. Ectopic production of parathyrin (PTH) occurs most often in tumors of the lung, kidney or lymphomas. However, tumors of the pancreatic islets, adrenal cortex, gonads, intestines and liver may produce PTH [110–112]. The resultant hypercalcemia must be differentiated from that associated with tumors in which bone metastases, vitamin D-like sterol production, vitamin D-enhancing factors, prostaglandin release, osteoclast-activating factors or parathyroid gland stimulation are the responsible factors. Indeed, tumor hypercalcemia is at least as frequent as primary hyperparathyroidism [113].

Pathology. The ubiquity of the APUD cells and the concept of malignant derepression back to a state of totipotentiality help explain the occurrence of ectopic PTH-secreting tumors. There are immunoreactive differences between normal PTH and that secreted by ectopic tumors [114]. While tumor PTH appears to be more potent in producing hypercalcemia than parathyroid PTH, their pharmacologic and biologic activities are similar. Parathyrin increases plasma calcium concentration, decreses plasma phosphate concentration, increases tubular excretion of phosphate, increases tubular resorption of calcium, increases bone remodeling by increasing the number and activity of osteoblasts and osteoclasts, increases bicarbonate excretion by the kidney, activates adenylate cyclase in cells of target tissues and increases gastrointestinal absorption of calcium by enhancing vitamin D synthesis [115].

Clinical presentation. Patients with ectopic PTH production may exhibit many of the primary effects of hypercalcemia including lethargy, fatigue, anorexia, constipation, polyuria and polydipsia. Secondary signs of hypercalcemia, such as bone resorption and renal calculi are rarely observed [116]. The symptoms may be easily confused with those of a preterminal state and patients sometimes present in the coma of hypercalcemia crises. Other clinical features related to the mechanical presence of the primary tumor itself are not usually obvious.

Diagnosis. The exocrine parameters related to calcium and phosphorus metabolism in ectopic tumors are similar to those of primary hyperparathyroidism and should include calcium, phosphorus, chloride, protein, albumin, globulin, alkaline phosphatase, creatinine, urea nitrogen, pH, uric acid and magnesium determinations. The tubular reabsorption of phosphate is usually less than 80%. Because of the heterogeneity of the molecular forms of parathyrin-like peptides, the usual laboratory immunoassay techniques will not always demonstrate elevated plasma levels. In fact, the measured immunocomponents of the PTH molecule may be undetectable. In such instances, the pharmacologic administration of phosphates to decrease the serum calcium levels will be followed by an elevation of the PTH concentration to normal levels; this diagnostic circumstance suggests that the hypercalcemia suppressed parathyroid release of parathyrin until the calcium was therapeutically reduced, a phenomenon typical of normal parathyroid glands. When the normal parathyroid glands respond in this way, a search should be made for an ectopic source of tumor parathyrin of different immunochemical characteristics. Because of variants of PTH elaborated by tumors, special assay techniques have been developed [117].

On the other hand, when PTH values are immunologically elevated using the usual assay for parathyrin, the hypercalcemia associated with ectopic PTH is often higher than that associated with comparable levels of parathyroid-produced PTH. This higher ratio may help in differentiating the source of excess parathyrin [118]. Selective venous assays of PTH may help localize the tumor but the more common techniques for detection of malignancies are more likely to be diagnostic. When a pancreatic tumor is suspected computerized tomography improves the diagnostic yield.

Treatment. Surgical excision of the tumor is the treatment of choice when possible. Alternatively, chemotherapy using streptozotocin has been reported to be effective for hypercalcemia associated with pancreatic islet cell carcinoma [119]. Hypercalcemia is treated by a variety of agents including saline and sulfate infusion, chelating agents and the administration of oral and intravenous phosphorus and mithramycin. Hemodialysis will also effectively reduce calcium levels.

Prognosis. Tumors that produce ectopic hormones are known for their more malignant course: those which manifest hypercalcemia are no exception and often eventuate in crises of stupor and renal failure.

3. OVERVIEW

It is clear from the descriptions of the syndromes caused by functioning tumors of the pancreas and gastrointestinal tract that there is a wide spectrum of clinical pictures running the gamut from asymptomatic pancreatic polypeptide tumors to the fulminating ulcerogenic tumors. Some syndromes such as those due to glucagonomas and even insulinomas may present in such a subtle way that they are easily overlooked as diabetic patients or 'nervous' patients, respectively. That such an array of endocrinopathies result from pathologic changes of cells which have a common embryologic origin is quite remarkable. The types of hormones, polypeptides and amines that are common to them vary tremendously in their biologic effects but only slightly in their molecular weights and amino acid residues. The actions of the amines are almost instantaneous where as polypeptide effects require at least minutes and symptomatic fluctuations can be detected clinically.

The cells that become dysplastic have common APUD cytochemical and embryologic characteristics. When pathologic abnormalities occur in cells which are native to their functional location, the resulting syndromes are called entopic; when the tumors arise in a locus with biologic effects foreign to that site, the syndrome is called ectopic. If it is accurately appreciated that the cells of origin of both entopic and ectopic functioning tumors are the same, namely APUD cells or their precursors, then the term ectopic is not necessarily applicable; functionally they 'appear to be ectopic' owing only to the fact that the abnormal cell has reverted to a precursor functional state. With a clear understanding of the APUD concept and the theory of ectopia, it should not be a surprise to discover that a pancreatic apudoma might elaborate serotonin and gastrin, or ACTH or parathyrin. Such bizarre revelations add to the clinical excitement of endocrinology and stimulate basic research and ultimately bring out the best in the surgical and medical management of more and more newly recognized syndromes.

The innovative thrust in the development of humoral assays, using radioimmunochemical techniques has revolutionized the diagnosis of endocrinopathies so that diagnostic and prognostic markers assist clinicians in their management of such patients. Even markers in asymptomatic patients at risk for development of familial endocrinopathies are just beginning to become significant as early detectors of tumors. A case in point is the assay for human pancreatic polypeptide for the pancreatic component of·the MEA, type

I syndrome. Because the most certain possibility for cure in most endocrino-pathies today is surgical excision, it is all the more important that diagnoses be made early, before metastases develop. There also is some consideration that dysplasias may progress from cellular hyperplasia to neoplasia, a possibility that also augurs for early detection and excision. Since diagnosis depends first upon clinical recognition of a possible syndrome with its general and systemic manifestations, certain specific observations of laboratory determinations of exocrine end-organ derangements should then prompt the more specific assays of the appropriate endocrine hormone. The two types of determinations should be made simultaneously to look for 'inappropriate' levels, such as glucose and insulin determinations or calcium and PTH values. In these ways early diagnoses are possible; further localization of tumors then requires the newer radiologic techniques of computerized tomographic scanning and selective angiography with selective venous humoral assays.

Finally, selective angiography is important also for intelligent administration of selective chemotherapy of non-resectable tumors. Present day experience with the use of both intra-arterial streptozotocin, as well as its intravenous administration, is demonstrating increasing therapeutic benefit for some patients even with hepatic metastases. Further innovations in receptor blockade, such as with cimetidine interruption of one of the receptors on the acid-secreting parietal cell, provide excellent palliation of the gastrin-secreting syndromes. Further developments in tumor chemotherapy and receptor modification will certainly enhance the surgical treatment of patients who develop neoplasms of endocrine cells.

REFERENCES

1. Friesen SR (ed): Surgical Endocrinology: clinical syndromes. Philadelphia: J.B. Lippincott, 1978.
2. Pearse AGE, Polak JM: Neural crest origin of the endocrine polypeptide (APUD) cells of the gastrointestinal tract and pancreas. Gut 12:783–788, 1971.
3. Friesen SR: APUD tumors of the gastrointestinal tract. In: Current problems in cancer, Hickey RC (ed.). Chicago: Year Book Medical Publishers, vol 1, No 4, October 1976.
4. Wermer P: Multiple endocrine adenomatosis; multiple hormone-producing tumours, a familial syndrome. Clin Gastroenterol 3:671–684, 1974.
5. Sipple JH: The Association of pheochromocytoma with carcinoma of the thyroid gland. AM J Med 31:163–166, 1961.
6. Schimke RN, Hartmann WH, Prout TE, Rimoin DL: Syndrome of bilateral pheochromocytoma, medullary thyroid carcinoma and multiple neuromas. N Engl J Med 279:1–7, 1968.
7. Friesen SR: The development of endocrinopathies in the prospective screening of two families with multiple endocrine adenopathy, Type I. World J Surg 3:753–764, 1979.

8. Bayliss WM, Starling EH: The mechanism of pancreatic secretion. J Physiol 28:325–353, 1902.

9. Zollinger RM, Ellison EH: Primary peptic ulceration of the jejunum associated with islet cell tumors of the pancreas. Ann Surg 142:709–728, 1955.

10. Edkins JS: On the chemical mechanism of gastric secretion. Proc Roy Soc, London 76:376, 1905.

11. Lubarsch O: Über den primären Krebs des Ileum, nebst Bemerkungen über das gleichzeitige Vorkommen von Krebs und Tuberkulose. Virchows Arch Path Anat 111:280, 1888.

12. Ransom WB: A case of primary carcinoma of the ileum. Lancet 2:1020, 1890.

13. Oberdorfer S: Ergebnisse der allgemeinen Pathologie und pathologischen Anatomie des Menschen und der Tiere 13:527, 1909.

14. Masson P: Carcinoid (argentaffin-cell tumors) and nerve hyperplasia of the appendicular mucosa. Am J Pathol 4:181–211, 1928.

15. Lembeck F: 5-Hydroxytryptamine in carcinoid tumors. Nature 172:910–911, 1953.

16. Pernow B, Waldenstrom J: Paroxysmal flushing and other symptoms caused by 5-hydroxytryptamine and histamine in patients with malignant tumors. Lancet 2:951, 1954.

17. Wilson H, Cheek RC, Sherman RT, Storer EH: Carcinoid tumors. In: Current problems in surgery, Ravitch MM (ed.). Chicago: Year Book Medical Publishers, vol 7 P 1, July 1970.

18. Moertel CG, Sauer G, Dockerty MB, Bagenstom AH: Life history of the carcinoid tumor of the small intestine. Cancer 14:901–912, 1961.

19. MacDonald RA: A study of 356 carcinoids of the gastrointestinal tract. Am J Med 21:867–878, 1956.

20. Sandler M, Karim SM, Williams ED: Prostaglandins in amine-peptide-secreting tumours. Lancet 2:1053–1054, 1968.

21. Roberts LJ, Marney SR Jr, Oates JA: Blockade of the flush associated with metastatic gastric carcinoid by combined histamine H_1 and H_2 receptor antagonists. N Engl J Med 5:236–238, 1979.

22. Kaplan EL: The carcinoid syndromes. in: Surgical endocrinology: clinical syndromes, Friesen SR (ed.). Philadelphia: J.B. Lippincott, 1978, pp 120–147.

23. Ibid.

24. Aune S, Schistad G: Carcinoid liver metastases treated with hepatic dearterialization. Am J Surg 123:715–717, 1972.

25. McDermott WV Jr, Hensle TW: Metastatic carcinoid to the liver treated by hepatic dearterialization. Ann Surg 180:305–308, 1974.

26. Murray-Lyon IM, Dawson JL, Parson VA, Rake MO, Blendis, LM, Laws JW, Williams R: Treatment of secondary hepatic tumours by ligation of hepatic artery and infusion of cytotoxic drugs. Lancet 11:172–175, 1970.

27. Feldman JM, Quichel KE, Marleck RL, Lebouty HE: Streptozotocin treatment of metastatic carcinoid tumours. Southern med J 65:1325–1327, 1972.

28. Costello C: Carcinoid tumor metastases. Prospective study of twenty-two patients. Am J Surg 130:756–759, 1975.

29. Frolich JC, Bloomgarden ZT, Oates JA, McGuigan JE, Rabinowitz D: The carcinoid flush. Provocation by pentagastrin and inhibition by somatostatin. N Engl J Med 299 19:1055–1057, 1978.

30. Godwin JD II: Carcinoid tumors. An analysis of 2,837 cases. Cancer 36:560–569, 1975.

31. Becker SW, Kalm D, Rothman S: Cutaneous manifestations of internal malignant tumors. Arch Dermatol Syph 45:1069–1080, 1942.

32. McGavran MH, Unger RH, Recant L, Polk HC, Kilo C, Levin ME: A glucagon-secreting

alpha-cell carcinoma of the pancreas. N Engl J Med 274:1408–1413, 1966.

33. Unger RH, Eisentraut AM, Lochner JV: Glucagon-producing tumors of the islets of Langerhans. J Clin Invest 42:987–988, 1963.

34. Wilkinson DJ: Necrolytic migratory erythema with carcinoid of the pancreas. Trans St John's Hosp Dermatol Soc 59:244–250, 1973.

35. Mallinson CN, Bloom SR, Warin AP, Salmon PR, Cox B: A glucagonoma syndrome. Lancet 2:1–5, 1974.

36. Higgins GA, Recant L, Finchman AB: The glucagonoma syndrome: surgically curable diabetes. Am J Surg 137:142–148, 1979.

37. Danforth DN Jr, Triche T, Doppman JL, Beazley RM, Perrino PV, Reçant L: Elevated plasma proglucagon-like component with a glucagon-secreting tumor. Effect of streptozotocin: N Eng J Med 295:242–245, 1976.

38. Valverde I, Lemon HM, Kensinger A, Unger RH: Distribution of plasma glucagon immunoreactivity in a patient with suspected glucagonoma. J Clin Endocrinol Metab 2, 5:804–808, 1976.

39. Sohier J Jeanmougin M, Lombrail P, Passa Ph: Rapid improvement of skin lesions in glucagonoma with intravenous somatostatin infusion. Lancet 1:40, 1980.

40. Nichols AG: Simple adenoma of the pancreas arising from an island of Langerhans. J Med Res 8:385, 1902.

41. Banting FG, Best CH: The internal secretion of the pancreas. J Lab Clin Med 7:251–266, 1922.

42. Harris S: Hyperinsulinism and dysinsulinism. JAMA 83:729, 1924.

43. Wilder RM: Clinical diabetes mellitus and hyperinsulinism. Philadelphia: Saunders, 1941.

44. Howland G, Campbell WR, Maltby EJ Rovinson WC: Dysinsulinism: convulsion and coma due to islet cell tumor of pancreas, with operation and cure. J Am Med Assn 93:674–679, 1929.

45. Whipple AO, Frantz VK: Adenoma of islet cells with hyperinsulinism. Ann Surg 101:1299–1335, 1935.

46. Marks V, Samok E: Insulinoma: natural history and diagnosis. Clin Gastroenterol 3:559–573, 1974.

47. Fajans SS, Floyd JC Jr, Vij SK: Differential diagnosis of spontaneous hypoglycemia. In: Endocrinology and diabetes, Dryston CJ, Shaw RA (eds). New York: Grune & Stratton, 1975, pp 453–472.

48. Edis AJ, McIlrath DC, Van Heerden JA, Fulton RE, Sheedy PF II, Service FJ, Dale AJD: Insulinoma — current diagnosis and surgical management. In: Current problems in surgery, Ravitch MM (ed). Chicago: Year Book Medical Publishers, XIII, 10, October 1976.

49. Kramer S, Marlina T, Marcus J: Metabolic studies in the malignant glucagonoma syndrome. Diabetes 25:370, 1976.

50. Curnow RT, Carey RM, Taylor A, Johnson A, Monad F: Somatostatin inhibition of insulin and gastrin hypersecretion in pancreatic islet cell carcinoma. N Engl J Med 292:1385–1386, 1975.

51. Schein PS, DeLellis RA, Kahn CR, Gorden P, Kraft AR: Islet cell tumors: current concepts and management. Ann Int Med 79:239–257, 1973.

52. Larsson LI, Hirsch MA, Holst JJ, Ingemansson S, Jensen SL, Kuhl C, Lundquist G, Rehfeld JF, Schwartz TW: Pancreatic somatostatinoma. Clinical features and physiological implications. Lancet 1:666–668, 1977.

53. Brazeau P, Wylie V, Burgus R, Ling N, Butcher M, Rivier J, Guilleman R: Hypothalamic polypeptide that inhibits the secretion of immunoreactive pituitary growth hormone. Science 179:77–79, 1973.

54. Unger RH: Somatostatinoma. N Engl J Med 296, 17:998–1000, 1977.

55. Ganda OP, Weir GC, Soeldner JS, Legg MA, Chick WL, Patel YC, Ebeid AM, Gabbag KH, Reichlin S: 'Somatostationoma': a somatostatin-containing tumor of the endocrine pancreas. N Engl J Med 296:963–967, 1977.

56. Krejs GJ, Orci L, Coulon JM, Ravazzola M, Davis GR, Raskin P, Collins SM, McCarthy DM, Baetens D, Rubinstein A, Aldor TAM, Unger RH: Somatostatinoma syndrome. Biochemical, morphologic and clinical features. N Engl J Med 301:285–292, 1979.

57. Kovacs K, Horvath E, Ezrin C, Sepp H, Elkan I: Immunoreactive somatostatin in pancreatic islet-cell carcinoma accompanied by ectopic ·ACTH syndrome. Lancet 1:1365–1366, 1977.

58. deNutte N, Somers G, Gepts W, Jacob M, Pipeleers D: Pancreatic hormone release in tumour-associated hypersomatostatinemia. Diabetologia 15:227, 1978.

59. Galmiche JP, Colin R, DuBois PM, Chayvialle JA, Descos F, Paulin C, Geffroy y: Calcitonin secretion by a pancreatic somatostatinoma. N Engl J Med 299:1252, 1978.

60. Kimmel JR, Hayden LJ, Pollock HG: Isolation and characterization of a new pancreatic polypeptide hormone. J Biol Chem 250:9369–9376, 1975.

61. Lin TM, Chance RE: Gastrointestinal actions of a new bovine pancreatic polypeptide (BPP). In: Endocrinology of the gut, Chey WY, Brooks FP (eds). Thorofare, N.J. chas. B. Slack, 1974.

62. Floyd JC Jr, Fajans SS, Pek S, Chance RE: A newly recognized pancreatic polypeptide; plasma levels in health and disease. Recent Prog Horm Res 33:519–570, 1977.

63. Larsson LI, Schwartz T, Lundquist G, Chance RE, Sundler F, Rehfeld JF, Grimelius L, Fahrenkrug J, Schaffelitzky de Muckadell O, Moon N: Occurrence of human pancreatic polypeptide in pancreatic endocrine tumors. Am J Pathol 85:675–684, 1976.

64. Tomita T, Kimmel JR, Friesen SR: Pancreatic polypeptide cell hyperplasia with and without watery diarrhea syndrome. J Surg Oncol (in press).

65. Polak JM, Adrian TE, Bryant MG, Bloom SR, Heitz PH, Pearse AGE: Pancreatic polypeptide in insulinomas, gastrinomas, vipomas and glucagonomas. Lancet 1 7955:328–330, 1976.

66. Friesen SR, Kimmel JR, Tomita T: Pancreatic polypeptide as screening marker for pancreatic polypeptide apudomas in multiple endocrinopathies. Am J Surg 139:61–72, 1980.

67. Bordi C, Togni R, Baetens D, Ravazzola M, Mallaisse-Lagae F, Orci L: Human islet cell tumor storing pancreatic polypeptide: a light and electron miscroscopic study. J Clin Endocrinol Metab 46:215–219, 1978.

68. Modlin IM, Lamers CB, Jaffe BM: Evidence for cholinergic dependence of pancreatic polypeptide release by bombesin — a possible application. Surgery 88, 1:75–85, 1980.

69. Lamers CBH, Diemel J Roeffen W: Serum Levels of pancreatic polypeptide in Zollinger-Ellison syndrome, and hyperparathyroidism from families with multiple endocrine adenomatosis type I. Digestion 18:297–302, 1978.

70. Huard GS, Stephens R, Friesen SR: Streptozotocin therapy for metastatic pancreatic apudomas. J Kansas Med Soc (in press).

71. Dragstedt LR, Oberhelman HA Jr, Smith CA: Experimental hyperfunction of the gastric antrum with ulcer formation. Ann Surg 134:332–342, 1951.

72. Gregory RA, Tracy HJ, French JM, Sircus W: Extraction of a gastrin-like substance from a pancreatic tumor in a case of Zollinger-Ellison syndrome. Lancet 1:1040, 1960.

73. Ellison EH, Wilson SD: The Zollinger-Ellison syndrome: reappraisal and evaluation of 260 registered cases. Ann Surg 160:512–530, 1964.

74. Grossman MI: Physiology and pathophysiology of gastrin. Clin Gastroenterol 3:533–538, 1974.

75. Modlin IM: Endocrine tumors of the pancreas. Surg Gynecol Obstet 149:751–769, 1979.

76. Friesen SR: Treatment of the Zollinger-Ellison syndrome — a twenty-five year assessment.

Am J Surg (in press).

77. McGuigan JE: The radioimmunoassay of gastrin. JAMA 235: 405–406, 1976.
78. DeVeney CW, DeVeney KS, Jaffe BM, Jones RS, Way LW: Use of calcium and secretin in the diagnosis of gastrinoma (Zollinger-Ellison syndrome). Ann Int Med 87:680–686, 1977.
79. Zollinger RM, Ellison EC, Fabri PJ, Johnson J, Sparks J, Carey LC: Primary peptic ulceration of the jejunum associated with islet cell tumor — twenty-five years experience. Ann Surg (in press).
80. Hofmann JW, Fox PS, Wilson SD: Duodenal wall tumors and the Zollinger-Ellison syndrome Arch Surg 107:334–339, 1973.
81. Friesen SR: Effect of total gastrectomy on the Zollinger-Ellison tumor. Observations by a second-look procedure. Surgery 62:609–613, 1967.
82. Wilson SD, Ellison EH: Total gastric resection in children with the Zollinger-Ellison syndrome. Arch Surg 91:165–173, 1965.
83. McCarthy DM, Olinger EJ, May RJ, Long BW, Gardner JD: H$_2$-histamine receptor blocking agents in the Zollinger-Ellison syndrome. Experience in seven cases and implications for long-term therapy. Ann Int Med 87:668–675, 1977.
84. McCarthy DM: The place of surgery in the Zollinger-Ellison syndrome. N Engl J Med 302:1344–1347, 1980.
85. Stadil F, Stage G, Rehfeld JF, Efsen F, Fischerman K: Treatment of Zollinger-Ellison syndrome with streptozotocin. N Engl J Med 294:1440–1442, 1976.
86. Wilson SD, Ellison EH: Survival in patients with the Zollinger-Ellison syndrome treated by total gastrectomy. Am J Surg 111:787–791, 1966.
87. Verner JV, Morrison AB: Islet cell tumor and a syndrome of refractory watery diarrhea and hypokalemia. Am J Med 25:374–380, 1958.
88. Chears WC Jr, Thompson JE, Hutcheson JB, Patterson CO: Pancreatic islet tumor with severe diarrhea. Am J Med 29:529–533, 1960.
89. Matsumoto KK, Peter JB, Schultze RG, Hakim AA, Franck PT: Watery diarrhea and hypokalemia associated with pancreatic islet cell adenoma. Gastroenterology 50:231–242, 1966.
90. Murray JS, Paton RR, Pope CE II: Pancreatic tumor associated with flushing and diarrhea. Report of a case. N Engl J Med 264: 436–439, 1961.
91. Espiner LA, Beaven DW: Nonspecific islet-cell tumor of the pancreas with diarrhea. Quart J Med 31:447–471, 1962.
92. Verner JV, Morrison AB: Endocrine pancreatic islet disease with diarrhea. Arch Intern Med 133:492–500, 1974.
93. Tomita T: Pathology of ulcerogenic and diarrheogenic tumors of the pancreas. Acta Path Jap 24:189–205, 1974.
94. Gagel RF, Costanza ME, De Lellis RA, Norkon RA, Bloom SR, Miller HM, Ucci A, Nathanson L: Streptozocin-treated Verner-Morrison syndrome. Arch Int Med 136:1429–1435, 1976.
95. Bloom SR, Polak JM, Pearse AGE: Vasoactive intestinal peptide and watery diarrhea syndrome. Lancet 2:14–16, 1973.
96. Jaffe BM, Condon S: Prostaglandins E and F in endocrine diarrheagenic syndromes. Ann Surg 184:516–524, 1976.
97. Jaffe BM, Kopen DF, DeSchryver-Kecskemeti K, Gingerich RL, Greider M: Indomethacin-responsive pancreatic cholera. N Engl J Med 297:817–821, 1977.
98. Kahn CR, Levy AG, Gardner JD, Miller JV, Gorden P, Schein PS: Pancreatic cholera: beneficial effects of treatment with streptozotocin. N Engl J Med 292:941–945, 1975.
99. Cushing H: The pituitary body and its disorders. Philadelphia: J.B. Lippincott, 1912.

100. Marks LJ, Roenbaum DL, Russfield AB: Cushing's syndrome and corticotropin-secreting carcinoma of the lung. Ann Intern Med 58:143–149, 1963.

101. Kyriakides GK, Silvis SE, Ahmed M, Vennes JA, Vogel SB: Gastrinoma associated with common bile duct obstruction and the ectopic production of ACTH. Am J Surg 137:800–802, 1979.

102. Joffe SN, Elias E, Rehfeld JF, Polak JM, Bloom SR, Welbourn RB: Clinically silent gross hypergastrinaemia from a multiple hormone-secreting pancreatic apudoma. Br J Surg 65:277–280, 1978.

103. O'Neal LW, Kipnis DM, Luse SA, Lacy PE, Jarett L: Secretion of various endocrine substances by ACTH-secreting tumors–gastrin, melanotropin, norepinephrine, serotonin, parathormone, vasopressin, glucagon. Cancer 21:1219–1232, 1968.

104. Smith LH: Syndromes due to ectopic hormone production. In: Surgical endocrinology: clinical syndromes, Friesen SR (ed). Philadelphia: J.B. Lippincott 1978.

105. Pavlatos F Ch, Smilo RP, Forsham PH: A rapid screening test for Cushing's syndrome. JAMA 193:720–723, 1965.

106. Hunt TK, Tyrrell JB: Cushing's syndrome: Hypercortisolism. In: Surgical endocrinology: clinical syndromes, Friesen SR (ed). Philadelphia: J.B. Lippincott 1978, pp 330–345.

107. Krieger DT, Amorosa L, Linick F: Cyproheptadine-induced remission of Cushing's disease. N Engl J Med 293:893–896, 1975.

108. Friesen SR, Allen MS: Malignant hyperparathyroidism of pancreatic and parathyroid origins. Bull Soc Internal de Chirurgie 5:439–441, 1975.

109. Powell D, Singer FR, Murray TM, Minkin C, Potts JT: Nonparathyroid humoral hypercalcemia in patients with neoplastic diseases. N Engl J Med 289:176–181, 1973.

110. Friesen SR, McGuigan JE: Ectopic apudocarcinomas and associated endocrine hyperplasias of the foregut. Ann Surg 182:371–385, 1975.

111. Kukreja SC, Hargis GK, Rosenthal IM, Williams GA: Pheochromocytoma causing excessive parathyroid hormone production and hypercalcemia. Ann Int Med 79:838–840, 1973.

112. Knill-Jones RP, Buckel RM, Parson V: Hypercalcemia and increased parathyroid hormone activity in a primary hepatoma. N Engl J Med 282:704–708, 1970.

113. Smith LH: Ectopic hormone production. surg Gynecol Obstet 141:443–453, 1975.

114. Riggs BL, Arnaud CD, Reynolds JC, Smith LH: Immunologic differentiation of primary hyperparathyroidism from hyperparathyroidism due to nonparathyroid cancer. J Clin Invest 50:2079–2083, 1971.

115. Rasmussen H: Parathyroid Hormone. Nature and mechanism of action. Am J Med 30:112–128, 1961.

116. Scholz DA, Riggs BL, Purnell DC, Goldsmith RS, Arnaud CD: Ectopic hyperparathyroidism with renal calculi and subperiosteal bone resorption. Mayo Clin Proc 48:124–126, 1973.

117. Benson RC Jr, Riggs BL, Pickard BM, Arnaud CD: Immunoreactive forms of circulating parathyroid hormone in primary and ectopic hyperparathyroidism. J Clin Invest 54:175–181, 1974.

118. Roof BS, Carpenter B, Fink DJ, Gordan GS: Some thoughts on the nature of extopic parathyroid hormones. Am J Med 50:686–691, 1971.

119. Dewys WD, Stoll R, Au WY, Salisnjak MM: Effects of streptozotocin on an islet cell carcinoma with hypercalcemia. Am J Med 55:675–684, 1976.

14. Epidemiology, Early Diagnosis and Treatment of Liver Cell Cancer

SUN TSUNG-TANG, TANG ZHAO-YOU and CHU YUAN-YUN

Liver cell cancer, arising from the hepatic parenchyma cells, may very likely be one of the commonest human cancers in the world. This is based on the fact that its occurrence is very frequent among densely populated areas, especially in the Far East and southern Africa [1–4]. Prognosis of this grave disease is still very poor. However, progress had been achieved in recent years of research on possible etiological factors, mechanism of carcinogenesis, early diagnosis and surgical treatment of liver cell cancer. Some aspects of the recent development will be reviewed here.

1. EPIDEMIOLOGY

1.1. Geographic Distributions

The pattern of incidence or mortality rate of liver cell cancer is characterized by its great variation in worldwide distribution and by the frequent occurrence in the densely populated areas of developing countries [1, 4, 5]. It had been stressed [1] that the true incidence of liver cell cancer was to a large extent incomplete. Cancer registries that provided reliable epidemiological data began to be established only recently in many developing countries. Besides, the lack of internationally accepted standardized classification of hepatic tumors in previous years also introduced difficulties in the identification of acinar type of liver cell cancer from cholangiocarcinoma. Therefore, the incidence rate in different areas can not be compared in strict quantitative terms. In spite of these difficulties, the general pattern of global incidence of liver cell cancer remained to be an established fact. This has been further substantiated by the recently published data of cancer epidemiology in China [4, 6], which demonstrate the wide variation in nationwide distribution and the relatively high incidence of liver cell cancer maintained in recent years.

J. J. DeCosse and P. Sherlock (eds.), Gastrointestinal cancer 1, 387-411. All rights reserved.

On a worldwide scale, the highest incidence of liver cell cancer was reported among the Shangaans of Mozambique. The age adjusted incidence rate reached around 100/100 000 per annum among males[1, 7], but recent data showed that the rate was declining. The average age-adjusted mortality rate of liver cell cancer in the mainland part of China was recently reported to be 10/100 000, being 14.5 among males and 5.6 among females[4]. Greece also has a relatively high frequency of this disease, and the mortality rates for men and women were reported to be 23.3 and 14.8 per 100 000 respectively[8]. This seemed to be followed by Switzerland[5], black people of the U.S.A., Romania[1], and Japan[9], being in the range of 2 to 10/100 000 per annum. The frequency of liver cell cancer is generally considered to be low in central and North Europe, in North America and in many countries of Latin America. In general, males are more prone to develop liver cell cancer than females, the ratio being 2:1 or more. In areas of high incidence, this ratio may exceed 3:1. The reason for the influence of sex is not yet clear.

As a result of enormous collaborative effort, the mortality rate of liver cell cancer in the whole mainland part of China has been mapped. This work was based on retrospective analysis of mortality data collected for 3 consecutive years[6]. The map shows that the geographical distribution of this disease is very uneven. The south east coastal regions have much higher frequency of occurrence than the north west inland areas. The areas where liver cell cancer is relatively prevalent are heavily populated. As a matter of fact, more than 90 000 people died from this disease each year in China. There are a few 'hotspots' where, as in Qidong county, the age adjusted mortality rate reached 76.3 among males, nearly 100 times higher than that of the lowest incidence areas. The identification of high incidence fields has facilitated the collaborative study on etiology, early diagnosis and control strategy of human liver cell cancer.

Pattern of geographical distribution of liver cell cancer and the analytical epidemiological studies thus followed among high incidence areas had offered in recent years valuable etiological clues to human liver cancers. Factors such as race, malnutrition, alcohol, parasites, metabolic disorders, liver diseases, viral agents and environmental chemical carcinogens, had been suggested in association with liver cell cancer. Many of them did not appear to play any important role[10]. Epidemiological studies in China also led to the same conclusions. For example, inhabitants of areas having a several fold difference in incidence are of the same ethnic group: hence, the racial factor is not significant. Malnutrition in the general sense is not a problem in the south east coastal regions of China where liver cell cancer is quite frequent. Areas of higher incidence do not coincide with endemic areas of schistosomiasis. There is no schistosomiasis in the hotspot of Qidong county. Consumption of alcohol is generally low in China, especially in the relevant areas including the hotspots mentioned.

Close association with chronic liver disease, including cirrhosis, appears to be a more general phenomenon[11]. However, the association seems to be pathogenically related, rather than a causal one. Cirrhotic patients are not equally likely to develop liver cell cancer subsequently. HB$_s$Ag positive patients with cirrhosis were found at about 4 times greater risk than comparable but HB$_s$Ag negative patients[12]. Individuals in the high incidence area having serological expression of active and persistent liver cell hyperplasia had a very high risk of developing the cancer[13]. Strong evidence accumulating in recent years has narrowed down the field of searching for relevant causal factors, and has identified the mycotoxins and the hepatitis B virus to be the most probable candidates as the etiological factors of human liver cell cancer. The list of candidates may well be expanded in subsequent years. Meanwhile, the possible role of host factors influencing the development of liver cell cancer also needs to be re-examined.

1.2. Hepatotoxins

Among substances having hepatocarcinogenic potential, the mycotoxins deserve special interest. The most important mycotoxins are the aflatoxins, elaborated by the strain of mould *Aspergillus flavus*, a common and widely distributed food spoilage fungus. Aflatoxin B$_1$ is the most frequently encountered member and possesses the highest hepatotoxicity. It may induce liver cancers in a wide variety of animals, including nonhuman primates, though considerable variation exists in susceptibility among different species[14, 15].

Strong evidence on the relationship between aflatoxin exposure and liver cell carcinoma incidence in human populations was obtained as a result of several field studies designed to obtain quantitative estimates of actual amounts of aflatoxin ingested by local inhabitants and then to compare them with the incidence of liver cell cancer in the same population group. Thus, investigations carried out in areas of Thailand[16], Kenya[17], Mozambique[18], and Swaziland[19] had obtained consistent results, demonstrating that the amount of aflatoxin B$_1$ ingested was directly correlated with the incidence of liver cancer. This approximately linear relationship[20], resembling the dose-effect curve obtained in experimental animals, offered very strong evidence supporting the concept that aflatoxins might be one of the major factors in the causation of human liver cell cancer. Increased exposure to aflatoxin B$_1$ had also been observed in the high incidence areas in China[21].

The epidemiological data just mentioned do not constitute proof of the causal nature of aflatoxins, but do justify an intervention trial. This appears to be further supported by the results obtained by feeding aflatoxin B$_1$ to monkeys[22]. Of the 45 animals fed, two female monkeys developed liver cell carcinoma after four to six years. Another three developed adenocarcinoma of the biliary system. Although these results came from one series of experiments, the difference with human situations in high incidence areas appeared to be impressive. The successive conduction of an intervention trial required the constant monitoring of the amount of aflatoxin ingestion on individual basis. This needs quantitative measurements of minute amounts of aflatoxin B_1 in a large number of biological samples. Recent developments using HPLC[23] and radioimmunoassays[24] for aflatoxins may provide a promising approach to that problem. Works along this direction are under way in several centers.

Other mycotoxins such as sterigmatocystin, luteoskyrin, cyclochlorotine and others had also been suggested for playing a possible role in the causation of liver cancer. Much work remains to be done to clarify their significance[25].

Nitrosamines are a group of potent and versatile chemical carcinogens. Currently available evidence suggests that people may be constantly exposed to variable amounts of N-nitroso compounds either directly from the environment, or after their formation in the alimentary tract. It constitutes a potential carcinogenic risk to humans. Nevertheless, field studies comparable to that on aflatoxins are generally lacking. It should be noted that studies done in the high incidence area. Qidong county, of China has revealed that nitrosamines, mainly diethylnitrosamine, were frequently detected in the salted vegetables used at home by local inhabitants, especially in those samples taken from the families of liver cell cancer patients[26].

1.3. Hepatitis B Virus (HBV)

For a long time, liver cell cancer was known to be closely associated with chronic liver disease, especially with cirrhosis. Since the discovery of Australia antigen by Blumberg, the identification of HBV, its association with hepatitis and liver cell carcinoma has made rapid progress. Work done in many centers over the world gave consistent results on the association of HBV infection with the development of liver cell cancer.

Three lines of strong evidence were collected. First, there is a close correlation in the geographical distribution of liver cell cancer and HBV infections. Cancer occurs frequently in the regions where chronic carriers are also prevalent[2, 3, 27]. Secondly, liver cell cancer patients very frequently had coexisting HBV infections, as shown by various markers of the infection[3, 27, 28]. This also included patients who were asymptomatic but had liver cell cancer at its early resectable stage[13]. The association appeared to be specific when compared with control groups of either normal people, patients with benign diseases or patients with non-hepatic malignancies.

Thirdly, prospective studies on patients with chronic liver diseases demonstrated that the HB_sAg positive group had a significantly higher risk than the HB_sAg negative group to develop liver cell cancer in the subsequent 3 to 3.5 years of follow up [12, 28]. Furthermore, prospective studies on 'healthy' chronic carriers of HBV and controls who were not carriers showed that significantly higher number of liver cell cancer patients developed in the carrier group during a follow-up period of about 4 years [29, 30]. Available evidence appears to be sufficiently strong to consider HBV to be a very probably candidate that might be etiologically related to human liver cell cancer.

Recent data indicate that two factors, one chemical and one viral, may play an important role in the causation of liver cell cancer, certainly not excluding other factors. Actually, increased exposure to aflatoxin and prevalence of chronic carrier of HBV were both observed in the endemic areas of liver cell cancer, as in Qidong field of China. They may act synergistically. This concept is also supported by the epidemiological data from Qidong. Based on the incidence rate of liver cell cancer [4], chronic carrier rate [29] and the positivity rate of HB_sAg in liver cell cancer patients [28] in the same population of Qidong, it has been calculated that the annual incidence rate among HB_sAg negative people is $17.1/10^5$ [see Table 1]. This value is quite high, suggesting increased exposure to the environmental carcinogens, although the role of other viral factors could not be excluded. However, when the factor of HBV infection is further added to the same population, the annual incidence rate of liver cell cancer increased to $206/10^5$. The addition of HBV infection to the local inhabitants further increases the risk 12 fold. In areas of lower incidence of liver cancer in China, the risk introduced by HBV infection appears to be higher than that found in the high incidence field. The interaction of various etiological factors remains an important issue for further investigation.

1.4. Host Factors

Even in the endemic areas where exposure to various oncogenic agents would be severe, only a very small portion of the population develop liver cell cancer. In Qidong, the carrier rate is around 17%, but 83% are not. Only a small percentage of the chronic carriers develop chronic liver disease, whereas the majority remain apparently healthy. Finally, only a certain proportion of the group having a background of liver disease develop liver cell cancer. Obviously, there are many ways through which the host factors might be expressed. The acquisition of a chronic carrier state appears to be the expression of tolerance. The latter was postulated to result from the cross-reactivity between a determinant on HB_sAg and a host antigen, preferentially a male-associated antigen [2]. It was also suggested to be an immunodeficiency to

Table 1. Liver cell cancer incidence among different groups in the Qidong county.

People group	Annual incidence
HB$_s$Ag negative population	$17.1/10^5$
HB$_s$Ag positive population	$206/10^5$
Low fluctuating AFP group*	$\sim 3\%$

* Among 233 persons having low level fluctuating AFP, 8 developed liver cell cancer in the second year of follow-up and 6 in the 3rd year (Chu Yuan-yun, unpublished data).

HBV which might be HLA-gene associated[31]. Another aspect of possible host influence is on the development of chronic liver disease. As shown in Table 1, the HB$_s$Ag positive population has a very high incidence of liver cell cancer. There are patients in the same region who exhibit low level fluctuating pattern of serum AFP, probably reflecting persistent hyperplasia of the hepatic cells[32]. They are mostly HB$_s$Ag positive, but show an extremely high probability of developing liver cell cancer, possibly reaching around 3% per annum. Even after correcting for age difference and others, a further increase of risk of about 3 fold is observed over the HB$_s$Ag positive local inhabitants. This probably reflects that a small percentage of people might be inherently susceptible to develop persistent liver cell hyperplasia in responding to the common assault from external causative factors.

For chemical carcinogenesis, the species and tissue specificity of tumor development might be explained in part by the heterogeneity of the monooxygenase system, concerning the amount and the specificity of the various groups of cytochrome p-450 species[33]. It is not inconceivable that the inherent difference in the capacity of metabolic activation of carcinogens and other processes might also be present among different individuals. Furthermore, case control studies carried out in the Qidong field suggested the presence of some genetic influence on the occurrence of liver cancer. Retrospective analysis of over 4000 members of families having liver cell cancer patients and comparable controls showed that the significantly higher cancer incidence among cancer families were correlated mainly with the common living environment (living together) and less so with consanguineous relationship[34]. These observations were also consistent with the concept that both environmental and host factors might be operative in the development of liver cell cancer, but the effect of environmental causative factors appeared to predominate.

1.5. Prevention Trials

Research on etiological aspect of liver cell cancer has justified the first stage of primary prevention, the intervention trials. Control of aflatoxin intoxication seems to present socio-economical problems but no serious technical ones. Besides the difficulty of affording large investment in developing countries, a change of living habit is also very difficult to achieve. For example, it is very hard in Qidong field to persuade local people to give up salted and pickled vegetables which have been a favorite food for generations. The control of hepatitis is easier to approach from the socio-economical side, but there are still many technical uncertainties. An effective vaccine against HBV appears to be on horizon [35], and encouraging results were observed in young children [36]. However, a safe and effective vaccination procedure, especially among the immunologically immature infants and very young children, still needs further substantiation. The control of the chronic carrier state of the mothers still poses a serious challenge to the medical field. Interferon appears to offer some promise in this respect [37], but there is still a long way to go even if the initial observations are confirmed. In spite of the difficulties just mentioned, field trials are justified. As a matter of fact, prevention studies in several areas, including the Qidong field where we have been participating, have already started. It might be expected that a real possibility of approaching the primary prevention of human liver cancer would be formed in the coming decade through cautiously controlled trials in the high incidence fields.

2.. EARLY DIAGNOSIS

Early diagnosis of liver cell cancer means the definition of the cancer at a stage during which proper intervention may lead to the cure of patients with high probability [38]. The diagnostic technology in detecting hepatic tumors has been refined significantly in recent years. Application of alpha fetoprotein (AFP) serology was proved to have potential in the early diagnosis of liver cell cancer in the high incidence areas of China [39–41]. This potential might be fully expressed if the highly probable candidates found through AFP assays could be further confirmed and their tumor mass be identified in size and location through other diagnostic techniques, preferably non-traumatic ones. Early diagnosis of AFP negative liver cancers is obviously hampered by the lack of suitable tumor markers which may permit first line detection as AFP has done for the positive counterparts.

2.1. AFP Serology

AFP is a normal foetal serum α_1 globulin, a glycoprotein with a molecular weight around 71 000. It is synthesized in the foregut and liver cells during embryonic life, but the synthesis is significantly depressed after birth. The production at high levels may be re-expressed in the malignant liver cells and in the embryonal cells of teratoblastomas [42]. It is the best characterized and the most specific member of the group of onco-foetal proteins.

It had been repeatedly stressed that AFP assays were useful for the diagnosis of clinical cases of liver cell cancer, especially for monitoring the therapeutic effect [43]. Its value in early diagnosis of liver cell cancer had been demonstrated in mass screening trials conducted in Qidong and Shanghai areas using sensitive techniques since 1973 [40, 41, 44]. The most impressive facts following these sero-surveys were the significant increase of survival rates as well as the appearance of a significant number of long-term survivors. A several fold increase of 3 year survival among patients detected in mass survey over those found in the clinic was observed (further discussed in 3.1). The presence of long-term survivals is exemplified by a group of 27 patients detected and operated in Qidong during 1974 and 1975. They have survived over 4 or 6 years after surgical resection, and resumed their normal work. They are still healthy and have shown no signs of recurrence. It should be noted that long-term survival in that high incidence area was a rare event before the introduction of a mass survey program. These facts demonstrate that an early stage of liver cell cancer does exist and may be identified through an AFP survey, at least in the areas studied.

The diagnostic task to differentiate those candidates for early liver cell cancer from other nonmalignant patients is rather difficult. Among the group of people having elevated serum AFP in the range of 25 to 400 ng/ml detected in mass screening, the patients with chronic liver diseases usually

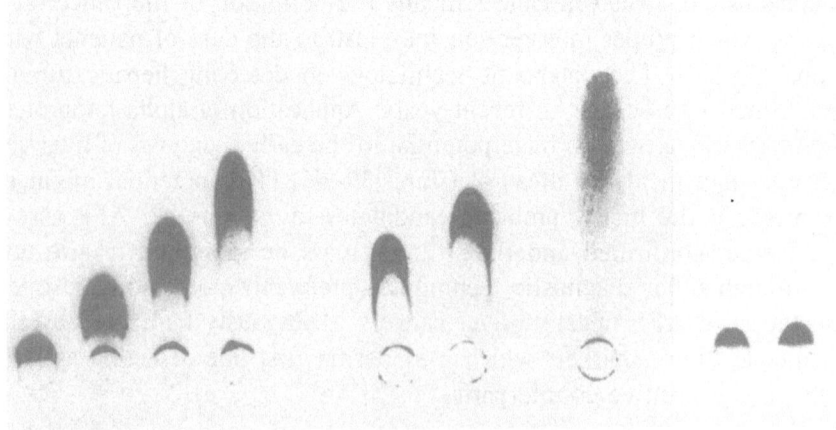

Figure 1. AFP pattern of early liver cell cancer patient before and after surgical resection. Serial AFP assayed by radio-rocket electrophoresis autography [39]. Wells from left, No. 1: normal serum, Nos. 2–4: Standard AFP, 125, 250, 500 ng/ml respectively. Nos. 5–7: patient sera before surgery, 2 wks between 5 and 6, 6 wks between 6 and 7. Surgery done soon after No. 7. Nos. 8, 9: 6 months and 1 yr after resection. The patient is still well, 6 years after operation.

outnumbered the candidates by a factor of several fold. The dynamic pattern of serum AFP obtained by sequential determinations of its concentration appeared to provide valuable information. As shown in Figure 1, there was a steady rise of serum AFP in the time course. The average doubling time in this case was found to be 30 days. After the surgical resection of localized liver cell cancer, the serum AFP fell sharply and mostly remained at the level of normal people. This particular patient is still well and has survived over 6 years after operation.

The steadily rising pattern in the range of 50 to 1000 ng/ml, having an average doubling time of 20 to 50 days in most cases, appears to be the most reliable serological expression of the presence of liver cell cancer, usually asymptomatic. Over 90% of cases presenting this pattern were found to be suffering from liver cancer [32, 40]. Analysis of the histological pictures of the surgical specimens taken from these patients showed that the rising pattern probably reflected the expanding mode of the tumor cell populations at this stage of malignant growth. The doubling time found in the high incidence areas of China appeared to be longer than the value reported in Africa [45], reflecting the slower growth rate of the cancer in China. The importance of the rising pattern had also been reported for the detection of liver cell cancer at a relatively early stage through continuous monitoring for AFP in patients with chronic liver disease [46].

The identification of the critical moment to start radical intervention on the patients on the basis of serological information appeared to be an important factor in deciding the outcome of the patients. The use of double diffusion and also countercurrent electrophoresis in the initial phase of the mass screening program in China found a significant number of asymptomatic patients. However, their survival rate was still low. Subsequent use of more sensitive techniques, such as reverse passive hemagglutination [47] and radiorocket electrophoresis autography [48] having a sensitivity of 50 ng/ml or less, has detected more patients at an earlier stage. Analysis was made to find out whether the level of AFP at which the surgery was performed would effect the survival of the patients, taking 1 μg/ml as the line of demarcation in accordance with the previous experiences. The group operated above 1 μg/ml had a relatively low 3 year survival rate, around 6% (4/64), thus confirming the results of previous studies. However, the group of patients operated below 1 μg/ml had a significantly higher 3 year survival rate, reaching around 40% (13/33) [32]. Twelve patients of the latter group are still healthy, having survived over five years after operation. This result also demonstrated that a significant percentage of liver cell cancer still remains in localized state when the serum AFP of the host has not exceeded the level of 1 μg/ml.

It was possible to detect the majority of liver cell cancer patients in a stage without apparent symptoms and find their AFP below the level of 1 μg/ml through regular surveys performed twice a year [44, 49]. However, the potential thus provided could not be fully utilized without the introduction of additional diagnostic techniques that might define the extent and location of the suspected cancer mass. As an example to illustrate this problem of a more general nature, let us analyze the remaining patients of the series of 33 patients just mentioned. The remaining 20 patients, 60% of the series, could not be successfully treated because of the following situations: 1) the tumor had already grown to a stage beyond resection; 2) the tumor could not be found during operation; and, 3) in a small number of patients, the tumor was situated in the 'forbidden areas' of liver. Hepatic angiography, computerized tomography and ultrasonography may offer opportunites [50] for addressing this problem. When this issue can be solved, a more complete strategy on early diagnosis of AFP positive liver cell cancer can be formulated and impact favorably on the survival of patients suffering from this dreadful disease in some populated areas, taking into consideration the capacity of surgical treatment.

2.2. Hepatoangiography

Angiographic characteristics of liver cell cancer have been thoroughly studied for years [51]. It is important to accumulate experience in the diagnosis and localization of small liver cell cancer. It should be further stressed that hundreds of patients with subclinical liver cancer were picked up by screening. Of these asymptomatic patients, only 26.7% showed a space-occupying lesion in liver scintiscan, and 20.6% showed positive features by conventional ultrasound [52]. Transumbilical hepatography has been tried, and the smallest tumor detected by this procedure and confirmed by operation was found to be 2.5×2.5 cm. However, it failed to show filling defect of small liver cancer in the right lobe in majority of cases [53]. Selective celiac or hepatic arteriography was claimed to be the modality of choice for the identification of small liver cell cancer [54–56]. Tumors as small as 1 cm in diameter have been demonstrated in the hypervascular type [55, 56]. Tumor vessels and tumor stains are two distinctive features of small liver cell cancer in selective arteriogram. The lower limit of detection by this technique was considered to be 1 cm. However, arteriography for tumors of hypovascular type and for tumors located in the left lobe was found to be unsatisfactory [57].

2.3. Ultrasonography

Both gray scale ultrasonography (B-scan) and computerized tomography (CT) provide a hopeful future for a non-invasive approach to the diagnosis and localization of small liver cell cancer [50]. Ultrasound is less expensive than CT. However, accuracy of B-scan seems to be less favorable than scintigraphy and angiography, being 72%, 85%, and 93% respectively in a series of cases reported [58]. Its potential in the detection of small liver cell cancer remains to be studied.

2.4. Computerized Tomography

Computerized tomography had been proved of value in demonstrating lesions in the liver [50]. Patients with suspected lesion in liver found by radionuclide scan had been subjected to CT examinations before invasive angiography [59]. It was commented that in the majority of liver cell cancer, the difference in densities between tumor and the surrounding parenchyma was so small that the relatively lucent area might easily be overlooked [50]. The accuracy for liver tumors with CT varied from 63.2% [60] to 93.8% [61]. The accuracy for CT, radionuclide scan, and arteriography was found to be 63.2%, 94.7% and 100% respectively [60]. Although the non-invasive feature of CT is very attractive, the large expense involved is a problem, especially for the developing countries. The exploration of the potential of using CT for the identification and localization of early liver cell cancer found in the field has been started by us recently. Preliminary results appear to be encouraging though problems still exist.

2.5. Radionuclide Imaging

Radionuclide scan remains a valuable tool for the localization in the clinical situations. Combined liver and gallium scan was claimed to have special value for detection of liver cell carcinoma [62]. Several studies comparing the effects of radionuclide scan, CT, and/or ultrasonography gave inconsistent results [58, 63, 64]. Since only 20% of the early liver cell cancer were demonstrated to have space-occupying lesions, the use of conventional radionuclide scan is of limited value in the early diagnosis of this cancer [55].

2.6. Tumor Markers other than AFP

Despite some advances achieved in the early diagnosis of AFP positive liver cell cancer, the early diagnosis of the AFP negative counterparts (10–50% of liver cell cancer in different areas of the world) remains a serious problem. Search for new tumor markers was one of the main topics in the recent International workshop on primary liver cancer held in Singapore. Several new markers were reported to be hopeful in the diagnosis of low level (<400 ng/ml of AFP) or AFP negative liver cell cancer. The positivity rate of several agents were reported as follows: novel gamma-glutamyl transpeptidase 32%, carcinoplacental alkaline phosphatase 32%, basic feto-protein 64% [65], hepatoma-liver antigen 58–67% [66]. Other markers studied including alpha$_1$ antitrypsin [67, 68], alpha$_1$ acid glycoprotein [68] and 5'-nucleotide phosphodiesterase (NPD) isozyme V test for human liver cancer [69] were also reported. Positivity rate of 5'-NPDase isozyme V up to 78.2% was found in 23 AFP negative liver cell cancer in Shanghai [70]. No data have yet been available for assessing the potential of using the above-mentioned markers for the early diagnosis of AFP negative liver cell cancer.

3. TREATMENT

Liver cell cancer is one of the most malignant cancers with grave prognosis. However, substantial progress, although far from adequate, has also been achieved in the field of treatment. Early detection, aggressive approach and multimodality treatment contribute to this progress.

3.1. Early Treatment of Mass Survey Patients and its Ultimate Outcome

It has been accepted that early detection and early treatment of subclinical cancer may be the principal approach to rescue patients dying from malignancies before breakthroughs are made in relevant basic research. In China, over 1000 patients with liver cell cancer were detected in AFP screening. Of these, more than 400 patients were found in the subclinical stage. More than 100 cases of small cancers were resected. Of these patients, a good number resume their original work without recurrence [71, 72]. In Japan, patients with small liver cell cancer have also been discovered by monitoring AFP in patients with chronic liver disease [46]. Resection of small liver cancers in 20 cases was reported in 1976 [73], and some survivors were observed.

3.1.1. Clinical Pattern of the Mass Survey Patients. The clinical stage distribution, the therapeutic pattern and the survival pattern have clearly changed with introduction of mass screening. The discovery of subclinical cases remarkably increases the role of surgical resection and improves the overall prognosis. Subclinical liver cell cancer only amounted to 0.4–0.9% in clinical cases [74, 75], but it went up to 44.7 to 71.2% in mass survey patients [52, 75]. In clinical patients, only 5.3 to 17.7% could be resected [74, 75], but it rose to 23.1–56.1% among the mass survey patients [52, 75, 76]. Results of a comparative study of pathologically proven 220 clinical and 66 mass survey patients in the same period showed that 1 year, 2 year and 3 year survival were 14.8, 7.4 and 5.5% in the clinical group, but increased to 64.2, 39.3 and 28.9% respectively in the mass screening patients [75]. The survival data of 117 patients in Qidong detected in mass survey and treated surgically were also very striking [76]. The survival pattern of clinical patients has been stable for several decades. The 3 year survival also amounted to 6% both in the United States during 1964–1969 [77] and in Japan during 1968–1977 [78]. It seems, therefore, that mass screening might be the principal approach to improve the prognosis of patients having liver cell cancer.

3.1.2. Comparison Between Surgical Resection and Conservative Treatment. Surgical resection is so far the curative treatment of choice. The priority of this modality is even more clearly demonstrated among mass survey patients. The longer the follow-up, the greater will be the difference. 79.1% vs 45.2% in 1 year survival, 67.8% vs 16.4% in 2 year survival and 61.6% vs 4.1% in 3 year survival were observed in the patients who received resection or conservative treatment respectively[75]. Similar results were also obtained in the Shangai group. The 1, 2, and 3 year survival rate of cases with tumor excision were 86.7, 75.0 and 57.1% respectively. The corresponding figures in the group treated by drugs were only 70.4%, 26.8% and 10.0%[52]. In another series with small liver cell cancer, the corresponding survival rate rose to 83.3%, 70.5% and 70.0% after resection[79]. The conclusion is to make every effort for radical resection of tumor in subclinical stage with compensated liver function.

3.1.3. Pathological Basis for Early Resection. A comparative study on the pathology of liver cell cancer in different groups revealed that the following factors may contribute to the improvement of survival after resection of the small liver cell cancer: 1) Well encapsulated tumor was observed in 85.0% of the small cancer group, 45.0% in the clinical group and none in the necropsies. 2) Tumor embolus in portal or hepatic vein occurred less frequently in the small liver cell cancer, being 30.0%, 70.0% and 100% in the corresponding groups. 3) The accompanied liver cirrhosis in small liver cell cancer was less severe. It was observed in 37.5%, 83.3%, and 94.7% among the corresponding groups. 4) Small liver cell cancers were mostly well differentiated[80]. Similar results were also reported from necropsy material in Japan[81]. Furthermore, a better immunological status was observed in patients with small liver cell cancer[79].

3.2. Surgical Resection

The history of surgical resection for liver cancer has progressed from the stage of anatomical basis, through the stage of physiological basis to the present stage of biological basis. Owing to the rapid growing knowledge on tumor immunology and cancer biology, some new concepts have been emphasized; early detection and radical resection, local resection for small tumors, multimodality treatment, second look operation, etc. During the last ten years, large series (over 80 cases) of resection for liver cell cancer were recorded[76, 82–89]. Efforts have been directed to further increase the resectability, decrease the operative mortality and prolong the survival.

3.2.1. Efforts to Increase Resectability. The relatively low resectability of liver cell cancer mostly resulted from the dissemination of malignant cells, the accompanying liver cirrhosis and the involvement of the portahepatitis. Early detection has been stressed to enable the dramatic increase of the rate of resection. The so-called 'bloodless hepatectomy' – vascular isolation with [90, 91] or without hypothermic perfusion [92] — has been employed. These new techniques have further increased the resectability of tumors located near the portahepatis and inferior vena cava. The cirrhosis present makes resection difficult, especially on the right lobe. Nevertheless, local resection or partial hepatectomy instead of typical right lobectomy for cancer in relatively early stage is usually helpful to increase the resectability and provides similar survival [93].

3.2.2. Efforts to Decrease Operative Mortality. Operative mortality for resection of liver cell cancer has decreased from 24% to around 10% or less [82, 87, 88] in recent years. Hepatic failure and hemorrhage are the two major causes of postoperative death. Efforts include: prior dissection of the hilum with ligation of lobar portal vein and hepatic artery [95]; and, finger fracture method and hepatic clamp [85] or temporary occlusion of the portahepatis [88] to control bleeding. Careful judgement of the extent of hepatic resection in right lobe on cirrhosis background is one of the key links to decrease operative mortality [93]. Resection in mass survey patients further decreases the operative death from 5.1% to 2.7% in one series [75] and from 8.6% to 0 in another [87].

3.2.3. Efforts to Prolong Survival after Resection. Analysis of the resected cases of liver cell cancer showed that early detection and curative resection were the two major factors influencing the probability of long-term survivals [82, 96]. Most favorable outcome was indicated by the rapid return to normal level of serum AFP, below 20 ng/ml. Reappearance of AFP was observed in 33.3% of a series after radical resection [79]. Second look operations were tried to remove the solitary lung metastasis or liver recurrence in selective cases, and encouraging results were recorded [97]. Postoperative multimodality treatment has also been emphasized.

3.3. Surgical Approach to Nonresectable Cases

Surgical management of nonresectable liver cell cancer has been a major issue for years. Intravascular infusion chemotherapy, dearterialization, cryosurgery, and laser irradiation have been employed.

3.3.1. Intravascular Infusion Chemotherapy. Intravascular infusion chemotherapy has been an essential form of treatment for nonresectable liver cell cancer since 1962 [98]. Based on the hypervascular nature of the cancer in most cases, transhepatic artery catheterization and chemotherapy infusion remains the most common procedure. However, portal vein catheterization via umbilical vein or mid-colic vein has also been reported [99]. 5-FU, FUDR, thiotepa, methotrexate, adriamycin [100, 101], mitomycin C, and actinomycin D are agents commonly used. The use of *Corynebacterium parvum* [102] and radioisotopes [103] have also been reported.

Some modifications have been developed: intermittent occlusion of hepatic artery by balloon [104], or by starch microsphere [105]; one shot chemotherapy through selective celiac or hepatic artery catheterization [106]; isolation perfusion chemotherapy [107]; and, hepatic artery infusion with whole liver irradiation [108]. In China, infusion chemotherapy in combination with Chinese medicinal herbs has been used [109, 110]. One patient survived for 6 years [110]. Complications including bleeding in the upper GI tract and arterial thrombosis in a transbrachial procedure [111] were observed. Prolongation of survival, fall of AFP and relief of symptoms in patients having good response were also observed [106, 109].

3.3.2. Dearterialization and Arterial Embolization. Hepatic dearterialization has been claimed as a useful palliative treatment for hypervascular nonresectable liver cancer [112–115]. Liver cell cancer derives most of its blood supply from the artery [116]. Ligation of hepatic artery resulted in necrosis of tumor, but collateral circulation was reestablished within 6 weeks [117]. The mortality rate after hepatic artery ligation is 6.7% [118] to 17% [114]. Renal failure resulting from massive tissue necrosis was reported to be the major cause of death [119]. This procedure is contraindicated in case of huge tumor, occupying over 70% of liver [120]. Blood gases were employed as a guide to the safety of hepatic artery ligation [121]. Patients having severe cirrhosis, decompensated liver function, portal vein occlusion, jaundice or ascites are also contraindicated. Intermittent occlusion has been designed to minimize the complication mentioned above [104, 105]. In a series of 22 cases receiving ligitation of the hepatic artery, 1 year survival amounted to 33.3% [109]. In another series of 60 cases, 19 survived over one year [118]. Arterial embolization by gel foam injection through selective hepatic arteriographic catheter offers similar palliative results. Regression of tumor, decline of AFP and prolongation of survival time were observed [122].

3.3.3. Cryosurgery and laser. Since 1974 cryosurgery has been employed for treatment of nonresectable liver cell cancer in China. It is indicated for localized tumor without severe liver cirrhosis. The 1, 2, and 3 year survival of 28 cases was found to be 58.3, 18.2 and 12.5% respectively. One patient survived 4 years and 2 months and died from pneumonia: autopsy revealed no recurrence in the area of cryosurgery [123]. Experimental study for laser evaporization of tumor has also been explored [124].

3.4. Conservative Treatment of Liver Cell Cancer

3.4.1. Radiation Therapy. In 1956 impressive results of radiotherapy were obtained; five of ten patients survived over one year[125]. In subsequent studies the effect observed was not encouraging[126, 127]. Of 43 patients, 22% survived over one year[127]. The present trend of radiotherapy has been its combination with chemotherapy and immunotherapy[118]. Anticoagulants might be of value for minimizing radiation hepatitis[128]. Longer survival was obtained after radiotherapy when compared with drug therapy[129]. Experiences accumulated led to the following opinion: in localized cancer without severe cirrhosis, radiotherapy may be an acceptable modality for non-resectable cases. In 178 cases of moderate stage during 1966–1975, 1 year survival was 37.1% and 5 year survival 5.1%. Accuracy of radiation field, a total dose over 4000 rads, combination with small dose of chemotherapy and Chinese medicinal herbs were considered to be important factors[130]. Internal radiation by intra-arterial or intravenous administration of radioactive isotopes ^{90}Y microsphere[103], colloidal ^{32}P[131], colloidal ^{198}Au[132] have also been reported.

3.4.2. Chemotherapy. The relatively low response rate of systemic chemotherapy in liver cell cancer has not been changed for a long time. The 1 year survival was 5.4% [74] and 12% [77] before the 1970s. Neither single agent nor combination therapy provided a satisfactory response[126, 133, 134]. Since 1975, adriamycin has been claimed to be a promising drug in the treatment of liver cancer[135–137]. Meanwhile, oral 5-Fu or its analog Ftorafur has also been reported to be useful[138, 139]. 35.7% of partial response was observed by using camptothecin suspension treatment in 263 cases, but the remission period was only 30–100 days[140]. Recently, Eckhardt[141] reviewed the literature and concluded: of drugs adequately tested, only methotrexate, adriamysin and 5-fluorouracil show activity against primary liver cancer. Adequately tested drugs showing no or marginal activity include actinomycin D, CCNU, methyl-CCNU, cyclophosphamide, and cytosine arabinoside.

3.4.3. Chinese Traditional Medicine. The one year survival rate after treatment with Chinese medicinal herbs was 11.7% in 205 cases of moderate stage, compared with 10.8% in the chemotherapy group[74]. It appeared to be more acceptable among patients accompanied by severe liver cirrhosis[142]. Results of 400 cases using a combination of Chinese traditional medicine and chemotherapy showed that lower incidence of bleeding (GI bleeding or rupture of tumor nodule) and longer survival were observed with appropriate combination of the two modalities[143].

3.4.4. Immunotherapy. Observations demonstrated that the cellular immunity of liver cancer patients was inversely related to the stage of development of the disease, as revealed by various immunological parameters [144, 145]. An array of immunotherapeutic agents, such as tumor cell vaccine, fetal liver cell, transfer factor, immune RNA, BCG, *C.parvum*, levamisole and others, have been tried for any beneficial effect on liver cell cancer. Only BCG had been adequately tested and proved to be of limited value to the patients [146, 147].

4. SUMMARY

Epidemiological studies have identified aflatoxins and hepatitis B virus to be the most probable candidates for etiological factors in human liver cell cancer, and have stressed the importance of host factors in determining the mode of response. Prevention trials on the basis of recent development have been planned and started in the high incidence areas.

Serological-survey studies have demonstrated the existence of an early stage of liver cell cancer having a high potential of being cured, and have formulated the serological basis for its early diagnosis among the AFP positive members. Further exploration for non-traumatic techniques capable of assessing small liver cancer in location and extent, as well as for new tumor markers of the AFP negative counterparts, will promote the development of a complete strategy for early diagnosis of liver cell cancer.

Liver surgery has been refined in recent years. Radical resection of the localized tumors among subclinical patients detected and diagnosed through AFP serology has significantly increased the survival rate and has led to the appearance of a considerable number of candidates for long-term survival. Facing the problems of possible early dissemination of tumor, severe cirrhotic background, possible location of tumor in 'forbidden areas', the lack of suitable marker among AFP negative tumors, and others, further improvement in survival and further reduction of iatrogenic complications remains a great challenge to medicine.

REFERENCES

1. Linsell CA: Epidemiology of liver cancer. In: Advances in Medical Oncology, research and education, vol IX: Digestive cancer, Thatcher N (ed). Oxford: Pergamon 1979, pp 61–68.
2. Blumberg BS, London WT: Hepatitis B virus and primary hepatocellular carcinoma; the relation of 'Icrons' to cancer. 7th Cold Spring Harbor conference on cell proliferation, 1979 (In press.

3. Szmuness W, Linsley F: The relationship between hepatocellular carcinoma and hepatitis B virus infection. 7th Cold Spring Harbor conference on cell proliferation, 1979. In press.

4. National Cancer Office of Ministry of Health, The People's Republic of China: Studies on mortality rate of cancer in China (in Chinese). Beijing: People's Health Publishing House, 1980.

5. Linsell DA, Higginson J: The geographic pathology of liver cell cancer. In: Liver cell cancer, Cameron HM, Linsell DA, Warwick GP (eds). Amsterdam: Elsevier Scientific, 1976, pp 1–16.

6. Editorial committee for atlas of cancer mortality: Atlas of cancer mortality in the People's Republic of China (in Chinese). Beijing: China Map Press, 1980.

7. Kew MC: Hepatocellular cancer in southern Africa. In: Primary liver tumors, Remmer H, Bolt HM, Bannash P, Popper H (eds). Lancaster: MTP Press, 1978, pp 179–183.

8. Trichopoulos D, Violaki M, Sparros L, Xirouchake E: Epidemiology of hepatitis B and primary hepatic carcinoma. Lancet 2:1038–1039, 1975.

9. Hirayama T: Strategy for cancer control in Asia. GANN Monogr Cancer Res 18:3–16, 1976.

10. Anthony PP: The background to liver cell cancer. In: Liver cell cancer, Cameron HM, Linsell DA, Warwick GP (eds). Amsterdam: Elsevier Scientific, 1976, pp 93–120.

11. Cameron HM: Pathology of liver cell cancer. In: Liver cell cancer, Cameron HM, Linsell DA, Warwick GP (eds). Amsterdam: Elsevier Scientific, 1976, pp 17–43.

12. Obada H: Hepatitis B virus and liver cancer and cirrhosis of the liver. Clinician 24:63, 1977.

13. Sun Zongtang, Wang Nengjun, Xia Qiujie, Wan Laiqi, Zhang Yulan: Pathological and serological investigation on early primary hepatocellular carcinoma and its liver disease background (in Chinese). Chin J Oncol 1:13–19, 1979.

14. Wogan GN: The induction of liver cell cancer by chemicals. In: Liver cell cancer, Cameron HM, Linsell DA, Warwick GP (eds). Amsterdam: Elsevier Scientific, 1976, pp 121–152.

15. Adamson RH, Correa P, Sieber SM, McIntire KR, Dalgard DW: Carcinogenicity of aflatoxin B1 in rhesus monkeys: two additional cases of primary liver cancer. J Nat Cancer Inst 57:67–78, 1976.

16. Shank RC, Gordon JE, Wogan CN, Nondasuta A, Subhamani B: Dietary Aflatoxins and human liver cancer III. Field survey of rural Thai families for ingested aflatomins. Food Cosmet Toxicol 10:61–84, 1972.

17. Peers FG, Linsell CA: Dietary aflatoxins and liver cancer: a population based study in Kenya. Br J Cancer 27:473–484, 1973.

18. Van Rensburg SJ, van der Watt JJ, Purchase IFH, Pereira Cautinho L, Markham R: Primary liver cancer rate and aflatoxin intake in a high incidence area. S Afr Med J 48:2508a-d, 1974.

19. Peers FG, Gilman GA, Linsell CA: Dietary aflatoxins and human liver cancer. A study in Swaziland. Int J Cancer 17:167–176, 1976.

20. Linsell CA, Peers FG: Fields studies on liver cell cancer. In: Origins of human cancer, Book A, Hiatt HH, Watson JD, Winsten JA (eds). Cold Spring Harbor Laboratory, 1977, pp 549–556.

21. Deng Nihun: Aflatoxins and liver cancer (in Chinese). Qidong Liver Cancer Res 1976, pp 36–39.

22. Sieber SM, Adamson Rh: Chemical carcinogenesis in non-human primates and attempt at prevention. In: Antiviral mechanism in the control of neoplasm, Chandra P (ed). New York: Plenum, 1978, pp 455–480.

23. Takahashi DM: High pressure liquid chromatographic determination of aflatoxins in wines and other liquid products. J AOAC 60:799–804, 1978.

24. Sun PS, Chu FS: A simple solid-phase radioimmunoassay for aflatoxin Bl. J Food Safety 1:67–75, 1977.
25. Preussmann R: Hepatocarcinogens as potential risk for human liver cancer. In: Primary liver tumors, Remmer H, Bolt HM, Bannasch P, Popper H (eds). Lancaster: MTP Press, 1978, pp 11–29.
26. Hu Yun-mei: Nitrosamines and liver cancer (in Chinese). Qidong Liver Cancer Res 1976, pp 45–50.
27. Nishioka K: Hepatocellular carcinoma and hepatitis B virus. In: Hepatitis viruses, Toshitsugu Oda (ed). University of Tokyo Press, 1978, pp 247–255.
28. Chou Lizhong: Hepatitis and liver cancer (in Chinese). Qidong Liver Cancer Res 1976, pp 31–35.
29. Lu Gianhua: Prospective study on HBsAg Positive and negative populations in Qidong county (in Chinese). To be published.
30. Beasley RP, Lin CC: Hepatoma risk among HBsAg carriers. Am J Epidemiol 108:247, 1978.
31. Simons MJ, Chen SH: Liver and pancreatic tumors, liver tumoroncogenesis. In: Advances in medical oncology, research and education, vol V: Digestive cancer, Thatcher N (ed). Oxford: Pergamon 1979, pp69–79.
32. Sun Zongtang, Chu Yuan-yan, Wang Laiqi, Xia Qiujie, Wang Nengjun, Zhang Yulan: Immunological approach to natural history, early diagnosis and etiology of human hepatocellular carcinoma (in Chinese). 7th Cold Spring Harbor Conference on cell proliferation, 1979. (In press.
33. Remmer H: Metabolism of carcinogens; its significance for the initiation of liver tumors. In: Primary liver tumors, Remmer H, Bolt HM, Bannasch P, Popper H (eds). Lancaster: MTP Press, 1978, pp 31–49.
34. Yu Zhan-Zhang: Primary hepatoma (in Chinese). In: Epidemiology, Geng Guan-ye (ed). Beijing: People's Health Publishing House, 1980, pp 638–654.
35. Millman I, Blumberg BS: Perspectives de la vaccination contre le virus de l'hepatite. Rev Prat 28:1943, 1978.
36. Maupas P, Gougeau A, Coursaget P, Drucker J, Barin F, Perrin J, Chiron JP, Denis F, Diop Mar, Summers J: HBV infection and hepatoma — epidemiological, clinical and virology study in Senegal. Perspective of prevention by active immunization. 7th Cold Spring Harbor Conference on cell Proliferation, 1979. To be published.
37. Stewart WE II: The interferon system. Berlin: Springer-Verlag, 1979.
38. Sun Tsung-tang, Wan Lai-che, Chang Yu-lan, Lu Cheng-hung, Hsia Chu-chieh, Li Fengming: Radio-rocket electrophoresis autography (RREA) through labelled antigen for AFP assay and its application in sero-epidemiological investigation on primary hepatocellular carcinoma. Chin Med J 92:17, 1979.
39. Coordinating Group for Research on liver cancer, China: Studies on human AFP (in Chinese). Res Cancer Control 4:277–286, 1974. Abstract form in: Int Cancer Congress, Florence, Abst. No. 3, p 492, 1974.
40. Coordinating group for research on liver cancer in Qidong: Experience on early diagnosis and surgical treatment of primary liver cancer (in Chinese). Res Cancer Control 1:1–5, 1975.
41. Coordinating group for research on liver cancer, China: Studies on human alpha-fetoprotein; further study in the application of AFP assay in mass screening for liver cancer (in Chinese). Nat Med J China 58:586–588, 1978.
42. Abelev GI: Alpha-fetoprotein in ontogenesis and its association with malignant tumors. Adv Cancer Res 14:295–358, 1971.
43. Alpert E: Assay summary on serum alpha-1-fetoprotein (AFP). In: Compendium of assays

for immunodiagnosis of human cancer, Herberman RB (ed). Amsterdam: Elsevier North-Holland, 1979, pp 35–39.

44. Chu Yuan-yun: AFP sero-survey and early diagnosis of liver cell cancer in the Qidong field (in Chinese). Chin J Oncol 3:35–38, 1981.

45. Purves LR: Alpha-fetoprotein and the diagnosis of liver cell cancer. In: Liver cell cancer. Cameron HM, Linsell DA, Warwick GP (eds). Amsterdam: Elsevier Scientific, 1976, pp 61–79.

46. Okuda K, Kotoda K, Obata H, Hayashi N, Nisamitsu T, Tamiya M, Kubo Y, Yakushiji FF, Nagata E, Jinnouchi S, Shimokawa Y: Clinical observation during a relatively early stage of hepatocellular carcinoma — with special reference to serum alpha-fetoprotein levels. Gastroenterology 69:226–234, 1975.

47. Lo Gin-han, Chu Yuan-yun, Cheng Ming, Chou Ai-ding, She Pin-van: Preliminary report on the use of haemaglutination test for serum AFP in mass survey of hepatocellular carcinoma (in Chinese). Res Cancer Control 1:6–12, 1975.

48. Sun Tsung-tang, Wang Lai-che: Radio-rocket electrophoresis autography in assaying serum AFP (in Chinese). Res Cancer Control 1:12–16, 1975.

49. Ji Zhen, Sun Zongtang, Wang Laiqi, Ding Guanshuo, Chu Peipei, Li Fengming: Characteristics of AFP serology in early PHC and the high risk group (in Chinese). Chin J Oncol 1:96–100, 1979.

50. Yeh HC: Ultrasonography and computed tomography of the liver In: Progress in liver diseases, vol VI, Popper H, Schaffner F (eds). New York: Grune & Stratton, 1979, pp 519–537.

51. Okuda K, Obata H, Kubo Y, Nakashima T: Early diagnosis and angiographic feature of hepatocellular carcinoma. In: Primary liver tumors, Remmer H, Bolt HM, Bannasch P, Popper H (eds). Lancaster: MTP Press, 1978, pp 149–164.

52. Shanghai Coordinating Group for Research on Liver Cancer, Shanghai, China (Tang Zhaoyou *et al.*): Diagnosis and treatment of primary hepatocellular carcinoma in early stage-report of 134 cases. Chin Med J 92:801–806, 1979.

53. Zhongshan Hospital, Shanghai First Medical College: Transumbilical hepatography for diagnosis of primary liver cancer (in Chinese). Nat Med J China 55:265–269, 1975.

54. Tang Zhaoyou, Yang Binghui, Zhou Xinda: Advances in early diagnosis of primary liver cancer in China (in Chinese). Chin J Oncol 1:233–235, 1979.

55. Tang Zhaoyou, Yu Yeqin, Zhou Xinda, Cao Yunzhen, Lu Jizhen: Small hepatocellular carcinoma IV diagnosis of small hepatocellular carcinoma (in Chinese). Acta Acad Med Primae Shanghai 5:118–125, 1978.

56. Okuda K, Nakashima T: Hepatocellular carcinoma: A review of the recent studies and developments. In: Progress in liver diseases, vol V, Popper H, Schaffner F (eds). New York: Grune & Stratton, 1979, pp 639–650.

57. Tang Zhaoyou: Screening and early treatment of primary liver cancer — with special reference to the eastern part of China. Annls Acad Med Singapore 9:234–239, 1980.

58. Kawasaki H, Sakaguchi S, Irisa T, Hirayama C: Value of B-scan Ultrasonography in the diagnosis of liver cancer — accuracy compared to scintigraphy and angiography. Am J Gastroenterol 69:436–442, 1978.

59. Sheedy PF, Stephen DH, Hattery RR, Stanson AW, Adson MA, MacCarty RL: CT and angiography in the evaluation of patients with suspected solitary hepatic mass lesions. J Computer assist Tomography 3:556, 1979.

60. Kusano S, Kubayashi T, Matsubayashi T, Ishiik, Shibata H, Kido Kido Y, Ohmiya H: Comuted tomography of the liver; the cross-sectional anatomy of the liver and its clinical usefulness in the diagnosis of the liver cancer. Acta hepatol Jap 19:299–312, 1978.

61. Stephens DH, Sheedy PF, Hattery RR, MacCarty RI: Computed tomography of the liver.

Am J Roentgenol 128:579–590, 1977.

62. Yeh SDJ, Benua RS: Gallium Scans For follow-up of patients with lymphoma and hepatoma. In: Medical radionuclide imaging, vol II. Vienna: International Atomic Energy Agency, 1977.

63. Bryan PJ, Dinn WM, Grossman ZD, Wistow BW, McAfee JC, Kieffer SA: Correlation of computed tomography, gray scale ultrasonography and radionuclide imaging of the liver in detecting space occupying process. Radiology 124:387–393, 1977.

64. Yeh SDJ, Watson RC, Benua RS: A comparison of radionuclide studies with early experience with CTT scans of the abdomen. In: Medical radionuclide imaging, vol I. Vienna: International Atomic Energy Agency, 1977, pp 463–475.

65. Hattori N: Immuno-biochemical diagnosis of hepatocellular carcinoma (HCC) with special reference to AFP-lower and negative cases with HCC. In: Abst of International Workshop on Primary Liver Cancer and Chronic Hepatitis. Singapore, 1979, p 23.

66. Oon CJ, Yo SI: Presence of a hepatoma-liver antigen in the sera of patients with primary hepatocellular carcinoma. Singapore Med J 20:317, 1979.

67. Thung SN, Berber MA, Sarno E, Popper H: Distribution of five antigens in hepatocellular carcinoma. Lab Invest 41:101–105, 1979.

68. Chio LF, Oon CJ: Changes in serum alpha 1 antitrypsin, Alpha 1 acid glycoprotein and beta 2 glycoprotein I in patients with malignant hepatocellular carcinoma. Cancer 43:596–604, 1979.

69. Tsou KC, Lo KW: Serum 5′-nucleotide phosphodiesterase isozyme V test for human liver cancer. Cancer 45:209–213, 1980.

70. Xin Hua Hospital: Serum 5′-nucleotide phosphodiesterase isozyme V and primary liver cancer (in Chinese). Personal communication, 1980.

71. Tang Zhaoyou: Treatment of primary liver cancer — with special reference to the eastern part of China. Annls Acad Med Singapore 9:251–255, 1980.

72. Hung Shunyou, Sa Yen-wen: Diagnosis, surgical effect and prognosis of small liver cell cancer, clinical analysis of 38 cases. Res Cancer Control, 1980. To be published.

73. Liver Cancer Study Group of Japan: Survey and follow-up study of primary liver cancer in Japan-report 3. Acta Hepatol Jap 17:460–465, 1976.

74. Shangai Coordinating Group for Liver Cancer Research, China (Tang Zhaoyou et al.): Primary liver cancer — a clinical analysis of 3,254 cases (from 11 provinces 21 hospitals in China) (in Chinese). Res Cancer Control 3:207–215, 1974.

75. Tang Zhaoyou, Yang Binghui, Tang Chenlong, Yu Yeqin, Lin Zhiying, Weng Huizhi: Evaluation of population screening for detection of hepatocellular carcinoma. Chin Med J 93:795–799, 1980.

76. Hung Shunyao: Surgical treatment of primary hepatoma. Report on 117 cases (in Chinese). Chin J Oncol 3:57–60, 1981.

77. Nat Cancer Inst: End results in cancer. Report No. 4. U.S. Department of Health, Education & Welfare. Public Health Service, 1972.

78. Liver Cancer Study Group of Japan: Survey and follow-up study of primary liver cancer in Japan-report 4. Acta Hepatol Jap 20:433–441, 1979.

79. Tang Zhaoyou, Yu Yeqin, Lin Zhiying, Zhou Xinda, Yang Binghui, Cao Yunzhen, Lu Jizhen, Tang Chenlong: Small hepatocellular carcinoma. Clinical analysis of 30 cases (in Chinese). Chin Med J 92:455–462, 1979.

80. Ying Yehying, Chai Weiyung: Small hepatocellular carcinoma. III. Pathology of small hepatocellular carcinoma (in Chinese). Acta Acad Med Primae Shanghai 5:111–118, 1978.

81. Okuda K, Nakashima T, Obata H, Kubo Y: Clinicopathological studies of minute hepatocellular carcinoma. Analysis of 20 cases, including 4 with hepatic resection. Gastroentero-

logy 73:109–115, 1977.

82. Tang Zhaoyou: Surgical resection of primary liver cancer (in Chinese). In: Primary liver cancer, Tang Zhaoyou (ed). Shanghai Sci & Technical press, 1980, chap 19.

83. Shanghai Coordinating Group for Research on Liver Cancer, China: Surgical resection of primary liver cancer — analysis of 258 cases (in Chinese). Res Cancer Control 3:215–218, 1974.

84. Foster JH, Berman MM: Solid liver tumors. Philadelphia: Saunders, 1977.

85. Lin TY: Results in 107 hepatic lobectomies with a preliminary report on the use of a clamp to reduce blood loss. Ann Surg 177:413–421, 1973.

86. Ong GB, Chan PKW: Primary carcinoma of the liver. Surg Gynecol Obstet 143:31–38, 1976.

87. Tang Zhaoyou, Qian Shiquang: Surgical treatment of primary liver cancer (material in Chitung county) (in Chinese). Jiangsu Med 11:501–505, 1977.

88. Wu Mongchao: Eighteen years experience in surgical resection of primary liver cancer (in Chinese). 9th Proc National Surgical Conference, China, 1978.

89. Balasegaram M: Hepatic resection for malignant tumors. Surg Rounds 2:14–26, 1979.

90. Fortner JG, Shiu MH, Kinne DW, Castro EB, Watson RC, Hawland WS, Beattie EJ: Major hepatic resection using vascular isolation and hypothermia perfusion. Ann Surg 180:644–652, 1974.

91. Yu Yeqin, Tang Zhaoyou, Zhou Xinda, Lin Zhiying, Lu Jizhen, Cao Yunzhen: Bloodless hepatectomy (in Chinese). Chin J Surg 18:146–147, 1980.

92. Offenstadt G, Huguet C, Gallot D, Bloch P: Hemodynamic monitoring during complete vascular exclusion for extensive hepatectomy. Surg Gynecol Obstet 146:709–713, 1978.

93. Yu Yeqin, Tang Zhaoyou, Zhou Xinda: Experience in hepatic resection of small hepatocellular carcinoma (in Chinese). Chin J Surg 16:266–268, 1978.

94. Foster JH: Survival after liver resection for cancer. Cancer 26:493–502, 1970.

95. Pack GT, Baker HW: Total right hepatic lobectomy. Ann Surg 138:253–258, 1953.

96. Cao Yunzhen, Tang Zhaoyou, Ying Yehying, Chai Weiyung: Factors influencing prognosis of primary liver cancerclinicopathological analysis of 224 cases (in Chinese). Nat Med J China 59:35–40, 1979.

97. Yu Yeqin, Tang Zhaoyou, Zhou Xinda: Second look operation on recurrence of liver cancer after resection (in Chinese). To be published.

98. Clarkson B, Young C, Dierick W, Kuchn P, Kim M, Berrett A, Clapp P, Lawrence W: Effects of continuous hepatic artery infusion of anti-metabolities on primary and metastatic cancer of the liver. Cancer 15:472–488, 1962.

99. Fortner JG, Pahnke LD: A new method for long term intrahepatic chemotherapy. Surg Gynecol Obstet 143:979–980, 1976.

100. Bern MM, McDermott W, Cady B, Oberfield Ra, Trey C, Clouse ME, Tullis JL, Parker LM: Intraarterial hepatic infusion and intravenous adriamycin for treatment of hepatocellular carcinoma MM a clinical and pharmacology report. Cancer 42:399–405, 1978.

101. Garnick MB, Ensminger WD, Israel M: Aclinical pharmacological evaluation of hepatic arterial infusion of adriamycin. Cancer Res 39:4105–4110, 1979.

102. Patt YZ, Wallace S, Hersh Em, Hall SW, Menachem YB, Granmayeh M, Mcbride Cm, Benjamin RS, Mavligit GM: Hepatic arterial infusion of Corynebacterium parvum and chemotherapy. Surg Cynecol Obstet 147:879–902, 1978.

103. Ariel IM: Tratment of inoperable primary pancreatic and liver cancer by the intraarterial administration of radioactive isotopes (Y^{90} radiating microspheres). Ann Surg 162:267–278, 1965.

104. El-Domeiri AA, Mojab K: Intermittent occlusion of the hepatic artery and infusion chemotherapy for carcinoma of the liver. Am J Surg 135:771–775, 1978.

105. Aronsen KF, Hellekant C, Holmberg J, Rothman U, Teder H: Controlled blocking of hepatic artery flow with enzymatically degradable microspheres combined with oncolytic drugs. Eur Surg Res 11:99–106, 1979.

106. Sawa Y: Treatment of hepatocellular carcinoma by one shet injection of anticancer agents through the hepatic artery. Acta Hepatol Jap 20:852–860, 1979.

107. Fortner JG et al.: Actinomycin D perfusion of the isolated liver for cancer. Bull Soc Int Chir 34:399, 1975.

108. Friedman Ma, Volherding PA, Cassidy MJ, Resser KJ, Wasserman TH, Phillips TI: Therapy for hepatocellular cancer with intrahepatic arterial adriamycin and 5-fluorouracil combined with whole liver irradiation: a northern California Oncology Group Study. Cancer Treat Rep 63:1885–1888, 1979.

109. Yu Yeqin: Surgical management of nonresectable primary liver cancer (in Chinese). In: Primary liver cancer, Tang zhaoyou (ed). Shanghai Sci & Technical Press, 1980, chap 21.

110. Department of Medicine, Ri Tan Hospital, Chinese Academy of Medical Sciences: Hepatic artery perfusion in treatment of advanced primary liver cancer (in Chinese). National Liver Cancer Conference, Shanghai, China, 1977.

111. Clouse ME, Ahmed R, Ryan RB, Oberfield RA, McCaffrey JA: Complications of long term transbrachial hepatic arterial infusion chemotherapy. Am J Roentgenol 129:799–803, 1977.

112. Riehoff WF, Woods AC: Ligation of hepatic and splenic arteries in treatment of cirrhosis with ascites. JAMA 152:687–690, 1953.

113. Nilson LAV: Therapeutic hepatic artery ligation in patients with secondary liver tumors. Rev Surg 23:374–376, 1966.

114. Almersjo O, Bengmark S, Hafström L, Leissner H: Results of liver dearterialization combined with regional infusion of 5-fluorouracil. Acta Chir Scand 142:131–138, 1976.

115. Nagasue N, Inokuchi K, Kobayashi M, Ogawa Y, Iwaki A, Yukaya H: Hepatic dearterialization for nonresectable primary and secondary tumors of the liver. Cancer 38:2593–2603, 1976.

116. Breedis C, Young G: The blood supply of neoplasm of the liver Am J Pathol 30:969–985, 1954.

117. Kim DK, Kinne DW, Fortner JG: Occlusion of hepatic artery in man. Surg Gynecol Obstet 136:966–968, 1973.

118. Balasegaram M: Management of primary liver cell carcinoma. Am J Surg 130:33–37, 1975.

119. Kim DK, Penneman R, Kallum B, Carrillo M, Scheiner E, Fortner JG. Acute renal failure after ligation of the hepatic artery. Surg cynecol Obstet 143:391–394, 1976.

120. Fortner JG, Kim DK, Barrett MK, Iwatsuki S, Papachristou D, McLaughlin C, Maclean BJ: Eight years experience with the surgical management of 321 patients with liver tumors. In: Adv Med Oncol Res & Education, Canonico A, Estevez O, Chacon R, Barg S (eds). Oxford: Pergamon, 1979, vol 9, pp 93–97.

121. Madden RE, de Blasi H, Zinns J: Blood gases as a guide to the safety of hepatic artery ligation for metastic carcinoma. In: Adv Med Oncol Res & Education, Canonico A, Estevez O, Chacon R, Barg S (eds). Oxford: Pergamon, 1979, vol 9, pp 87–91.

122. Yamada R, Nakatsuka H, Nakamura K, Sato M, Tamaoka K, Takemoto K, Kobayashi N, Itami M, Ono T, Minakuchi K, Yamaguchi S, Tamaki M: Superselective arterial embolization in unresected hepatoma. Nippon Igaku Hoshasen Gakkin Zasshi 39:540–543, 1979.

123. Zhou Xinda, Tang Zhaoyou, Yu Yeqin et al.: Cryosurgery for liver cancer: experimental and clinical study (in Chinese). Chinese J Surg 17:480–483, 1979.

124. Zhou Xinda, Yu Yeqin, Tang Zhaoyou et al.: Experimental study of laser hepatic ausgery

(in Chinese). Acta Acad Med Primae Shanghai 7:216–221, 1980.

125. Ariel IM: The treatment of primary and metastatic cancer of the liver. Surgery 39:70–91, 1956.

126. Geddes EW, Falkson G: Malignant hepatoma in the Bantu. Cancer 25:1271–1278, 1970.

127. El Domeiri AA, Huvos AG, Goldsmith HS, Foote FW: Primary malignant tumors of the liver. Cancer 27:7–11, 1971.

128. Lightdale CJ, Wasser J, Coleman M, Brower M, Tefft M, Pasmantier M: Anticoagulation and high dose liver radiation. Cancer 43:174–181, 1979.

129. Yin Weibai *et al.*: Nonsurgery treatment of primary liver canceranalysis of 60 cases (in Chinese). Nat Med J China 49:499–502, 1963.

130. Yu Erxin: Radiation therapy of primary liver cancer (in Chinese). In: Primary liver cancer, Tang Zhaoyou (ed). Shanghai Sci & Technical Press, 1980, chap 22.

131. Grady ED, Molan TR, Grumbley AJ, Larose JH, Cheek WV: Internal hapatic radiotherapy: II. Intra-arterial radiocolloid therapy for hepatic tumors. Am J Roentgenol 124:596–599, 1975.

132. Nelson BM, Andrews GA, Watson EE: Histopathologic studies of the liver following intravenous colloidal 198Au therapy. Radiology 127:239–247, 1978.

133. Yang Binghui, Tang Zhaoyou: Chemotherapy of primary liver cancer (in Chinese). In: Primary liver cancer, Tang Zhaoyou (ed). Shanghai Sci & Technical press, 1980. chap 24.

134. Link JS, Batemen JR, Paroly Ws, Durkin WJ, Peters RL: 5-Fluoreuracil in hepatocelluler carcinoma: report of twenty-one cases. Cancer 39:1936–1939, 1977.

135. Olweny CLM, Toya T, Katongole-Mbidde E, Mugerwa J, Kyalwazi SK, Cohen H: Treatment of hepatocellular carcinoma with adriamycin. Preliminary communication. Cancer 36:1250–1257, 1975.

136. Falkson G, Moertel CG, Lavin P, Pretorius FJ. Carbone PP: Chemotherapy studies in primary liver cancer — a prospective randomized clinical trial. Cancer 42:2149–2156, 1978.

137. Hepatoma & Liver Study Research Group, Singapore: Clinical studies in Asian patients with irresectable primary hepatocellular carcinoma treated by adriamycin and prednisolone alone or in combination with 5-fluorouracil, vincristine and prednisolone. Singapore Med J 19:192, 1978.

138. Smart CR, Townsend LB, Rusho WJ, Eyre HJ, Qualiana JM, Wilson ML, Edwards CB, Manning SJ: Phase 1 study of Ftoraful, an analog ML, Edwards CB, Manning SJ: Phase 1 study of Ftoraful, an analog of 5-fluorouracil. Cancer 36:103–106, 1975.

139. Kennedy PS, Lehane DE, Smith FE, Lane M: Oral fluorouracil therapy of hepatome. Cancer 39:1930–1935, 1977.

140. Institute materia Medica, Academia Sinica, Shanghai, China: Treatment of primary liver cancer by intravenous administration of camptothecin suspension (in Chinese). 4th National Cancer Congress, China, 1977.

141. Eckhardt S: Chemotherapy of primary liver cancer. J Toxicol Environ Health 5:395–400, 1979.

142. Shanghai Coordinating Group for Cancer Research, China: Primary liver cancer — analysis of 1,200 cases (in Chinese) Shanghai Med 9:3–8, 1973.

143. Liver Cancer Research Unit, Zhongshan Hospital, Shanghai First Medical College, Shanghai (Tang Zhaoyou *et al.*): Experience in combination treatment of Chinese traditional medicine and western medicine of primary liver cancer. (in Chinese). Res Cancer Control 5:96–104, 1977.

144. Dairo Kan *et al.*: Cellular immunity in hepatocellular carcinoma Acta Hepatol Jap 19:175, 1978.

145. Lin Zhiying, Tang Zhaoyou: Delayed hypersensitivity reaction to old tuberculin and the

prognosis of primary carcinoma of the liver (in Chinese). Acta Acad Med Primae Shanghai 6:103–110, 1979.
146. Liver Cancer Research Unit, Zhongshan Hospital, Shanghai First Medical College, Shanghai, China: Active immunotherapy on primary liver cancer (in Chinese). Res Cancer Control 3:336–339, 1975.
147. Lin Zhiying, Tang Zhaoyou: Immunostatus and immunotherapy of primary liver cancer (in Chinese). In: Primary liver cancer, Tang Zhaoyou (ed). Shanghai Sci & Technical press, 1980, chap 25.

15. Chemotherapy of Pancreatic, Colorectal and Gastric Cancer

JOHN R. NEEFE and PHILIP S. SCHEIN

1. ADENOCARCINOMA OF THE PANCREAS

1.1. Epidemiology and Natural History

Pancreatic cancer currently represents the fifth leading cause of cancer death in this country; its toll is surpassed only by lung, colon and rectum, breast, and prostate cancer[1]. The only therapeutic modality with the potential for cure is surgery, and even with surgery the cure rate is exceedingly low. Most patients present with localized or regional disease but an attempt at resection is warranted in only a minor fraction because of involvement of major abdominal structures[2]. Gudjonsson *et al.*[3] have analyzed 100 patients from their own institution and reviewed a number of series in the literature. They calculate from their own patients a median survival of $5\frac{1}{2}$ months from the time of first symptoms, a median survival of four months from the time of histologically confirmed diagnosis, a one year survival of 10% and a five year survival of 1% (a single patient who survived eight years with a palliative bypass procedure but without resection). They estimate from review of the literature that 80% of patients with carcinoma of the pancreas come to abdominal exploration; however, only 10–15% of these are resected for cure. Fewer than 1% survive five years, and many institutions have failed to record their first five year survival.

1.2. Staging

The development of a staging system usually depends on variables of presentation which determine prognosis. Since the prognosis of pancreatic cancer is uniformly grim, staging has not been of very great practical importance. It is worthwhile, however, to delineate certain groups of patients, particularly in understanding drug trials. Patients are inoperable if they have evidence of distant metastasis but no evidence of biliary or intestinal obstruction. Patients are resectable for cure if they have tumor confined to the

J. J. DeCosse and P. Sherlock (eds.), Gastrointestinal cancer 1, 413-444. All rights reserved.
Copyright © 1981 Martinus Nijhoff Publishers, The Hague/Boston/London.

pancreas without involvement by local extension of neighboring vascular or other vital structures and without evidence of distant metastasis or lymph node involvement. Patients with locally advanced disease have involvement by direct extension into neighboring vital structures or lymph nodes and no evidence of distant metastasis. Patients with advanced disease have evidence of distant metastases, often to the liver.

1.3. Importance of Histological Diagnosis

It has been claimed that diagnosis of pancreatic cancer can be made by observation at laporatomy. Since biopsy of the involved pancreas may lead to fistula formation, hemorrhage, pancreatitis, and abscess in up to 10% of cases and even an occasional death [4] many surgeons are reluctant to establish the diagnosis histologically. As a consequence, patients without cancer in the operative specimen have undergone a needless aggressive resection. If diagnosis of cancer carries a therapeutic implication in a given patient — either resection, radiotherapy, or chemotherapy, none of which is risk-free — histological diagnosis must be made. This will also ensure proper identification of benign pancreatitis, the occasional lymphoma or mucinous cystadenocarcinoma, each of which has a very different natural history from the usual pancreatic carcinoma. At laporatomy, patients with tumor restricted to the pancreas can be biopsied with an acceptably low risk of complications [5]. An alternative to open biopsy is percutaneous fine needle aspiration with ultrasound guidance [6, 7]. Although this procedure requires a skilled cytopathologist, the reported morbidity is negligible and the false negative rate is only about 20%. Tissue diagnosis has also been accomplished by endoscopic aspiration biopsy through a flexible fiberoptic duodenoscope [8] or by cytology of pancreatic juice obtained by cannulation of the main pancreatic duct via a duodenoscope [9].

1.4. General Considerations in Chemotherapy of Pancreatic Cancer

Despite the obvious need for effective systemic therapy, only a few anticancer drugs have undergone adequate trials in patients with advanced but measurable disease [10, 11]. Several reasons account for this. The widely held concept that this tumor is resistant to chemotherapy and radiotherapy dampens investigator enthusiasm for pursuing new trials. This concept in turn traces from difficulties in identifying measurable parameters of disease and from the fact that the disease is rapidly progressive and debilitating. Modern methods of delineating masses including ultrasound and computed tomography have not yet been fully accepted as reproducible enough to allow actual measurement of pancreatic masses. Most patients with measurable disease must therefore have huge, palpable abdominal masses or large defects by radionuclide scan of the liver. Measurable disease is far advanced, and the concomitant of far advanced disease is pain, anorexia, malabsorption, malnutrition and weight loss; obstructive jaundice and hepatic dysfunction impair the patient's tolerance of many chemotherapeutic agents. Most adequate studies of drug activity in pancreatic cancer have been biased against detection of drug activity by heavy reliance on difficult patients such as these; reports of low activity may reflect more the rapidly progressive nature of the disease than any intrinsic resistance to chemotherapy.

1.5. The Therapeutic Activity of Single Anti-Cancer Agents (Table 1)

5-Fluorouracil (5-FU) has been studied more extensively than any other drug in pancreatic cancer. The range of reported responses in various series is wide, but Carter et al. [12] found an overall response rate of 28% in 212 patients collected from various series. Even this low response rate is probably an overestimate, as current trials with carefully defined criteria of response report rates of under 20% [13].

The value of various modes and schedules of administration of 5-fluorouracil has been debated. Stolinsky et al. compared oral 5-FU at 15 mg/kg weekly to the same dose given intravenously in 30 patients with advanced measurable pancreatic cancer. The response for the group receiving intravenous 5-FU was 21%, but none of the patients receiving oral 5-FU responded [14].

The anti-cancer antibiotic mitomycin C has activity as a single agent comparable to 5-FU. In a relatively small number of patients collected from several series, 27% responded to mitomycin C [12]. This drug was initially given in a loading course of small intravenous doses at daily intervals; this appeared to be well tolerated until it was realized that there is a serious delayed and cumulative myelosuppression commonly resulting in chronic

Table 1. Activity of single agents in adenocarcinoma of the pancreas*.

Drug	Responders/total patients	Response rate % [†]
5-FU	60/212	28
Mitomycin C	12/44	27
Streptozotocin	8/22	36
Adriamycin	2/15	13
Methyl CCNU	3/34	9
BCNU	0/31	0
Actinomycin D	1/28	4
Methotrexate	1/25	4
Chlorambucil	4/6	—
Cyclophosphamide	1/2	—

* References: see text.
[†] Where total patients were greater than 10.

marrow hypoplasia [15]. This problem with mitomycin C may be ameliorated if the drug is given in single doses at about 6 week intervals when one can document recovery of peripheral blood counts from previously observed maximum suppression. When used in this fashion, mitomycin C has been an effective and acceptably safe component of combination regimens.

Chloroethylnitrosoureas have been tested in patients with pancreatic cancer. 1,3 Bis (2 chloroethyl)-1-nitrosourea (BCNU) showed no activity in a trial at the Mayo Clinic. Thirty-one patients were studied, and 22 of these had received no prior therapy [16]. The analogs of BCNU — CCNU and methyl CCNU — were also tested by Moertel and colleagues. A small number of responses to both agents was observed. A larger series of 34 patients studied by the Eastern Cooperative Oncology Group resulted in a 9% response rate to methyl CCNU [17].

Streptozotocin is a naturally occurring nitrosourea with toxicity for the pancreatic islet beta cell in animals [18]. This apparent predilection of streptozotocin for pancreatic tissue has provoked clinical trials of the single agent activity of this drug. An overall response rate of 36% has been observed in collected series of small numbers of patients [12, 19–21]. It seems unlikely that this response rate would be borne out in larger series of consecutive patients, but streptozotocin does have the advantage of relatively mild myelosuppressive properties.

There are few data on alkylating agents in pancreatic cancer. Occasional responses have been reported.

Like streptozotocin, the enzyme inhibitor of protein synthesis, L-asparaginase, seems to have some predilection for pancreatic tissue in that it produces pancreatitis in man. It has been tested for activity against two continuous cell lines derived from pancreatic carcinoma (MiA Pa Ca-2 and PANC-1) and it did result in significant growth inhibition [22]. No therapeutic activity has been reported in clinical trials, however.

A series of Phase II studies was undertaken by the Gastrointestinal Tumor Study Group in an attempt to identify single agents active in pancreatic carcinoma. Sixty-six consecutive patients with measurable advanced disease were treated with doxorubicin (Adriamycin), methotrexate, or actinomycin D as single agents with random assignment to one of the treatment groups [23]. Fifteen of 25 assigned to Adriamycin received the drug as initial therapy and two of these responded for a response rate of 13%. None of the previously treated cases responded. One patient responded to each of the other agents.

Overall, the single agent data are not very encouraging in pancreatic carcinoma, and new agents with activity remain an urgent need. 5-FU, streptozotocin, mitomycin C, and Adriamycin thus far seem to offer the greatest promise and have formed the basis of combination therapy.

1.6. Combination Chemotherapy

The earliest randomized studies of combination chemotherapy failed to demonstrate any superiority to 5-FU administered as a single agent [24, 25]. In part, the discouraging results in the early studies may have been a consequence of (a) small numbers of patients, (b) combination regimens of drugs without any significant activity as single agents, and (c) the debilitated condition of many patients at the time of entry into the studies. Recent reports have been more encouraging, and Table 2 presents a selected list of combination regimens that have been used in carcinoma of the pancreas.

Most combinations have employed 5-FU with a nitrosourea or 5-FU with mitomycin C. Kovach *et al.* in a randomized study compared 5-FU by continuous infusion with BCNU alone and with the combination of 5-FU plus BCNU. Eighty-two patients with advanced pancreatic carcinoma were randomized to one of these three treatment regimens. Of the patients treated with 5-FU alone, 16% responded, but 0 of 21 cases responded to BCNU alone. Ten of 30 patients treated with the combination responded. However, there was no survival benefit when patients treated with the combination were compared with either of the single agent groups [25].

Lokich and Skarin administered 5-FU and BCNU in combination [26]. They obtained 27% objective responses, and responding patients had a longer median survival than nonresponders.

Buroker and colleagues studied two regimens of 5-FU administered by continuous intravenous infusion [27]. The first regimen involved addition of mitomycin C and the second regimen involved the addition of methyl CCNU. One hundred and forty-four patients with advanced measurable pancreatic carcinoma were randomized to one of these treatment arms. The combination of 5-FU and mitomycin C produced a response rate of 30%,

Table 2. Combination chemotherapy for advanced pancreatic cancer: collected experience of selected regimens*.

Combination	Responders/total patients	Response rate %
5-FU + BCNU	14/45	31
5-FU + methyl CCNU	9/113	8
5-FU + mitomycin C	22/72	30
5-FU + mitomycin C + streptozotocin	15/49	31
5-FU + Adriamycin + mitomycin C	16/42	38
Cyclophosphamide + vincristine + methotrexate	6/23	26

* References: see text.

which was statistically superior to the 17% response rate observed with the other combination.

The Eastern Cooperative Oncology Group studied the combination of 5-FU and methyl CCNU in 41 patients with advanced measurable pancreatic carcinoma. Four of 41 responded for an objective response rate of 10% [28].

The three drugs with the highest reported activities as single agents are streptozotocin, 5-FU, and mitomycin C. The Vincent T. Lombardi Cancer Research Center of Georgetown University studied a combination of these three drugs (SMF) in 23 consecutive patients with advanced measurable pancreatic cancer [29]. Forty-three percent of the patients showed an objective response and one patient with biopsy proven hepatic metastases showed a complete response. This patient remains alive and free of clinical evidence of disease more than four years from initiation of SMF therapy. The median survival of all cases was six months, but responders achieved a median survival of 10 months, whereas nonresponders survived only three months. The majority of patients in this study were of good performance status i.e. asymptomatic or symptomatic but ambulatory. Only three of 23 patients were bedridden greater than 50% of the time. The good performance status of the patients in this trial stands in contrast to other treatment series, and the results of this trial demonstrate what can be accomplished with such patients.

The results of the SMF regimen at the Vincent T. Lombardi Cancer Research Center have been confirmed [30]. Sixteen patients were treated with a similar regimen in which 5-FU was given as a loading course, 500 mg/m^2/day IV $\times$ 5; streptozotocin was given 300 mg/m^2/day IV $\times$ 5; and mitomycin C was given 10 mg/m^2 IV on day 1. The cycle was repeated every eight weeks. An objective response was recorded in 31% of the patients treated, and the three drug combination was superior to the two drug combination of 5-FU and streptozotocin.

The nausea and vomiting produced by the streptozotocin as well as the renal toxicity associated with this drug motivated a search for other combinations which might circumvent these problems. The Vincent T. Lombardi Cancer Research Center initiated a pilot study of the FAM regimen in which streptozotocin was replaced by Adriamycin. This regimen is also given in 56 day cycles, and the doses and scheduling are shown in Table 3. Appropriate modifications of dose and schedule were made when necessary. Twenty-seven patients with advanced measurable carcinoma of the pancreas were available for response evaluation. Ten of the 27 patients obtained a partial response for a response rate of 37%. The results with the FAM regimen have been confirmed by other centers [31].

The three drug combination of 5-FU, mitomycin C and hexamethylmelamine was tested in 15 evaluable patients [32]. Six patients (40%) had objective

Table 3. FAM chemotherapy for pancreatic and gastric cancer.

	Day of 56-day cycle							
	1	8	15	22	29	36	43	50
5-FU 600 mg/m² i.v.	X	X			X	X		
Adriamycin 30 mg/m² i.v.	X				X			
Mitomycin C 10 mg/m² i.v.	X							

tumor regressions. The combination of 5-FU, methyl CCNU, and streptozo-tocin, tested by the Eastern Cooperative Oncology Group, resulted in a 7% response rate, and was not superior to 5-FU plus methyl CCNU[28]. The Central Oncology Group compared a three drug combination of 5-FU, strep-tozotocin, and tubercidin with 5-FU alone[33]. There was no benefit of the three drug combination over 5-FU alone. The three drug combination of Adriamycin, BCNU, and the 5-FU analog ftorafur was tested in 19 patients with pancreatic carcinoma[34]. Twenty-six percent of the patients achieved partial remissions. This would not appear to be superior to results achievable with 5-FU alone, and, moreover, a significant myelotoxicity was observed with this three drug combination.

Twenty-three patients were treated with the combination of cyclophos-phamide, vincristine, and methotrexate. Twenty-six percent of the patients responded[35]. Although the response rate appeared to be no better than that reported for 5-FU alone, the responders in this study had a strikingly long duration of response.

In summary, regimens of combination chemotherapy are beginning to show encouraging results in selected patients with advanced carcinoma of the pancreas. Patients with normal liver function, good nutrition, good perfor-mance status, and with modest tumor burden can now be expected to respond 40% of the time to the FAM combination of 5-FU, Adriamycin, and mitomycin C. With careful monitoring and appropriate dosage adjustments, these drugs can be administered with a minimum of toxicity.

1.7. Combined Modality Treatment of Locally Advanced Carcinoma of the Pancreas

Traditionally, it has been believed that carcinoma of the pancreas is not susceptible to radiotherapy, either because of intrinsic radioresistance of the tumor cells or because of limited radiation tolerance of adjacent structures. However, Haslam *et al.* [36] had suggested that regional irradiation, 6000 rads, in several courses separated by 2 week rest periods, could provide effective palliation. A report from the Mayo Clinic [37] also suggested that 3500 to 4000 rads of regional irradiation in two courses separated by a rest period could be enhanced significantly by the addition of intravenous 5-FU in daily doses on the first three days of the course of radiation. The Gastrointestinal Tumor Study Group, compared in a randomized fashion, regional irradiation at two dosage levels with or without 5-FU in patients with locally advanced pancreatic cancer [28]. The first arm of the study consisted of 6000 rads of irradiation in three split courses of 2000 rads in 2 weeks separated by 2 week rest intervals. This arm was subsequently dropped from the study when it was apparent that the regimen produced significantly inferior survival. The other two arms involved split courses of 4000 or 6000 rads combined with intravenous 5-FU at 500 mg/m^2 on the first three days of each course of irradiation and continued weekly after radiation.

The early results indicated that the combined modality regimens of radiotherapy and chemotherapy were superior to radiotherapy at the higher dose alone. The median time to progression with high dose irradiation alone was 13 weeks compared to 28 weeks with 4000 rads plus 5-FU and 32 weeks with 6000 rads plus 5-FU. It was very unlikely that the result could be attributed solely to the toxicity of high dose irradiation, since the same dose of irradiation in combination with chemotherapy produced a much longer median survival period. When the combined modality data were corrected for certain prognostic determinants of survival, the corrected median survival for 4000 rads plus 5-FU was 31 weeks. The corrected median survival for 6000 rads plus 5-FU was 39 weeks, but this difference was not statistically significant [39].

Fast neutron radiotherapy has a theoretical advantage over conventional photon therapy in that it does not require oxygen for effectiveness. It may be more appropriate therapy for poorly vascularized tumor masses with anoxic centers [40]. The Vincent T. Lombardi Cancer Research Center in cooperation with Mid Atlantic Neutron Therapy Association attempted to take advantage of this theoretical advantage by combining 15 MEV fast neutron therapy with or without 5-FU on the first and last three days of radiotherapy. Thirteen patients had measurable disease and partial responses were reported in 46% of these patients. 5-FU at higher doses in combination with fast neutron therapy was excessively toxic. Fast neutron therapy alone or in combination with the lower doses of 5-FU was quite well tolerated. Whether 5-FU added anything to the radiotherapy could not be ascertained due to the small number of patients. However, the two longest survivors did receive 5-FU.

2. COLORECTAL CANCER

2.1. Epidemiology and Natural History

Cancer of the colon and rectum taken together is the second leading cause of cancer death among both males and females and accounts for 12–15% of all deaths in the United States from cancer. 112 000 new cases of colorectal cancer appeared in the United States in 1979, and 52 000 individuals died of this disease [1]. About one half of patients with large bowel cancer develop disseminated disease, and these patients invariably die of their disease. Despite extensive investigations of therapeutic approaches used successfully in other malignancies, the static survival statistics for colorectal cancer during the past three decades demonstrate the lack of real progress in this disease. No curative therapy is available for the patient with disseminated colon cancer, and available palliative therapy is characterized by the modest proportion of patients responding, the limited duration of response, and the marginal impact of response on survival.

2.2. The Therapeutic Activity of 5-FU

Response rates for single drugs used for the treatment of advanced cancer of the colon are summarized in Table 4. Many of these data were tabulated by Wasserman et al. [41] from collected series. The extensive Mayo Clinic expe-

Table 4. Activity of selected single drugs in adenocarcinoma of the colon*.

Drug	Responders/Total patients	Response rate %
5-FU	454/2107	21
Ftorafur	9/84	11
Mitomycin C	35/218	16
Streptozotocin	5/33	15
BCNU	17/128	13
CCNU	7/75	9
Methyl CCNU	18/148	12
Chlorozotocin	6/34	18
Vincristine	0/26	0
Cyclophosphamide	15/71	21
Melphalan	19/110	17
Methotrexate	19/111	17
Actinomycin D	7/48	15
Adriamycin	8/92	9
Hydroxyurea	16/151	10

* References: 41 and others noted in text.

rience, which may be more representative, generally yielded lower objective response rates [42].

Since its development in 1957, 5-fluorouracil (5-FU) has remained the standard drug for colon cancer, and no other drug has thus far proved superior [43]. Carter and colleagues collected over 2000 patients from various series and calculated an overall response rate of 21% [41]; among these series the range of reported response rates was quite large [44].

One approach to improving the response rate of 5-FU has been to optimize the method of administration. Substantial toxicity was seen with the original 'loading course' administration, which involved rapid intravenous injection of 15 mg/kg/day for five days followed by four half doses every other day. Nausea, vomiting, stomatitis, and bone marrow suppression were observed in 50–90% of patients, and toxic deaths have been observed [44, 45]. Other methods of administration have included continuous intravenous infusion lasting hours to days, rapid intravenous injection on a weekly schedule, and the 'loading course' with lower doses of drug [44, 46–48]. A 5 day 'loading course' of 12 mg/kg/day was compared with a 96 hour continuous infusion of 30 mg/kg/day [49]. The infusion resulted in less marrow suppression and a numerically superior response rate without improved duration of survival. Other studies have confirmed the advantage of infusion in terms of bone marrow suppression but have failed to support the suggestion of therapeutic advantage [44–48]. However, this advantage of the infusion method of administration might be useful in combination therapy.

In early studies of oral 5-FU dramatic response rates, especially of hepatic metastases, were reported [48, 50, 51]. Subsequently, oral and intravenous 5-FU have been compared in controlled trials involving patients with colon cancer [52, 53]. These trials have shown a superiority of intravenous administration both in response rate and in response duration; no advantage of oral 5-FU was observed in the management of liver metastases. Inconsistent absorption appears to account for the inferiority of the oral route [54].

Four methods of administration of 5-FU were compared in a randomized controlled trial of 141 evaluable patients with advanced measurable adenocarcinoma of the colon [53]. Treatment one consisted of five intravenous doses of 12 mg/kg/day followed by half doses every other day to toxicity or to a total of 11 half doses. Then weekly doses of 15 mg/kg were given. Treatment two consisted of weekly intravenous doses of 15 mg/kg. Treatment three consisted of 500 mg/day intravenously for four days followed by 500 mg weekly. Treatment four was orally administered, 15 mg/kg/day for six days and then 15 mg/kg once weekly. The 'loading course' (treatment one) produced a superior response rate of 33%. This result was statistically significant. However, the patients receiving this regimen also experienced increased toxicity including severe or life-threatening marrow suppression in 18%.

Response duration and patient survival were statistically superior in this group.

5-FU has a well-defined response rate and a median remission duration of four to five months in patients with colon cancer, yet there is little evidence that a patient responding to 5-FU will survive longer than he would have survived otherwise. Our own experience at the Lombardi Cancer Research Center of Georgetown University is that occasional patients responding to 5-FU enjoy many months of useful remission. The original Mayo Clinic experience showed a definite prolongation of median survival when a group of patients responding to 5-FU was compared to nonresponders in an untreated historical control series [44]. It is not necessary to treat to toxicity with 5-FU in order to obtain a response [44], and it may be concluded that 5-FU offers a significant chance of benefit for the responder at the price of an acceptable risk of toxicity for the non-responder. Intravenous administration of 5-FU is the preferred mode of administration. Intensive schedules of administration such as the 'loading course' probably offer a higher likelihood of response, but this schedule is more toxic and is relatively inconvenient for outpatient management.

Ftorafur is a 5-FU analogue that is slowly metabolized *in vivo* to release the active drug. It has been employed as a slow release form of 5-FU with the hope that it might be similar in its pharmacokinetics to the continuous infusion method of 5-FU. Limiting toxicity has been to the central nervous system with lethargy and nervousness the prominent manifestations [55, 56]. Myelosuppression has been minimal. Buroker *et al.* studied 84 previously untreated patients with advanced colon cancer. The drug was administered at a dose of 2.25 g/m^2/day for five days in 3-week cycles. The response rate of 11% does not suggest any superiority of ftorafur to 5-FU [51].

2.3. The Therapeutic Activity of Other Anti-Cancer Drugs

A 12-16% response rate has been observed for mitomycin C in advanced colon cancer [41, 42, 58]. However, the duration of response has been less than three months, and toxicity, primarily in the form of chronic myelosuppression, limits the usefulness of this drug.

A response rate of 10-15% has been observed with the chloroethyl nitrosoureas, BCNU, CCNU, and methyl CCNU [41, 42]. Methyl CCNU appeared to be as active as 5-FU in one controlled trial [59]. For this reason, and also because methyl CCNU is administered orally, it has come to be the preferred nitrosourea in colon cancer. In studies at the Lombardi Cancer Research Center, chlorozotocin, a new nitrosourea, produced responses in 18% of 34 patients with a median remission duration of 19.5 weeks [60]. Many drugs including cyclophosphamide, methotrexate, hexamethylmelamine, actinomycin D, Adriamycin, and hydroxyurea have reported response rates of less than

20% [41] and have not proved useful in colon cancer. Vincristine, which has been widely used in combinations of drugs for colon cancer, has negligible activity as a single agent [41]. L-PAM (melphalan) was reported to produce a 20% response rate [61], but DiBenedetto *et al.* observed only a 4% response rate in previously treated patients [62]. Baker's antifol (BAF) was studied at the Mayo Clinic in 28 patients with cancer of the colon, including 14 who had been previously treated with other anti-cancer therapy. An objective response rate of 18% was observed at a dose of 250 mg/m^2/day on three consecutive days. Four of the five responders were previously treated [63]. Padilla *et al.* noted a 10% response rate in 29 previously treated patients with colon cancer [64]. Dibromodulcitol was studied in 16 patients who had been previously treated. The drug was administered in six week cycles at a dose of 180 mg/m^2/day for 10 consecutive days. A response rate of 12.5% was observed, but significant hematologic toxicity occurred [65].

Recent trials of other newer agents include rubidazone [66], metronidizole [67], chromomycin A$_3$ [68], cytembena [69], pyrazofurin [70], cytosine arabinoside [71], and maytansine [72], vindesine [73, 74], 2,2' anhydro a beta-D arabinofuranosyl-5-fluorocytosine [75], anguidine [76], VP-16-263 [77], and diglycoaldehyde [77]. None of these agents appear to have significant activity for colorectal cancer.

2.4. Combination Chemotherapy

Cancer chemotherapy has yielded the greatest benefits when individually active cytotoxic drugs have been brought together in combinations with additive antitumor affects and nonoverlapping toxicities. This approach has not been particularly effective in cancer of the colon because few drugs have important single agent activity. Many combinations have been tried (Table 5); although improved response rates have occasionally been observed with combination therapy, no combination has significantly improved overall survival.

A 20% response rate was obtained through the use of the earliest combination of 5-FU, BCNU and mitomycin C [78]. However, Falkson *et al.* compared 5-FU with the combination of 5-FU, BCNU, vincristine, and DTIC in a randomized trial. The 43% response rate yielded by the combination was not significantly different from the 25% response rate with 5-FU alone [79]. In a report from the Mayo Clinic, a similarly high response rate of 43% was obtained with the combination 5-FU, vincristine, and methyl CCNU; controls randomized to 5-FU alone had 19.5% response rate [80]. The results with the three drug combination were confirmed by Falkson and Falkson in a randomized study and in an uncontrolled trial at the Lombardi Cancer Research Center [81, 82]. The experience of some others with the combination was not

Table 5. Combination chemotherapy of adenocarcinoma of the colon: collected experience with selected regimens*.

Combination	Responders/total patients	Response rate %
5-FU + methyl CCNU	107/561	19
5-FU + methyl CCNU + vincristine	87/403	22
5-FU + vincristine + methyl CCNU + streptozotocin	10/28	36
5-FU + methyl CCNU + daunomycin	6/38	16
5-FU + Adriamycin + mitomycin C	15/113	13
Mitomycin C + cyclophosphamide + methotrexate	4/14	29
Cyclophosphamide + vincristine + methotrexate	4/20	20

* References: see text.

as favorable [66, 83, 84], and a subsequent report from the Mayo Clinic involving a larger number of patients revealed an overall objective tumor regression rate revised downward to only 27% [85].

Because of the suggestion that the three drug combination of 5-FU, vincristine, and methyl CCNU might be useful in colon cancer and because vincristine alone is not active in this disease, the two drug combination without vincristine has been tested by a number of groups. The Central Oncology Group observed a 37% response rate, while randomized controls receiving methyl CCNU alone responded only 7% of the time [86]. The Southwest Oncology Group also found the two drug combination to be useful. In a randomized phase III trial of 5-FU compared with 5-FU plus methyl CCNU, the combination resulted in a 32% response rate [87]. However, other studies have not confirmed these results, and the overall response rate of 561 patients treated with 5-FU and methyl CCNU in eight series is 19% [83, 85-91]. Efforts to increase the efficacy of the 5-FU plys methyl CCNU regimen have included alterations in the dosage and scheduling of 5-FU. Administration of 5-FU by continuous infusion did not result in improved response rates [91, 92] although Vaughn *et al.* recently reported a 47% response rate including four complete responses in a small number of patients receiving infusional 5-FU at a high dose plus mitomycin C [93]. The Southwest Oncology Group substituted ftorafur for 5-FU with a similar rationale, but the substitution did not improve the response rate [94].

Kemeny *et al.* at the Memorial Sloan-Kettering Cancer Center attempted to ameliorate the gastrointestinal intolerance of the 5-FU, methyl CCNU, vincristine combination by administering the nitrosourea in smaller doses for five consecutive days ($30 \, mg/m^2/day \times 5$). They compared this schedule with the usual regimen in which methyl CCNU is administered in a single dose on day one. The response rates of the two schedules were identical and disappointingly low, although the new schedule was tolerated better [95]. These investigators have recently added streptozotocin to produce a four drug combination, MOF-streptozotocin [96]. 5-FU was administered at a dose of $300 \, mg/m^2/day$ for five consecutive days; methyl CCNU was given at a dose of $30 \, mg/m^2/day$ for five consecutive days; 1 mg of vincristine was given every five weeks; and streptozotocin was given at a dose of $500 \, mg/m^2$ weekly. The MOF-streptozotocin combination was compared to MOF without streptozotocin in a prospectively randomized controlled trial; the 36% response rate for the four drug combination in 28 patients was significantly superior to the response rate for MOF without streptozotocin.

Other single agents with activity against colon cancer have been added to the basic combination of 5-FU plus methyl CCNU, but improved response rates have not resulted. The Eastern Cooperative Oncology Group added DTIC or vincristine plus DTIC, and also tested 5-FU with hydroxyurea. None of these combinations was superior to the response to be expected from 5-FU alone [83]. The Cancer and Leukemia Group B added daunomycin to the two drug combination without advantage [97]. The addition of Baker's antifol yielded no improvement [98].

Other combinations which have shown no activity greater then 5-FU alone include mitomycin C with cyclophosphamide and methotrexate [99], 5-FU and melphalan [90, 100], 5-FU with cyclophosphamide and CCNU [101, 102], 5-FU cyclophosphamide and methotrexate [102], ftorafur and mitomycin C [56], 5-FU and streptozotocin [103], 5-FU with Adriamycin and mitomycin C [104, 105], 5-FU with Adriamycin, mitomycin C, and cytosine arabinoside [106], 5-FU plus anguidine [107], and 5-FU plus thymidine [108, 109].

At the present time there is no irrefutable evidence that any combination of drugs is superior in colon cancer to 5-FU alone. Although some studies suggest that the addition of methyl CCNU with or without vincristine may be advantageous, even with the combination, responses are partial, response duration averages not more than four to five months, and no impact on survival has been shown. There is currently some enthusiasm for the four drug combination MOF-streptozotocin, but a final assessment must await further data.

2.5. Chemotherapy after 5-FU Failure

Even more difficult than the choice of initial chemotherapy in colon cancer is the choice of second line therapy for the patient who has progressive tumor growth while receiving 5-FU. Mitomycin C is unsatisfactory as a single agent

even in the previously untreated patient. The nitrosoureas occasionally produce responses in patients progressing on 5-FU, but the response rate is lower
than in previously treated patients. At the Mayo Clinic 10% of 112 patients
progressing on first line chemotherapy responded to one of the nitrosoureas [110]. Of the 33 patients progressing on prior chemotherapy, 15% responded to the naturally occurring nitrosourea, streptozotocin [111]. In a study
of the Eastern Cooperative Oncology Group, 7% of 205 patients who had
received prior 5-FU responded to one of various two drug combinations
containing methyl CCNU [83]. Isolated responses have been reported in previously treated patients with melphalan [112], Baker's antifol [113], and with
the combination cyclophosphamide plus vincristine plus methotrexate [114].

2.6. Perfusion of the Liver with Chemotherapy

The liver represents the predominant site of involvement in many patients
with metastatic cancer. Infusion of chemotherapy, usually 5-FU, directly into
the liver via an hepatic artery catheter has its theoretical justification in
evidence that metastases to liver derive most of their blood supply from the
hepatic artery [115–118]. Moreover, 5-FU is metabolized to less toxic products
via the liver, and intra-arterial administration of this drug allows greater
delivery of cytotoxic drug to a major site of metastases with minimal systemic
toxicity.

Ansfield reported 419 patients in whom a catheter was placed in the hepatic
artery usually from a transbrachial approach. In most patients, 5-FU was
infused continuously at a rate of 20 mg/kg/day for four days and then at
15 mg/kg/day for 15 days. Subsequently 5-FU was administered intravenously on a weekly basis. 293 patients were considered evaluable, and 55%
of these were considered to have responded with measurable reduction in
liver size [119]. Many of the patients responding had shown progressive disease previously while receiving intravenous 5-FU. Buroker et al. described a
35% objective response rate in 21 colon cancer patients who has previously
failed adequate trials of intravenous 5-FU. All received 5-FUDR, an analogue
of 5-FU, by continuous infusion at 0.3 mg/kg/day via a portable pump [120].
Similar results have been reported by others [121]. Major toxicity consisted of
gastro-intestinal side effects in about 10% of patients and myelosuppression
in less than 5%. Problems related to the catheter included cracking of the
catheter and infection at the sight of insertion, but such problems were
observed in fewer than 10% of patients [122].

The value of hepatic perfusion was determined in a randomized comparison
of intra-arterial 5-FU with intravenous 5-FU conducted by the Central Oncology Group [123]. Intraarterial 5-FU was given at a dose of 20 mg/kg/day for
14 days followed by 10 mg/kg/day for 7 days. Systemic 5-FU was given as a
'loading course' of 12 mg/kg/day for 4 days and 6 mg/kg/day every other

day for four doses. All patients subsequently received intravenous 5-FU weekly. The response rate was 23% with intravenous administration and 34% with hepatic perfusion. The duration of response was also greater with intraarterial 5-FU. However neither difference was statistically significant.

A variety of other chemotherapeutic drugs either singly or in combination have been delivered via an hepatic artery catheter [124–126].

Hepatic artery infusion, particularly with 5-FU, offers a significant chance of palliation of liver metastases, even in the patient who has previously developed progressive disease while receiving intravenous 5-FU. The toxicity of such therapy is generally acceptable, but it involves considerable expense and inconvenience to the patient. It remains unproven that patient survival or well-being is improved, and this approach should be reserved for very carefully selected patients, preferably in the setting of a clinical study.

2.7. Adjuvant Chemotherapy for Colorectal Cancer

Many patients with resectable colon cancer, even those with no evidence of residual disease at the time of surgery, subsequently die of disseminated disease. Patients with B_2 lesions (extension of tumor through the tunica muscularis) or C lesions (involvement of adjacent mesenteric lymph nodes) in the Astler-Coller modification of the Dukes' staging scheme have five year survivals of about 50% and 30% respectively, despite complete absence of clinically detectable disease at the conclusion of primary surgery [127]. There is a great need for an additional adjuvant therapy for these patients to reduce the unacceptably high relapse rate and improve the cure rate.

Adjuvant trials in colon cancer have emphasized the use of 5-FU, the single drug with the most important activity in advanced cancer of the colon. The Veterans Administration Surgical Adjuvant Group studied several schedules of adjuvant 5-FU, but no clearcut benefit was obtained with any schedule. In one trial, 5-FU was given at 12 mg/kg/day intravenously for five consecutive days in six to eight week cycles. Therapy was continued for 18 months or until recurrence was noted, and results were compared to those in a concurrent untreated matched control population. Five year survival for the treated group was 49% and for the control group was 45%, but this difference was not significant [128]. The Central Oncology Group attempted to improve this result with more aggressive administration of adjuvant 5-FU. In this trial 5-FU was administered until toxicity was noted, and weekly maintenance was continued for one year. A small survival benefit was noted in the treated population, but this difference was not statistically significant [129]. In summary, the available evidence does not support the use of 5-FU as a single drug in the adjuvant treatment of patients with colon cancer resected for cure and with a high risk of recurrence.

The Gastrointestinal Tumor Study Group initiated a prospectively randomized multi-institutional trial of adjuvant therapy in colon cancer. The trial consisted of four arms: 1) a control group receiving no treatment; 2) a group receiving combination chemotherapy with 5-FU and methyl CCNU; 3) a group receiving adjuvant immunotherapy with methanol extracted residue (MER) of BCG (attenuated tuberculosis mycobacteria); and, 4) a group receiving both the chemotherapy with 5-FU and methyl CCNU and the immunotherapy with MER. This study remains coded at the time of writing, but results may be available in the near future.

A recent report concerned the adjuvant infusion of 5-FU through an umbilical vein catheter. After surgery with curative intent, both high and low risk patients were randomized to receive 5-FU and heparin for 7 days or no therapy. Some toxicity was noted in the treatment group including one treatment related death, but the early results suggested a very substantial benefit in the treated group [130]. Further followup will be necessary before this study can be interpreted unequivocally, and confirmation from other centers would be desirable.

In summary, there is no evidence to dictate the use of adjuvant therapy for the patient with resected cancer of the colon and a high risk of recurrence.

2.8. Immunotherapy of Colon Cancer

There has been great interest in the possible role in cancer therapy of agents that have been used in experimental models to heighten specific immune responses. It has seemed obvious to many that immunological factors are extremely important in oncogenesis and this belief has been strengthened by the extensive publicity surrounding animal experiments in which 'immune stimulants' have led to tumor eradication and some clinical studies involving human patients in which immunotherapy seemed to be of benefit. In September, 1979, the International Registry on Tumor Immunotherapy of the National Cancer Institute listed more than 25 studies with at least one immunotherapy arm in colorectal cancer. The agents under investigation included BCG, MER, C. parvum, levamisole, tumor vaccines, and other immunological or quasi-immunological agents. No benefit has resulted in randomized controlled trials to date [131-133]. Although the rationale for immunotherapy remains attractive, it is clear that our knowledge of the phenomena of tumor immunology is too meager at the present time. It seems likely that breakthroughs at the level of clinical immunotherapy must await important breakthroughs at the fundamental research level.

2.9. Radiation Therapy of Colorectal Cancer

Radiation therapy has been studied most extensively in patients with cancer of the rectum. The bowel below the peritoneal reflection cannot be mobilized for excision with wide margins and this limits the effectiveness of resection in rectal cancer. Moreover, the pattern in rectal cancer of lymphatic drainage and progress by local spread is such that advanced disease frequently can be encompassed within a radiation port [134]. Preoperative radiotherapy in patients subsequently receiving resection with curative intent and displaying no evident residual disease after surgery conferred an apparent survival advantage in a large nonrandomized study [135]. However, this result was not confirmed in subsequent randomized studies [136–138]. Surgeons have preferred postoperative radiotherapy since preoperative radiation delays resection, interferes with staging at surgery, and exposes some patients with very limited disease to extra morbidity. Several cooperative studies involving postoperative radiotherapy have been established, but final results will not be available for several years. Thus the role of radiotherapy in rectal cancer and, by inference, in colon cancer is undefined and any potential benefit is unproven. Significant palliation in a high proportion of patients with advanced disease has been achieved in specific situations such as painful metastases of liver, nerve or bone and local complications in the rectum including tenesmus, bleeding, and mucus discharge [134, 139].

2.10. Summary

5-FU remains the standard chemotherapy of unresectable cancer of the colon or rectum. 5-FU has a clearcut but low response rate of about 20%, and when a response is achieved it can be expected to last for four or five months. Patients who respond to 5-FU occasionally live many months with normal activity, and this observation provides the justification for offering 5-FU to patients with advanced disease despite the absence of proof that 5-FU prolongs survival of the total treated population. Oral administration of 5-FU is inferior. Intensive 'loading course' administration of 5-FU probably results in higher response rates, but this advantage is balanced by increased toxicity and an inconvenient schedule. Consequently, a weekly or intermittent schedule of IV administration is frequently employed. Combinations of drugs including 5-FU, particularly the two drug combination of 5-FU and methyl CCNU have seemed to be superior to 5-FU alone in some trials but not in others. Current interest centers around the four drug combination of 5-FU, vincristine, methyl CCNU, and streptozotocin, but the advantage of this combination remains to be proved. In no study of chemotherapy of colon cancer has a survival benefit been demonstrated for the entire study group.

Chemotherapy of the patient who has developed progressive disease while on first line chemotherapy is totally inadequate at present, and only a few agents have detectable response rates in this setting. Infusion of 5-FU into the hepatic artery may reduce hepatic metastases in patients who have previously received intravenous 5-FU, but the method is quite complicated and expensive, and the advantages do not justify its routine use.

Radiotherapy offers useful palliation in certain clinical situations. Immunotherapy has no defined role in the routine treatment of colorectal cancer.

3. GASTRIC CANCER

3.1. Epidemiology and Natural History

Early in this century gastric cancer was the leading cause of cancer death in the United States. For unknown reasons, the incidence of this disease has declined dramatically, until the number of new cases predicted for 1979 was about the same as for carcinoma of the pancreas — 23 000 [1]. In contrast to carcinoma of the pancreas, a significant number of patients with stomach cancer are cured by primary surgery; nevertheless, the majority of patients, estimated to be 14 000 in 1979, die of disseminated disease.

3.2. The Therapeutic Activity of Single Drugs in Advanced Gastric Carcinoma

Table 6 summarizes the single agent activity of selected drugs for advanced carcinoma of the stomach. As in other gastrointestinal malignancies, the most extensive experience has been gained with 5-FU, and Comis and Carter calculated an overall 21% response rate in 392 patients from collected series [140]. Mitomycin C has been associated with a partial response rate of 30%, but this figure is probably inflated by overly optimistic results from early reports [141]. A more realistic response rate may be 24%, and the average duration of response is less than three months. Adriamycin has

Table 6. Activity of drugs used alone in gastric cancer*.

Drug	Responses/total patients	Response rate %
5-FU	84/392	21
Mitomycin C	24/98	24
BCNU	6/33	18
CCNU	1/35	3
Methyl CCNU	1/28	4
Adriamycin	7/27	26
Chromomycin A_3	53/152	35
Mithramycin	3/11	27
Cytosine arabinoside	3/11	27
Mechlorethamine	4/25	16
Chlorambucil	3/18	17
Hydroxyurea	6/31	19
Vinblastine	3/16	19
DTIC	2/15	13

* References: see text.

significant activity as a single agent in advanced gastric cancer, with a response rate of 26% in the small number of patients reviewed by Wasserman *et al.* [41], and higher response rates in some other series [141]. The nitrosoureas, particularly BCNU, have a modest response rate, less than 20% [41, 141]. Some other drugs, including alkylating agents, vinblastine, cytosine arabinoside, hydroxyurea and DTIC, produce occasional responses [41, 141].

3.3. Combination Chemotherapy for Advanced Gastric Carcinoma

Among the major gastrointestinal malignancies, stomach cancer has appeared to be relatively more responsive to chemotherapy. This reputation has led to considerable interest in combination chemotherapy, and it now seems clear that regimens containing Adriamycin may provide significant benefit to the patient with gastric cancer. Some selected regimens are listed in Table 7.

Early trials conducted by the Mayo Clinic and by the Eastern Cooperative Oncology Group [142, 143] have suggested that a combination of 5-FU with a nitrosourea could result in response rate and survival superior to that obtained with 5-FU alone. However, Kingston *et al.* [144] were unable to confirm the efficacy of the combination of 5-FU and methyl CCNU.

Because other drugs including mitomycin C and Adriamycin seem to have greater activity as single agents in gastric cancer than nitrosoureas, a number of trials have evaluated combinations of these agents. The Eastern Cooperative Oncology Group compared Adriamycin alone with the combination of 5-FU plus mitomycin C and with the combination of 5-FU plus methyl CCNU. The single agent activity of Adriamycin was confirmed with a response rate of 22%, and the best arm was the 5-FU plus mitomycin C group, which achieved a response rate of 32% [145]. In contrast to these results is the report of the randomized trial of the Southwest Oncology Group in which 5-FU was given in a continuous 96 hour infusion with either mitomycin C or methyl CCNU [146]. In this study, the combination with

Table 7. Combination chemotherapy of advanced gastric cancer: collected experience with selected regimens*.

Regimens	Responders total patients	Response rate %
5-FU + methyl CCNU	31/155	20
5-FU + mitomycin C	23/96	24
5-FU + mitomycin C + cytosine arabinoside	3/18	17
5-FU + Adriamycin + methyl CCNU	15/37	41
5-FU + Adriamycin + mitomycin C	49/134	37

* References: see text.

mitomycin C was superior, but a response was seen in only six of 43 patients. The difference between the two studies may be related to differences in the scheduling of drug administration. Early reports from Japan[147] and from the Memorial Sloan Kettering Cancer Center[148] had suggested the combination of 5-FU, mitomycin C, and cytosine arabinoside might be very effective in advanced gastric cancer with an objective response rate as high as 55%. The Gastrointestinal Tumor Study group was unable to confirm this optimistic estimate of activity; of 18 previously untreated patients, only 17% responded to this combination[149].

Extensive and persuasive data are now accumulating to indicate the importance of Adriamycin in combination chemotherapy of advanced gastric carcinoma. The FAM regimen (Table 3) has now been evaluated in a number of patients from several centers. The Lombardi Cancer Research Center had initially recorded a 50% objective response rate with this combination in 36 patients[150]. In a recent update of this study with 61 patients, an overall partial response rate of 43% was observed[151]. Even more impressive was a statistically significant survival benefit for the responders as compared with the non-responders — 13 months vs 3.5 months. FAM has been well tolerated, but mild to moderate myelosuppression has been dose-limiting. These results have been confirmed by Bitran et al. [31], who observed an impressive 55% response rate in a small number of patients with advanced gastric cancer. A randomized trial of the Southwest Oncology Group has provided further confirmation[152]. In this study patients were randomized to receive FAM or to receive the same three drugs in sequence. A total of 123 patients were considered evaluable, and 40% of those treated with FAM responded, a result superior to those obtained with the sequential regimen. Bernath et al. studied the combination of the FAM drugs with a nitrosourea and observed a response rate comparable to those previously reported for FAM alone[153].

Several studies of a nitrosourea in combination with 5-FU and Adriamycin have been reported. Lacave et al. compared 5-FU, Adriamycin, and methyl CCNU to the two drug combination of 5-FU and methyl CCNU[154]. Of the patients receiving this three drug combination, 36% responded as compared with 9% of the other group. Levi et al. observed a 52% response rate in 35 patients treated with the three drug combination of 5-FU, Adriamycin, and BCNU[155]. The Gastrointestinal Tumor Study Group compared Adriamycin as a single agent with the three drug regimen also including 5-FU and methyl CCNU. Four of 17 patients responded to Adriamycin alone, whereas seven of 15 responded to the three drug combination[149].

Currently, it is of great importance to compare three drug regimens with the two drug combination of 5-FU and Adriamycin alone. In addition, it would be important to compare in a randomized trial the two three-drug combinations FAM and FAMe (5-FU, Adriamycin, and methyl CCNU). Both of these questions are currently being evaluated in a phase III study of the Gastrointestinal Tumor Study Group.

Other combinations currently of interest include *cis*-platinum diaminedichloride. A preliminary report of a combination of this drug with anhydro-ara-5-fluorocytidine describes three responses among five previously untreated patients [156].

3.4. Adjuvant Chemotherapy After Surgical Resection for Cure

Patients with no known residual carcinoma after surgical resection for cure remain at high risk for recurrence. Such patients are excellent candidates for adjuvant chemotherapy with drugs known to be active in gastric carcinoma in an attempt to improve the surgical cure rate. Published studies to date have been inconclusive with regard to the value of adjuvant chemotherapy, however. The earliest reports involved short-term administration of single agents [157–160]. A more recent report by Nakajima *et al.* suggested a possible benefit to a short course of combination chemotherapy followed by long-term oral 5-FU [161].

The Gastrointestinal Tumor Study Group initiated a randomized trial (protocol 8174) in patients with no known residual disease after surgery for gastric carcinoma. The control group received no therapy, and the treatment group received long-term 5-FU plus methyl CCNU. Accrual to this trial continues at the present time and no data will be available for several years.

No data are now available to support or reject the hypothesis that adjuvant therapy with an Adriamycin containing regimen, such as one of the combinations known to be effective in advanced disease, increases disease-free interval after surgery or five year survival rate.

3.5. Combined Modality Radiotherapy Plus Chemotherapy in Locally Advanced Gastric Cancer

Locally unresectable or locally advanced gastric cancer is, by definition, tumor remaining after surgery and confined to the stomach, local lymph nodes, local omentum, and/or local peritoneum. Such disease should be contained within an area of 20×20 cm and would permit a radiation field sufficiently small that radiation could be delivered to all areas of known disease with acceptable gastrointestinal toxicity. Efforts to define optimal treatment for such patients are ongoing at the present time.

An early trial from the Mayo Clinic suggested that radiation plus 5-FU produces a significant benefit in comparison to radiation alone in terms of mean survival [162].

The Gastrointestinal Tumor Study Group proceeded from this result to attempt to assess a combined modality radiation therapy plus combination chemotherapy in comparison with combination chemotherapy alone. The chemotherapy group received 5-FU plus methyl CCNU. The combined modality group received two courses of 2500 rads over three weeks, and the courses were separated by a 2-week rest period. Intravenous 5-FU was given for the first three days of each radiation course. After the completion of radiotherapy, the group received maintenance chemotherapy with the same regimen of 5-FU plus methyl CCNU. Initially, this study suggested a substantial advantage for combination chemotherapy without radiotherapy in terms of longer survival and diminished toxicity [163]. In a more recent evaluation of follow up data the survival advantage for the group receiving chemotherapy alone remains: the median survival for the group receiving chemotherapy was 70 weeks, while the median survival for the group receiving combined modality therapy was 36 weeks [164]. However, the proportion of long-term survivors may be greater in the group receiving radiotherapy. The final conclusions from this study must await further observation of the remaining patients.

3.6. Summary

A number of anticancer drugs including 5-FU, Adriamycin, mitomycin C, and methyl CCNU have significant activity against gastric cancer. Combination chemotherapy can be expected to confer a significant benefit to as many as 40% of patients with advanced disease. A combination regimen including Adriamycin is optimal, and excellent results have been obtained at several institutions with the combination of 5-FU, Adriamycin, and mitomycin C (FAM). It is tempting to treat the patient with no known residual disease after surgery with adjuvant chemotherapy, such as one of the combination regimens active in advanced disease. However, data are not yet available to demonstrate that such adjuvant therapy either increases disease-free interval after surgery or increases five year survival rate. The optimal treatment of the patient with locally advanced unresectable gastric cancer remains controversial. The use of combination chemotherapy is appropriate.

Whether radiotherapy should be offered in addition is unclear. Combined modality therapy in this setting will certainly entail significant toxicity, but it is possible that the final analysis will show a larger number of long-term survivors among those patients receiving both radiotherapy and chemotherapy.

REFERENCES

1. American Cancer Society. Cancer facts and figures, 1979. New York.
2. McDermott MV, Bartlett MK: Pancreaticoduodenal cancer. N Engl J Med 248:927–931, 1953.
3. Gudjonsson B, Livstone EM, Spiro HM: Cancer of the pancreas: diagnostic accuracy and survival statistics. Cancer 42:2494–2506, 1978.

4. Isaacson R, Weiland LH, McIlrath DC: Biopsy of the pancreas. Arch Surg 109:227–230, 1974.

5. Brooks JR: Operative approach to pancreatic carcinoma. Semin Oncol 6:357–367, 1979.

6. Hancke S, Holms HH, Koch F: Ultrasonically guided percutaneous fine needle biopsy of the pancreas. Surg Gynecol. Obstet 140:361–364, 1975.

7. Beazley RM: Percutaneous needle biopsy for diagnosis of pancreatic cancer. Semin Oncol 6:344–346, 1979.

8. Tsuchiya R, Henmi T, Kondo N et al.: Endoscopic aspiration biopsy of the pancreas. gastroenterology 73:1050–1053, 1977.

9. Kawanishi H, Pollard HM: Endoscopic evaluation of cancer of the pancreas. Semin Oncol 6:309–317, 1979.

10. Levin B, ReMine WH, Herman RE et al.: Cancer of the pancreas. Am J Surg 135:185–191, 1978.

11. MacDonald JS, Widerlite L, Schein PS: Biology, diagnosis and chemotherapeutic management of pancreatic malignancy. Adv. Pharmacol. Chemother. 14:107–141, 1977.

12. Carter SK, Comis RL: Adenocarcinoma of the pancreas, prognostic variables, and criteria of response in cancer therapy. In: Response in cancer therapy: prognostic factors and criteria of response, Staquet MJ (ed). New York: Raven Press, 1975, pp 237–253.

13. Reitemeier RJ, Moertel CG, Hahn RG: Comparative evaluation of palliation with fluorometholone (NCSA-33001), 5-fluorouracil (NSC-19893), and combined fluorometholone and 5-fluorouracil in advanced gastrointestinal cancer. Cancer Chemother. Rep 51:77–80, 1967.

14. Stolinsky DC, Pugh RP, Bateman JR: 5-Fluorouracil (NSC-19893) therapy for pancreatic carcinoma: comparison of oral and intravenous routes. Cancer Chemother Rep 59:1031–1033, 1975.

15. Moertel CG, Reitemeier RJ, Hahn RG: Therapy with mitomycin-C. In: Advanced gastrointestinal cancer/clinical management and chemotherapy, Moertel CG, Reitemeier RJ (eds). New York: Harper & Row, 1969, pp 168–175.

16. Moertel CG: Therapy of advanced gastrointestinal cancer with the nitrosoureas. Cancer Chemother. Rep 4:27–34, 1973.

17. Douglass HO Jr, Lavin PT, Moertel CG: Nitrosoureas: useful agents for treatment of advanced gastrointestinal cancer. Cancer Treat Rep 60:769–780, 1976.

18. Rakieten N, Rakieten ML, Nadkarni MV: Studies on the diabetogenic action of streptozotocin (NSC-37917). Cancer Chemother Rep 29:91–98, 1963.

19. Dupriest RW, Hintington M, Massey WH et al.: Streptozotocin therapy in 22 cancer patients. Cancer 35:358–367, 1974.

20. Stolkinsky DC, Sadoff L, Braunwald J et al.: Streptozotocin in the treatment of cancer. Cancer 30:61–69, 1972.

21. Broder LE, Carter SK: Streptozotocin: clinical brochure. Therapy Evaluation Program, National Cancer Insitute, Bethesda, Maryland.

22. Yunis AA, Arimura CK, Russin DJ: Human pancreatic carcinoma (MIA PaCa^{-2}) in continuous culture: sensitivity to asparaginase. Int. J. Cancer 19:128–135, 1977.

23. Schein PS, Lavin PT, Moertel CG et al.: Randomized phase II clinical trial of Adriamycin in advanced measurable pancreatic carcinoma: a Gastrointestinal Tumor Study Group report. Cancer 42:19–22, 1978.

24. Reitermeier RJ, Moertel CG, Hahn RG: Combination chemotherapy in gastrointestinal cancer. Cancer Res 30:1425–1428, 1970.

25. Kovach JS, Moertel CG, Schutt AJ, Hahn RG, Reitermeier RJ: A controlled study of combined 1,3-bis (2-chloroethyl)-1-nitrosoureas and 5-fluorouracil therapy for advanced gastric and pancreatic cancer. Cancer 33:563–567, 1974.

26. Lokich JJ, Skarin AT: Combination therapy with 5-fluorouracil (5-FU) and 1,3-bis (2-chlorethyl)-1-nitrosourea (BCNU) for disseminated gastrointestinal carcinoma. Cancer Chemother Rep 56:653-657, 1972.
27. Buroker T, Kim PN, Heilbrun L et al.: 5-FU infusion with mitomycin C (MMC) vs 5-FU infusion with methyl CCNU (Me) in the treatment of advanced upper gastrointestinal cancer. Proc ASCO 19:310, 1978.
28. Horton J, Gelber R: Trials of single agent and combination chemotherapy in advanced cancer of the pancreas. Proceedings ASCO 21:420, 1980.
29. Wiggans, G, Woolley PV, Macdonald JS et al.: Phase II trial of streptozotocin, mitomycin-C and 5-fluorouracil (SMF) in the treatment of advanced pancreatic cancer. Cancer 41:387-391, 1978.
30. Aberhalden RT, Bukowski RM, Groppe CW et al.: Streptozotocin (STZ) and 5-fluorouracil (5-FU) with and without mitomycin-C (Mito) in the treatment of pancreatic adenocarcinoma. Proc ASCO 18:301, 1977.
31. Bitran JD, Desser RK, Kozloff MF, Billings AA, Shapiro, CM: Treatment of metastatic pancreatic and gastric adenocarcinomas with 5-fluorouracil, Adriamycin, and mitomycin-C (FAM). Cancer Treatment Rep 63:2049-2051, 1979.
32. Brown JC, Bruckner HW, Storch J, Schamberlain J, Pressmen PI: Combination chemotherapy for pancreatic cancer. Proc ASCO 21:420, 1980.
33. Awrich A, Fletcher WS, Klotz JH, Minton JP, Hill GJ II, Aust GJ, Grage TB, Multhauf BP: 5-FU versus combination therapy with tubercidin, streptozotocin, and 5-FU in the treatment of pancreatic carcinomas: COG Protocol 7230. J Surg Oncol 12:267-273, 1979.
34. Hall SW, Benjamin RS, Murphy WK, Valdivieso M, Bodey GP: Adriamycin, BCNU, ftorafur chemotherapy of pancreatic and biliary tract cancer. Cancer 44:2008-2013, 1979.
35. Costanzi JJ, Panettiere FJ, Wolma FJ: Combination chemotherapy for advanced pancreatic carcinoma. Texas Med 75:50-51, 1979.
36. Haslam JB, Cavanaugh PJ, Stroup SL: Radiation therapy in the treatment of irresectable adenocarcinoma of the pancreas. Cancer 32:1341-1345, 1973.
37. Moertel CG, Childs DS, Reitemeier RJ et al.: Combined 5-fluorouracil and supervoltage radiation therapy of locally unresectable gastrointestinal cancer. Lancet 2:865-867, 1969.
38. Moertel CG, Lokich JJ, Schein PS et al.: An evaluation of high dose radiation and combined radiation and 5-fluorouracil therapy for locally unresectable pancreatic carcinoma. Proc ASCO 17:244, 1976.
39. The Gastrointestinal Tumor Study Group. A multi-institutional comparative trial of radiation therapy alone and in combination with 5-fluorouracil for locally unresectable pancreatic carcinoma. Annls Surg 189:205-208, 1979.
40. Catterall M: A report of three years' fast neutron therapy from the medical research council's cyclotron at Hammersmith Hospital, London. Cancer 34:91-95, 1974.
41. Wasserman TH, Comis RL, Goldsmith M, Handelsman H, Penta JS, Slavik M, Soper WT, Carter SK: Tabular analysis of the clinical chemotherapy of solid tumors. Cancer Chemother Rep 6:399, 1975.
42. Moertel CG: Clinical management of advanced gastrointestinal cancer. Cancer 36:675-682, 1975.
43. Heidelberger C: Fluorinated pyrimidines, a new class of tumor inhibitory compound. Nature 179:663-666, 1957.
44. Moertel CG, Reitemeier RJ, Hahn RG: Therapy with the fluorinated pyrimidines. In: Advanced gastrointestinal cancer, Moertel CG, Reitemeier RJ (eds). New York: Koeber, 1969, pp 86-107.
45. Moertel CG: Clinical management of advanced gastrointestinal cancer. Cancer 36:675-682,

J.R. NEEFE and P.S. SCHEIN

1975.

46. Carter SK: Large bowel cancer — The current status of treatment. J Nat Cancer Inst 56:3–10, 1976.
47. Jacobs EM, Reeves WJ, Wood DA, Pugh R, Braunwald J, Bateman JR: Treatment of cancer with weekly intravenous 5-fluorouracil. Cancer 27:1302–1305, 1971.
48. Leone LA: The chemotherapy of colorectal cancer. Cancer 34:972–976, 1974.
49. Seifert P, Baker LH, Reed ML, Vaitkevicius VK: Comparison of continuously infused 5-fluorouracil with bolus injection in treatment of patients with colorectal adenocarcinoma. Cancer 36:123–128, 1975.
50. Khung CL, Hall TC, Piro AJ, Dederick MM: A clinical trial of oral 5-fluorouracil. Clin Pharmacol. Ther 7:527–533, 1966.
51. Lahiri, SR, Boileau G, Hall TC: Treatment of metastatic colorectal carcinoma with 5-fluorouracil by mouth. Cancer 28:902–906, 1971.
52. Bateman J, Irwin L, Pugh R et al.: Comparison of intravenous and oral administration of 5-fluorouracil for colorectal carcinoma. Proc Am Assoc Cancer Res 16:242, 1975.
53. Ansfield R, Klotz J, Nealon T, Ramirez G, Minton J, Hill G, Wilson W, Davis H, Cornell G: A phase III study comparing the clinical utility of four regimens of 5-fluorouracil. Cancer 39:34, 1977.
54. Hahn RG, Moertel CG, Schutt AJ, Bruckner HW: A double-blind comparison of intensive course 5-FU by oral vs intravenous route in the treatment of colorectal carcinoma. Cancer 35:1031–1035, 1975.
55. Valdivieso M, Bodey GP, Gottlieb JA, Freireich EJ: Clinical evaluation of ftorafur. Cancer Res 36:1821, 1976.
56. Buroker T, Wojtaszak B, Dindogru A, DeMattia M, Baker L, Groth C, Vaitkevicius VK: Phase II trial of ftorafur with mitomycin C versus ftorafur with methyl CCNU in untreated colorectal cancer. Cancer Treatment Rep 62:689, 1978.
57. Buroker T, Padilla F, Groppe C et al.: Phase II evaluation of ftorafur in previously untreated colorectal cancer. A Southwest Oncology Group Study. Cancer 44:48, 1979.
58. Comis RL, Carter SK: A review of chemotherapy in gastric cancer. Cancer 34:1576–1586, 1974.
59. Moertel CG: Therapy of advanced gastrointestinal cancer with the nitrosoureas. Cancer Chemother. Rep. (Part 3), No. 3, 4:27–34, 1973.
60. Hoth D, Butler T, Winokur S, Kales A, Woolley P, Schein P: Phase II study of chlorozotocin. Proc Am Assoc Cancer Res Am Soc Clin Oncol 19:381, 1978.
61. Carter SK, Freidman M: Integration of chemotherapy into combined modality treatment of solid tumors. II. Large bowel cancer. Cancer Treatment Rev 1:111, 1974.
62. DiBeneditto J, Moayeri H, Evans JT, Mittleman A: Phase II study of melphalan in colorectal carcinoma. Cancer Treatment Rep 62:1401, 1978.
63. Cashmore AR, Skeel RT, Makulu, Dr, Gralla EJ, Bertino, JR: Pharmacology of a new triazine antifolate in mice, rats, dogs and monkeys. Cancer Res 35:17, 1975.
64. Padilla F, Correa J, Buroker T, Vaitkevicius VK: Phase II study of Baker's antifol in advanced colorectal cancer. Cancer Treatment Rep 62:553, 1978.
65. Biermann WA, Catalano RB, Engstrom PF: A positive Phase II study of dibromodulcitol in previously treated patients with advanced colorectal carcinoma. Proc Am Assoc. Cancer Res 20:341, 1979.
66. Joss RA, Goldberg RS, Yates JW: Combination chemotherapy of colorectal cancer with 5-fluorouracil, methyl-1, 3-cis (2-chloroethyl)-1-nitrosourea, and vincristine. Med. Pediatr. Oncol 7:251–255, 1979.
67. Frytak S, Moertel CG, Childs DS, Schutt AJ, Albers JW: Phase II study of metronidazole therapy for advanced colorectal carcinoma. Cancer Treatment Rep 62:483, 1978.

68. Moertel CG, Schutt AJ, Hahn RG, Marciniak TA, Reitemeier, RJ: Phase II study of chromomycin A_3 (NSC 58514) in advanced colorectal cancer. Cancer Chemother Rep 59:577–579, 1975.

69. Moertel CG, Schutt AJ, Hahn RG, Marciniak TA, Reitemeier, RJ: Phase II study of cytembena (NSC 104801) in advanced colorectal cancer. Cancer Chemother Rep 59:581–583, 1975.

70. Creagan ET, Rubin J, Moertel CG, Schutt AJ, O'Connell MJ, Hahn RG, Reitemeier RJ, Frytak S: Phase II study of pyrazofurin in advanced colorectal carcinoma. Cancer treatment Rep 61:491, 1977.

71. Cullinan SA, O'Connell MJ, Moertel CG, Schutt AJ, Hahn RG, Reitemeier RJ, Frytak S, Rubin J: Phase II study of cytosine arabinoside in advanced large bowel cancer. Cancer Treatment Rep 61:1725, 1977.

72. O'Connell, MJ, Shani A, Rubin J, Moertel CG: Phase II trial of maytansine in patients with advanced colorectal carcinoma. Cancer Treatment Rep 62:1237, 1978.

73. Corroll DS, Kemeny NE: Vindesine DVA in the treatment of patients with metastatic colorectal carcinoma. Proc Am Assoc Cancer Res 20:195, 1979.

74. Bedikian AY, Valdivieso M, Bodey GP, Freireich EJ: Phase II evaluation of vindesine in the treatment of colorectal and esophageal tumors. Cancer Chemother Pharmacol 2:263–266, 1979.

75. Kemeny N, Yagoda A, Burchenl JH: Phase II study of 2,2' anhydro-1-beta-D-arabinofuranosyl-5-fluorocytosine in advanced colorectal carcinoma. Cancer Treatment Rep 62:463, 1978.

76. Diggs CH, Scoltock MJ, Wiernik PH: Phase II evaluation of enguidine (NSC-141537) for adenocarcinoma of the colon or rectum. Cancer Clin Trials 1:297–299, 1978.

77. Douglass HO Jr, Lavin PT, Evans JT, Mittelman A, Carbone, PP: Phase II evaluation of digycoaldehyde, VP-16-213, and the combination of methyl-CCNU and beta-2'-deoxythioguanosine in previously treated patients with colorectal cancer: an Eastern Cooperative Oncology Group Study (EST-1275).

78. Moertel CG, Reitemeier RJ, Hahn RG: Combination chemotherapy in advanced gastrointestinal cancer. Cancer Res, 30:1425–1428, 1970.

79. Falkson G, Van Eden EG, Falkson HC: Fluorouracil, imidazole carboximide dimethyltriazeno, vincristine and bis-cholorethylnitrosourea in colon cancer. Cancer 33:1207–1209, 1974.

80. Moertel CG, Schutt AJ, Hahn RG, Reitemeier RJ: Therapy of advanced colorectal cancer with a combination of 5-fluorouracil, methyl-1, 3-cis (2-chlorethyl)-1-nitrosourea and vincristine. J Nat Cancer Inst 54:69–71, 1975.

81. Falkson G, Falkson HC: Fluorouracil, methyl-CCNU, and vincristine in cancer of the colon. Cancer 38:1468–1470, 1976.

82. Macdonald JS, Kisner DF, Smythe T, Woolley PV, Smith L, Schein PS: 5-Fluorouracil (5-FU), methyl-CCNU and vincristine in the treatment of advanced colorectal cancer. Phase II study utilizing weekly 5-FU. Cancer Treatment Rep 60:1597–1600, 1976.

83. Engstrom P, MacIntyre J, Douglass H Jr, Carbone P: Combination chemotherapy of advanced bowel cancer. Proc Am Assoc Cancer Res Am Soc Clin Oncol 19:384, 1978.

84. Kemeny N, Yagoda A, Golbey R: Randomized study of 2 different schedules of methyl CCNU (MeCCNU), 5-fluorouracil (5-FU), and vincristine (VCR) for metastatic colorectal carcinoma. Proc Am Assoc Cancer Res Am Soc Clin Oncol 18:336, 1977.

85. Moertel CG: Chemotherapy of gastrointestinal cancer. N Eng J Med 299:1049, 1978.

86. Posey L, Morgan LR: Methyl CCNU versus methyl CCNU and 5-fluorouracil in carcinoma of the large bowel. Cancer Treatment Rep 61:1453, 1977.,

87. Baker LH, Talley RW, Matter R, Lehane DE, Ruffner BW, Jones SE, Morrison FS,

Stephens RL, Gehan EA, Vaitkevicius, VK: Phase III comparison of the treatment of advanced gastrointestinal cancer with bolus weekly 5-FU vs. methyl-CCNU plus bolus weekly 5-FU: a Southwest Oncology Group Study. Cancer 38:1-7, 1976.

88. Lokich JJ, Skarin AT, Mayer RJ, Frei E: Lack of effectiveness of combined 5-fluorouracil and methyl CCNU therapy in advanced colorectal cancer. Cancer 40:2792–2796, 1977.

89. Buroker T, Kim PN, Heibrun L: 5-FU infusion with mitomycin in C vs. 5-FU infusion with methyl CCNU in the treatment of advanced colon cancer: a Phase III study. Proc Am Assoc Cancer Res Am Soc Clin Oncol 18:271, 1977.

90. Berman R, Giles GR, Malhutra A, Bird GG, Gajjar, PD, Bunch, GA, Hall R: Randomized trial of melphalan plus 5-fluorouracil (5-FU) versus methyl CCNU plus 5-FU in patients with advanced colorectal cancer. Cancer Treatment Rep 62:457, 1978.

91. Kane RC, Cashdollar MR, Bernath AM: Treatment of advanced colorectal cancer with methyl CCNU plus 5 day 5-fluorouracil infusion. Cancer Treatment Rep 62:1521–1525, 1978.

92. Buroker T, Kim PN, Groppe C, McCracken J, O'Bryan R, Panettiere F, Coltman C, Bottomley R, Wilson H, Bonnett J, Thigpen T, Vaitkevicuis VK, Hoogstraten B, Hellrum L: 5-Fluorouracil infusion with mitomycin vs. 5-FU infusion with methyl-CCNU in the treatment of advanced colon cancer. A Southwest Oncology Group Study. Cancer 42:1228, 1978.

93. Vaughn CB, Brady P, Chinn BJ, Daversa GC, Parzuchowski JS: Combination chemotherapy in advanced gastrointestinal malignancy. Oncology 37:57–61, 1980.

94. Buroker T, DeMattie M, Baker L, Groth C, Vaitkevicius VK, Wojtasak B, Dindognu A: Phase II trial of ftorafur with mitomycin-C versus ftorfur with methyl-CCNU in untreated colorectal Cancer. Cancer Treatment Rep 62:689, 1978.

95. Kemeny N, Yagoda, A, Braun D Jr, Golbey R: A randomized study of two different schedules of methyl-CCNU, 5-FU, and vincristine for metastatic colorectal carcinoma. Cancer 43:78–82, 1979.

96. Kemeny N, Yagoda A, Golbey R: A prospective randomized study of methyl-CCNU, 5-fluoruracil, and vincristine (MOF) vs. MOF plus streptozotocin (MOF-Strep) in patients with metastatic colorectal carcinoma. Proc Am Soc Clin Oncol 21:417, 1980.

97. White LA Jr, Perry MC, Kardinal CG, Kennedy BJ, Weiss, RB, Carey RW: Phase II study of 5-fluourouracil, methyl-CCNU, and daunorubicin in colorectal cancer. A Cancer and Leukemia Group B Study. Cancer Treatment Rep 63:215–217, 1979.

98. Shaw MT, Heilbrum LK: Baker's antifol (BAF) in combination with methyl-CCNU and 5-fluorouracil (5-FU) for the treatment of metastatic colorectal cancer. Proc Am Assoc. Cancer Res 20:300, 1979.

99. Presant CA, Ratkin G, Klahr C: Phase II study of mitomycin C, cyclophosphamide, and methotrexate in drug-resistant colorectal carcinoma. Cancer Treatment Rep 62:549, 1978.

100. Presant CA, Ratkin G, Klahr C: Phase II trial of 5-fluorouracil plus melphalan in colorectal carcinoma. Cancer Treatment Rep 62:461, 1978.

101. Bedikian AY, Staab R, Livingston R, Valdivieso M, Burgess MA, Bodey GP: Chemotherapy for colorectal cancer with 5-fluorouracil, cyclophosphamide, and CCNU: comparison of oral and continuous IV administration of 5-fluorouracil. Cancer Treatment Rep 62:1603, 1978.

102. White DR, Richards FD, Muss HB, Cooper MR, Spurr CL: Therapy of advanced colorectal carcinoma with 5-fluorouracil and cyclophosphamide in combination with either CCNU or methotrexate. Cancer 45:662–665, 1980.

103. Seligman M, Bukowski RM, Groppe CW, Weick JK, Hewlett JS, Greenstreet RL: Chemotherapy of metastatic gastrointestinal neoplasms with 5-fluorouracil and streptozotocin. Cancer Treatment Rep 61:1375, 1977.

104. Haller DG, Woolley PV, MacDonald JS, Smith LF, Schein PS: Phase II trial of 5-fluorouracil, Adriamycin, and mitomycin-C in advanced colorectal cancer. Cancer Treatment Rep 62:563, 1978.
105. Kessinger MA, Foley JF, Lemon HM: Adriamycin, mitomycin-C, and 5-fluorouracil in combination for advanced colorectal adenocarcinoma previously treated with 5-fluorouracil. Cancer Clin Trials 2:317–319, 1979.
106. Davis S, Park YK: Chemotherapy for colorectal cancer with a combination of 5-fluorouracil, mitomycin-C, Adriamycin, and cytosine arabinoside: a pilot study. Cancer Treatment Rep 62:1557–1559, 1978.
107. Murphy WK, Valdivieso M, Burgess MA, Bodey GP: Chemotherapy of advanced colorectal cancer and other malignancies with 5-fluorouracil (5-FU) and anguidine (ANG). Proc Am Assoc Cancer Res 20:419, 1979.
108. Woodcock TM, Martin DS, Damin LA, Kemeny NE, Young CW: Combination clinical trials with thymidine and fluorouracil: a phase I and clinical pharmacologic evaluation. Cancer 45:1135–1143, 1980.
109. Vogel SJ, Presant CA, Ratkin GA, Klahr C: Phase I study of thymidine plus 5-fluorouracil infusions in advanced colorectal carcinoma. Cancer Treatment Rep 63:1–5, 1979.
110. Moertel CG, Schutt AJ, Reitemeier RJ, Hahn RG: Therapy for gastrointestinal cancer with the nitrosoureas alone and in drug combination. Cancer Treatment Rep 60:729, 1976.
111. Douglass HO, Lavin PT, Moertel CG: Nitrosoureas: useful agents for the treatment of advanced gastrointestinal cancer. Cancer Treatment Rep 60:769, 1976.
112. DiBenedetto J, Moayeri H, Evans JT, Mittelman A: Phase II study of melphalan in colorectal carcinoma. Cancer Treatment Rep 62:1401, 1978.
113. McCreary RH, Moertel CG, Schutt AJ, O'Connell MJ, Hahn RG, Reitemeier RJ, Rubin J, Frytak S: A phase II study of triazinate (NSC 139105) in advanced colorectal carcinoma. Cancer 40:9, 1977.
114. Taylor SG, Desai SA, DeWys WD: Phase II trial of a combination of cyclophosphamide, vincristine, and methotrexate in advanced colorectal carcinoma. Cancer Treatment Rep 62:1203, 1978.
115. Ackerman NB, Lien WM, Kondi ES, Silverman NA: The blood supply of experimental liver metastases. 1. The distribution of hepatic artery and portal vein blood to 'small' and 'large' tumors. Surgery 66:1067–1072, 1969.
116. Mann JD, Wakim KG, Baggenstoss AH: The vasculature of the human liver — a study by injection-cast method. Proc Mayo Clin 28:227–232, 1953.
117. Healey JE: Vascular patterns in human metastatic liver tumors. Surg Gynecol Obstet 120:1187–1194, 1965.
118. Bierman HR, Byron RL, Kelley KH, Grady A: Studies on blood supply of tumors in man; III. Vascular patterns of liver by hepatic arteriography in vivo. J Nat Cancer Inst 12:107, 1951-1952.
119. Ansfield FJ, Ramirez G, Davis HL, Wirtaneu GW, Johnson RO, Davis TE, Esmaili M, Bryan GRT, Manolo FB, Bordeu EC: Further clinical studies with intrahepatic arterial infusion with 5-fluorouracil. Cancer 36:2413, 1975.
120. Buroker T, Samson M, Correa J, Fraile R, Vaitkevicius VK: Hepatic artery infusion of 5-FUDR after prior systemic 5-fluorouracil. Cancer Treatment Rep 60:1277, 1976.
121. Oberfield RA, McCaffrey JA, Polio J, Clouse ME, Hamilton T: Prolonged and continuous percutaneous intra-arterial hepatic infusion chemotherapy in advanced metastatic liver adenocarcinoma from colorectal primary. Cancer 44:414–423, 1979.
122. Ansfield FJ, Ramirez G: The clinical results of 5-FU intrahepatic arterial infusion in 528 patients with metastatic cancer to the liver: In: Progress in clinical cancer, vol 7. Ariel IM (ed). New York: Grune & Stratton, 1978.

123. Grage TB, Vassilopoulos PP, Shingleton WW, Jubert AV, Elias, EG, Aust JB, Moss SE: Results of a prospective randomized study of hepatic artery infusion with 5-fluorouracil versus intravenous 5-fluorouracil in patients with hepatic metastases from colorectal cancer: a Central Oncology Group Study. Surgery 86:550–555, 1979.

124. Kinami Y, Miyazaki J. The superselective and the selective one shot method for treating inoperable cancer of the liver. Cancer 41:1720, 1978.

125. Misra NC, Jaiswal MSD, Singh RV, Das B. Intrahepatic arterial infusion of combination of mitomycin C and 5-fluorouracil in treatment of primary and metastatic liver carcinoma. Cancer 39:1425, 1977.

126. Douglass CC: Improved survival in liver metastases from colorectal carcinoma following periodic arterial infusions with mitomycin-C, 5-fluorouracil, adriamycin, velban and vincristine. Proc Am Assoc Cancer Res 20:431, 1979.

127. Hoth DF, Petrucci PE. Natural history and staging of colon cancer. Seminars in Oncology; Colon cancer, vol. III, No. 4, 1976.

128. Higgans GA Jr, Humphrey E, Juler GL, LeVeen HH, McCaughan J, Keehn RJ: Adjuvant chemotherapy in the surgical treatment of large bowel cancer. Cancer 38:1461-1467, 1976.

129. Grage TB, Hill GJ, Cornell GN, Frelick RW, Moss SE: Adjuvant chemotherapy in large bowel cancer: demonstration of effectiveness of single agent chemotherapy in a prospectively controlled, randomized trial. Rec Res Cancer Res. 68:222–230, 1978.

1J0. Taylor I, Rowling J, West C: Adjuvant cytotoxic liver perfusion for colorectal cancer. Br J Surg 66:833–837, 1979.

131. Moertel CG, O'Connell MJ, Ritts RE, Schutt AJ, Reitemeier, RJ, Hahn RG, Frytak SK, Rubin J: A controlled evaluation of combined immunotherapy (MER-BCG) and chemotherapy for advanced colorectal cancer. In: Immunotherapy of cancer: present status of trials in man, Terry WD, Windhorst D (eds). New York: Raven Press, 1978, p 573.

132. Engstrom PF, Paul AR, Catalano RB, Mastrangelo MJ, Creech RH: Fluorouracil versus fluorouracil + BCG in colorectal adenocarcinoma, In: Immunotherapy of cancer: present status of trials in man, Terry WE, Windhorst D (eds). New York: Raven Press, 1978, p 587.

133. Gough IR, Clunie GJ, Bolton PM, Dury M, Burnett W: A trial of 5-fluorouracil and corynebacterium parvum in advanced colorectal carcinoma. Dis Colon Rectum 22:223–227, 1979.

134. Gunderson LL: Radiation therapy: results and future possibilities. Clin Gastroenterol 5:743, 1976.

135. Quan SH: Preoperative radiation for carcinoma of the rectum. NY State J Med 66:2243, 1966.

136. Stearns MW, Deddish MR, Quan SH, Learning RH: Preoperative roentgen therapy for cancer of the rectum and rectosigmoid. Surg Gynecol Obstet 138:584, 1975.

137. Higgins GA, Conn JH, Jordan PH, Humphrey EW, Roswit B, Keehn RJ: Preoperative radiotherapy for colorectal cancer. Ann Surg 181:624–631, 1975.

138. Roswit B, Higgins GA, Keehn RJ: Preoperative irradiation for carcinoma of the rectum and rectosigmoid colon: report of a National Veterans Administration randomized study. Cancer 35:1597, 1975.

139. Kligerman MR: Radiation therapy for rectal carcinoma. Semin Oncol 3:407, 1976.

140. Comis RL, Carter SK: Cancer 34:1576-1586, 1974.

141. Woolley PV, MacDonald JS, Schein PS: Chemotherapy of malignancies of the gastrointestinal tract. Progr. Gastroen 3:671, 1977.

142. Kovach JS, Moertel CG, Schutt AJ, Hahn RG, Reitemeier RJ: A controlled study of combined 1,3-bis-(2-chloroethyl)-1-nitrosourea and 5-fluorouracil therapy for advanced gas-

tric and pancreatic cancer. Cancer 33:563, 1974.

143. Moertel CG, Mittelman JA, Bakemeier RF, Engstrom P, Hanley J: Sequential and combination chemotherapy of advanced gastric cancer. Cancer 38:678, 1976.

144. Kingston RD, Ellis DJ, Powell J, Brookes VS, Waterhouse JA, Hurst MD, Smith JA: The West Midlands gastric carcinoma chemotherapy trial: planning and results. Clin Oncol 4:55, 1978.

145. Moertel CG, Lavin RT: Phase II-III chemotherapy studies in advanced gastric cancer. Cancer Treatment Rep 63:1863–1869, 1979.

146. Buroker T, Kim PN, Groppe C, McCracken J, O'Bryan R, Pannettiere F, Costanzi J, Bottomley R, King GW, Bonnet J, Thigpen T, Whitecar J, Hass C, Vaitkevicius VK, Hoogstraten, B, Heilbrun L: 5-FU infusion with mitomycin-C vs. 5-FU infusion with methyl-CCNU in the treatment of advanced upper gastrointestinal cancer. A Southwest Oncology Group Study. Cancer 44:1215, 1979.

147. Ota K, Kurita S, Nishimura M, Ogawa M, Kamei Y, Imai K, Ariyoshi Y, Kataoka K, Murakami MO, Oyama A, Hoshino A, Amo H, Kato T: Combination therapy with mitomycin-C, 5-fluorouracil and cytosine arabinoside for advanced cancer in man. Cancer Chemother Rep 56:373, 1972.

148. DeJager RL, Magill Gb, Golbey RB Krakoff IH: Combination chemotherapy with mitomycin C, 5-fluorouracil, and cytosine arabinoside in gastrointestinal cancer. Cancer Treatment Rep 60:1373–1375, 1976.

149. The Gastrointestinal Tumor Study Group. Phase II-III chemotherapy study in advanced gastric cancer. Cancer Treatment Rep 63:1971, 1979.

150. MacDonald JS, Wolley PV, Smythe T, Ueno W, Hoth D, Schein PS: 5-Fluorouracil, Adriamycin and mitomycin-C (FAM) combination chemotherapy in the treatment of advanced gastric cancer. Cancer 44:42, 1979.

151. MacDonald JS, Schein PS, Woolley PV, Boiron M, Gisselbrecht, C, Brunet R, Lagarde C: 5-Fluorouracil (5-FU), Mitomycin-C (MMC) and Adriamycin (ADR) FAM combination chemotherapy results in 61 patients with advanced gastric cancer. Proc Am Soc Clin Oncol 20:434, 1979.

152. Panettiere F, Heilbrun L: Comparison of two different combinations of Adriamycin, mitomycin-C and 5-FU in the management of gastric carcinoma. A SWOG study. Proc AM. Soc. Clin Oncol 20:315, 1979.

153. Bernath AM, Thornsvard CT: Treatment of advanced gastric carcinoma with BCNU, Adriamycin, 5-FU, and mitomycin-C (BAFMI). Proc Am Soc Clin Oncol 20:312, 1979.

154. Lacave AJ, Brugarolas A, Buesa JM, Garcia Moran M, Perez Ricarte P, Garcia Muniz L, Astudillo A, Urrutia C: Methyl-CCNU (Me), 5-Fluorouracil (F), Adriamycin (A) (MeFA) versus MeF in advanced gastric Cancer. Proc Am Soc Clin Oncol 20:310, 1979.

155. Levi JA, Dalley DM, Aroney RS: Improved combination chemotherapy in advanced gastric cancer. Br Med J 2:1471, 1979.

156. Magill GB, Golbey RB, Burchenal JH: Combined anhydro-ara-5-fluorocytidine (AAFC) and cis-platinum diamminedichloride (PPD) therapy in gastric and pancreatic carcinoma. Proc Am Soc Clin Oncol 19:353, 1978.

157. VASAG — Veteran's Administration Cooperative Surgical Adjuvant Study Group. Use of thiotepa as an adjuvant to surgical management of carcinoma of the stomach. Cancer 18:291, 1965.

158. Hattori T, Ito I, Katsvr H, Hirata K, Iizuka T, Abe K: Results of combined treatment in patients with cancer of the stomach: Palliative gastrectomy, large dose mitomycin-C, and bone marrow transplantation. Gann 57:441, 1966.

159. Serlin O, Wolhoff JS, Amadeo JM, Keehn RJ: Use of 5-fluorodeoxyuridine (FUDR) as an adjuvant to surgical management of carcinoma of the stomach. Cancer 24:223, 1969.

160. Nakajima T, Fukami A, Ohashi I, Kajitani T: Long-term follow-up Study of gastric cancer patients treated with surgery and adjuvant chemotherapy with mitomycin C. Int J Clin Pharmacol Biopharm 16:209–216, 1978.

161. Nakajima T, Ota H, Takagi K, Kajitani T: Combination of multidrug therapy (i.v.) and Long-term oral chemotherapy as an adjuvant to surgery for gastric cancer. J Jpn Soc Cancer Ther 15th Cong. 226, 1977.

162. Moertel CG, Childs DS, Reitemeier R, Colby MY, Holbrook MA: Combined 5-fluorouracil and supervoltage radiation therapy of locally unresectable gastrointestinal cancer. Lancet 2:865, 1969.

163. Schein PS, Childs D: For GITSG. A Controlled randomized evaluation of combined modality therapy (5000 rads, 5-FU+MeCCNU) vs. 5-FU+MeCCNU alone for locally advanced gastric cancer. Proc. Am Soc Clin Oncol 19:C–329, 1978.

164. Schein PS, Novak J: For the Gastrointestinal Tumor Study Group. Combined modality therapy (XRT-chemo) versus chemotherapy alone for locally unresectable gastric cancer. Proc Am Soc Clin Oncol 21:419, 1980.